Improving U
Mental Health

Improving University Mental Health

Jane Morris
University of Aberdeen

CAMBRIDGE
UNIVERSITY PRESS

CAMBRIDGE
UNIVERSITY PRESS

Shaftesbury Road, Cambridge CB2 8EA, United Kingdom

One Liberty Plaza, 20th Floor, New York, NY 10006, USA

477 Williamstown Road, Port Melbourne, VIC 3207, Australia

314–321, 3rd Floor, Plot 3, Splendor Forum, Jasola District Centre, New Delhi – 110025, India

103 Penang Road, #05-06/07, Visioncrest Commercial, Singapore 238467

Cambridge University Press is part of Cambridge University Press & Assessment, a department of the University of Cambridge.

We share the University's mission to contribute to society through the pursuit of education, learning and research at the highest international levels of excellence.

www.cambridge.org
Information on this title: www.cambridge.org/9781911623830

DOI: 10.1017/9781911623847

First published 2024

A catalogue record for this publication is available from the British Library.

Library of Congress Cataloging-in-Publication Data
Names: Morris, Jane, 1951- author.
Title: Improving university mental health / Jane Morris, University of
  Aberdeen.
Description: Cambridge, United Kingdom ; New York, NY : Cambridge
  University Press, 2023. | Includes bibliographical references and index.
Identifiers: LCCN 2023016937 (print) | LCCN 2023016938 (ebook) |
  ISBN 9781911623830 (paperback) | ISBN 9781911623847 (epub)
Subjects: LCSH: College students–Mental health–Great Britain. |
  College students–Mental health services–Great Britain.
Classification: LCC RC451.4.S7 M678 2023 (print) | LCC RC451.4.S7
  (ebook) | DDC 362.1968900835–dc23/eng/20230623
LC record available at https://lccn.loc.gov/2023016937
LC ebook record available at https://lccn.loc.gov/2023016938

ISBN 978-1-911-62383-0 Paperback

Contents

Foreword

When I became Principal of Newnham College, Cambridge in the autumn of 2019, people asked me what had changed since I had been a student there many years before. I said I was struck by how much more conversation there was around mental health. I was pleased to find a real openness about the topic, and to see students with long-term mental illness supported to thrive and achieve their potential. I noted the fact that one in ten students visited the university counselling service in any one academic year. When I became a member of the steering group overseeing a strategic review of mental health within the University of Cambridge at the end of 2020, those conversations deepened. As Dr Jane Morris' book makes clear, university mental health is multi-faceted. The subject can feel overwhelming for institutions, staff and students. Resources –in terms of both funding and trained professionals – are tight, and need to be used effectively, whilst demand only ever seems to increase.

I was fortunate enough to speak with Jane in the autumn of 2021 when she gave a series of three interactive talks on student mental health as part of the programme to celebrate the 150th anniversary of Newnham College, where Jane was also a student many years ago. This book feels like a way of enabling many more people to talk with Jane through the proxy of its pages. There is no easy blueprint here and not everyone will agree with everything, but we will all be much better able to engage. For university mental health policies to work well, all those involved have to listen to the particular student populations with which they work and to the latest evidence on how best to do that.

This handbook brings together a wide range of research and experience in a readable way. Jane covers promotion of well-being and of good mental health. She considers how to respond effectively to poor mental health and to long term mental illness, and the ways both impact differently on different groups. She challenges us and provides us with hope and practical ways forward. My hope for this thorough and insightful handbook is that it will enable not just more but better conversation and action around university mental health.

Alison Rose
Principal
Newnham College
Cambridge

Acknowledgements and Thanks to Contributors

This book could not have been written without the help of literally hundreds of people who generously contributed personal stories – some of them very moving and some quite distressing. Noreen Ahktar spurred me on to still write after COVID struck and completed the first of a series of literature searches to motivate me. Karen Sinclair of Cornhill Library conducted more searches and uncomplainingly pursued all my requests. Meanwhile, senior academics and staff at the Royal College of Psychiatrists and in UK universities gave their blessing for students and staff to participate in the work.

Many current students met me individually or more often in groups, and particularly over Zoom and Teams during the COVID lockdown. I heard from academic and pastoral staff, both current and retired, from school and college students and their teachers in state and private sectors, and from parents, grandparents and other family members of those involved in university life. I met with so much enthusiasm for the project that I was persuaded to persist even when I felt tempted to abandon the effort.

A number of the people I approached put me in touch with others whom they wanted to 'bear witness'. Others – often the same people – agreed to read and comment on the various drafts of particular chapters. I have already acknowledged specific expertise and advice at the end of Chapter 11, but most contributors offered ideas across the range of the book. My thanks to all of them. Some have offered their experiences on an anonymous basis, others have given explicit permission for their names to be listed. I have tried not to omit anyone, but if anyone feels overlooked, this is almost certainly because I am not sure I have your consent. Privacy in matters of mental health is even more sensitive than for other health matters, and not only because of stigma.

Thanks to all these people:

Presenters and delegates at Westminster Higher Education Conferences, particularly those who spoke on behalf of bereaved parents
Academic and pastoral staff and students at Newnham College, Cambridge
Aberdeen medical and nursing students
Students at the universities of Glasgow, Edinburgh, St Andrews, and Heriot-Watt
Mental health mentors
Amna Ahktar
The late Pam Alexander
Amy Atkinson-Ward
Barbara Arnold
Chris Ayton
John Callender
Carol Cooper
Perry Crofts
Elrika Erasmus

Alice Flatman
Peter Flatman
Tom Flatman
Wendy Hirsch
Mihiri Jayaweera
Sophie Rui Qi Koh
Rebecca Lawrence
Serrie Meakins
Carol Millard
Bill Morris
Jacqui Nicholson
Valerie Rees
Richard Ribchester
Alison Rose
Anne Schumacher
Oluchi Ugochuwu

I am also indebted to the staff at Cambridge University Press for their thorough professionalism, good communication skills and engagement in the work.

Introducing This Handbook

University life has always fascinated me. My own experience of going to university was intense and positive, but many of the people I have met professionally have – perhaps by definition – described painful or damaging experiences. I was the first person in my family to get a university degree, and since that time I have been the daughter, sister, cousin, mother, aunt, friend, colleague and teacher of students and staff in a large variety of higher education institutions across the UK. I have observed a kaleidoscope of shifts and changes in different institutions and faculties, across the UK and over half a century.

More students than ever are now disclosing a psychiatric diagnosis. The report 'Student Mental Well-Being in Higher Education' (Universities UK, 2015) found that the proportion of students who declared a mental health condition doubled from 0.4% in 2007–8 to 0.8% in 2011–12. By 2018/2019, 4.3% of UK students (5.3% of females and 2.8% of males) disclosed a mental health condition to their higher education institutions (The Insight Network, 2020). This may not indicate increased rates of mental illness so much as increased willingness to seek support, as universities made concerted efforts to facilitate and normalise disclosure. One international study found that a fifth of university students (from 21 different countries though not the UK) had a mental health issue. Four fifths of these students had been diagnosed before they started at university (Auerbach et al., 2016). More recently, the Dunedin Birth Cohort Study found that by age 18, half of the population meets criteria for at least one diagnosable mental disorder (Caspi et al., 2020).

In my long career as a psychiatrist, I have developed a long-term interest in the welfare of students and other young people. I've worked variously in child and adolescent mental health services, adolescent and adult eating disorders services, trauma clinics, and liaison and psychotherapy settings, and have taught and supervised counsellors and mental health mentors in different universities. This is a single-author text not because I claim specific expertise in every key topic, but because the most successful aspects of my career have involved making connections and building networks. The intention is that each chapter (or in some cases a small group of two or three chapters) should stand alone. Readers can plunge into whichever topic they most need to consider, without having to start with this introduction and read through to the end of the book. I have avoided too much repetition by signposting readers to other relevant chapters within the text.

Since Cambridge University Press first invited me to write a handbook called *Improving Student Mental Health* the title has evolved further. There were already several excellent handbooks from the United States, where a great deal of research is focussed, but where the legal, welfare and cultural context is different. We decided to specifically address the UK experience, whilst obviously drawing on relevant research and experience from across the globe.

As I began to write, and to realise the importance of a 'whole university approach' to well-being and mental health, I asked for a further change in title, to 'University' rather than 'Student' mental health. In fact, this is a convenient clarification too, as US English tends to use the word 'student' to include children and teenagers attending school, as well as those in higher education.

I have devoted Chapter 13 to consideration of the roles and needs of academic and teaching staff in terms of mental health, but virtually all the chapter topics raise issues of staff responsibilities and vulnerabilities. I addressed Chapter 4 to the roles and concerns of parents and families, to validate their important stake in shaping university health. Alumni are also becoming increasingly important as investors in the financial and cultural health of their former institutions, and all taxpayers and voters in the UK are, to some extent, stakeholders in our universities.

I am glad I rejected the title 'Student Mental Health' because it now seems not only exclusionary but also somewhat condescending. It might imply that students are the objects of concern, and that mental health is something for others to address. We have seen a huge rise in the power of people with 'lived experience' of health conditions in the design of support and services. Collaborative work is a way to recognise the expertise and strengths as well as the vulnerabilities of the student age group as well as their experience of mental health and ill health.

It is important also to challenge the dichotomy of 'us', the adults and professionals who are 'unflawed and powerful' and 'them', the students and patients who are 'vulnerable and young'. I was a patient before I even thought of becoming a doctor, and as a psychiatrist I am even more aware of my own psychological vulnerability. We are all likely to develop a diagnosable mental disorder at some point in our lives (Caspi et al., 2020), whether we may be politicians, vice chancellors, professors, parents, domestic staff, secretaries or students.

At the same time, this book constantly has to debate the question of whether young adults should be expected to shoulder full adult responsibilities, or whether we are buying too much into what Terri Apter (2008) called 'the myth of maturity'. A university is like a laboratory or a gym where young as well as mature adults can experiment in building their own society under carefully controlled conditions. Sometimes the question arises as to how much outside control is beneficial both in its own right, to enhance health and learning, and to protect against unhealthy outside influences.

Finally, I even questioned using the optimistic word 'improving' in the title. The book was commissioned just before the world unexpectedly went into lockdown. I became distracted from the project by my desire to join emergency clinical activity during the pandemic. When I returned to the book, I was appalled by the consequences of COVID and lockdown, particularly for university students. The group of people at lowest physical risk from COVID was obliged to pay the highest psycho-social penalty. The worst restrictions overshadowed the very years when they had expected to live out a major life transition.

As we emerged from the worst self-isolation, waiting lists for psychiatric services for young people had ballooned and there has been talk of a 'mental health pandemic' to follow the COVID pandemic.

I returned to my writing, fearful that existing research would be inadequate to the plight of the universities. Subsequent global and political events have added further concerns. The aspiration to 'improve' matters seemed arrogant. Even restoration to previous levels of mental health sounded ambitious. As we have moved into a 'new normal' though, it feels reasonable to return to the idea of 'improvement' even if this is from a new and lower baseline than before.

The commonest question from potential readers has been 'who is the intended audience?' If you are reading these words, then the answer is 'you are!' Those readers who are seeking a series of simple answers to the multitude of mental health dilemmas posed in university life will come away disappointed. I am disappointed myself and would have loved to come up with a series of training manuals on 'How to be a Mentally Healthy Student', 'How to be the Perfect University Parent', 'How to Behave at all Times as an Effective Director of Studies', and especially 'How Ministers of Health and Education Can Legislate for Mentally Healthy Universities'.

Individuals and institutions are too diverse in terms of populations and resources, research is both inconclusive and constantly obliged to deal with new challenges and developments. Improvements seem to come about through dialogue and experiment, rather than as a series of getting right answers right away. Each chapter emerged as providing an overview of the overview of the context with vignettes to bring the topic to life. I tried to find examples of good practice and good progress as well as examples of unmet needs. I have concluded each chapter with 'practice points', which are comments and suggestions to different groups of readers.

This book has emerged as a basic overview of the state of UK university mental health in the 2020s. I hope it will inform those who need to get the best out of the provision that is there, and stimulate debate and action from all who have power to make improvements.

References

Apter, T. E. (2002). *The myth of maturity: What teenagers need from parents to become adults*. New York: WW Norton & Company.

Auerbach, R. P., Alonso, J., Axinn, W. G., et al. (2016). Mental disorders among college students in the World Health Organization world mental health surveys. *Psychological Medicine*, 46(14), 2955–70.

Caspi, A., Houts, R. M., Ambler, A., et al. (2020). Longitudinal assessment of mental health disorders and comorbidities across 4 decades among participants in the Dunedin birth cohort study. *JAMA Network Open*, 3(4), e203221.

The Insight Network (2020). *University student mental health survey 2020*. The Insight Network. www.diginbox.com

Universities UK (2015). *Student mental wellbeing in higher education: Good practice guide*. www.m25lib.ac.uk/wp-content/uploads/2021/02/student-mental-wellbeing-in-he.pdf

Building a New Sense of Belonging

The Transition from School to University

Chapter 3 will address the challenges of the transition when the student has a pre-existing mental disorder. It is recommended that this chapter is read before Chapter 3. Both chapters may be considered alongside Chapters 14–16, which describe different mental conditions as they affect young students, and Chapter 18, which outlines mental health treatment services both within universities and in the NHS.

Schools and parents work hard to prepare young people for university life, and universities themselves have designed outreach and engagement programmes to attract students and promote retention and completion of courses. The beginning of university life is recognised as so important that there are learned journals devoted entirely to the first year. By the very nature of transition, neither school nor university can manage the whole process, nor even link up around each individual student to recognise their unique backgrounds and needs. Some reports and surveys on the topic have names that highlight both the liberation and daunting risks involved – *Reality check* (Unite Students & Higher Education Policy Institute, 2017), *Betwixt spaces* (Palmer et al., 2009) and *Finding our own way* (Harris, 2019).

Students as 'Transition Aged Youth'

The expression 'transition aged youth' originated in US health and foster-care systems to describe young people from 16 to 25 years old who were at risk of serious disturbance as a result of becoming too old for children's services and having to make their way in the world as vulnerable adults. The term is now used more often to refer to everyone in the age range. It has taken on a similar meaning to the term 'emerging adults'. However, emerging adulthood was the period of life from 19 to 29 years of age, proposed by Jeffrey Arnett (2000) as a time young people experience a normal discrete developmental phase involving the exploration of life possibilities. Meanwhile, in her book *The myth of maturity*, Terri Apter (2002) coined the term 'thresholders' to describe this developmental phase, without setting any chronological age definitions upon it.

Whatever we call it, this is a time when we face more adult challenges without having yet mastered the tools and cognitive maturity of adulthood. Neuroimaging scan studies demonstrate that in this period of development there are changes in the structure, connectivity and function of brain tissue itself which extend well into our twenties (Giedd, 2008).

This chapter focusses on the most common route into university life: a young person in their late teens coming straight from school (or from a gap year), probably moving away from home to university accommodation, after attending a day school from the family home. International students may have the even greater challenges of a change of culture and of studying in a second language. Mature students may have already mastered many of the obvious tasks of youthful transition, but still have to manage change. Students from other minority groups, including those with pre-existing disorders and disabilities, will also face a different range of challenges. These challenges will be considered in more detail in later chapters.

The late adolescent brain is still experiencing the instability of accelerated development. This makes it more sensitive to psychosocial stressors, recreational drug and alcohol use and sleep disruption. Half of all mental disorders have emerged by early adulthood, and there are substantial delays in treatment provision. Untreated or inadequately treated mental illness is associated with progression to more chronic and complex disorders, self-destructive behaviours, addictions and drop out from education and work. An influential *Lancet* article (Duffy et al., 2019) points out that

> taken together, the transition to university coincides with a high-risk period for maladaptive coping, onset of psychopathology, and academic failure; a corollary is that it also represents an important window of opportunity for prevention and timely intervention.

Thinking about the Nature of Transition

Anthropology, sociology, psychotherapy and related disciplines have studied and reflected deeply on the nature of transition. One characteristic of transitions is their tendency to cluster, so that we generally face social, physiological, geographical and interpersonal changes all at once. This is a classic transition cluster, often played out against the background of parental transitions into menopause, retirement and ageing, and losses and bereavements in the grandparents' generation. Individual students and whole family systems have adjustments to make.

Some Life Transitions
- Starting school
- Moving from primary to secondary school
- Experiencing relationship breakups and bereavements in adult family members
- Leaving the family home to live more independently
- Becoming a university student
- Leaving university
- Physical transitions: puberty, pregnancy, menopause, illness, disability
- Moving to/from another country with different health and medico-legal systems
- Starting work
- Changing occupation and losing a job
- Relationship challenges, break-ups and divorce
- Co-habitation, partnerships and marriages
- Bringing children into the family
- Retirement
- Family bereavement
- Some consider birth and death to be transitions rather than the start and end of life.

Transitions are unavoidable and potentially refreshing milestones in life for everyone concerned. They are often marked with ceremonials and rituals that allow society to acknowledge, digest and celebrate the changes involved. Throughout the animal kingdom, one of the ways young creatures become adults is by challenging their elders to the point of retaliation. They are thrown out of the family den in exasperation, as ageing parents defend themselves against the growing dominance of the younger generation.

Some of this aggression between the generations persists in human initiation rites in which the new adults' strength and courage are tested in almost sadistic challenges. Such instincts may still be with us alongside the urge to continue to nurture and protect our young. There's a tension between the view that 18-year-olds should 'learn the hard way' and the alternative view that sees them as still essentially needy children.

Young people's rates of progress may differ from one transitional area to another. For instance, social skills and confidence may develop at a different rate to the achievement of economic independence. Students need to take on new skills and responsibilities in self-care, group living and budget management and have to negotiate with a range of organisations and services as independent adults. They also have to adjust to new patterns of studying and learning and to a new social environment.

The move away from the family and local community offers freedom to explore new sexual and social roles, which can be thrilling but also worrying. Rejections are devastating without a secure network to cushion the blow. Ironically it is also difficult to return home and juggle the different expectations appropriate to home and university settings.

The founders of Interpersonal Psychotherapy (Klerman & Weissman, 1994) observed that 'transitions' were among the most common triggers of major depression. Their model explores two aspects of the transition – the work of mourning what has been lost, and the reconstruction of a scaffolding of relationships that approximately substitutes for what has been lost, whilst also leaving behind relationships which were harmful or outgrown. This can be a helpful way to envisage the work of managing transitions. It certainly IS hard work. Students often need help in processing healthy grief and mourning, and in finding opportunities to form good new attachments. We also need to take care not to overburden those in transition with too many demands at the same time. The drunken, overcrammed 'Freshers' Week' may have been replaced to some extent by more thoughtful, less intoxicated induction courses, but these are still overstuffed with information. It's hard for students to recognise and store what might be relevant for future times of need.

At a societal level we facilitate transitional adjustments with ceremonials and observances that bring communities together for solidarity. In his 1909 work *Les rites de passage*, French anthropologist van Gennep (1909/1960) writes of three phases to be negotiated: divestiture (separation and loss), liminality (being on the threshold with a foot in each camp) and investiture (settling in to a new sense of belonging). In practice, most of the well-recognised life transitions have an even earlier phase – that of anticipation and preparation, which is both constructive and anxiety-provoking. This anticipatory phase provides a unique context for each student. Previous experiences of navigating life changes are important, too. We seem a little hypnotised by societal expectations of going to university and forget that we have some control over when and how the process is managed. We are not obliged to send all the young people of the tribe out into the wilderness together at the magically appointed time to endure initiation rites. Readiness can be considered and nurtured.

This book urges not only a whole-university approach to the mental health of each individual student, but also a course-long, and even lifelong approach to the development of coping skills. For many young people, their whole university career represents the transitional stage between child-like dependency and the independence they are expected to assume on leaving higher education to make their way as adults in the world.

Preparation, Pacing, Practicalities and People

For all but the most sublimely resilient students, arrival at university is too late to start the process of preparation. Is going to university really a 'leap'? A leap of faith, or an act of bravado? Are students 'finding their own way' like babes in the wood, rejected from their home and wandering in the wild? Such metaphors matter because it matters how we conceptualise going to university. Expectations are important when they drive self-fulfilling prophecies; if hopes are dashed and core beliefs shaken the trauma can be damaging. As in all of life, we are healthiest when our expectations and beliefs are a little skewed towards the positive side of reality.

One study (Denovan & Macaskill, 2016) explored a range of psychological strengths shown individually to influence stress and subjective well-being. Optimism emerged as a key factor for new students to adjust to university and buffered the impact of stress on well-being throughout the academic year. It is really hard, though, to tease out whether the students' optimism was itself the determining factor, or whether it was rather a consequence of these individuals' health and strength. The same study noted that 'academic self-efficacy' was another feature that corresponded with life satisfaction and positive affect. Perhaps the healthiest way to improve a student's optimism is to help them find realistic causes for such optimism. Many of the effective interventions around student transitions to university seem to achieve precisely that. It's a good start if the young person is actively choosing university rather than succumbing to pressure to follow the crowd. In today's UK, about half of all young people and the majority of those who stay on at school after age 16 go to university. Sixth forms and higher examinations are all focussed on university entry. It can be tacitly assumed that everyone who gets good enough grades will apply, and that not doing so is a failure rather than a positive choice. But there are other options.

Readiness for University
Organisational skills – time management, prioritising
Academic and independent study skills
Accommodation – healthy and comfortable and secure environment
Financial resources and ability to budget – see Chapter 9
Social skills – making, keeping and shedding friends
Interpersonal support – network people/services to turn to (e.g., doctor, dentist)
Sexual awareness and skills
Self-care in terms of eating, sleeping, exercise
Social media skills
Ability to manage alcohol and drug culture
Resources to manage disorder, disability, etc.
Psychological resilience – optimism, resourcefulness, emotion regulation, distress tolerance

Schools, families and individuals themselves may form an idealised attachment even before attending a university open day, certainly before applying. If they then fail to get the grades needed, there's an assumption they will feel humiliated and resentful. There's even a myth that certain institutions are populated entirely by students who are bitter they didn't get into Oxbridge (as the Universities of Oxford and Cambridge are collectively known). Research does not in fact find that students who entered their first choice of university are happier. An incidental finding from a study of student finance (Richardson et al., 2017) was that those who got their first-choice university had more severe depression scores and greater alcohol misuse than those who got their back-up choice. Perhaps we're not very good at identifying the universities that will allow us to thrive.

Teachers, parents and friends can all help the young person assess whether they are mature enough for university at this stage. It's not a binary choice. There are other options in terms of both work and play, and within education there is also further education at college on either a part- or full-time basis, or the option of an extra year at school – or at a different school. Within the world of work there are apprenticeships, internships and vocational training posts, as well as voluntary work and a whole range of opportunities for gap years. University is often grasped with relief by students and their families alike as a way to postpone the world of work – or the world of not enough congenial, available, work – whilst the young person gains some maturity. For some young people, though, the university environment does not nurture their maturity, and in fact demands more of them than is yet possible.

For those who do opt for university, the question of which institution to apply for is too often a purely academic competition, with each student seeking to attend the most 'prestigious' to which their grades will grant entry. The process can seem almost political – some young people deliberately selecting less popular courses to gain entry to a prestigious university where their preferred subject is oversubscribed. Many schools, in both state and private sectors, offer extra mentoring and coaching for Oxbridge candidates only, and parents purchase tutoring if they have the money to do so. For some families this is a magnified repeat of the secondary school entrance competition, whilst for many in deprived areas it is an unaffordable or irrelevant process.

Karen was a precociously bright 17-year-old with a scholarship to study classics at the University of Oxford. She also had severe obsessive–compulsive disorder and would sometimes wash herself until her skin was bleeding. After months of successful treatment, she would invariably relapse, usually having stopped taking medication and dropped out of psychological treatment for one reason or another. Finally, she admitted that she was terrified of leaving home. She felt even younger than her 17 years, and the protected patient role felt safer than the thought of 'having to' take part in sex, drugs and rock and roll. She said her raw skin provided a visible 'excuse for not getting on with life'. She decided to take a gap year – this consisted of studying Hebrew at the local college whilst living at home with parents and younger siblings. During this time, she cooperated fully with her medication and therapy and began to socialise, mostly with her sisters' contemporaries. At the end of the year, she opted to attend a local university, but planned to reapply to take a higher degree at the University of Oxford in the future.

Many teachers are of course aware of specific universities that have delivered good pastoral and well-being support to their former students, or the reverse. The knowledge comes from personal experience and word of mouth. They pass on anecdotes about which universities display arrogance and lack of flexibility, and which are understanding and compassionate. One teacher described a bright student who had been in a secure mental health unit for a year before joining her school. She could have chosen to attend a Russell Group university, but opted for a less famous institution, which had reassured her of the accommodation and pastoral support she would receive. Another teacher praised a university which gave a student an extra 2 years to complete their degree in the context of mental health struggles.

Teachers and students confirm that for all concerned, there can be undue focus on high pressure academic competition, at the expense of balanced preparation of each individual to mature at their own pace in all dimensions of their life. The quest for academic excellence is entirely honourable and students who thrive on fast paced intellectual study need institutions where this is the norm. More balanced attention to psychosocial maturity and readiness, together with better matching of individuals to their working or learning environment could provide better academic results as well as healthier people.

We need better ways to compare universities on their approach to well-being and mental health, beyond specific anecdotes shared between teachers. Making a university's track record on well-being and mental health more prominent in the university search, and supported by data collected on this issue, could empower better-informed decisions about where to study. The University Mental Health Charter, launched by Student Minds in 2018, could help with this. support this objective. It was co-produced with charities and higher education bodies to provide recognition to institutions that demonstrate good practice in student and staff mental health and well-being. This could particularly help young people with mental health issues and/or disabilities, and those who are sensitive, vulnerable or less socially confident, to make more informed decisions about where to study and live.

Throughout childhood and schooldays, written records and verbal information about the child are passed from adult to adult, without the child having much responsibility for this. Suddenly at age 18 the individual is expected to become the agent of responsibility. Only rarely will a schoolteacher have a counterpart in the university with whom they can share the profile of concerns and expectations of the student, and mental health clinicians may not have identified counterparts in adult services in other geographical areas who will communicate about mental disorders. Written records are less likely to be read in a large organisation where the student is a stranger, than in a small institution in which the child was already known.

Ideally, the move to independent living should be 'piloted' before leaving home. There are a range of ways to do this. The best schools change their teaching styles gradually so that by the sixth form they avoid 'spoon-feeding' to achieve higher grades. Instead, there is a move to showing the young person how to structure and carry out their own research, how to organise assignments rather than setting specific homework for one night, and encouragement of peer support in learning.

Nick and Jesse complained that their sixth form history teacher wasn't doing what he was paid to do. Their previous teacher had told them what they needed to learn to get top marks, and they had practically memorised the textbook and tested each other on questions from past papers. They liked to 'push for perfection'.

But Mr Hill sent them off to libraries and scholarly databases to do their own research, suggested they mark each other's essays, and asked them to study widely, beyond the demands of the syllabus. The freedom to study what interested them was confusing and destabilising at first. Neither of them chose history as their university course, but as a result of Mr Hill's methods, both found themselves better prepared than others for the way they were expected to study when they become undergraduates.

Socially, adult family members, friends and mentors can shift relationships between teenager and adult to a more equal footing, and of course the teenager can practise spending more time away from home. Within the home the young person can be expected to take on more financial responsibilities, household chores and work contributions.

Wise parents and teachers encourage affiliations to organisations that transcend the local level, whether they are political, musical, artistic, technical or voluntary groups. There's particularly strong evidence for thriving of students with religious affiliations, and such groups often provide a sort of extended family when their members leave home. Holiday camp experiences, such as outward-bound adventures, build confidence in taking on new challenges and demonstrate that it is possible to bond with other people in a short time – useful to build social confidence, even though the group may not be going on to the same university as the young person.

Many young people plan a 'gap year' before, during or after studying for a degree. The individual can sample a variety of voluntary or paid activities, catching up on developmental tasks and sheltering for a while from academic and other stressors. However, ambitious long-haul travel projects can threaten the physical as well as psychosocial well-being of anyone who is already vulnerable to mental or physical disorder, particularly when foreign health systems are difficult to access or prohibitively expensive.

How Institutions Manage the Transition Process for Students

The sort of joint working that occurs between secondary schools and their 'feeder' primaries simply cannot apply to universities, which may welcome students from hundreds of different establishments. It may though be possible for representatives of an individual student to advocate for and support that individual from before the start of university and to then continue until they have made the adjustment to the new situation. Such supporters may be called mentors or transition coaches – there are a variety of role titles – and the role is often informal or else restricted to identified high risk students.

During the overlap period the student is supported to explore and explain the differences in the ways of working between the two environments and get to know key peers and members of staff. Then the student can be 'weaned off' the extra support. Most existing mentorship arrangements suffer from the drawback that they only move into action when the student has actually started at the university. Mental Health Mentorship is applied for in advance but the first meeting with the mentor is not until the first term has started. The 'university families' scheme, whereby each first-year student may be allocated a trained volunteer 'parent student' is also unlikely to start until the student arrives, and summer schools rarely reach so far back that they overlap with school.

School teachers tell researchers of their concern that universities will not meet their pupils' needs for teaching and pastoral care. Senior school pupils are often invited to open days or special events mounted by universities. This sort of outreach attracts bright and interested pupils to apply to the specific institution. There is rarely a bridging role that can understand the young person's situation while they are still at school and home, then reach forward to support the young person for a while – from a term to a year – as a new student.

The word 'mentor' has all manner of informal as well as official meanings. This makes it a useful non-stigmatising term, but also a confusing one. The 'university parents' idea is elegant in that it encourages students to seek and then deliver support on a peer-to-peer basis. This formalises and protects what can sometimes be a natural process and fosters maturity and kindness without too much regulation. Most 'parents' will have been at school themselves only recently and so understand the contemporary realities of transition. Groups of 'university parents' could usefully hold stalls for prospective students at open days to promote a philosophy of kindness and accessibility that transcends individuals.

Ideally, buddying or mentorship would be set up before the student arrives. As things are, the first face-to-face interpersonal contacts for most new university students are the peers they meet in halls and shared houses. Students will often have participated in social media groups before arrival, too. These first attachments are incredibly influential, bonding people together at a time of maximum vulnerability. Universities are missing a trick by allowing relatively random contacts to take precedence over considered induction. Immature peer-led induction can lead new students into high-risk cultures of substance misuse, scorn for diversity and difference, and gender-based disparagement.

Experience of using Zoom and similar platforms during Lockdown means that technological communication is no longer the preserve of students in their social time. One-to-one and group meetings can be held before students arrive in university accommodation. Staff can meet students to discuss their roles and expectation of students.

Living the Process: Feeling Homesick

Moving away from home to university brings additional stresses at the same time as taking away supportive people and structures. This is a recipe for anxiety. 'Nostalgia' – from the Greek word for home – and homesickness, are universal experiences. Even Odysseus, the great warrior, experienced homesickness. Modern soldiers, facing death and life-changing injury, yearn not for safety but for 'home'. Bowlby (1969) and his contemporaries examined the consequences of the disordered attachments that occurred when young children were sent to hospital without their parents, or away to boarding schools. At the other end of life, old people in nursing homes grieve the loss of home and family.

Taking on new challenges can involve a 'manic defence' that also serves the purpose of distracting the new students from the less openly acknowledged business of mourning the passage of childhood. Even when the student is aware of their struggles, they may be too ashamed to acknowledge them. Whilst this is an almost universal painful experience, frequently self-limiting and part of a healthy adjustment process, we should not disqualify it as 'just' homesickness.

'By the time I went to university I had felt sick OF home for some time. I was exhilarated to find myself at the beautiful university of my choice, with a wide choice of intelligent and beautiful friends and three long years ahead to explore my chosen subject and many extracurricular options. I woke each morning to the joy of a new day ahead. So, I was astonished to find myself crying into my pillow most nights, yearning for home, grieving for the loss of my secure childhood, the existence where I was a protected child in a cocoon of unconditional love.'

Some time ago, a longitudinal study examined the effects of the transition to university for students living on campus or at home (Fisher & Hood, 1987). All students experienced some increase in psychological disturbances and 'absent-mindedness' but the symptoms were significantly worse for those who reported homesickness. In these days of electronic communication, we might expect a reduction in reports of homesickness, but there may also be a risk that when parents and students connect several times each day, this can diminish the student's ability to engage fully in university life and to move on in their transition.

The more vulnerable the young person, the more important it is to respect the therapeutic value of a strong attachment in bridging transitions. When feelings are not acknowledged, maturity may be thwarted at this hurdle and the student damaged by unaddressed fear and isolation.

> Julie's mother had a chronic disabling illness and depended on her daughter for emotional as well as practical support. Her father worked long hours to bring financial security to the family, leaving Julie to 'mother' her younger brother She left her prestigious school and studied at a local college which gave her more flexibility to be at home. She achieved high marks and was urged by family and teachers alike to take up her Oxbridge scholarship.
>
> Terms were short, though academically intense, and Julie returned home every weekend. She spent far more of the year caring for family than living in college. She had always been the uncomplaining 'strong one' in the family. She felt excluded by the rich young women on her stair, who partied and studied, apparently without any responsibilities. This made her angry, but she couldn't find anywhere to express this.
>
> Gradually, she became exhausted and depressed. Her marks suffered, though never to the point of failure. It was only some years later, when she embarked on a master's degree elsewhere, that a perceptive tutor noticed that she seemed depressed and encouraged her to seek support. She was treated for major depressive disorder and wondered whether she might never have fallen ill if her difficulties had been picked up sooner, and helpfully addressed.

One key task in the transition to adulthood is that of developing close friendships and relationships to compensate for reduced emotional dependence on parents. The family left behind, especially parents and younger siblings, must also adjust to the loss of the new student. Healthy families can usually find their own compensations and progressions, so that the student feels there is a secure base they could still rely on, rather than a sense that bridges have been burned behind them. Where the student has been a young carer, the loss of practical and emotional care may be too great to tolerate. Transition may not be possible, and the student is split painfully.

Induction Strategies: Drawing the Student into the New Culture

The term 'Welcome Week' has widely replaced 'Freshers Week' to imply an experience that provides more structure, less alcohol, and a focus on making connections and exploring common interests, rather than partying. Induction courses and summer schools are more extended versions of Welcome Week, before the university term begins. These can usefully target prospective freshers identified as needing more information, skills and networks to flourish in university life. Vulnerable minorities such as 'first generation' students and those with pre-existing mental disorders are sometimes offered specific inductions. However, these miss the substantial proportion of students who haven't disclosed – or even yet developed – a disorder.

Universities, unlike most primary and secondary schools, are the size of city states, with sub-groups such as faculties, courses, year groups, societies, residences, colleges and cohorts. Young adults pass through a sort of initiation from being relatively passive recipients of adult care, to being agents of their own well-being, subject to the supports of their chosen groups and to the rulings of the broader university councils and courts. As they emerge from adolescence into adult life, they are empowered to bring their own contributions to the structures that serve them. They can actually build the sense of their own belonging and participate in shaping the community in which they live.

Alternative approaches to either academic or social inductions are outdoor orienta-tion programmes such as that reported by Hill (2018) in the US, and similar in content to such courses offered by secondary and even primary schools in the UK. Residential outdoor expeditions can form an integral part of courses such as geography or archae-ology, and often constitute part of the motivation for selecting such courses. Other disciplines have incorporated short trips to outdoor centres as part of 'reading week' or revision preparation before examinations. The mix of physical activity, immersion in nature, supportive company, and being provided with catering, is a powerful stress reducer.

Hill's analysis identified major themes related to resilience, well-being and readiness for college. Even students who mostly disliked physical activity were enabled to develop connections, feel welcome in the university community, understand more about univer-sity life, and develop confidence in themselves and their abilities.

The Importance of Friends

The feeling of 'belonging' mediates student academic success and retention (Thomas, 2012). Interpersonal relations are generally essential for satisfying this need to belong, although the built environment has a role too, as does a university's reputation and academic record Goodenow (1993) described belonging as 'the sense of being accepted, valued, included, and encouraged by others (teacher and peers) in the academic class-room setting and of feeling oneself to be an important part of the life and activity of the class'.

The *What works?* projects (Advance HE, 2020) used retention rates as a pragmatic outcome measure, and found some interventions achieved 10% improvements through a focus on:

- supportive peer relations;
- meaningful interaction between staff and students;
- developing knowledge, confidence and identity as higher education learners;
- educational experiences relevant to interests and future goals.

In contrast with what students predicted, they found that the contribution of the academic experience in making students feel part of the university community was substantially more than that of the social experience. Effective interventions started pre-entry, with an emphasis on engagement and an overt academic purpose.

The situation is complex and dynamic, though. It may be that whilst an overt focus on academic matters is most effective, it is the beneficial social spin-off that mediates flourishing. A study of the outcomes of a pre-entry programme found that benefits for participants consisted of higher academic self-efficacy at the start of the academic year (Pennington, 2018). However, it was 'in-group social identity' that predicted satisfaction at the end of the academic year.

As Brown and Murphy (2020) point out, finding new friendships is the main source of anxiety for new students. Their concern focuses primarily on new living companions rather than on academic course mates. Students felt that they would need to decide quite early on who they got on with, so they could plan who to live with in their second year of university. These concerns are realistic. The second year is indeed a time of immense challenge, not least because of the traditional move out of halls, and research also suggests many benefits for those who can make early friendships.

Most research into the first year is published in US journals drawing on US student samples so may not be directly applicable to UK students. However, over half of students surveyed in the United States and Canada reported feeling "very lonely" in the past 12 months (American College Health Association, 2016). A Canadian study examined the number of friendships reported by new students at a large university, without evaluating the quality or nature of those relationships (Klaiber et al., 2018). Three years later, students who made more friends in their first term reported healthier physical exercise and diet, as well as lower tobacco, alcohol and marijuana consumption. Good social integration had both direct and indirect influences on health. The students appeared to actively support each other in healthier behaviours, and to jointly set realistic healthy norms.

Klaiber et al. (2018) point out that existing interventions to improve students' health commonly focus on one specific health behaviour and are not strikingly effective. They suggest that interventions targeting students' social adjustment, rather than any one specific health behaviour, may be more effective.

The realistic concern to create a new friendship group can be experienced as sheer desperation to 'fit in'. Young students, even more than the rest of us, are keenly sensitive to the need to impress their peers as capable. When still at school they were able to confide worries and concerns to close friends. In the early weeks at university, though, they prefer to get support from staff instead of peers. Untested peers, they told research-ers, might 'ruin your social reputation' by spreading the information to other students as gossip.

This demonstrates how uniquely vulnerable students feel in the first term, except for the minority who have come with an established friendship group. Some do use the strategy of turning back, through phone or other media, to parents or friends from home. This can feel safer, but too much reliance on previous supports risks retarding the formation of new relationships and even of preventing progress in transitioning.

How Do UK Students Cope? Alcohol Oils the Transition

The Canadian study (Kleiber et al., 2018) suggests that a wide friendship group can reduce alcohol consumption. In the UK, unfortunately, there is evidence that current norms and pressures of student culture actually increase the misuse of alcohol and other substances. Students use alcohol to relieve social anxiety and to fit into a culture where high levels of intoxication are normalised. Not drinking can result in social exclusion. The consequences of alcohol use for students' mental health and well-being are discussed further in Chapter 6. Meanwhile it is important to be aware that the culture is anticipated even before arrival at university, and that individual interventions are limited and socially prejudicial to those individuals.

Even before arrival at university, students are exposed to social media expectations of 'partying', where social anxieties are numbed by intoxication and students feel pressured to plunge into the sex, drugs and rock and roll of student cliché. At present there is little evidence of real change at an institutional level. Attempts to change such behaviour at an individual level are rarely successful.

A qualitative study by Brown and Murphy (2020) vividly illustrates the situation through analysis of detailed interviews with 23 first-year students. The students described their pre-arrival concern over new peer relationships and how this was subsequently relieved by drinking together. This experience confirmed their expectation that alcohol was beneficial, which in turn increased the behaviour. Drinking – or even the expectation of drinking – worked as a cure for anticipatory anxiety, then the act of drinking with peers reduced anxiety in the actual company of others. The rituals of drinking included going out or coming together in student accommodation, having a glass to hold and occupy one's hands, and the act of drinking as a reason for being there. These seemed at least as important for some students as the experience of being intoxicated, but they didn't appear to find communal tea drinking, for example, as an acceptable alternative.

For this group, alcohol felt like the ideal – or perhaps the only – solution for successful transition. Those who drank little or no alcohol said it was a real challenge to make social connections. They had to make careful plans and prepare avoidance tactics to try to both meet others and resist the pressure to drink. It was a distressing and lonely experience to be sober in a crowd of heavily intoxicated others.

The new students' previous drinking experiences were highly variable, but the expectation of the centrality of alcohol to university social activity was universal. The official message from university authorities and student unions was that alcohol was not promoted, but local retailers were free to promote alcohol use, and drinking and 'partying' dominates the informal narrative of student leisure activities. Participants in this study seemed discount the risks of alcohol-related harms in the context of social benefits. They behaved as if the risks were entirely acceptable, much as we would expect to discount the risks to life and health of travelling on the roads, in the light of the desirability of getting around.

Regulation of student alcohol use in such a context seems futile. Staff told the researchers 'there's nothing you can do about that'. It may be true that there are limits to the effectiveness of interventions by individual staff members. Universities and even wider communities will need to work together at a systemic level.

Some students reported taking steps to reduce [. . .] pre-arrival concerns, going online to either Facebook groups linking students from the same residences or the chat site 'Student Room', where current and previous students post information on halls, social activities in the area and other aspects of university life. This generally involved planning drinking events, with previous residents suggesting 'big pre-drinks' sessions to meet housemates and break the ice on arrival. Online groups like this were identified as helpful in starting to create an image of campus life and also providing opportunities for development of social connections.

(Brown and Murphy, 2020)

Incomplete Transitions

Students' first-year experience is seen as a high-priority research area, not least because of the consequences of student attrition and failure for university reputations and finances (Wilcox, 2005). Virtually all UK universities deploy interventions to help embed students, and enhance retention during the transitional period.

Retention and reduction of dropout are important for university finances but not necessarily good proxies for healthy connectedness. The loss of intellectually gifted but unhappy scholars is an academic and reputational loss to all, but we need to consider the best interests of an individual student. Sometimes there is a mismatch between the way of life demanded by a university or course, and the readiness of the student to engage with it, and they shouldn't be coerced into living with the discomfort for three or four miserable and expensive years.

Students at highest risk, including the risk of suicide, include those who are obliged to leave their course in an unplanned way, a phenomenon uncomfortably described as 'dropping out'. Whether this occurs because of financial breakdown, academic failure, mental or physical illness, family tragedy or some mixture of these, there is likely to be a huge emotional component to the experience. Even when there is a sense of relief, families as well as the student, are likely to experience disappointment, shame, embarrassment, a sense of loss and even despair.

When Does It All Settle Down?

Preparation and transition do not end with the arrival of the student on their new campus. Questions of readiness and pacing should be asked at each stage in higher education – some graduates rush straight into higher degree courses when they might be better served by taking a break from academia. Much is made of the challenges faced by older students, moving back into education after a gap, but in practice these individuals often thrive and relish the educational experience more than younger students, who are too preoccupied with day-to-day survival to truly enjoy their studies.

There is evidence that the acute stressors of the first term recede. Gall's (2000) sample of 68 first-year students found that as time passed there was steady improvement in most aspects of adjustment. In this study, women showed greater vulnerability to the transition into university life, despite having more resources. A much larger study of over 4000 students at a UK university examined self-reported anxiety symptoms over the course of first year (Cooke et al., 2006). Moving from home to university was associated with increased self-reported symptoms. Reported psychological well-being fluctuated throughout the year but did not return to pre-university levels.

Further transitions emerge too. It's important not to focus so much on the first year that we overlook the needs of students returning to the second year. Andrews and Wilding (2004) assessed the mental health of UK undergraduates a month prior to starting university and in the middle of the second year. At the second assessment, 20% of students with no previous mental health symptoms had clinical levels of anxiety and 9% had clinical levels of depression. Financial difficulties made a significant independent contribution to depression, whilst relationship difficulties independently predicted anxiety.

Macaskill (2013) found that on admission, 13% of students had a mental health condition. The figure dropped a little by the end of first year but peaked in the middle of the second year to more than 23% of students before dropping to 19% for mid-third-year students. Student Minds (2014) highlighted the challenges of transitioning from living in university accommodation or in private, shared accommodation with other students, and fixed tenancy agreements make it hard for students to move elsewhere if they are unhappy living with their housemates. Also, for second-year students, the university induction and support systems are less structured than those for first-year students, their lecturers and support tutors may have changed, the novelty of university life may have worn off, they are accumulating student debt, and there is more pressure to perform academically, given that often the second and third years determine the degree grade.

It seems that the whole of university life is a continuous 'transitional' experience or at least one of repeated transitions. In the third or final year, the transition into the wider world brings loss of 'student' role status, choices to be made about careers or further study, financial adjustments from living on loans to earning a salary and even repaying debts, and often further geographical moves.

An interesting 2012 study (Richardson et al., 2012) examined the well-being of Australian first-year students. It compared the characteristics of "thriving" students with those who described themselves as "just surviving". Close social relationships, good time management and organisational skills, and effective coping strategies were the key differences. For instance, one 'thriving' student said she made a point of pairing something stressful, such as exam revision, with spending time with friends, in a study group. The healthier students tended to be much more focused on taking action to deal with the stress, allowing them to relax afterwards, whereas 'just surviving' students used passive and avoidant strategies, which left them feeling worse. One implication of this finding is that those who struggle may need to be approached with assertive help rather than expected to make use of available generic information that is available and to reach out for the support they need. 'Just surviving' students may not (yet) be experiencing a diagnosable mental disorder. They could benefit from straightforward skills: keeping a diary, attending some clubs and activities, combining friendship and study, and learning to recognise and manage feelings.

Practice Points

Awareness for All

- Life transitions cluster in the age group in which young people commonly go to university.
- Students' lives are in constant transition. This is exhilarating and stimulating provided there is a secure base still available.
- All transitions increase the risk of depression and other mental illnesses, particularly if they are not managed supportively.
- An incomplete transition may be necessary and beneficial but 'dropping out' can also raise the risk of mental illness and even suicide.

Schools and Families

- Students, and their supporting family, friends and teachers, should embark on the transition process early on.
- Well-being and pastoral support need to be a more prominent factor when choosing universities. Charter recognition can help with this.

Students Preparing for University Life

- Induction courses and summer schools can usefully target prospective freshers identified as needing more information, skills and networks to flourish in university life.
- Powerful peer influences often start on social media and in university accommodation before term begins.
- Caution is needed to challenge social media expectations of student life.

Students Arriving at University

- Interpersonal connections are rightly identified by prospective students as key to thriving.
- The experience of 'homesickness' is normal and not trivial. It can be managed by getting to know the new environment, learning life skills, becoming involved in university activities and making new friendship groups.
- Students are expected to use alcohol to facilitate socialising. This is discussed further in Chapter 6.

Mentorship in Universities: Formal and Informal

- Young people value having a single contact who knows them well, who they can raise concerns with and visit for advice.
- Informal mentoring relationships are valuable. Friends and mentors from schooldays can reach into university life to provide age-appropriate support.
- More formal mentoring is particularly important for those vulnerable to mental illness.

At the Institutional Level

- The culture of alcohol and other substance misuse still has to be addressed.
- Students are at particular risk of loneliness and anxiety during the frenetic early weeks of the first term, when new relationships have yet to reach trustworthy levels. Educational institutions and accommodation providers should work together to bridge this gap.
- Universities should sign up to the UK Mental Health Charter to ensure they are providing students with a psychological environment in which education can be effective.

References

Advance HE (2020). *What works? Student retention and success change programme.* www.advance-he.ac.uk/guidance/teaching-and-learning/student-retention-and-success/what-works-student-retention-and-success-change-programme

Andrews, B. & Wilding, J. M. (2004). The relation of depression and anxiety to life-stress and achievement in students. *British Journal of Psychology*, 95 (4), 509–21.

Apter, T. E. (2002). *The myth of maturity: What teenagers need from parents to become adults.* New York: WW Norton & Company.

Arnett, J. J. (2000). Emerging adulthood: A theory of development from the late teens through the twenties. *American Psychologist*, 55(5), 469.

Bewick, B., Koutsopoulou, G., Miles, J., Slaa, E. & Barkham, M. (2010). Changes in undergraduate students' psychological well-being as they progress through university. *Studies in Higher Education*, 35(6), 633–45. www.doi.org/10.1080/03075070903216643

Bowlby, J. (1969). *Attachment Vol. I of Attachment and loss*. New York: Basic.

Brown, R. & Murphy, S. (2020). Alcohol and social connectedness for new residential university students: Implications for alcohol harm reduction. *Journal of Further and Higher Education*, 44(2), 216–30. www.doi.org/10.1080/0309877X.2018.1527024

Cooke, R., Bewick, B. M., Barkham, M., Bradley, M. & Audin, K. (2006). Measuring, monitoring and managing the psychological well-being of first year university students. *British Journal of Guidance & Counselling*, 34(4), 505–17.

Denovan, A. & Macaskill, A. (2016). Stress and subjective well-being among first year UK undergraduate students. *Journal of Happiness Studies*, 18(2), 505–25. www.doi.org/10.1007/s10902–016-9736-y

Duffy, A., Saunders, K. E. A., Malhi, G. S., et al. (2019). Mental health care for university students: A way forward? *Lancet Psychiatry*, 6(11), 885–7. https://doi.org/10.1016/S2215-0366(19)30275-5

Elgàn, T. H., Durbeej, N. & Gripenberg, J. (2019). Breath alcohol concentration, hazardous drinking and preloading among Swedish university students. *Nordic Studies on Alcohol and Drugs*, 36(5), 430–41. https://doi.org/10.1177/1455072519863545

Fisher, S. & Hood, B. (1987). The stress of the transition to university: A longitudinal study of psychological disturbance, absent-mindedness and vulnerability to homesickness. *British Journal of Psychology*, 78, 425–41.

Gall, T. L., Evans, D. R. & Bellerose, S. (2000). Transition to first–year university: Patterns of change in adjustment across life domains

and time. *Journal of Social and Clinical Psychology*, 19(4), 544–67.

Giedd, J. N. (2008). The teen brain: Insights from neuroimaging. *Journal of Adolescent Health*, 42(4), 335–43.

Goodenow, C. (1993). Classroom belonging among early adolescent students: Relationships to motivation and achievement, *The Journal of Early Adolescence*, 13(1), 21–43.

Harris, A. (2019). *Finding our own way*. Centre for Mental Health. www.centreformentalhealth.org.uk/sites/default/files/2019-01/CentreforMH_FindingOurOwnWay.pdf

Hill, E., Posey, T., Gomez, E. & Shapiro, S. L. (2018). Student readiness: Examining the impact of a university outdoor orientation program. *Journal of Outdoor Recreation, Education, and Leadership*, 10(2), 109–23.

Hughes, G. & Smail, O. (2014). Which aspects of university life are most and least helpful in the transition to HE? A qualitative snapshot of student perceptions. *Journal of Further and Higher Education*, 39(4), 466–80. https://doi.org/10.1080/0309877X.2014.971109

Klaiber, P., Whillans, A. V. & Chen, F. S. (2018). Long-term health implications of students' friendship formation during the transition to university. *Applied Psychology: Health and Well–being*, 10(2), 290–308. https://doi.org/10.1111/aphw.12131

Klerman, G. L. & Weissman, M. M. (1994). *Interpersonal psychotherapy of depression: A brief, focussed specific strategy*. London: Jason Aronson Inc.

Macaskill, A. (2013). The mental health of university students in the United Kingdom. *British Journal of Guidance & Counselling*, 41(4), 426–41.

Palmer, M., O'Kane, P. & Owens, M. (2009). Betwixt spaces: Student accounts of turning point experiences in the first–year transition. *Studies in Higher Education*, 34 (1), 37–54.

Pancer, S. M., Hunsberger, B., Pratt, M. W. & Alisat, S. (2016). Cognitive complexity of expectations and adjustment to university in the first year. *Journal of Adolescent*

Research, 15(1), 38–57. https://doi.org/10 .1177/0743558400151003

Pennington, C. R., Bates, E. A., Kaye, L. K. & Bolam, L. T. (2018). Transitioning in higher education: An exploration of psychological and contextual factors affecting student satisfaction. *Journal of Further and Higher Education*, 42(5), 596–607. https://doi.org/ 10.1080/0309877X.2017.1302563

Richardson, A., King, S., Garrett, R. & Wrench, A. (2012). Thriving or just surviving? Exploring student strategies for a smoother transition to university. A practice report. *The International Journal of the First Year in Higher Education*, 3 (2), 87–93. https://doi.org/10.5204/intjfyhe .v3i2.132

Richardson, T., Elliott, P., Roberts, R. & Jansen, M. (2017). A longitudinal study of financial difficulties and mental health in a national sample of British undergraduate students. *Community Mental Health Journal*, 53, 344–52. https://doi.org/10 .1007/s10597-016-0052-0

Royal College of Psychiatrists (2021). *Mental health of higher education students.* www .rcpsych.ac.uk/docs/default-source/ improving-care/better-mh-policy/college-reports/mental-health-of-higher-education-students-(cr231).pdf

Stroebe, M., Schut, H. & Nauta, M. (2015). Homesickness: A systematic review of the scientific literature. *Review of General Psychology*, 19(2), 157–71. https://doi.org/ 10.1037/gpr0000037

Student Minds (2014). *Grand challenges in student mental health.* www.studentminds.org.uk/ uploads/3/7/8/4/3784584/grand_challenges_ report_for_public.pdf

Thomas, L. (2012). *Building student engagement and belonging in higher education at a time of change: Final report from the What Works? Student retention and success programme.* London: Paul Hamlyn Foundation.

Unite Students & Higher Education Policy Institute (2017). *Reality check: A report on university applicants' attitudes and perceptions.* www.hepi.ac.uk/wp-content/ uploads/2017/07/Reality-Check-Report-Online1.pdf

Universities UK (2015). *Student mental wellbeing in higher education: Good practice guide.* www.m25lib.ac.uk/wp-content/ uploads/2021/02/student-mental-wellbeing-in-he.pdf

Van Gennep, A. (1960) *The rites of passage.* (Vizedom, M. B. & Caffee, G. L., Trans.). London: Routledge. (Original work published 1909)

The Transition to University for New Students with Pre-Existing Mental Conditions

This chapter will address the challenges of the transition when the student already has a known pre-existing mental disorder. Many of the issues involved will of course be the same as for any new student, so readers who have plunged directly into this chapter may like to read the preceding chapter first.

The transition from school to university is recognised as a time when most young people need support to prevent extreme mental stress and make the most of their academic and psychosocial opportunities. For those who have already been diagnosed with a mental illness, the need for protection is more obvious, but the means of providing it is not always straightforward.

We are all likely to develop a diagnosable mental disorder at some point in our lives. The Dunedin Birth Cohort Study found that by age 18, half of the entire population meets criteria for at least one diagnosable mental disorder (Caspi, 2020). About 70% of UK students are between age 17 and 25. This age range is a high-risk period for the onset of schizophrenia, bipolar disorder and common mental disorders such as anxiety and depression. Some in the age group are affected by conditions with onset in childhood or early adolescence, such as attention deficit hyperactivity disorder (ADHD), anorexia nervosa and obsessive–compulsive disorder. Others may be vulnerable to experiencing these conditions in future.

A study from the World Health Organization World Mental Health Surveys estimated that only a fifth of university students (from 21 different countries though not the UK) had a mental health issue. Four fifths of these had been diagnosed before they started at university (Auerbach et al., 2016). Certainly, more students than ever are now disclosing a psychiatric diagnosis. The report 'Student Mental Well-Being in Higher Education' (Universities UK, 2015) states that over 5 years the proportion of students who declared a mental health condition doubled from 0.4% of the student population in 2007–8 to 0.8% in 2011–12. It is impossible to say whether this increase represented higher rates of mental disorder or – perhaps more likely – greater willingness to disclose, as universities made concerted efforts to facilitate and normalise disclosure.

When Lily applied for a teacher training course, she anguished about whether to disclose her ADHD and anxiety issues. She would have liked to have support and consideration of the extra difficulties they caused her, but she was afraid that any 'mental illness' would disqualify her for working with children, or at least that she would be seen as a less competitive candidate than someone who was 'perfect and capable'. The form did not state that such information would be kept confidential from academic staff or those deciding on allocation of places. Her parents advised her to say nothing.

At the time of writing (2021), students can disclose a mental health condition under the 'disability/special needs' section of the UK's standardised Universities and Colleges Admissions Service (UCAS) application form. Not all young people with mental health problems identify as having a 'disability', though. Those who do may well be cautious about disclosure in this context. UCAS is in the process of *launching its new Application Management Service to replace the current Apply service*. It has reviewed the 'disability' question and supporting text, to allow students with mental health issues to alert their chosen university or college to any concerns or support needs they may have. UCAS plans to review the acceptability of this system in partnership with young people.

It is essential to describe who will and who will not have access to the disclosure, and what protection is then afforded to such information. Indeed, this applies to declarations and disclosures on all such forms, whether applications for university, for employment, and for treatment or support. Students of professions such as medicine, nursing, teaching and the law tell us they are particularly apprehensive about the potential risks of making a declaration (See Chapter 19).

Disclosure of a disability or mental health condition does not usually result in stigma and discrimination, despite the mythology that exists, but it might not automatically guarantee effective support either. A number of factors interfere with provision of appropriate help. These factors include difficulties in managing to juggle the academic timetable alongside dealing with treatment for a mental health condition (Royal College of Psychiatrists, 2011) and a lack of advice before their transition between services and locations (Akinrogunde, 2016).

Information about a disclosed disability is protected by the Equality Act and the Data Protection Act. It is sensitive personal information and should not be passed onto anybody else without the individual's permission, or exceptionally, in the case of a formal legal requirement. Universities and colleges have policies outlining which members of staff will be told about a student's disability. With the student's consent, this might include the disability adviser, the personal tutor, examinations officer and individual lecturers.

Communicating the presence of a mental disorder to the university is only part of the difficult process of ensuring transfer of appropriate care. Sometimes the nature of the mental disorder makes the experience of change particularly hard to tolerate. People who are high on the autistic spectrum rely heavily on predictability and control in order to feel safe. Those with obsessive conditions and eating disorders can also suffer from heightened anxiety when their compulsive rituals are linked to particular environments. Chapters 14–18 explore in more detail how different mental disorders are manifested and managed at university. In terms of the transition process, those vulnerable to all significant mental conditions benefit from early and thorough planning.

The day I turned 18 everything changed. Not only was it fairly daunting – the prospect of being an adult – but also my treatment was to be changed. The problem lay with the fact that I was not able to make changes on my own without support but was encouraged under an adult service to take responsibility for myself, make the changes independently and not rely on my parents.

(Patient A, Royal College of Psychiatrists College Report)

Throughout childhood and schooldays, written records and verbal information about the child are passed from adult to adult, without the child having much responsibility for this. Suddenly at age 18 the individual is expected to become the agent of responsibility. Only rarely will a schoolteacher have a counterpart in the university with whom they can share the profile of concerns and expectations of the student, and mental health clinicians may not have identified counterparts in adult services in other geographical areas. Written records are less likely to be read in a large organisation where the student is a stranger, than in a small institution in which the child was already known.

Most existing mentorship arrangements suffer from the drawback that they only move into action when the student has actually started at the university. For instance, mental health mentorship is applied for in advance, but the first meeting with the mentor does not occur until the first term has started. It is disappointing too that such input is often confined to attending appointments, as if at a clinic. Community based coaching could usefully involve eating together, walks and visits to key venues, grappling with electronic timetables, and exploring society options.

The latest edition of the Royal College of Psychiatrists (2021) College Report on the Mental Health of Students in Higher Education summarises longstanding systemic problems and makes a series of helpful recommendations. They include the advice that

> the student going to university should be advised to contact and meet the mental health or disability advisor at their intended place of study to discuss any support that may be required and to consider applying for Disabled Students' Allowance.

The following website provides an estimate of whether the student is likely to be eligible for DSA:

www.surveymonkey.co.uk/r/HE-support-checker

Guidance on the application process is available at:

https://diversityandability.com/dsa-find-your-way/

It is often overlooked that mental illness, like physical illness, can involve students in extra financial expense too, and this can be recognised and alleviated to some extent. The Disabled Students' Allowance (DSA) is a government-funded allowance designed to ensure that students who have a longer-term health condition or 'disability' are not disadvantaged in accessing their university studies. When a student discloses their mental health disorder to the university, this generally sets off the process of inviting them to apply for DSA.

The allowance is not a loan and is not financially means tested. The amount received depends on individual needs. Students with longer-term mental health conditions as well as those with physical disabilities are eligible for DSAs. A formal psychiatric diagnosis is not required, but the student must provide evidence, for instance in the form of a general practitioner (GP)'s or psychiatrist's letter. Dual or multiple diagnoses, including for instance autism, ADHD, visual or hearing impairments, dyslexia or epilepsy, are taken into account in deciding the level of allowance needed.

Graduate students as well as undergraduates are eligible, provided that their course is longer than 12 months, and distance learning courses are included. Whilst international students may not be formally eligible, some universities can help them to access equivalent funding. Further details about applications and the financial context of mental health are described in Chapter 9.

For many students with mental health problems, the greatest benefit to receiving DSA is being able to access one-on-one support from a specialist mental health mentor, which can continue, usually with the same professional, for the length of the university course.

A Not-So-National Health Service

We might imagine that once a person is a patient within the National Health Service (NHS), treatment would automatically continue, making allowances for the fact that we get older or move about within the UK. However, the system is in fact managed within separate health trusts and boards, to the extent that budgets are allocated locally rather than nationally, and medical records – even electronic records – are unavailable outside those boundaries. Moreover, for those with long-term conditions, even within local services there is a major change to be negotiated when a young patient becomes an adult.

Fortunately, GPs have responsibility for our lifelong care, so long as we remain within their catchment area. However, this is not the case for the specialist secondary care providers to whom GPs refer us. For short-term disorders, continuity is less important, and we may hardly notice that we are directed for treatment in accordance with our age. In the management of longer lasting conditions though, it can be disturbing to discover that our service is unable to provide treatment once we reach a certain age. When the condition is a mental illness, and the treatment depends so strongly on a trusting therapeutic relationship, the enactment of a strict boundary at age 18 can set back recovery.

There has been great variation in the age at which paediatric services move their patients up to adult services, but in mental health services, the cut off is at 18. Patients and families tell us that the transition from child and adolescent mental health services (CAMHS) all too often feels like a withdrawal of treatment, requiring a re-referral to adult services, involving a return to the GP, justifying further specialist treatment in the face of partial recovery, and returning to waiting lists.

For those who then do manage to access psychiatric treatment, the style of working is usually strikingly different in adult services from what was experienced in CAMHS. Sometimes there is an unfortunate culture split between the different services. Adult services may be seen (with some justification) as impoverished, situated in unattractive premises, and less family friendly, with clinicians who lack training in the needs of transition aged youth, and rely heavily on prescribing medication rather than providing psychological therapies. Conversely, CAMHS services may be seen as being 'precious' and as fostering unhelpfully dependent and 'entitled' attitudes in young patients and their families. Several institutions have launched recommendations and initiatives to enact transition as a move within a treatment setting, but with limited success so far, partly because the culture divide remains unaddressed., and partly because geographical divisions are so hard to surmount.

Well-intentioned plans to do away with the transition entirely, or to delay the age at which it occurs may not resolve problems of geography. In England, the NHS 2019 Long Term Plan included a commitment 'to extend current service models to create a comprehensive offer for 0-to-25-year-olds', and similar commitments are part of the Scottish Government plans. A more youth-focussed approach to the care of the student age group is welcome, but clinicians and managers alike feel overwhelmed by the complexities of resource transfer and retraining. They point out that the transition would still be an obstacle at age 25 rather than 18, and that for most young people there are already geographical and life changes around age 18 that have to be negotiated, particularly the bureaucratic obstacles involved in geographical moves.

> ...my home specialist services did all they could to transfer care smoothly and ahead of time but were constantly told nothing could be set up until I had arrived at university and registered with a new GP, and then despite my history and letter from my specialist consultant urging a rapid referral to specialist services, I still had to go through the referral process from GP to CMHT [community mental health team] to specialist services, which takes months and then you are on a waiting list to get treatment too...
>
> (Hambly & Byrom, 2014, cited in CR208)

As well as transitioning from CAMHS to adult mental health services, young patients simultaneously experience the transition from sixth form or college to university, from home to university accommodation, and very often from one geographical health board or trust to another. A report by the Joint Commissioning Panel for Mental Health (2013) found that nearly a third of teenagers lose their support during these transitions and a further third experience an interruption in care.

The 'transition', when it occurs, is not even a stable one. Access to the new local health services is only possible during term time, and during university vacations students may return home, work elsewhere or even go abroad. Treatment is usually suspended during vacations. The result is repeated mini-transitions, with massive disruption to treatment. Such difficulties may defeat even the most highly motivated student when seeking mental health treatment.

There may be ways for services to deliver care on a more flexible basis. Some clinicians already offer telephone contact outside term time, and since the COVID lockdown, telemedicine and video-consultations have become more normal. It would be dangerous to imagine that all care can be safely delivered by remotely, but it might allow geographically mobile students (and others) to select a base service that could then reach out to them when they are not at their registered address. Meanwhile, NHS financial arrangements need to be examined and updated to provide realistically for a mobile population.

When students move away from home for university, they have to register with a new GP, which takes time and can result in disruption or delayed treatment if the new mental health service insists on GP registration as a prerequisite for admission to the services. Some students who are still recovering from mental disorders choose to attend a university in their home town to allow them access more parental support and even to live at home. Such choices are not available to remote and rural dwellers, though. The key role of the GP in facilitating access to all health services was highlighted in the previous chapter. When a student has a pre-existing mental health condition it is even more imperative.

> Jake moved away to study at a university a hundred miles from home. He moved in with an aunt and uncle and telephoned their GP practice to register. He was told the list was full, then on contacting a neighbouring practice was told to present with a photo ID at 11 a.m. the next

morning. Each day a limited number of registrations was permitted, and after 2 weeks, Jake was still not one of those. He was now in trouble for missing a great many lectures and had run out of his obsessive–compulsive disorder medication. When he finally spoke with his relatives about the situation, they let him know he could consult with their own doctors on a temporary basis, and his uncle wrote to the local MP to highlight the problem.

Pros and Cons of Delaying the Start of University

It is a pity to have to advise young people to curb their adventures at this stage of life. Some students do choose, though, to delay taking up a place at university for a year or so to allow extra time to plan and link services, as well as to undertake further treatment and to make up for the developmental delays caused by a period of illness. There is a balance to be struck between rights of people to progress through education if academically possible (expecting the institution to provide care), and on the other hand the rights of a university to expect people to recover as much as possible before going to university (or perhaps dropping out at times of acute illness and returning when well).

Most families and services have good intentions in terms of planning, but many struggle with the time required for such planning, the difficulties in co-ordinating timetables of pressured CAMHS and adult services, the rigidity of patient care pathways, which may insist on local GP registration before a referral or transfer can be accepted, and the relatively short time available between a student finding out which university will accept them, and their arrival on campus.

Universities do expect to make provisions for people living with stable long-term disabilities but not necessarily for medium-term episodes of illness. They are not hospitals providing full nurture. Sometimes, students may be able to access the academic curriculum despite serious illness, but miss out on the broader experience of university life. The goal of attending university is not merely to emerge with a certificate!

The option of delaying the start of university – in contrast with the active choice of taking a 'gap year' – is a complicated one. Adolescents are acutely sensitive to peer pressure and to 'belonging'. Many of them will have moved through previous transitions as a 'tribe'. The moves from class to class, then from primary to secondary school are often made, and celebrated, as a whole group. Nurseries often have extremely close relationships with primary schools, and 'feeder' primary schools with high schools. Adults understand that those children who move alone from school to school or even within school, require extra support.

Jilly suffered from anorexia nervosa and spent most of her teens in and out of hospital. The hospital school provided excellent tuition – she managed to sit higher examinations and achieve high grades. At age 18 she was transferred to an adult inpatient unit. There was no school, but occupational therapists arranged with the local university for her attend some classes and complete assignments from the ward. She threw herself into her studies with her characteristic perfectionism and did well. She was able to feel proud of her achievement, at a time when her self-esteem was otherwise low, but a few years later, now recovered, working and starting her own family, she spoke of her degree as 'just a piece of paper' and wished she had enjoyed the independence and social experiences others enjoyed at university.

The move from school to university is different in that it rarely involves more than a small group making the same move together. However, there is usually ceremonious acknowledgement of a communal leaving and moving forward. The prize-givings, leavers' balls and parties, farewells to teachers, and parental involvement in all these celebrations can be painful for people who are not moving positively forward to university or to gap year adventures.

Kit had a severe depressive breakdown, and despite getting good grades and a place at her chosen university, was 'persuaded' to take a year out to recover more. She experienced a further drop in self-esteem and blamed her parents for holding her back. She worked weekdays in a local supermarket. This left her free to spend many weekends with friends in student halls – none of them at her future university. She always said, 'that should have been me'. She was horrified to find she would be starting her course with two pupils from the year below at school, and resolved to avoid them. It distressed her that her younger sister would start university in the same year, although the sister then opted to take her own year out, to travel.

Kit recovered well, regained confidence, and finally left for university, now with savings accrued from working and living rent-free at home. She was able to continue part-time work at a branch of her local supermarket and certainly appreciated the financial and social advantages of having the job. She was referred to the local psychology service, and continued to take a low dose of medication, but declined to take up her right to a mental health mentor. She was amazed to find there was no noticeable age gap between her and her peers, nor had she lost her academic skills in her 'year out'. She was open about her illness and used the fact she was on medication as a reason to not drink heavily or use drugs. Her group of friends respected that choice.

Kit now admitted privately that if she had rushed to take up her place straight after school she might have had to drop out and re-start.

For students who are not mentally healthy enough to proceed to university, it is particularly difficult if they do not even have a deferred place to look forward to. The sense of a stalled transition is depressing. One strategy is to find ways to value the unplanned time for its own sake and fill it productively. Options include short-term paid or voluntary jobs, mastering a new skill or language, or conceptualising the time as a retreat. Ambitious plans for an adventurous 'gap year' can be more dangerous than university though, if the mentally unwell young person travels far from home.

Janys had severe anorexia nervosa from age 12. She was treated and achieved a normal weight, although she exercised compulsively and made herself sick when not supervised. She worked hard and achieved the high grades required for university, but opted to take a gap year first to visit an aunt in Hong Kong. Now that she was 18, CAMHS treatment came to an end and she did not keep appointments offered in adult services, telling her family that she was still on a waiting list.

She had already lost a lot of weight when she left for Hong Kong and by the time she arrived, after a few stopover visits on the journey, her relatives were horrified by her visible emaciation. They were unable to access appropriate treatment for her, so insisted she return home. After a second long journey, during which she ate nothing, her parents were devastated by her appearance, but could not persuade the family doctor to admit her to hospital against her will. By the time she became frightened enough to accept admission she had suffered irreversible organ damage and tragically died.

An enquiry found that the GP should have invoked the Mental Health Act to admit her to hospital sooner.

When a Student Leaves University in a Planned or Unplanned Way

The end of a student's university career may be a particularly high-risk transition for vulnerable students. Even those who have achieved their hoped-for degree face yet another major life change, often with a student debt to pay off. They may not yet have settled employment, and their accommodation arrangements will probably come to an end unless they and their flatmates have plans to stay in the university city. Friendships and life partnerships forged over the past few years have to survive dispersion at the end of higher education. A growing proportion of young people return to the family home, and most become once more fairly dependent on family support. Students who do not have the backstop of a stable family home to provide financial and emotional cushioning may be obliged to sacrifice career plans in order to earn money and find accommodation urgently.

University mental health and other support services are dedicated to students and staff enrolled in the institution. When individuals leave, they may be at increased risk, but no longer have access to these facilities. Careers services do help students look to the future but do not address the full range of needs faced by those young adults who return to the world outside academia.

Students at highest risk, including the risk of suicide, include those who are obliged to leave their course in an unplanned way, a phenomenon uncomfortably described as 'dropping out'. Whether this occurs because of financial breakdown, academic failure, mental or physical illness, family tragedy or some mixture of these, there is likely to be a huge emotional component to the experience. Financial penalties are inevitable too, in terms of course fees and accommodation rent, which continue to the end of the year or term in many cases, as well as any student debt already accumulated. Even when there is a sense of relief, families as well as the student are likely to experience disappointment, shame, embarrassment, a sense of loss and even despair.

For students suffering from mental disorder, it can be impossible and often unwise to make important decisions about the future, but hard to tolerate a period of uncertainty and insecurity. Rebuilding a social and work life requires energy and support. This support often falls to parents and partners of the student who has left. It is crucial that they be provided with the information and resources to provide this care. Both GP registration and any secondary mental health care may need to be transferred back to the home services.

In many ways the situation resembles the transition to university but in reverse. Sadly, it is neither accompanied by happy anticipation nor by a programme analogous to 'Freshers' Week' or 'Welcome Week', yet a package of resources for students leaving university, with a period of permitted overlap of services, and meetings with family and carers where appropriate, might start to address some of the associated risks.

Society is waking up to the risks when vulnerable people leave institutions – whether the armed services, prisons, or the workplace. Pre-retirement courses have been developed to examine the financial, physical and psychosocial aspects of later life. Something similar could usefully follow final examinations for graduating students, perhaps with a modified package of support being made available to students who are obliged to leave university in an unplanned way. A period of grace might need to be offered to allow counselling or other support services to continue beyond the student's leaving date to ensure that the ending is properly prepared and enacted, and to put post-discharge plans into place. The concept of a 'transition mentor' might be particularly helpful in such circumstances particularly for those students without good family support, or for international students returning to their country of origin.

Think Student, Think Family

The Royal College of Psychiatrists' Report (2021) supports bereaved parents in calling for better communication with families when students are mentally ill.

- *Think Student, Think Family! Parents and other family members are usually the most important part of a student's network of support, especially undergraduates. They can be an invaluable source of information in relation to assessment and diagnosis. There are of course situations where the family is the main source of the student's mental health problems and involving them may not be appropriate.*

- *Anyone who is involved in helping mentally troubled students, should, wherever appropriate, seek the consent of the student to engage families in the processes of assessment and treatment. Families should be given a point of contact that they can utilise to communicate concerns about the student.*

> Jim fell ill with a psychotic episode and had to return to his parents' home to recover. He was too ill to contact academic staff to explain why he could not submit work. His father was refused any contact with his tutors 'for reasons of confidentiality' but Jim was sent repeated emails warning him of consequences if he did not send assignments, and then informing him he had failed his course. When he recovered sufficiently to access his emails he was devastated, and experienced a further setback in his mental state. His parents asked medical staff to advocate for Jim with the university.

Family should have rights to information and support commensurate with the responsibilities placed on them and the burden experienced by them. Extreme insistence on 'confidentiality' is not based on firm legal principles, although it is often implied that this is so. Students, staff, parents and university officials should regularly review and discuss guidance around autonomy and confidentiality. The blanket withdrawal of all information about the student is simply unnecessary unless the student has given explicit instructions that this should be the case. There are different levels of privacy, with different boundaries. It is rare that an individual should be left with information to which no one else is privy. Professional organisations have guidance on how to ensure communication and discussion can be protected from widespread availability whilst extending far enough to provide safety and planning.

Staff in universities and in adult health services may find it inconvenient to have to deal with parental interventions and impractical to do so in the way expected of schools and of CAMHS. The development of individual autonomy is also a laudable aim. However, the sudden switch is not suitable for all young people as they turn 18. They may have only just left home, be living with strangers and may have developed psychological difficulties. We all tend to regress to a less mature stage of development when ill or stressed, and benefit from the people around us communicating on our behalf until we recover.

Family, or extended family, can helpfully provide emotional nurturing, respectful advice and practical assistance. Family anxiety can sometimes come across as over-protective or intrusive or even attacking, when in fact it is a mixture of love and loss. Sometimes the extreme anxiety of a parent is in fact a realistic risk assessment by someone who knows the student well, and should be respected.

The Royal College of Psychiatrists (2017) provides a checklist for supporting transitions from CAMHS to adult services. Relationships between services even in the same health trust or board are not always optimal or able to transfer care smoothly. When the patient is moving to a university away from home, CAMHS in one area may struggle to plan ahead and set up arrangements with colleagues in adult services in the new place of residence. Over-stretched mental health services with long waiting lists find it stressful to prioritise referrals from outside the usual catchment. The student is suddenly expected to take on more agency, at the very time when parental advocacy drops away. Affirmative action has to come from those with an investment in the health of the young person.

Checklist for Good Practice

- Awareness
- Early identification and notification
- Involve family and carers
- Flexible timing
- Close links between services
- Transition coordinator
- Provide good information
- Clear protocols and pathways
- Patient-centred transition plan
- Multidisciplinary discharge planning meeting
- Overlap period of joint working
- Respect for attachment and therapeutic alliances

(Lamb et al., 2008, cited in CR208)

Even with the most ideal service transfers, the young person has to simultaneously cope with intellectual, social and geographical changes. The practical, organisational, and emotional work involved in moving away to university is undeniably greater for a student with a disorder or disability. It is the nature of disorders – and their treatment – to put many maturational tasks on hold. This makes it particularly important to take the necessary time to prepare the student for the next stage in their life.

Practice Points

Families, Schools and Prospective Students

- Consider starting university later to allow time for transfer bureaucracy and to allow the recovering student to reach a higher level of maturity.
- Time out between school and university has many benefits. However, adventurous gap year projects in foreign countries pose significant dangers to young people with mental conditions.

- A university close to home may be the best choice to allow gradual weaning from family support.
- Students, and their supporting family, friends and teachers, should embark on the transition process early on if there is a pre-existing mental illness, and take time to ensure that everything is in place – this takes far longer than you might expect.
- Academic studies can be therapeutic and contribute to recovery and self-esteem. However, academic success is not a guarantee of mental health. High levels of competitiveness actually threaten both success and mental well-being.
- Well-being and pastoral support are important factors in choice of a university for people with pre-existing mental illness. UK Mental Health Charter recognition can help with this.

Arrival at University

- All new students should register with a local GP. Students with pre-existing conditions may benefit from special arrangements to plan this in advance. Services in the university may decline to take on a patient who is not registered with a catchment GP.
- More formal mentoring is particularly important for those vulnerable to mental illness. Mental Health Mentoring is available for students alongside psychiatric services (not as a substitute for these).
- Students with pre-existing mental illness may be particularly vulnerable to using alcohol to 'self-medicate' but may also have increased risk of harm from culturally 'normal amounts of alcohol, sometimes because of prescribed medication. They may also be at risk of prescribed medication having a street value and being appropriated or diverted to other students. Open discussion of this with mentors and clinicians should be sympathetic and supportive rather than accusatory.

NHS Services, GPs and University Support Services

- Institutions need to work together to improve overlap and reduce risk of vulnerable students falling through the gaps. These gaps occur in the transition from school to university and again when the student leaves their course – particularly if this is unplanned.
- Induction courses and summer schools can usefully target prospective freshers identified as needing more information, skills and networks to flourish in university life.
- Telemedicine might allow geographically mobile students (and others) to select a 'base' service that then reaches out when they are away from their registered address.
- NHS financial arrangements need to be examined and updated to provide realistically for a mobile population.

References

Akinrogunde, M. (2016). *Do university students receive the health information and support they need?* [Unpublished research project report] UCL/Universiteit Utrecht.

Auerbach, R. P., Alonso, J., Axinn, W. G., et al. (2016). Mental disorders among college students in the World Health Organization world mental health surveys. *Psychological Medicine*, 46(14), 2955–70.

Caspi, A., Houts, R. M., Ambler, A., et al. (2020). Longitudinal assessment of mental health disorders and comorbidities across 4 decades among participants in the Dunedin birth cohort study. *JAMA Network Open.* 3(4), e203221. http://doi.org/10.1001/jamanetworkopen.2020.3221

Joint Commissioning Panel for Mental Health (2013). *Guidance for commissioners of mental health services for young people making the transition from child and adolescent to adult services.*

Royal College of Psychiatrists (2011). *Mental health of students in higher education (CR166).* www.rcpsych.ac.uk/docs/default-source/improving-care/better-mh-policy/college-reports/college-report-cr166.pdf

Royal College of Psychiatrists (2017). *Managing transitions when the patient has an eating disorder: Guidance for good practice (CR208).* www.rcpsych.ac.uk/docs/default-source/improving-care/better-mh-policy/college-reports/college-report-cr208.pdf

Royal College of Psychiatrists (2021). *Mental health of higher education students (CR231).* www.rcpsych.ac.uk/docs/default-source/improving-care/better-mh-policy/college-reports/mental-health-of-higher-education-students-(cr231).pdf

Unite Students (2018). *The leap: Making the move to university.* www.unite-group.co.uk/sites/default/files/2018-06/The%20Leap%20White%20Paper%20FINAL.pdf

Universities UK (2015). *Student mental wellbeing in higher education: Good practice guide.* www.m25lib.ac.uk/wp-content/uploads/2021/02/student-mental-wellbeing-in-he.pdf

The Roles of Parents and Carers

There is a risk that only parents of students will read this chapter, but it is not addressed only to them. Parent power is a growing force in UK universities that may be troublesome if not engaged with respectfully. The role of the student's family – their parents and other carers – in the mental health of a university student, involves at least a three-way relationship. The attitudes of university authorities and staff, families themselves, and of course the students, all interact.

The intention is that this chapter can be read alone, so there is some overlap with the material in other chapters. Where it would be helpful to explore further detail of particular issues, this is indicated. The chapters on mental health services and on different mental health conditions are the obvious companion chapters to this one.

The most obvious source of parent power in universities is the financial one. Students are expected to pay fees and there are further expenses for accommodation, sustenance and entertainment, usually away from home. This, as well as the respect young people still show for their parents' views, gives parents considerable power in terms of the choice of university. As a result, higher education publicity and information is aimed beyond the individual student and is addressed also to supportive adults such as school teachers and advisors, and above all, parents.

The ubiquity of social media and other forms of electronic communication means that today's families are in much more frequent communication than in the days of the weekly telephone call from a shared phone booth (or in my case the weekly letter home scribbled on the backs of concert programmes and posted in the series of stamped addressed envelopes provided by my father). Faster travel allows visits in both directions several times each semester, rather than students not seeing their families during term time. It is far easier for parents to know what is going on at their child's university as well as with their individual student child, although it is still usually impossible to interact with teaching staff and get direct feedback as they did with schoolteachers.

Perhaps most important, in terms of mental health, is the observation that students generally seem less competent and socially mature than used to be the case. This book frequently makes reference to the concept of 'transition aged youth' or 'emerging adulthood' as a recognisable developmental stage that was not acknowledged until quite recently. In fact, even the concept of 'adolescence' was described by Anna Freud (1958) as 'the Cinderella of psychoanalysis' as recently as 1958. This further concept may generate useful research into how we only gradually mature towards relative autonomy.

There has been increasing focus on the population known as *transitional aged youth* (TAY). Although variably defined, TAY typically refers to the span from older adolescence (e.g., 15–16 years old) to young adulthood (24–26 years old). . . .Some critical developmental steps occur during the transitional years, reflecting changing neurobiology, the tasks of separation and individuation, and the influences of pre-existing and concurrent mental health and substance use issues.

Parents with TAY sustain high burdens of care, particularly for those with very common unmet needs. Indeed, psychopathology and substance abuse are the leading cause of disability worldwide and constitute 45% of disease burden in youth 10 to 24 years of age.

(Wilens & Rosenbaum, 2013)

There are other reasons why students may seem less mature these days. For instance, there has huge increase in the student population relative to the total population. Many young people who would have previously been regarded as too vulnerable to cope with university life are now being encouraged to apply and are doing so successfully.

In the context of opposing claims for and against greater parental involvement, this chapter will examine how families best support students' well-being during their time in higher education. At the same time, it will examine the implication that today's students might benefit from a slightly tougher love, to promote autonomy and maturity. It will cover issues of confidentiality, communications, financial and emotional support through the undergraduate degree course. Finally, it will consider how parents may be involved in the less well-researched transition that occurs when students leave university, whether that is as a successful graduate, or, more worryingly, when this is unplanned or unchosen.

Most research and discussion has focussed on the caring parents of young undergraduate students, but this chapter will also consider students who do not have a family around them to provide care, and those – students and staff members too – who themselves have significant caring roles, either for children or for loved ones with disabilities.

Choice of University

At the start of adolescence, children's secondary education is generally chosen and arranged by their parents, with consideration of the child's own opinions. By the end of secondary school, the young person probably expects to choose and manage their own application to university. Some families have traditions or expectations that cannot fail to influence the choice, even if they are not explicitly discussed. Depending on personality, a young person may actively seek to emulate relatives in attending particular institutions or study particular disciplines. Others may explicitly shun the 'family business' and forge their own individual path.

These influences are not necessarily malign, and are certainly not the only external forces at work. Schools may have a vested interest in sending as many pupils as possible to prestigious institutions, young peers may have formed their own opinions of the 'coolest' or best places to be a student, the universities' marketing strategies obviously exert a pull, and the young person may have visited older friends and relatives at university and formed attachments towards or dislike of certain places. Geographical location is a major consideration for many, and understandably, as with the transition to secondary school, many students aspire to make the move in the company of their friendship group.

> Jeanette's parents were liberal academics who had 'bent over backwards' to give their only child freedom and autonomy. She excelled almost effortlessly at her comprehensive school, where no one aspired to the Oxbridge colleges her parents had attended. They carefully refrained from proposing these as options for her.
>
> Jeanette picked her course and institution to fit in with her friendship group at school, but found to her dismay that she was the only one to get the required grades. She was lonely in halls, and disillusioned with her choice of subject.
>
> Her parents became worried when she returned home every weekend, and encouraged her to stay in halls to build a new friendship group, but she experienced this as a rejection. She decided to leave university for good halfway through her first term.
>
> After a year of casual jobs, she asked her parents to help and advise her in applying for the local university. They were saddened to think that their neutral stance had felt uncaring rather than liberating. Ironically, Jeanette moved away to study for a higher degree in her mother's own area of expertise, and embarked on a career in academia.

Parents and carers can provide perspective and wisdom to the young person, not by suggesting certain choices, but by explicitly drawing attention to the different influences affecting the student's choices. Adults can point out considerations that a young person may not have considered, such as the university's record on pastoral care, or the particular facilities for sport or music performance. They also have an important potential role in helping the young person manage disappointment or triumph in being accepted or rejected by universities, holding their nerve if they are involved in the process of 'clearing' (for students who do not achieve the grades required by universities that initially offered them a place) and reaching an acceptance of the options they have.

Changes in Family Roles When the Student Leaves Home

The early chapters of this book are deeply concerned with the experience of a student's transition to university life. One characteristic of transitions is their tendency to cluster, so that we generally face social, physiological, geographical and interpersonal changes all at once. For the young student, there is often continuing physical growth and further brain development beyond the teenage years and well into the twenties. They will have only just attained the age of legal maturity, with the rights and responsibilities that come with that milestone. As they leave school, they often leave the family home, further explore sexuality and friendships, and form new primary relationships. Less remarked is the background transition cluster experienced by the family they leave behind. Parents may be living with menopause, retirement, ageing and revaluation of the marital relationship. The grandparents' generation is likely to be dealing with illness, loss and bereavements, and any siblings left in the home may also be struggling with the major changes going on around them. Whole family systems have adjustments to make.

Students benefit from being able to trust the remaining family members to thrive without them, despite missing their company and contribution. Meanwhile, parents, grandparents and younger siblings need to manage their loss in ways that do not hold the young person back, but do justice to the shift in relationships that has occurred. In many ways, the loss and the transition are more symbolic than practical, given that university terms are shorter than school terms, and most students spend many weeks each year back in their original homes. Symbolism is crucial, though, to managing mental health.

If at all possible, families should avoid adding to the cluster of inevitable transitions at the same time. Preserving continuity as much as possible allows people to adjust to new roles against a secure background, and to digest changes in manageable chunks.

It is understandable that parents living in a large family home may be eager to 'downsize', perhaps even to free up money to help fund the student. However, one student said

> Sometimes it feels as if they have burned the bridges behind me, as I don't have my own bedroom to go back to now… and there is such a fuss about the move that my leaving for uni has been completely upstaged.

Even more poignantly, parents whose marriage has been uncomfortable might decide to delay separation until the child leaves home, tolerating a distressing situation for the sake of their child's well-being. Some students experience extreme guilt, as they wonder if they could have prevented the divorce by staying at home. They may be distracted from university life by powerful anger at one or both parents, or by concern as to whether a vulnerable parent will cope alone.

Javier, a first-year student, was distraught to discover that his father had moved out and was living with another woman. His mother told him they were selling the family home, finances became chaotic, and Javier was obliged to approach student services when he could not pay hall rent.

Over the course of the term, he drank heavily, broke up with his girlfriend and fell behind with his studies. His father became worried that he ignored all calls and messages, although he knew his son was angry with him. He visited in person and found Javier in a smelly, darkened room, unwashed, unfed, hung over and incoherent.

His response was to call Javier's mother. They were uncomfortably aware that it had taken this breakdown to bring the parents together to address the effects of their separation on their son.

All these complicated family dynamics can impact a young person's ability to learn and to enjoy university life. By no means all students will succumb to a frank breakdown or develop a mental disorder as a result of such stresses, but their well-being is shaken. Students with a vulnerability to mental illness or those who are high on the autism spectrum may be more profoundly disturbed by extra life changes.

The Empty Nest

Society now broadly recognises the parental experience of 'empty nest' syndrome, and associates it specifically with children leaving home for university. It is no longer classically linked with children leaving home for work, or at the time of marriage, which now tends to come later in young people's lives and to be less strikingly associated with any severance of relationships with parents. Fathers, as well as mothers, admit to feeling the sense of grief and loss. The chef Gordon Ramsay, for instance, was open about his experience in an interview reported in The Guardian (Moorhead, 2018).

The experience, though, is far from having the finality of a death, and brings benefits too. Parents can celebrate their own success in bringing a child up to the point of legal maturity, and welcome the extra freedoms and opportunities. Often, indeed, the student becomes more appreciative of family life and the contribution of parents, and developing adult child–to–adult parent relationships can be gratifying. The moment of leaving home is symbolically momentous, but equally important are the shifts in mutual expectations that form and settle over subsequent years. Apter (2002) says, 'leaving home is a stop-start transition and does not mark true independence from parents, emotionally or financially'. Suddenness of changes in external expectations are not well-matched by corresponding shifts in maturity.

As a psychiatrist who has worked both in child and adolescent mental health services (CAMHS) and in adult services, I observe a sudden exclusion of parents from the care of young adults, in contrast with the assertive expectation that they will be involved intensively in their children's therapy, right up to age 18. Parental engagement in the work and care transforms the burden on a hard-pressed NHS, and has often been demonstrated to yield better outcomes than inpatient hospital treatment (Diamond & Josephson, 2005). A university is not, of course, a mental health service. However, when a student is struggling with mental illness, then if they are willing, involving parents in partnership with NHS and university support services, using telemedicine platforms where necessary, may offer more effective care than is a present the case. Indeed, the Royal College of Psychiatrists recommends that, in the case of students with mental illness, 'Think student, think family!' (Royal College of Psychiatrists, 2021).

Whilst parental participation is welcome in supporting students with mental illness, a broader policy of bringing parents into campus life in general, in the way they participate in school life, would alter the ethos and atmosphere of higher education institutions. Unnecessary overinvolvement of parents in university life risks infantilising the culture for all. On the one hand, there needs to be consideration of how far universities should be in dialogue with all parents and providers. On the other hand, there is the important issue of ensuring that when a student becomes worryingly incapacitated – whether for physical or mental health reasons – parents and other supporters have appropriate communication and involvement. This minority group of students is important, but it would be a mistake to focus policy for all students on the needs of this group.

Ecclestone and Hayes (2009) savagely criticise views of school pupils and students as necessarily mentally fragile. Writing with alarm about the 'dangerous rise of therapeutic education', and using this term to describe the focus on managing emotional distress within the curriculum, the authors say such assumptions are partly responsible for the very distress and helplessness they seek to remedy (Ecclestone & Hayes, 2009). Furedi (2017) warns against 'The medicalisation of the university', writing that 'the university risks becoming a de facto clinic where students are the patients.' However, Meyer (2019) restores a balance to the discourse, acknowledging the harms of casting student distress and emotional difficulties as 'disabilities' but also regretting an 'ideological insistence on adulthood at 18'. She emphasises the observations of Apter (2002) on 'the maturity myth', pointing out the normal healthy need for young adults to have emotional, practical and financial support as they negotiate developmental challenges.

We may be able to learn from models and structures used in the United States, where universities have long functioned as commercial institutions catering for the demands of fee payers and donors such as parents and alumni. Another difference there is the existence of different tiers of student life. There are undergraduate colleges, attended while the student is still in their late teens, and then graduate schools where adult scholars form a university community. Anecdotally, I have heard many accounts from friends, family members and acquaintances, in which a 17- or 18-year-old has experienced a thoroughly miserable university career, but then relished the subsequent opportunity to undertake a master's degree or doctorate. In contrast, those of us who delayed starting university until we were just a little older often had happier stories. In some cases, students and parents spoke highly of the greater pastoral supports and structures available in Colleges of Further Education, possibly because these have the experience of catering for students under age 18.

Discussing Whether to Disclose a Mental Health 'Disability'

As earlier chapters have emphasised, under the Equality Act 2010, institutions must make reasonable adjustments for applicants and students with disabilities. The Act says that

a person has a disability if they have a physical or mental impairment which has a substantial and long-term effect on their ability to carry out normal day to day activities.

Not every mental health disorder will qualify but even when it does not, institutions are still obliged to deliver reasonable support under the concept of 'duty of care' already described, and in terms of contract law depending on what the institution has offered in their publicity and promotional material, as discussed earlier. The Act provides for rights and benefits that are mostly focussed on the individual who declares that they have a 'disability', so it would appear obvious that students should disclose their eligibility. Venville (2013) investigated attitudes towards this and confirmed that most staff members expected students to disclose their illness and considered reluctance to do so as tantamount to failure to take full responsibility for their education.

Estimates suggest that fewer than half of those eligible do so, even though the proportion of 'disabled' students who declare a mental health condition has steadily increased (Universities UK, 2015). Parents may need to overcome their own prejudices to properly support the new student to make their own individual decision about this. Young people are far less embarrassed by the notion of mental health than their elders. There are even youth subcultures that regard distress, self-harm and contact with psychiatric services as badges of belonging or even of pride. On the whole, though, young people tend to respect any sense of family shame their parents may feel, and to protect them by not acknowledging their own needs.

For both students and parents using the word 'disability' might feel like an emotional catastrophe, rather than a box to be ticked, though it is hard to suggest any alternative. Students often remark that they think of 'disability' as at a matter involving wheelchairs, or at least confining a person to their own homes if not to an institution. They say that describing themselves in such a way diminishes the idea that they have of themselves (Venville, 2013). Their parents may share this view, perhaps finding the idea that their child is 'disabled' as a matter of shame or criticism of their own parenting. Other parents may pressure the young person to 'disclose' a disability in order to get extra supports, without realising that the student may interpret their attitude as a lack of confidence in their abilities and strengths.

> Janys told her mental health mentor,
>
> No one resents Marie, because her disability puts her in a wheelchair. They spent thousands of pounds installing a ramp into the science block and building a low bench for her practical classes. No one else envies her the ramp or the low bench.
> But I have to have extended deadlines for my assignments and extra time in exams. They all want those, and they think I'm cheating.

By the time a child is ready for university, the parents' role in decision-making should have shifted from being the proxy decision makers, to being the providers of perspective. Parents might want to clarify that for them, some issues are 'non-negotiable' (for instance, parents might decide they can only provide funding if the student studies in the UK), but in others cases they will support the student's own plans and decisions even if they disagree with them (for instance choice of degree course, or whether or not to declare a mental health disability). Conversations about such issues can be sensitive and need to be very private and well-timed. It is helpful to spend some time acknowledging the problems of wording – in particular definitions of 'disability' and safeguards to 'confidentiality'.

Information about a disclosed disability is protected by the Equality Act and the Data Protection Act. It is sensitive personal information and should not be passed onto anybody else without the individual's permission, or exceptionally in the case of a formal legal requirement. Universities and colleges have policies outlining which members of staff will be told about the student's disability. With the student's consent, this might include the disability adviser, the personal tutor, examinations officer, and individual lecturers.

As a general principle, we might want more students to disclose, to provide a more accurate measure of what services are needed, and to normalise attitudes to mental illness. For the individual student, though, the situation is more nuanced. This book contains a number of cases, all based on real situations, where students and their friends and carers have benefitted from communicating their mental 'disability' so that it can be managed as well as possible. In contrast, it also includes narratives of students who had made their vulnerability known either privately to university authorities or more publicly, and who later regretted doing so – for instance, the young medical students 'M' and 'N' who are described in Chapter 19.

I have found it most helpful in speaking with students to leave aside any general principal of whether they 'should' or 'should not' disclose, and hear from them exactly how their needs will be met pragmatically if they do or do not make the decision to disclose. Parents are in a particularly good position to observe how their child's mental health condition can affect their life and what treatments, adjustments and supports allow them to be their best self. At school, they may have been automatically provided with time to attend hospital, with recorded lessons to catch up on what they missed, and facilities to sit examinations in a small room with an individual invigilator. The young person may assume that such facilities will automatically happen at university, when in fact they require special dispensation. Parents and students may also like to look at Chapter 18 to explore what facilities can be offered by universities, over and above those of the NHS. Making a disclosure of need can speed up access to these and begin the process of financing supports, modifications and mentorship for the student.

A young person who has recently recovered from an episode of mental illness commonly assumes that it is cured and finished. University will be a fresh, healthy start. This is impossible to predict. It can be heartbreaking to suggest that what was seen as a successfully treated episode of illness was in fact a 'disability' with the chronic lifelong consequences that term suggests. Young people with acknowledged lifelong physical conditions, such as diabetes or inflammatory bowel disease, also have to come to terms with them, as do their parents. However, the onset of those physical disorders is more often at a younger age. In contrast, mental illnesses that then recur through life commonly start in late adolescence, so that they have to be dealt with when there are big normative life changes going on too.

Confidentiality in Disclosing a Mental Disability

Parents as well as students can be assured that – contrary to some urban myths – disclosure to UCAS and to university authorities does not publicise the student's 'disability' or vulnerability to the whole university community or make it public knowledge. However, the nature of the supports provided for the student may make it likely that staff and peers will guess that there is a disclosed condition of some sort.

This absolutely does not mean, though, that the student is obliged to 'come out' as having a condition, and should not feel obliged to spend time as a representative or campaigner for mental health. Some young people do speak of wanting to 'give back' or to influence service development after an experience of mental health treatment, or may regard sharing and discussing their experience as an important stage in recovery. But this is separate from choice about privately disclosing potential support needs, either on a UCAS form, or at a later stage in university life.

It is essential to describe who will and who will not have access to the disclosure, and what protection is then afforded to such information. Indeed, this applies to declarations and disclosures on all such forms, whether applications for university, for employment, and for treatment or support. Students of professions such as medicine, nursing, teaching and the law tell us they are particularly apprehensive about the potential risks of making a declaration (see Chapter 19).

Disclosure does not usually result in stigma and discrimination, despite the mythology that exists, but it might not automatically guarantee effective support either. Obstacles include difficulties in managing to juggle the academic timetable alongside dealing with treatment for a mental health condition, and a lack of advice before the transition between services and locations (Royal College of Psychiatrists, 2021).

Supporting Homesick Students

Previous chapters have discussed the almost inevitable experience of a degree of 'homesickness' when people go through major transitions like the move to university. The emotional pain is a tribute to the value of the home environment and family relationships that have been left behind, and an acknowledgement that the young person has still not built a new sense of security in terms of the built and interpersonal environment around them. Today's electronic communications may both mitigate the separation and simultaneously slow down the work of building new attachments. Greater ease of transport too, may make the temptation to spend time back home a much greater one than in the past, and it can be tempting for parents feeling their own 'empty nest' distress, to seize every opportunity to enjoy their child's company rather than facilitate painful separation.

How to Help and Support

Developmentally, university represents an important transition between childhood and adulthood with young people expected, and expecting, to take far more responsibility for all aspects of their lives. Some embrace this challenge, others find it hard. The University of Oxford offers a strong support network, which includes tutors, college welfare teams, peer supporters, chaplains, college nurses, doctors and the Counselling Service. If your child is having a particularly hard time the most natural thing to do is to encourage them to come home where you can look after them, but we suggest you think carefully about when it is really in their interest to return home. In the face of problems, the desire to regress can be very powerful.

Being able to phone or go home can be a really important way of gaining some perspective or simply taking some time out. But, developmentally, one of the most important ways in which you can support your child is to encourage them to remain at the University and to make use of the help available to them here.

You may be able to help by reminding them of the support available and helping them to see getting help as a positive step. But be careful not to push too hard. Counselling (or other help) will be more effective if the student has chosen it for themselves.

www.ox.ac.uk/students/welfare/parents

It is important not to assume that all apparent 'homesickness' is benign and normal, particularly if the young person has a history of mental health problems. Delays in transfer of treatment and appropriate supports can be harmful in these cases, and it may take parental support to ensure the student has the promised and necessary facilities. Other reasons for student distress early in the year include financial delays and difficulties. Again, these may snowball if not addressed appropriately.

By the start of second or third year, parents may have become accustomed to the student's term time absence, and assume they have settled into their own university life. A young person may in fact struggle with the move out of halls into smaller and less central accommodation, with the loss of the group of peers, and perhaps the graduation and moving away of older students who had befriended them in first year. For some students, there are changes of subject too. University life can be seen as a continuous series of new transitions, all demanding adjustment and resilience.

Families can be helpful by speaking openly about the challenges, and so normalising them. It can be hard to find the balance between expecting young people to tolerate a healthy amount of discomfort and intervening to prevent damage. The approach suggested by the University of Oxford and Imperial College London (*see boxes*) is to encourage students to explore and use all possible university resources rather than fall back on home solutions. Some parents may find that visiting the student in their new 'home' is a better option than bringing them back to the family home. Parents can help the struggling student to explore the city and campus, make the accommodation as attractive and comfortable as possible, and facilitate new resources rather than retreating into old ones.

Legal Aspects of University Care: 'Duty of Care' and 'In Loco Parentis'

University staff, as well as parents, often ask what exactly is meant by the term 'duty of care'. There is no simple answer. All universities are legally expected to provide a 'duty of care' to students to deliver teaching and general pastoral support. This is not closely defined in specific operational terms, though. In the case of any formal legal challenges, there would be discussion about what could 'reasonably', rather than ideally, be seen as the standard of care expected of higher education institution. Institutions are expected to act 'reasonably' to protect the health, safety and welfare of their students and staff (Jones-Davies, 2019).

Documents such as the mental health charter (Hughes & Spanner, 2019) could be used as a benchmark for expectations of 'reasonable' practice, although they seek to institute excellent rather than merely acceptable practice. It is what happens in practice that creates the general 'norm'. Some sort of pastoral care is certainly expected, but many universities offer more than this. Lawyers point out, though that promising more than a minimum level of pastoral care opens a university up to more complaints and legal challenges if it is in breach of what is promised. The relationship between university and student, unlike school and pupil, is a contractual one, and effectively a 'consumer' contract. Contract law and other consumer legislation could be invoked if a university fails to deliver what it has promised in terms of pastoral support, or if it excludes a student on any grounds – for instance fitness to study – in ways it did not clearly declare up front to the student.

The term 'in loco parentis' means 'in the place of a parent'. The stereotypical view of this is that university authorities in loco parentis would treat students as if they were younger children, with paternalistic controls and protections There are good legal reasons for universities disputing the idea that they might be in loco parentis in this way, and there are developmental and societal reasons why this would be inappropriate too. It's important to remember that in real life, the role of a good parent is flexible, and adapts to the growing maturity of the 'child'. Such a concept would be even more confusing, though, than the idea of 'duty of care'.

In practice, it would be impossible for an institution as large as a university to provide 'parental' support, or for any agency to learn an individual's history and personality in the way parents can. Legally, the in loco parentis expectation could demand the same levels of individually-tailored support as that achieved by schools. This would require smaller, better-staffed units of higher education. The collegiate model of the Universities of Oxford and Cambridge perhaps comes closest to fitting that model.

We are likely to discard legally enforced in loco parentis obligations, but we can hold onto the principle of providing healthy, family-sized groups around students. University residences provide the opportunity to meet a manageable number of people, though most residents are first year undergraduates, rather than the mixture of young students and older scholars living in Oxbridge Colleges. Some universities have followed the St Andrews model in explicitly provide a family model around the new student, appointing volunteer older students as 'mothers' and 'fathers'.

Finance

Chapter 9 of this book examines financial aspects of university life, and in particular their close association with mental well-being and mental disorder. Most undergraduates rely on a patchwork of funding sources for their studies. Loans, grants and part-time paid work are rarely the complete financial solution, and students – where they are fortunate enough to have a supportive family – use the 'bank of mum and dad' while they are at university. Save the Student's (2021) most recent annual survey found that 66% students cited this as a major source of their income, ahead of loans, grants and part-time job income.

Even where cash does not necessarily change hands from parent to student, most young people are able to rely on a family home where they can stay during vacations, and to which they can return when they have no other accommodation. Some students opt to attend a university in their own home town and to remain living at home for at least part if not all of their university course. They may be expected to contribute to household expenses when able to do so, but the terms of residence at home are generally flexible and supportive, and effectively save the young person many thousands of pounds.

Jinevra was the eldest of four children in a family who encouraged to attend her local university. She was charged no rent and was provided with quite generous living expenses, as she always had when at school. The family assumed she would continue to provide informal 'baby-sitting' for her younger siblings, and now that her university timetable involved shorter hours than school, it was assumed that she would be available at home most of the time. When she went out to evening events, her parents expected her to let them know where she would be, with whom, and when she would return.

Jinevra complained of loneliness and envied her friends who had gone away from home. It took courage to broach the topic with her parents, but they agreed to a more formal arrangement about limiting childcare and giving her greater flexibility in terms of going out. Her father encouraged her to spend time studying in the library and the student union building rather than at the kitchen table, and this made an enormous difference to feeling that she was part of the university community. She appreciated the fact that she would have a smaller loan to pay off than some of her peers, but considered moving into a shared flat for her second year at university, to experience the independence she craved. She asked her parents to teach her about mortgage payments, household bills and other financial issues, so that she would be prepared rather than protected, financially.

All families stop receiving Child Benefit when the young person leaves secondary level education or training, or turns 18 and is no longer considered as 'dependent'. Families on low incomes can also lose several hundreds of pounds each month in Universal Credit. This can feel like a sudden and unwelcome reduction in family income. Financial arrangements for students whose parents are separated can also be subject to legal changes as a result of their passing their 18th birthday, and there may be a distressing lack of clarity and onset of conflict about financial support

Students may be deemed adults for legal purposes, but in terms of the amount of student loans granted to them by the Government, they are considered to be financially provided for by their parents. The think tank, the Higher Education Policy Institute has called the parental contribution for undergraduates 'a hidden nasty in the system'. The maintenance loan is assessed according to household income, but there is no legal compulsion for parents to pay it. It seems unjust, inconsistent and confusing to hold people to adult responsibilities without adult rights to a full student loan. It may be that the state cannot realistically meet such an expense without a period of preparation, but this would be a fair aim for the future.

The student maintenance loan is awarded to cover living expenses including accommodation, utilities, food, transport, entertainment and leisure activities. Students who choose to live at home receive less, and the highest amount is given to students living away from home and studying in London. The maintenance loan is means-tested so that the annual household income is taken into account. Low-income households are not theoretically expected to pay any money towards their child's university living expenses, then there is a sliding scale according to family income.

Household income is not taken into consideration for 'independent students' and 'estranged students'. To be eligible as an 'independent student', undergraduates must be age 25 or over or married or in a civil partnership. Students under age 25 who have no contact with parents, may be able to apply as 'estranged students'. Those who spent at least 13 weeks in the care of the local authority before age 16 may be able to apply as care leavers.

Students Who Do Not Have Supportive Families

Financial and practical support from parents brings mental and emotional benefits to students, as well as providing a general sense of security, a reliable reference point that is hard to replace. Some students will have spent time in the care system. Others have experienced a complete breakdown in the relationship with their parents, or have a difficult relationship, which could potentially break down later, during their time at university (*see box*). Sadly, family estrangement is becoming a more prevalent reality in modern society (Conti, 2015), but at least it is more widely recognised, and more students are managing to enter university despite not having family support behind them.

The Office for Students (2020) limits the status of estrangement in higher education to students between 18 and 24 years old and stipulates that estrangement means no communicative relationship with either living biological parent, a definition also shared by the Student Loans Company (2016).

Estranged students report a number of characteristic problems, common to their estranged status, but they often have extra complex concerns reflecting the history behind their estrangement. These may involve ethnicity, race, class, gender and sexuality, adding further to their sense of being 'different' from their peers at a time when belonging to a peer group feels essential (Taylor & Costa, 2019).

> Estranged students are one of these disadvantaged groups, who are studying without the support of their parents or a corporate parent. They may have been missed by the care system, or the care system didn't have a remit to intervene. We commonly work with LGBT+ students who have been rejected by family, abuse survivors, students who have been rejected by new step-parents after re-marriage or those who have different morals, values and beliefs to their immigrant parents. All have no entitlement to corporate parenting of any kind from a local authority or other agency.
>
> (Rouncefield-Swales & Bland, 2019)

Accounts of student life show that 'estranged students' are up to three times more likely to drop out of university, as well as being less likely to achieve high grades (Bland, 2018). They often become homeless over the summer months and have to stay in their student accommodation over the Christmas period. Stand Alone, a UK charity, has worked to increase awareness of, and support for, those experiencing estrangement, but find that 68% of their beneficiaries still feel their family circumstances are stigmatised. (Rouncefield-Swales & Bland, 2019).

I'm more focussed on surviving after graduating than on graduating ... I spend more time worrying about it than focussing on my uni work. I have lost sleep and the situation has been a massive source of stress.

A lot of my friends were able to move back home when they graduated and could save money/take time finding a good job and preparing for it. I knew I needed a job within a week of graduation or I was screwed, and even then I bought a tent with the full intention of living in it for at least the first month of my employment because my housing situation was so dire.

Student experiences quoted by UCAS (www.ucas.com/advisers/toolkits/adviser-toolkit-supporting-students-individual-needs/supporting-students-estranged-their-parents)

Difficult relationships with parents and families are associated with increased mental health difficulties in adult life as well as with suicide (Alm et al., 2019). One benefit of asking students to provide the name of a next-of-kin or other supporter, is that those who struggle to identify such a person can be flagged up as potentially more vulnerable. Drawing their attention to this aspect of their support system is an opportunity for them to identify themselves as 'estranged students' if they wish, and receive help. The UCAS website contains useful material about this scheme and lists universities who have signed up to the 'Stand Alone Pledge' to provide financial and other support to students in this position.

Communication between Parents and the University

What Can I Do If I'm Worried about Them?

Please try to discuss any concerns with them directly, and encourage them to access support from the University. If you have any serious concerns, please contact the Student Services Centre – we can make contact and help them to access further support provided by the University. Please note that we cannot provide specific details about your son/daughter without their explicit consent.

You can find out more about the action we will take to support students living in our halls on our Residence Life Support and Guidance pages.

www.keele.ac.uk/parents/waysyoucansupportthemduringtheirstudies/
#what-can-i-do-if-i'm-worried-about-them?-

The privilege of belonging to a caring family cannot be taken for granted, but is currently still the norm for young undergraduates. It clearly brings with it very striking financial and other advantages, including benefits to mental health and well-being. Both scholarly literature and media accounts tend to be critical of the standard of communication between universities and students' families.

Who's Here to Help?

- Their Personal Tutor – an academic member of staff in their department.
- Residential support teams – providing 24/7 care in our halls of residence
- Independent professional advisers – staff from the advice centre.
- Their 'parents' – student volunteers from the Union's mentoring scheme.

- The Student Financial Support team – offering advice on funding and budgeting.
- The Student Counselling and Mental Health Advice service – offering sessions with counsellors and workshops.
- Student Mental Health Advisers – offering support and advice to students affected by mental health difficulties.
- Study Mentors: Mental Health – providing support to help students keep on track with academic work.
- Nightline volunteers – working on this confidential overnight telephone listening service.

Our Student Support Zone website contains information on all of our student support services, alongside a wide range of practical guidance.

If you have any concerns about your child during their time at Imperial, please urge them to access some of the support available.

www.imperial.ac.uk/parents/student-support/personal-support/

I have not found any examples in the literature or anecdotally where students and their families have complained of over-involvement. It is important to avoid infantilising young adults, but in practice we may be expecting and demanding too much independence rather than too little. This is particularly likely to be the case when the student is vulnerable to mental illness.

The Royal College of Psychiatrists (2021) makes a strong recommendation to 'improve communication with families – think student, think family!' The College's report acknowledges that 'there are of course situations where the family is the main source of the student's mental health problems, and involving them may not be appropriate', and urges that 'anyone who is involved in helping mentally troubled students should, wherever appropriate, seek the consent of the student to engage their family in the processes of assessment and treatment. Families should be given a point of contact they can use to communicate concerns about the student'.

Parents and in fact the general public are of course free to browse much of each university's website, and several institutions have helpful webpages addressed explicitly towards parents, carers and guardians. Some focus on helping parents guide the prospective student through selection and application processes. Increasingly, university websites now provide excellent information on what support facilities students can be encouraged to access, and information on how parents or others who are concerned about a student will be listened to within the boundaries of confidentiality. Some even include documents that can be completed to communicate concerns, with email addresses and telephone numbers for emergency contacts.

Balancing Care with Confidentiality, Privacy and Autonomy

The Human Rights Act 1998, which incorporated the European Convention on Human Rights into UK law, recognises the importance of confidentiality under Article 8 of the Convention. Article 8 also protects the right to family life. In a situation where the individual is clearly 'competent' and does not wish for information to be shared with their family, their right to confidentiality is likely to outweigh any wish of the family to be informed, except in the case of extreme life or death circumstances. However, there is no legal reason to withhold information if the individual agrees to it being shared. Universities have tended to assume that students would withhold permission.

The 2019 Higher Education Policy Institute (HEPI)/Advance HE Student Academic Experience Survey asked over 14 000 UK undergraduates for their views on a range of aspects of university life, and for the first time included a question about contact with parents. It found that 66% wanted their parents to be contacted by the university 'in the event of extreme circumstances' and 15% in the event of any circumstance that aroused concern (Neves & Hillman, 2019). It would be wrong to assume, therefore, that students are most likely to want their families to be kept in the dark. Failure to keep the family informed of a dangerous situation could potentially be seen as an interference with the vulnerable person's human rights, actionable under the 1998 Act.

Medico-Legal Issues: The Concept of Mental Capacity

Within law and legal scholarship there are different models of legal personality and legal capacity. The most prominent models emphasise individual rationality, distilled into the medico-legal concept of 'mental capacity'. This medico-legal concept of 'mental capacity' refers to the ability to make particular decisions. In those areas where a person is found to lack 'mental capacity', specially appointed third parties may make decisions on their behalf in their best interests, within legally scrutinised structures. England and Wales, Scotland, and Northern Ireland have their own separate mental health legislation, but with broadly similar principles.

Evidence from the HEPI/Advance HE survey and the campaigns of parents bereaved by suicide are gradually changing the climate of communication between universities and families. Universities no longer presume that students require an absolute embargo on information sharing. Students are often given opportunities and encouragement to declare and review their preferences. They can provide contact details of their chosen 'emergency contact' at registration and can review and modify their choices at regular intervals. The universities of Bristol, Northumbria, Worcester and Brunel were among the first to implement 'opt-in policies', with others starting to follow suit.

At registration, students can choose to 'opt-in' so that we can contact your nominated emergency contact in the event of a significant concern about your welfare. This is the Student Emergency Contact Procedure. Regardless of whether you have opted-in, as part of the Student Agreement we can contact your emergency contact in the event of an emergency.

If a member of staff takes the view that a student is at risk of harming themselves or others, they are obliged under their duty of care to override confidentiality. This may mean that we cannot discuss our intention to share information with you before doing so.

www.bristol.ac.uk/students/support/wellbeing/policies/
student-services-confidentiality-statement/

Where there are extreme welfare concerns and emergencies, it is already a legal expectation that risk-reducing information should be shared with or without consent, as the Bristol website explains *(see box)*. There is no need for legal changes to allow this, as UK and international law already have the necessary provisions. Some authorities may need to change their habitual practice within the scope of existing law. The need to prioritise safety over confidentiality becomes even more relevant where the individual temporarily experiences a loss or reduction of decision-making capacity as a result of their mental state.

Qualitative research demonstrates the importance of relationships with parents, trusted clinicians, teachers and friends, that provide the necessary 'support and guidance' for the development of autonomy across adolescence and emerging adulthood (Series, 2015). Our legal systems themselves are evolving to reflect our growing understanding of the power of trusted, beneficent relationships in helping people to accept interventions that have to be imposed on them when they are too disabled to agree to them. A new approach to legal 'personality' is being developed, emphasising relationships of support as well as individual choice.

There is no legal guidance, however, on communication between university authorities and students' families when concerns are less extreme. This needs to take the form of agreements between university and student, or more appropriately between the vulnerable student and all the members of the support team around that student. For instance, a mental health mentor, general practitioner (GP), psychiatrist and parents may need to hold regular reviews of student progress, but without leaking unnecessary personal details beyond that network of care.

One situation, which can give rise to appropriate concerns, occurs when a student fails to attend classes or submit assignments. Electronic record-keeping makes it a straightforward matter for universities to keep track of such situations. They may then be able to contact the student concerned and offer support. However, if they are unable to make contact, or if the student merely provides defensive excuses, there is a dilemma about what action should be taken. It may be experienced as punitive rather than supportive to let parents know the student is not managing their coursework, and under current codes of practice, would probably not amount to an emergency situation justifying invocation of the student's emergency contact details. For a student already supported within university support services, there is an appropriate adult who can be informed and take action, but a student not known to services may have no one except their GP involved in their care, and this is unlikely to be a situation GPs would regard as warranting unsolicited intervention.

Another situation where there is little legal guidance on the rights of parents and families is the rare but tragic case of student suicide. Natalie Day, herself a bereaved parent, describes how after the death, details of what happened were kept from the family. Fellow bereaved parents told her that before their child's death 'everything was kept private from us, all for the sake of confidentiality, which seems to have been more important than safety. Even if we had gone to them, they wouldn't have had a discussion with us because he was an adult'. They question how much this is genuine protection of the student's right to confidentiality and how far it is a defensive refusal to communicate (Day, 2022).

Another concern flagged by Day is the likelihood that without adequate support from professionals and parents, 'the onus may fall upon the peers or immediate social circle of the student at risk'. Like colleagues, I have often been approached by worried students asking how they can help friends and fellow students who worry them and appear to have serious mental health struggles. Occasionally of course, this is a euphemistic way to ask to be directed to services themselves, but mostly it represents a serious problem, especially when the friend has begged them not to tell anyone else. Sometimes a student in the grip of a mental illness can end up behaving in a way that induces guilt and anxiety in friends. They can end up in well-meaning collusion with maladaptive coping strategies. A student's obsessive–compulsive disorder may compel flatmates to undertake cleaning or other rituals. A girlfriend or boyfriend may imply that leaving the relationship would trigger suicide.

Becoming the unofficial and isolated carer for a fellow student is damaging to a young person's own mental health, and an obstacle to the academic and social activities university has to offer. It is very different from the experience of being part of a supportive group sharing the care and concerns with others, including professionals. If parents suspect that their student child has been put in the role of an isolated lay carer for a friend or fellow student, they can help by urging the student to confide in a staff member, and by encouraging the unwell friend to seek formal help rather than rely on peers.

Students Who Are Themselves Carers

There are situations where the loss of the young person who is leaving home to become a student profoundly destabilises the family unit. Some students will have cared for parents or other family members with physical or mental health disabilities. In these cases, younger siblings and others left behind may find the extra burden intolerable, or the student may be so concerned about the family situation that they are unable to focus on their university studies or social activities. Young adult carers are four times more likely than other students to drop out of higher education and are amongst the under-represented and disadvantaged groups targeted in the National Strategy for Access and Student Success in Higher Education in the UK (Kettell, 2020).

Mental health problems are very likely for this group of students, but their plight is not so much a mental disorder, situated in their own neurological make up, as a mental injury, a series of traumatic wounds and demands that can exhaust and depress them. Readers may wish to turn back to the case of 'Julie' in Chapter 2, for a description of the conflicting demands of university life and functioning as a young carer.

The Carers Trust (2015) has made a particular study of the difficulties experienced by students, and also by university staff, who have caring responsibilities. They describe how even applying to college and university can be difficult for carers, faced with difficult considerations, such as whether or not they can move away from the person they care for to study, and whether they will be able to cope financially. Multiple demands on carers' time makes it difficult for them to attend all classes and meet coursework deadlines. Socialising may be too expensive in terms of both time and finance, even to contemplate. Student carers find it hard to reach out for support and are all too often unaware of its existence. However, when they do explain their predicament, those hearing them may also be unaware of any resource.

> If young adult carers know what support there is at university, the more likely they are to access it. There is certainly a need for a support worker/funding at university to provide essential support with the massive transition that young adult carers face when going to university. I did not think that I would be able to go to university. However, after knowing my parents would be able to cope and I could come home at weekends – that encouraged me to go. But I will admit it was incredibly hard to live away from home and that Student Services need to support young adult carers more.
>
> Alex, young carer, cited in Supporting Students with Caring Responsibilities Ideas and Practice for Universities to Help Student Carers, Carers Trust, 2015

A recent review of the literature on students who are carers (Runacres et al., 2021) confirmed that caring responsibilities have a negative impact on student carers' physical and mental health, university performance and financial status. It found that many universities had rigid rules and policies that did not suit the needs of student carers. Whilst studies examined the consequences of having to be a carer on the student's academic life, very little research examined the impact of studying on the student's ability to provide care. There was also very little demographic information or detail on the caring duties performed.

The review authors conclude that young adult carers require much greater flexibility from universities in terms of deadlines and timing. Perhaps part time studying would be more realistic for this group of students. Studying at a home-based university may be essential, even though the student will inevitably miss out on the freedoms and adventures of those who leave home.

The UCAS website contains useful advice for young carers (www.ucas.com/under graduate/applying-university/individual-needs/students-caring-responsibilities#). It suggests advance planning and discussion with potential universities. Prospective students are encouraged to describe their caring situation even before applying to a university, let alone after being accepted. UCAS provides useful links to such supports as the Carers Trust, and remarks that the provisions at different universities can be utterly different. Carers have legal rights to be supported, academically and financially, and these rights can be usefully invoked. Students can be supported to do so when they contact groups with experience in meeting their needs (available from the Carers Trust website).

Students and Staff Who Are Themselves Parents

Students and university staff whose caring responsibilities are for dependent children experience many of the barriers and obstacles experienced by other carers, but with the important benefit that they are a much larger and more acknowledged group. Moreover, childcare is now recognised and protected by legal measures. It may be that universities could apply some of the structures that help parents to support people who are caring for elderly or disabled people. Assistance to pay for alternative carers, or for attendance at day centres, could free up study time for the academic. Flexible carer's leave, analogous to parental leave, might allow both young parents and young carers to benefit from the fulfilment brought by higher education.

From a mental health point of view, it is worth remarking that the transition to parenthood is a time of increased vulnerability to mental illness, particularly in women. Hard-working academics and their loved ones, whether students or hard-pressed staff members, may struggle to distinguish a frank treatable mental disorder from the symptoms of exhaustion or 'burnout'. This is crucial – a mental disorder can be treated with medication and/or therapy, whilst environmentally-induced distress requires attention to the circumstances involved. Parental leave, for instance, tends to be associated only with permanent or longer-term contracts, thus disenfranchising the many university staff on short contracts.

When a Student Leaves University in a Planned or Unplanned Way

Services for students enrolled in the institution come to an end when students leave university. Yet the end of a student's university career may be a particularly high-risk transition. Even those who graduate face yet another major life change, often with a student debt to pay off. They may not yet have settled employment, and their accommodation arrangements will probably come to an end unless they and their flatmates have plans to stay in the university city. Friendships and life partnerships forged over the past few years have to survive dispersion at the end of higher education.

A growing proportion of young people returns to the family home, and most become once more fairly dependent on family supports. As we have seen, students without the backstop of a stable family home and financial and emotional cushioning may anticipate homelessness and hardship, so that it is hard to focus on studying for finals. Those who are obliged to leave their course in an unplanned way, are at highest risk of emotional and social adversity, including the risk of suicide (Stanley et al., 2009). Families as well as the student experience disappointment, shame, embarrassment, loss and even despair.

For students with mental disorder it can be impossible and often unwise to make important decisions about the future. It is especially hard, though, for young people tolerate uncertainty and insecurity. Rebuilding a social and work life requires energy and support. This will inevitably fall to parents and partners of the student who has left their course, and it is crucial that they be provided with the information and resources to provide this care. Both GP registration and any secondary mental health care may need to be transferred back to the home services, and in many ways the situation resembles the transition to university but in reverse. Sadly, it is neither accompanied by happy anticipation nor by a programme analogous to 'Freshers' Week' or 'Welcome Week', yet a package of resources for students leaving university might start to address some of the associate risks.

We are finally waking up to the risks experienced when leaving institutions – whether the armed services, prisons, or the workplace. There has been discussion and development of pre-retirement courses to examine the financial, physical and psychosocial aspects of later life. Something similar could usefully follow final examinations for graduating students, perhaps with a modified package of supports being made available to students who are obliged to leave university in an unplanned way. A period of grace might need to be offered to allow counselling or other support services to continue beyond the student's leaving date to ensure that the ending is properly prepared and enacted, and to put post-discharge plans into place. The concept of a 'transition mentor' might be particularly helpful in such circumstances particularly for those students without good family supports, or for international students returning to their country of origin.

Practice Points

Parents

- New concepts of 'transition aged youth', 'emerging adults' and 'thresholders' acknowledge that the undergraduate student age group is still considerably reliant on family of origin.
- Parents of university students now expect to have greater participation in the lives of their children, and financial realities give them considerable power in influencing their children's choices.
- Student experience of transition into university life, and parental 'empty nest' experience, are receiving greater validation. It is less recognised that university life is series of transitions. That bringing the greatest risk may be the transition OUT of university, especially if unplanned.

Governments and Finance Providers

- From age 18 students are held to adult responsibilities without adult rights to an independent student loan, or legal compulsion on their parents to provide finance they are deemed able to provide. Parents are expected to provide finance with little feedback or power over the resource they are asked to finance. Society needs to work towards a more equitable model of student finance.

University Authorities and Support Services

- While respecting principles of confidentiality, privacy and autonomy, existing law permits more communication than usually practised at present, and is moving towards legal recognition of the need to make choices within supportive relationships.
- Universities are experimenting with ways to ensure that where parents are supportive, they can be consulted about students who are at risk, whilst respecting principles of privacy and confidentiality.
- There may be value in developing a 'leavers' programme', analogous to 'Freshers' Weeks'.
- A specific package of supports is needed to support students who leave in an unplanned way.

Students without Supportive Families

- At present 'estranged students' and those who are themselves carers encounter financial, academic and social obstacles to a successful university experience.
- Prospective students in this position are recommended to research in advance which universities will best provide the financial and other supports integrate them healthily into academic life and to link with national charities such as Carers Trust and Standalone, for support and advocacy through and beyond the duration of the course.

References

Alm, S., Brolin Låftman, S. & Bohman, H. (2019). Poor family relationships in adolescence and the risk of premature death: Findings from the Stockholm birth cohort study. *International Journal of Environmental Research and Public Health*, 16(10), 1690.

Apter, T. E. (2002). *The myth of maturity: What teenagers need from parents to become adults.* New York: WW Norton & Company.

Bland, B. (2018). It's all about the money: The influence of family estrangement, accommodation struggles and homelessness on student success in UK higher education. *Widening Participation and Lifelong Learning*, 20(3), 68–89.

Carers Trust (2015). *Supporting students with caring responsibilities: Ideas and practice for universities to help student carers access and succeed in higher education.*

Conti, R. P. (2015). Family estrangement: Establishing a prevalence rate. *Journal of Psychology and Behavioral Science*, 3(2), 28–35. https://doi.org/10.15640/jpbs.v3n2a4

Day, N. (2022). Supporting students: The parents' perspective. In Mallon, S. & Smith, J. (eds) *Preventing and responding to student suicide.*

Diamond, G. & Josephson, A. (2005). Family-based treatment research: A 10-year update. *Journal of the American Academy of Child & Adolescent Psychiatry*, 44(9), 872–87.

Ecclestone, K. & Hayes, D. (2009). *The dangerous rise of therapeutic education*. Routledge.

Freud, A. (1958). Adolescence, *The Psychoanalytic Study of the Child*, 13(1), 255–78.

Furedi, F. (2017). The medicalisation of the university. *Policy: A Journal of Public Policy and Ideas*, 33(4), 48–51.

Hughes, G. & Spanner, L. (2019). *The university mental health charter*. Leeds: Student Minds. www.studentminds.org.uk/uploads/3/7/8/4/3784584/191208_umhc_artwork.pdf

Jones-Davies, S. (2019). The legal position: obligations and limits. In Barden, N. & Caleb, R. (eds) *Student mental health and wellbeing in higher education: A practical guide* (pp 18–39).

Kettell, L. (2020). Young adult carers in higher education: The motivations, barriers and challenges involved – A UK study. *Journal of Further and Higher Education*, 44:1, 100–12.

Meyer, D. (2019). The student life cycle: Pressure points and transition. In Barden, N. & Caleb, R. (eds) *Student mental health and wellbeing in higher education: A practical guide* (pp 63–84).

Moorhead, J. (2018, 25 October). *How to cope with empty-nest syndrome – without being gutted by grief*. The Guardian www.theguardian.com/lifeandstyle/2018/oct/25/how-to-cope-empty-nest-syndrome-children-move-out-gordon-ramsay

Neves, J. & Hillman, N. (2019). *Student academic experience survey 2019*. HEPI/Advance HE.

Office for Students (2020). *Estranged students*. www.officeforstudents.org.uk/advice-and-guidance/promoting-equal-opportunities/effective-practice/estranged-students/

Rouncefield-Swales, A. & Bland, B. (2019). *Transitioning out of higher education: Barriers and challenges for students estranged from their families*. www.standalone.org.uk/wp-content/uploads/2020/01/Standalone-report-v3-1.pdf

Royal College of Psychiatrists (2021). *Mental health of higher education students (CR231)*. www.rcpsych.ac.uk/docs/default-source/improving-care/better-mh-policy/college-reports/mental-health-of-higher-education-students-(cr231).pdf

Runacres, J., Herron, D., Buckless, K. & Worrall, S. (2021). Student carer experiences of higher education and support: A scoping review. *International Journal of Inclusive Education*, 1–18.

Save the Student (2021). *Student money survey 2021: Results*. www.savethestudent.org/money/surveys/student-money-survey-2021-results.html

Student Loans Company (2016). www.practitioners.slc.co.uk/estrangement/

Series, L. (2015). Relationships, autonomy and legal capacity: Mental capacity and support paradigms. *International Journal of Law and Psychiatry*, 40, 80–91.

Stanley, N., Mallon, S., Bell, J. & Manthorpe, J. (2009). Trapped in transition: Findings from a UK study of student suicide. *British Journal of Guidance & Counselling*, 37(4), 419–33.

Taylor, Y. & Costa, C. (2019). *Estranged students in higher and further education*.

UCAS *Supporting students estranged from their parents*. www.ucas.com/advisers/toolkits/adviser-toolkit-supporting-students-individual-needs/supporting-students-estranged-their-parents

Universities UK (2015). *Student mental wellbeing in higher education: Good practice guide*. www.m25lib.ac.uk/wp-content/uploads/2021/02/student-mental-wellbeing-in-he.pdf

Venville, A., Street, A., Fossey, E. (2013). Student perspectives on disclosure of mental illness in post-compulsory education: Displacing doxa. *Disability & Society*, 29(5), 1–15.

Wilens, T. E. & Rosenbaum, J. F. (2013). Transitional aged youth: A new frontier in child and adolescent psychiatry. *Journal of the American Academy of Child & Adolescent Psychiatry*, 52(9), 887–90. https://doi.org/10.1016/j.jaac.2013.04.020

Healthy Bodies, Body Image Concerns, Eating Disorders

Chapter 5

This chapter considers the importance of nutrition, physical activity and sleep 'hygiene' in the lives of students. For some students, physical and mental health have a lower priority than successful socialising, pleasure seeking and of course, studying. For many young people, body image concerns are high priorities. Increasing numbers of young people experience body image concerns so compelling that they cause obsessive efforts to avoid a fat or flabby body or to build lean muscle. The behaviours and preoccupations interfere with mental and social health as well as exposing the affected students to worrying physical consequences.

Some students imagine that they are seeking a 'healthy' body, when in fact they are damaging their health by misinterpreting what their body really needs or taking an exaggerated and distorted perspective. This takes us to a discussion of the so-called eating disorders. These are fairly diverse mental illnesses, usually characterised by obsessive body concern, but superimposed on different psychological characteristics and personality traits. The student age group is at particularly high risk for these conditions.

Health as a Matter of Social Connection

The ability to eat, sleep and exercise alongside peers facilitates a better social life at university, and things work both ways – a healthy social group improves student health. A Canadian study (Klaiber et al., 2018) found that the number of friends a student makes during the transition to university can predict their self-reported health and healthy eating several years later. Friendship formation during the first term was associated with healthier exercise and diet, and lower tobacco, alcohol and marijuana consumption 3 years later.

The authors allude to previous work showing how health-related behaviours are linked to social integration. 'Social norms' theory explains how a person who sees others making healthy eating choices is more likely to follow their example. Good social support can further affect physical health by providing soothing experiences that protect us from stress at the same time as modelling healthy behaviours.

This book observes repeatedly that the sense of belonging in itself, and particularly the power of belonging to a healthy group, improves mental health for us all. Students find themselves in a developmentally distinct group setting, however. They have more power than ever before to choose and influence their group, but it is a new group, and one they must form rapidly almost from scratch. In comparison with school and family life, the new group is fairly independent of adult input, so that anyone seeking to influence the group's behaviour from outside – authorities and well-wishers alike – may be resisted unless they are respectful and collaborative.

Provision of financial and administrative support through student unions and societies can be a way to exert more welcome influence. Another is to directly modify the university environment so that timetable structures encourage meal breaks, sports afternoons, adolescent sleep patterns. Most universities do well in providing societies, sports halls, stadia and a favourable climate for participation in physical activity.

'A Healthy Mind in a Healthy Body': Nutrition

People in affluent countries – and particularly poor people within affluent countries – are vulnerable to the concerning medical and emotional consequences of obesity. Unfortunately, campaigns to address this have not even slowed down the inexorable rise of the obesity epidemic in the UK. Young students will start university having received oversimplified messages in the classroom, in the community and in the media, equating nutritional health with low calorie intake and low body weight. There is even some evidence that anti-obesity messages are triggering eating disorders in vulnerable children and adolescents (Tan et al., 2019).

There are some balanced messages that apply to students wherever they may be in the weight spectrum. All can benefit physically and psychologically from taking regular meals that are not over processed and include plenty of vegetables. Eating at recognised mealtimes and in a social setting is associated with well-being and even with academic success (Dunbar, 2017). For adolescents living at home, a whole body of research in the UK and elsewhere has found that the more often they participated in family dinners, the less likely they were to experience substance use, risky sexual activity, depression, suicidal behaviour, antisocial behaviours, violence, school problems, and eating disorders of all sorts (Fulkerson et al., 2006).

When such students leave home, they lose this reassuring opportunity to touch base regularly with trusted loved ones. It is no longer easy to reconstruct the habit of social mealtimes outside the home. The old-fashioned practice of eating together at the same time every night in student residential halls has almost vanished even from Oxbridge. University catering can no longer accommodate large academic communities, particularly in the evenings. Once students move out of residential halls, usually at the end of the first year, they are more than ever responsible for feeding themselves. New students are often given special cookery books and advice on cheap meals, but there is also a fatalistic expectation they will patronise fast food outlets and pizza deliveries.

Most state secondary schools provide minimal domestic science instruction and many leave pupils to fend for themselves at lunchtime rather than seeing the school dining room as social and nutritional education in practice. Those of us who live near a secondary school observe swarms of uniformed teenagers spending a lot of money on over-packaged snack food, which is eaten in the street in all weathers. Hopefully, the common practice of skipping breakfast and lunching this way is then redeemed somewhat by participation in a family dinner most nights. This is far from being the norm in many family households, where commonly each individual in the family demands a different meal choice, and children's packed timetables of activities mean everyone eats at different times.

At university it is harder to replicate evening meal rituals. The most canny students teach themselves to prepare good food well and economically, and the more sociable and assertive students manage to share cooking and eating with friends, hallmates and flatmates. Eating and drinking are important social activities, but it is easier to go along with the prevailing norms – ordering in beer and pizza – than to set up something old fashioned and sensible like a rota for preparing evening meals together.

As a psychiatrist specialising in eating disorders, I have obviously seen a disproportionate number of students who are badly nourished and whose lives are handicapped by being unable to enjoy normal healthy eating, so it is heartening to read that 'a large group of students consumed nutritionally favourable and health-promoting diets and do not appear in need of dietary intervention' (Sprake et al., 2018). This conclusion was drawn from a study of students at five diverse UK universities and was unusual in analysing the nutritional composition of students' diets rather than relying on simplistic measures of nutritional health, such as weight or body mass index. The authors discovered four major dietary patterns that occurred in all the different universities: 'vegetarian', 'snacking' (dominated by biscuits, cakes, milk- and cream-based desserts, confectionery, crisps, pizza and fizzy drinks), 'health-conscious' and what they called 'convenience, red meat and alcohol'.

The 'health-conscious' pattern had the most favourable micronutrient profile. There was a concerning tendency for male students to have the 'convenience food, red meat and alcohol' style of eating. This was also associated with higher weekly food spending. Less healthful dietary patterns were positively associated with lifestyle risk factors such as smoking, low physical activity and take-away consumption. The combination of poor diet and associated lifestyle behaviours during the crucial physical and psychosocial transition to adult life may have long-term consequences (Sprake et al., 2018).

Previous explorations of student dietary behaviour have tended to focus on the widespread concern in American universities about the so-called Freshman 15, which describes the 15-pound weight gain said to typically occur to first-year college students. This does not seem to be such a prominent finding in the UK, however. A study of students in 23 UK universities found that overall there was an average weight gain of 1.34 kg, with 25% students actually losing weight across their first year (Vadeboncoeur et al., 2016).

The authors also point out that under 17% of these students met national criteria for being overweight or obese at the start of the year, which is only half the national average for their age group (30%–36%). Examination of healthy growth charts demonstrates that young people in their late teens have not finished the physical growth curve and would expect to gain weight – and in some cases height – beyond age 18. Another important finding, from a broader review of the evidence (León et al., 2022) is that the leading behaviours associated with unwanted student weight include the consumption of fizzy drinks and of alcohol. What students drink may be as important in their nutrition as what they eat.

For many years now, the UK has witnessed campaigns to include 'healthy eating' in school curricula, and public interventions to label foods and restaurant menus with calorie and other nutritional information. It is disappointing, then to find that university students may not be in possession of accurate or useful nutritional information. A survey of London University students found that fewer than half of them reached a good level on a questionnaire designed to assess their knowledge of dietary recommendations, nutrient sources of foods, healthy food choices and diet–disease relationships (Belogianni et al., 2022).

When Jenny went to high school mother gave her money each day to buy lunch from the local bakery. Like her friends, she often bought cakes and fizzy drinks rather than the cheese sandwich she told her mother about.

When the domestic science teacher in the second year spoke to the class about 'healthy' and 'unhealthy' food choices, Jenny realised that all her favourite lunches were 'unhealthy'. She changed back to eating sandwiches, but worried that cheese was high in fat. She began discarding the cheese from the centre of the sandwich, to the mockery of her friends. She was already slim and now became very thin.

As winter came, and Jenny started to feel the cold, she stopped going out of school with friends at lunchtime and chose to hug the radiators with a book rather than eating.

Some nutritionists see universities as 'a setting in which dietary behaviours are open to change and large groups of young adults can be reached, representing an appropriate target for health promotion efforts' and recommend 'efforts to promote student engagement in cooking and food preparation' (Sprake et al., 2018). This approach, though, accepts the status quo of a toxic food environment within which people are obliged to make individual efforts to protect their own health. So far, this has not been strikingly successful, even with public information and education. Pragmatically, environmental interventions may do more to change the behaviour of those who most need the change.

Advanced cooking skills are no guarantee of health. The majority of my most malnourished anorexic patients were obsessed with cookery. They endlessly watched cookery programmes on television, read cookbooks and recipes, and prepared elaborate, high-calorie dishes and banquets, which they pressured other people to eat. Many simple meals require little or no cooking, or can be produced healthily, economically and at scale in institutional kitchens.

Good nutrition is more about the discipline of eating roughly the right amount, regularly, and not too much of it sugar or alcohol. Eating with others is a way of pacing nutritional intake and getting a feel for the range of portion sizes healthy peers require. Mealtimes are a pleasant informal way to check in with each other, to notice if anyone is troubled or unexpectedly absent, and a way to socialise without having to think up a specific reason to do so – or to necessarily drink alcohol.

Obesity experts and nutritionists are already taking an interest in changing living environments to promote healthier nutrition. University campuses and halls would be in a position to pioneer and monitor such experiments. Rather than setting up yet more healthy eating campaigns and awareness workshops, universities might provide a more traditional eating environment, where student eat together regularly, with meals prepared from healthy raw ingredients, respecting economic and ecological concerns. It is a model that is disappearing from institutions such as schools, hospitals and universities too, and would require considerable effort to reconstruct. The evidence quoted at the start of this section (Dunbar, 2017) that eating at recognised mealtimes and in a social setting is associated with well-being and academic success might make us feel that such efforts would be worth trying.

Eat, Sleep, Repeat

Attending to our primitive biological rhythms improves the function of brains and bodies. 'Sleep hygiene' is a striking example of this. Sleep interacts with nutrition and the intake of caffeine and alcohol, as well as responding to physical activity patterns. Too little sleep makes it hard to learn and remember and in extremes can mimic psychotic illness. Sleep deprivation is notoriously used as a method of torture.

Over the life span our body clock alters, and teenagers notoriously become 'night owls' both naturally, in response to their hormones, and socially to participate in nightlife. Some become dysregulated to the extent that they miss classes or work shifts, become out of step with the community, and experience constant fatigue, even depression. Even mild sleep deprivation has been associated with significant health and educational concerns: increased risk for accidents and injuries, impaired learning, aggression, memory loss, poor self-esteem, and changes in metabolism, so secondary schools, particularly in the United States, have experimented with later starts to the academic day, and found overall evidence of benefits (Marx et al., 2017). A study based in a UK university found that students had longer sleep and healthier sleep quality when university first lectures started later. The earliest lecture start time that afforded sufficient sleep duration for students was 10 a.m. (Swinnerton et al., 2021).

Sleep is particularly sensitive to light and dark, which of course varies by seasonality up here in Northern Europe. Students and staff may be sensitive to 'seasonal affective disorder' and there have been reports of lower scores in exams and tests taken in winter months than in the summer. Our sleep patterns have been more rudely disturbed in modern times by artificial lighting, shift work, long-haul travel, and most recently by internet-based activities, which observe no single time zone and can occupy students on social media or gaming sites all through the night.

Students may have already developed habits of keeping their electronic devices switched on through the night, and feel an even greater need for 'connectivity' when they move away from home. At the same time, they are now deprived of restraining parental influences and the knowledge they will be woken and sent to school in the morning. Student halls are notoriously noisy places, and buildings could benefit from better soundproofing as well as clear regulations about quiet times. University libraries may be open all night, facilitating the dubious practice of 'all-nighters' to meet academic deadlines. However, students who do work late (or very early) at least have the option of a quiet and comfortable study environment.

Physical Activity and Sedentary Behaviour at University

Physical activity, both incidental and deliberate, also appears to be a largely positive contribution to physical health, longevity and positive mental health. It can be effective in preventing and treating depression and anxiety disorders. Exercise stimulates nerve-building processes, reduces inflammation and improves resilience to stress, as well as promoting self-esteem, self-efficacy and social support (Kandola et al., 2019).

Unfortunately, UK university students as a whole appear to have fairly high levels of sedentary behaviour (Rouse & Biddle, 2010) and inadequate levels of exercise and physical activity (Aceijas et al., 2016). 89% students said they did not use the university gym due to lack of time (40%), price (30%), and embarrassment (11%). Female and Black students had lower activity levels. Both underweight and obese women students reported taking less exercise as did disabled men. Financial and academic pressures were also often cited as reasons for less physical activity (Aceijas et al., 2016).

One study involved interviews with European students to collect their suggestions for improving physical activity in students. One chimed with a criticism I have heard from many UK students. He suggested that sports should be made more welcoming and attractive to students who are less fit or at least not elite athletes. There is often a sense that university sports are only for highly skilled competitive participants who offer prestige to the institution. Being part of a team for fun and good company has benefits for all abilities. Other students suggested that some 'sports time' could be incorporated as part of the curriculum, on a non-obligatory basis. The students also urged provision of 'university bike schemes' whereby they could subscribe into a programme allowing them to use designated bicycles owned by the university.

A piece of research from the UK highlighted a complicating factor in the relationship between student physical activity and improved mood (El Ansari et al., 2011). The study confirmed that fewer than half of the students in the seven UK universities sampled met criteria for healthy levels of activity. Physically active students, in the study were significantly more likely to perceive their health as good, to have higher health awareness, and to be male. There was, as expected, a relationship between higher activity and lower levels of depression, but this effect was diminished for the students who believed they were overweight and had poor body image. The study authors recommend that when we encourage depressed students to be more physically active, we should consider the need to incorporate 'effective components to enhance body image perception'. This is much more easily said than done. Such interventions require considerable specialist expertise and are all too easily undermined by influences in society such as social media, and engrained prejudices.

Body Image and Social Media

In 2020, 71% of respondents to the Girlguiding (2020) Girls' Attitudes Survey said they experienced online harms, above all body confidence issues. The biggest worry was comparisons with other girls' bodies, especially how they looked in photographs and the number of 'likes' their photographs received. The more visually dominated social media such as Instagram and Snapchat are particularly powerful in leading to poor body image and negative self-concept.

In biological, evolutionary terms, appearance is a signal to potential mates that healthy breeding is possible, so it is likely that young people will automatically be highly sensitive to physical appearance. Historically, young women have been particularly pressured by society likely to conflate body image and self-worth. There is evidence though that social media amplifies this to dangerous levels. Further discussion of the mental health consequences of social media use can be found in Chapter 8. This chapter will focus on the particular consequences for body image and development or maintenance of eating disorders.

Followers of the influencer Oenone Forbat (personal communication) tell her that an insidious 'diet culture' permeates most media platforms. Pressures and advice can arrive unasked for within the social media site. When people do actively search online for ways to lose weight, they open floodgates to a torrent of advice from the diet and gym industries, personal monitoring gadgets, quack remedies, dangerous weight loss drugs, pro-anorexic advice and bizarre concepts like 'thinspiration', 'fitspiration', 'thigh gaps' and the rest. Even the opposing jargon and images of the 'body positive' movement maintain the focus on bodily appearance, even if they glorify more diverse bodies.

Social media goes a step further than older media. They may have presented repeated images of thin attractive people as an implied standard to aspire to, but they did not provide the same opportunities for people to post their own images in public and invite feedback. People with obsessive body image concerns often engage in 'body checking' where they repeatedly weigh and measure and even pinch their bodies, keeping the obsession prominent in their consciousness. They may also make comments designed to elicit reassurance from others, such as 'does this make me look fat?' including statements of distress designed to be contradicted such as 'I've gained pounds over the winter'. This feeds the obsession, so treatment has to support people to disengage from such behaviours. It is certainly harder to avoid them when online. For young people who are vulnerable to an eating disorder, it is a good principle to minimise online time as much as possible and disable weight monitoring apps.

There is growing evidence that social media use and competitiveness can predispose people to eating disorders, trigger their onset and certainly maintain them (Mabe et al., 2014, Ferguson et al., 2014). Treatment and prevention strategies might benefit from identifying differences between helpful and harmful behaviour within the electronic environment.

In the past, patients with severe eating disorders would be separated from their mobile phones on admission to hospital. Now that mobile phones are permitted in hospital wards – and even seen as a human right – clinicians have to hold explicit discussion of how phones are 'feeding' the disorder. Patients are encouraged to uninstall those apps and sites that increase body checking and measurement, weight tracking, calorie counting, exercise monitoring and competitive comparisons with others with the same preoccupations.

When a Lifestyle Choice Becomes a Mental Disorder

The disorders known as 'eating disorders' occur when the person's self-image becomes completely dependent on their body image. Students with eating disorders often set themselves high standards in other areas of life too. They can be perfectionists, with a strong work ethic. This makes it all the more wasteful when they sacrifice their other ideals in the quest for a lean body.

Eating disorders can start at any age but typically begin in mid-adolescence. Students may arrive at university already battling an eating disorder, or may develop a condition during their university studies. In Western countries about 1% of women and 0.5% of men will have a diagnosed eating disorder over their lifespan, with the highest concentration of those in their teens and twenties. We should treat these figures with caution, as they are usually based on national registers. Studies that enquire about people's symptoms in the community (rather than looking at how many people received treatment) suggest that about half of people who meet criteria for an eating disorder do not receive any treatment.

Despite the misleading name, far more than eating behaviour is disordered. A whole raft of obsessional concerns and behaviours grows up around the extreme concern to be as lean as possible. This can end up dominating the whole of life, pushing other values lower down the list of priorities. Tragically, even relationships with loved ones can be sacrificed in the service of avoiding weight gain.

This obsession with body image is linked to modern culture and is the psychological concern common to the range of so-called eating disorders, but these disorders can take many overlapping and mutating forms even in the same person, over time. Modern genetic research does suggest, though, that there are distinct groups of disorder, and whilst it can be hard to assess which category we are dealing with, different treatment approaches are needed for the different types of eating disorder.

There are two main reasons for differentiating between the different eating disorders. One is the importance of treating the severe starvation that occurs in anorexia nervosa, because severe malnutrition affects brain and mind function in extraordinarily powerful ways. This has been known since Ancel Keys' (1946) post-war Minnesota Starvation Study.

Some observations about the abnormal mental and behavioural symptoms of people with anorexia nervosa, including brain scans, may reflect the consequences of starvation rather than of the mental disorder itself. I have seen young people recover from many of the symptoms of starvation, stop feeling depressed, see their bones gradually strengthen, regain their fertility and become socially confident again. This can take months and years to achieve, but it is remarkable how much recovery is possible.

In fact, proponents of family-based treatment (Lock & Le Grange, 2015) observe that weight restoration alone can be sufficient treatment for some teenagers with anorexia nervosa. The sooner treatment is provided, the more likely a full recovery and the lower the rate of mortality. This is vital, because anorexia nervosa has the highest mortality rate of all psychiatric disorders and is a leading cause of death in the student age group (Franko, 2018). More than half of these tragic deaths come from the fatal consequences of severe starvation or from the high-risk behaviours used to reduce weight.

The Psychosocial Consequences of Starvation

In the 1940s, a famous study examined the effects of deliberate 'semi-starvation' in healthy young, student-age men, conscientious objectors, who volunteered to live on campus at the University of Minnesota to be minutely monitored while they lost and then regained a significant amount of weight. They also kept highly illuminating personal diaries of the experience.

During the starvation phase these previously sociable, intellectually curious young men lost interest in friendships and sexual activity, stopped bothering with academic courses for which they had enrolled, became obsessed with food, cookery and food-related items and issues, and withdrew into themselves. Their eating behaviour slowed down and became ritualised, and they regarded other people with suspicion and hostility.

During the 'refeeding' phase, there was a lot of loss of control of appetite with binges, and some men induced vomiting. Many became emotionally disturbed, some profoundly so, with deliberate self-harm observed in previously mentally stable individuals.

However, a substantial number of deaths in eating disorders result from suicide or accidental deaths following non-suicidal deliberate self-harm. Starvation is not the only cause of death, nor is it the only difference between the different eating disorders. Some people who achieve temporary low weights, and most of those who do not, have different personalities and emotional characteristics from people with 'classic' anorexia nervosa. These reflect both environmental experiences and strong genetic underpinnings. (Watson et al., 2019).

Anorexia nervosa, then, is diagnosed when a person deliberately loses a significant amount of weight, usually for body image-related reasons. Adolescents may not lose weight but fail to gain weight – and even height – as expected. The weight losing has features of obsessive–compulsive experience. 80% people with anorexia nervosa experience other obsessive–compulsive symptoms at some point. Large-scale population studies show that people with anorexia nervosa and their close relatives have increased rates of autism spectrum disorder (Koch et al., 2015).

Cases of compulsive self-starvation have been reported throughout history and in all geographical areas of the globe, although not always associated with the body image concern we associate with today's anorexia nervosa diagnosis. They are disorders of extreme control. In contrast, bulimia nervosa and binge eating disorder only became common and well recognised in the late twentieth century. By definition these are only diagnosed in people of normal weight or above, and represent weight-losing efforts in people who have other psychological vulnerabilities from those who develop anorexia nervosa. They are character-ised by a sense of being out of control. The loss of control is a result of dysregulation.

In both bulimia nervosa and binge eating disorder, patients try to restrict their diet but find themselves bingeing on large amounts of food, not typically the kind of food they would consume in public. If they then use 'compensatory behaviours such as making themselves sick or using laxatives, then they are diagnosed as having bulimia nervosa. If not, then they are diagnosed with binge eating disorder. Both diagnoses have only been commonly recognised in the later quarter of the twentieth century.

The pressures of modern life certainly encourage dysregulated lifestyles. It is all too easy for individuals away from home and in a chaotically transitional stage of develop-ment to let go of traditional mealtimes, bedtimes and routines. There is also good news, however. Whilst anorexia nervosa can be highly resistant to treatment, the disorders of dysregulation respond very well to therapies such as cognitive behavioural therapy, which support the person to re-structure their life.

For students with binge eating disorder there is the extra challenge that they are more likely to be overweight than those with other eating disorders. If they try to lose weight without first attending to their eating disorder, the eating disorder may become much worse, and without lasting benefits to the overweight condition. However, complete recovery from binge eating disorder is unlikely to reduce body weight significantly, at least initially. This understandably leads impatient young people to renew their efforts at counter-productive dieting and relapsing into binge eating.

Treatment for bulimia nervosa and binge eating disorders involves reinstating healthy routines and eradicating the binges and associated purging behaviour. This is the essential groundwork for recovery. However, these disorders are associated with mood and anxiety disorders (Vögele et al., 2018), higher prevalence of substance misuse (Root et al., 2010) and other disorders of impulsivity and lack of control (Kim et al., 2018). These often need to be addressed in their own right. One study of European university students with bingeing and purging disorders also found a significant associ-ation with poorer academic grades (Serra et al., 2020). This provides extra motivation to treat students with these conditions.

Students at Particularly High-Risk for Eating Disorders

The different genetic as well as environmental contributions to different eating disorders mean that different preventative and treatment strategies may apply to different groups, although there are certainly some common factors. It is almost a cliché to observe that anorexia nervosa and bulimia nervosa are more common among female than male individuals (Hoek, 2006), but this should not blind us to the growing problems of eating disorders in men. There are also higher rates of disordered eating among sexual minorities, particularly in transgender people (Calzo et al., 2017).

Childhood deprivation and trauma are important risk factors for many mental disorders, and appear to be associated with increased risk of binging and purging symptoms but less so for purely restricting anorexia nervosa (Groth et al., 2020).

One US study followed hundreds of healthy girls to examine predictive factors for eating disorders and found that low mood and poor interpersonal relationships were risk factors for developing all eating disorders (Stice et al., 2017). The same study found that girls who pursued a thin body ideal, those with high levels of body dissatisfaction, and those who engaged in dieting, and unhealthy weight control behaviours were at highest risk for bulimia nervosa and binge eating disorders. Girls who were naturally thin and lean were at risk for developing anorexia nervosa even before they engaged in deliberate weight losing behaviour.

It is not surprising that actors, fashion models and others who work in or train for professions where physical appearance is central to the speciality, have increased risks of developing eating disorders. Athletes of all genders may also experience pressures to conform to an idealised appearance, if they compete in skating, gymnastics or other artistic displays. These groups, like dancers, have the double challenge of looking a certain way whilst maintaining levels of energy and strength that may not be compatible with a thin or fragile appearance. Even athletes whose appearance is not critical to their performance are vulnerable to obsessive compulsive body control behaviours, which have much in common with the more typical eating disorders.

There is considerable evidence of such disorders amongst elite and aspiring athletes, but we still do not know to what extent such activities attract participants who are already predisposed to develop such disorders rather than being the primary causes of developing an eating disorder (Stoyel et al., 2020). Athletic coaches have told me that the most successful athletes prioritise their physical performance over everything else, including their longer-term health. It is a moot point as to whether this is Is a valid, mature decision and how far a young student may be acting under the influence of a disorder or a strong social influence. Society is rightly horrified by revelations of frank physical and sexual abuse within sports and athletics. The risks of a pervasive body control culture need to be further described and debated.

Judith studied linguistics but was rarely seen in lectures or classes. She found her hall of residence to be too loud and messy and frequently retreated back to her family home at weekends. She spent most of her time in the library studying or sitting in the library café with mugs of black coffee and an open book. She was an emaciated figure, always dressed in many layers of black clothes even in summer.

She presented immaculate coursework, so it was a surprise when suddenly she stopped returning assignments. She was found almost moribund in her bedroom and spent months in hospital. She was diagnosed with anorexia nervosa, depressive disorder and probable ASD.

She was obliged to gain weight, and as she became better nourished, clinicians were amazed and delighted to observe that her depression lifted and a much more sociable, humorous personality emerged. The strange rituals and exclusions that were so noticeable at the dining table melted away too and she began to eat like a healthy person.

Her parents said they were seeing Judith's personality again as it had been when she was a child. They dreaded Judith reverting to restricting her eating in case they 'lost her again'.

Students who are high on the autistic spectrum are observed to have increased vulnerability to eating disorders. Gillberg (1983) has argued that many cases of severe anorexia nervosa represent underlying autism. It has been suggested that for some young people – especially women with autism – weight losing becomes a 'special interest', and there has been much interest in the observed cognitive style of patients with anorexia nervosa, though this is sometimes an effect of starvation (Li et al., 2022). Neurodiversity is discussed in more detail in Chapter 10. An important implication is that treatment services for students with anorexia nervosa should be guided by principles of respect for autistic functioning styles.

Perhaps the greatest risk for developing an eating disorder, and certainly the greatest risk of resulting permanent physical damage, is to young people with insulin-requiring diabetes. This sort of diabetes, commonly diagnosed in childhood, resulting from the body's failure to produce its own insulin. Without insulin, the glucose from our food stays in our blood stream and damages our bodily organs Eventually, without insulin altogether, we would die.

Taking too little insulin results in insidious damage to eyes, kidneys, nerves and other organs. In the short term, symptoms of injecting too little insulin include having to pass urine often and at night, constant thirst, mental vagueness and weight loss. This side effect of weight loss can be extremely tempting to a young person, and can become habit forming. The student with diabetes who wants to lose a little weight can do so without dieting, exercising or making themself sick. Among young people with diabetes, 30% to 40% admit that they omit or reduce insulin with the intention of losing weight (Hasken et al., 2010). As a result, the consequences of poorly managed blood sugar appear in these patients far earlier than in people who use insulin effectively, and blindness, organ failure and even premature death are tragically common.

We cannot assess a person who requires insulin by the standard criteria for eating disorders. The usual behaviours involved are only relevant to a person without diabetes. The term 'diabulimia' is commonly used, but is not officially included in formal diagnostic classifications. This should not mean that patients are denied specialist treatment.

Students with other conditions that require medication may either overuse or underuse their prescribed treatment because of its effects on their weight. This means that people with epilepsy, thyroid conditions, bowel disorders and cystic fibrosis, for instance, are at increased risk both from the eating disorder and from the consequences of the untreated physical condition.

What Is It Like to Be a Student with an Eating Disorder?

Jayne was not significantly overweight but felt like 'a very uncool kid'. She wore nondescript spectacles and no makeup. She faded into the background in social situations. Her friend Carol took the lead in giving them both 'makeovers' when they went to university together. They exchanged their glasses for contact lenses, dyed each other's hair, followed a different diet each week, and spent hours in the university gym.

Jayne weighed herself many times a day She had rules about only eating if her weight was below a certain number. She did more and more repetitions in the gym 'to turn her fat to muscle', and pinched her flesh under her clothes to keep up pressure on herself to 'tone up'.

The friends attracted more attention socially, but Jayne found herself sometimes completely unable to stop herself bingeing. The more she tried to restrict what she ate, the worse her loss of control. She was too ashamed to confide in Carol. To her horror, the size of her secret night time binges increased, and so did her weight. She knew the dangers of self-induced vomiting, but thought it could be a temporary solution, until her weight came back to normal.

Everything spiralled out of control with larger binges and more desperate purging, more exhaustion after gym sessions, and increased shame, despair and loneliness. It was the dentist who broke the vicious cycle when she examined Jane's tooth enamel. 'I wonder whether you might have an eating disorder', she remarked.

Jayne was amazed by the change in her life after a course of specialist cognitive behavioural therapy. She had more choices, and more time to exercise them, and her weight remained steady.

In the early stages of an eating disorder, people can feel exhilarated and pleased at the prospect of taking control of their body image. Later, the demands for the disorder become damaging and exhausting. They turn out to be tantamount to a full-time job, where the student has to work hard to prevent the terrifying prospect of weight gain alongside all the other demands of university life. Restricting food and drink is socially difficult, whilst the 'compensatory behaviours' and repeated 'body checking' result in fatigue and discomfort as well as requiring efforts to conceal them from others. Compulsive and competitive accessing of social media sites is a powerful maintaining factor. All this has to be prioritised over pleasurable and useful experiences, and over attainment of full academic potential. For those who were previously depressed, mood usually resists antidepressant treatments. Those who were not depressed before the condition took hold usually become so.

At school Jim was a keen footballer. The coach was ambitious and brought in a programme of extra training nights and 'healthy diet advice' to families. The team reached the top of the schools' league. At the same time, Jim was studying for exams that would decide his university place. He deliberately ended the relationship with his girlfriend and stopped all partying and socialising.

For a while, he felt in control of the challenges in his life, but started to find his grades falling and his energy levels dropping. Even football was a chore. His mother insisted on taking him to the doctor because of his low mood. The doctor immediately noticed Jim's striking weight loss. She referred him to a dietitian, and with his mother's enthusiastic cookery and family encouragement, the situation was reversed, at least physically. Jim stopped playing soccer and was accepted by his first choice of university.

He had been warned not to join sports societies, and set himself to study hard and get a first-class degree. He started to feel discomfort with his weight gain, though, and felt flabby rather than well-nourished. He began to go for solitary runs each evening between the end of lectures and the start of his long sessions in the library. Running left him feeling so much better that after a while he could not bear to miss a single day. His weight dropped in the absence of his mother's cooking.

One November night he was knocked over by a car while out running in the dark. He was not badly hurt, but his weight loss was again discovered and addressed, and he was treated first in a medical ward, then in a specialist eating disorders service. In this case body image concern appeared to have arisen after his initial weight loss and regain. In therapy, he had to address both fears of weight gain and his self-destructive levels of perfectionism and competitiveness.

Staff and fellow students sometimes ask me how they can tell if someone has an eating disorder, and whether they should say anything. Often the student's social withdrawal is a more telling sign than more specific behaviours, but people sharing accommodation are more likely to notice avoidance of eating or signs of bingeing and purging.

I have all too often heard young people say 'they *accused* me of having anorexia', or 'how can I ask her about this when I don't have *proof*?' It is important for both patients and those who care for them to remember that an eating disorder is an illness rather than a crime. Lay people are not expected to come to an accurate diagnosis, but rather to express concern if someone's symptoms appear to be causing them harm or damaging quality of life for others. Likewise, it is not healthy for a friend or sibling to take on the task of getting a person to eat, to gain weight or to refrain from bingeing or over-exercising. The healthiest and kindest attitude to take is to encourage the person to seek professional help, perhaps even offering to accompany them to the doctor's surgery, or to the counselling service.

Prevention and Treatment of Eating Disorders

In this world of endemic body image preoccupation, and valid concerns about obesity, the speciality of eating disorders is still relatively starved of good evidence but there is worldwide research in progress to discover effective prevention and treatment. In the UK, National Institute for Health and Care Excellence (2017) updated its eating disorders guideline in 2017, whilst in Scotland, the Scottish Intercollegiate Guidelines Network (2022) published new guidance in 2022.

A large number of prevention programs are under development and evaluation. Many have been found to improve participants' *knowledge*, and sometimes reduce known risk factors, but there is little evidence so far that they actually reduce development of diagnosed eating disorders. There is good evidence that prompt referral and treatment are beneficial. Specialist intervention in the first 3 years has the best prognosis (Stice et al., 2017) and evaluation of the First Episode and Rapid Early intervention for Eating Disorders service suggests early treatment reduces the need for later, more costly interventions (Fukutomi et al., 2020).

In an extreme situation, where an individual with an eating disorder is at risk of their life because of extreme weight loss or suicidal mood, it is important to act to save life in the first instance. This does not require going through the usual referral processes to go on a waiting list for therapy. Life threatening emergencies are prioritised by clinical services. Admission to a medical rather than psychiatric ward may be needed in the first instance, depending on the state of expertise and specialism in different parts of the country. It is also important to know that UK mental health legislation allows compulsory treatment when the illness is of a nature or degree that there are risks to health or safety. Any fully registered medical doctor can detain patients for brief periods. For longer periods, psychiatrists approved under the relevant legislation must be involved.

In a medical emergency, weight gain may not be the goal of urgent treatment. Rest, warmth, protection from infection and intravenous correction of blood chemicals may be life saving.

When life has been saved, longer-term treatments for eating disorders combine input to support emotion regulation, distress tolerance, body image acceptance and interpersonal skills alongside weight gain when needed. Effectively the patient is exposed to a normal healthy weight and learns to tolerate this without using weight loss as the automatic response to stress and distress. This is commonly delivered in the form of 'enhanced' cognitive behavioural therapy.

Certain medications have demonstrated benefits in supporting recovery from the different eating disorders. There is long experience of using certain antidepressant medications at the higher end of the dose range in the treatment of bulimia nervosa. Anorexia nervosa may respond to small doses of the drug olanzapine (Attia et al., 2019). In the United States, binge eating disorder has been treated using amphetamine-based drugs similar to those prescribed for attention deficit hyperactivity disorder, but such prescribing is not licensed for this purpose in the UK.

There is still uncertainty as to the precise mechanisms of effective treatment, but treatment is known to be effective: access to specialist eating disorders services is associated with better outcomes. Overall, around 50% of people with anorexia nervosa recover fully (Murray, 2019). Recovery from bulimia nervosa is widely considered to be more likely than from anorexia nervosa. At 9-year follow up, almost 70% of people with bulimia nervosa had recovered (Eddy et al., 2017).

Treatments for eating disorders rely crucially on strong therapeutic relationships, which may need to be maintained as far as possible over months and years. These relationships may be repeatedly interrupted when treatment has to span child and adult services, or when patients are discharged from specialist wards. Management of such crucial transitions is discussed further in a Royal College of Psychiatrists (2017) report. The short courses of counselling offered in university services do not offer a suitable model for such treatment, but provision of mental health mentors across a student's degree course can provide useful continuity if the mentor is integrated into the eating disorders team treating the patient.

True recovery involves more that the valuable but limited move to tolerating a healthy weight. Those who achieve genuine recovery experience a refocussing of values, a new wisdom and maturity that are utterly life changing for the former patient and their family and friends.

Summary

Most students benefit from the physical resilience of youth and the reserves of health invested in them through a childhood of care from families schools and welfare state. As a result, they often continue to function surprisingly well physically, despite paying scant respect for self-care, nutrition, activity, sleep and biological rhythms. Their mental, emotional and social health may be adversely affected, though. Students are more likely to be motivated to change their behaviour to enjoy potential improvements in interpersonal relationships and in personal confidence, than to do so out of fear of longer-term physical damage.

Practice Points

Parents and Families

- There are demonstrable benefits in having routines around regular social mealtimes, and ensuring young people get adequate sleep and physical activity.

- Good enough nutrition is important but obsessive attention to calories is not. Being able to eat a range of foods makes it easier for students to nourish themselves economically and participate in social eating.
- An adolescent with an existing eating disorder is likely to become much more vulnerable to relapse after the transition to university unless this is carefully managed.

Schools

- Parent and carer groups regularly report that eating disorders were triggered by 'healthy eating' messages from schools. The healthiest prevention programmes focus on overall healthy self-respect and self-image.
- All the same advice as that provided to families, with additional care to challenge obsessive and extreme attitudes.
- School canteens and cafeterias could provide a healthier food environment than sending children out into the streets at snack and mealtimes. Commercial food and drink outlets cannot be trusted to be the main influence on children's food choices.
- Classes in food preparation and consumption could helpfully focus on nutritional value and social participation rather than calorie counting and weight loss. However, didactive teaching needs to be backed up with practice, whereby nutritious economic food is eaten sociably on the school premises.
- Sports, athletics, dancing and physical activities should not be only competitive events for the prestige of a school; they are needed by all pupils as part of a healthy physical and mental lifestyle.

University Students and Staff

- Students should be helped to remember the cost and nutritional quality of what they drink as well as what they eat.
- Regular routines and adequate sleep contribute to good grades and better relationships.
- Physical activity, including outdoor activity is important for physical and mental health, and not just a competitive activity.
- Those who are concerned a peer may have an eating disorder should be careful to express concern rather than 'accusation' and support the person to seek medical help.

University Authorities

- A gradual return to high quality institutional staff and student dining rooms would be an investment in the intellectual and social well-being of the institution.
- Student timetables should be restructured where possible so that lectures start after 10 a.m. to allow for adequate sleep.
- Investment in sports and physical activity should span all students, not only elite performers.
- Universities will inevitably host many young people with eating disorders, given the demographic involved. Every university should identify a local specialist eating disorders service for young adults and build links with this. In the absence of such a

service, campaigns and joint working between the university and NHS may be able to set up such resource.

- Eating disorders can affect people of any age. Staff as well as students may experience these conditions and should be offered services where their privacy is protected. They may be uncomfortable in therapy groups shared by their students.

Clinicians – Doctors, Counsellors, Mental Health Specialists

- Pathways for the assessment and early treatment of eating disorders should already be in place and staff training in recognition, referral and support need to be provided in all universities.

References

Aceijas, C., Bello-Corassa, R., WaldhäuslN, S., Lambert, N. & Cassar, S. (2016). Barriers and determinants of physical activity among UK university students: Carmen Aceijas. *European Journal of Public Health*, 26(suppl_1), ckw174.255.

Attia, E., Steinglass, J. E., Walsh, B. T., et al. (2019). Olanzapine versus placebo in adult outpatients with anorexia nervosa: A randomized clinical trial. *American Journal of Psychiatry*, 176(6), 449–56.

Belogianni, K., Ooms, A., Lykou, A. & Moir, H. J. (2022). Nutrition knowledge among university students in the UK: A cross-sectional study. *Public Health Nutrition*, 25 (10), 2834–41.

Calzo, J. P., Blashill, A. J., Brown, T. A. & Argenal, R. L. (2017). Eating disorders and disordered weight and shape control behaviors in sexual minority populations. *Current Psychiatry Reports*, 19(8), 1–10.

Dunbar, R. I. M. (2017). Breaking bread: the functions of social eating. *Adaptive Human Behavior and Physiology*, 3(3), 198–211.

Eddy, K. T., Tabri, N., Thomas, J. J., et al. (2017). Recovery from anorexia nervosa and bulimia nervosa at 22-year follow-up. *The Journal of clinical psychiatry*, 78(2), 17085.

El Ansari, W., Stock, C., Phillips, C., et al. (2011). Does the association between depressive symptomatology and physical activity depend on body image perception? A survey of students from seven universities in the UK. *International journal of environmental research and public health*, 8(2), 281–99.

Ferguson, C. J., Muñoz, M. E., Garza, A. & Galindo, M. (2014). Concurrent and prospective analyses of peer, television and social media influences on body dissatisfaction, eating disorder symptoms and life satisfaction in adolescent girls. *Journal of youth and adolescence*, 43(1), 1–14.

Franko, D. L., Tabri, N., Keshaviah, A., et al. (2018). Predictors of long-term recovery in anorexia nervosa and bulimia nervosa: Data from a 22-year longitudinal study. *Journal of psychiatric research*, 96, 183–8.

Fukutomi, A., Austin, A., McClelland, J., et al. (2020). First episode rapid early intervention for eating disorders: A two-year follow-up. *Early Intervention in Psychiatry*, 14(1), 137–41.

Fulkerson, J. A., Story, M., Mellin, A., Leffert, N., Neumark-Sztainer, D. & French, S. A. (2006). Family dinner meal frequency and adolescent development: Relationships with developmental assets and high-risk behaviors. *Journal of Adolescent Health*, 39 (3), 337–45.

Gillberg, C. (1983). Are autism and anorexia nervosa related? *The British Journal of Psychiatry*, 142(4), 428.

Girlguiding UK (2020). *Girls attitudes survey.* www.girlguiding.org.uk/globalassets/docs-and-resources/research-and-campaigns/girls-attitudes-survey-2020.pdf

Groth, T., Hilsenroth, M., Boccio, D. & Gold, J. (2020). Relationship between trauma history and eating disorders in adolescents.

Journal of Child & Adolescent Trauma, 13 (4), 443–53.

Hasken, J., Kresl, L., Nydegger, T. & Temme, M. (2010) Diabulimia and the role of school health personnel. *Journal of School Health*, 80(10), 465–69.

Hoek, H. W. (2006). Incidence, prevalence and mortality of anorexia nervosa and other eating disorders. *Current opinion in psychiatry*, 19(4), 389–94.

Kandola, A., Ashdown-Franks, G., Hendrikse, J., Sabiston, C. M. & Stubbs, B. (2019). Physical activity and depression: Towards understanding the antidepressant mechanisms of physical activity. *Neuroscience & Biobehavioral Reviews*, 107, 525–39.

Keys, A. (1946). Human starvation and its consequences. *Journal of the American Dietetic Association*, 22(7), 582–7.

Kim, H. S., von Ranson, K. M., Hodgins, D. C., McGrath, D. S. & Tavares, H. (2018). Demographic, psychiatric, and personality correlates of adults seeking treatment for disordered gambling with a comorbid binge/purge type eating disorder. *European Eating Disorders Review*, 26(5), 508–18.

Klaiber, P., Whillans, A. V. & Chen, F. S. (2018). Long-term health implications of students' friendship formation during the transition to university. *Applied Psychology: Health and Well-being*, 10(2), 290–308 https://doi.org/10.1111/aphw.12131

Koch, S. V., Larsen, J. T., Mouridsen, S. E., et al. (2015). Autism spectrum disorder in individuals with anorexia nervosa and in their first-and second-degree relatives: Danish nationwide register-based cohort-study. *The British Journal of Psychiatry*, 206 (5), 401-7.

León, E., Tabares, M., Baile, J. I., Salazar, J. G. & Zepeda, A. P. (2022). Eating behaviors associated with weight gain among university students worldwide and treatment interventions: A systematic review. *Journal of American College Health*, 1–8.

Li, Z., Halls, D., Byford, S. & Tchanturia, K. (2022). Autistic characteristics in eating disorders: Treatment adaptations and impact on clinical outcomes. *European Eating Disorders Review*, 30(5), 671–90.

Lock, J. & Le Grange, D. (2015). *Treatment manual for anorexia nervosa: A family-based approach*. Guilford publications.

Mabe, A. G., Forney, K. J. & Keel, P. K. (2014). Do you "like" my photo? Facebook use maintains eating disorder risk. *International Journal of Eating Disorders*, 47(5), 516–23.

Marx, R., Tanner-Smith, E. E., Davison, C. M., et al. (2017). Later school start times for supporting the education, health, and well-being of high school students: a systematic review. *Campbell Systematic Reviews*, 13(1), 1–99.

Murray, S. B. (2019). Updates in the treatment of eating disorders in 2018: A year in review in *Eating Disorders: The Journal of Treatment & Prevention*. *Eating Disorders*, 27(1), 6–17.

National Institute for Health and Care Excellence (2017). *Eating disorders: Recognition and treatment*. www.nice.org .uk/guidance/NG69

Root, T. L., Pinheiro, A. P., Thornton, L., et al. (2010). Substance use disorders in women with anorexia nervosa. *International Journal of Eating Disorders*, 43(1), 14–21.

Rouse, P. C. & Biddle, S. J. H. (2010). An ecological momentary assessment of the physical activity and sedentary behaviour patterns of university students. *Health Education Journal*, 69(1), 116–25.

Royal College of Psychiatrists (2017). *Managing transitions when the patient has an eating disorder: Guidance for good practice (CR208)*. www.rcpsych.ac.uk/docs/ default-source/improving-care/better-mh-policy/college-reports/college-report-cr208 .pdf

Scottish Intercollegiate Guidelines Network (2022). *Eating disorders*. SIGN. sign.ac.uk/ our-guidelines/eating-disorders

Serra, R., Kiekens, G., Vanderlinden, J., et al. (2020). Binge eating and purging in first-year college students: Prevalence, psychiatric comorbidity, and academic performance. *International Journal of Eating Disorders*, 53(3), 339–48.

Sprake, E. F., Russell, J. M., Cecil, J. E., et al. (2018). Dietary patterns of university students in the UK: A cross-sectional study. *Nutrition Journal*, 17(1), 1–17.

Stice, E., Gau, J. M., Rohde, P. & Shaw, H. (2017). Risk factors that predict future onset of each DSM–5 eating disorder: Predictive specificity in high-risk adolescent females. *Journal of Abnormal Psychology*, 126(1), 38.

Stoyel, H., Slee, A., Meyer, C. & Serpell, L. (2020). Systematic review of risk factors for eating psychopathology in athletes: A critique of an etiological model. *European Eating Disorders Review*, 28(1), 3–25.

Swinnerton, L., Moldovan, A. A., Mann, C. M., Durrant, S. J. & Mireku, M. O. (2021). Lecture start time and sleep characteristics: Analysis of daily diaries of undergraduate students from the LoST-Sleep project. *Sleep Health*, 7(5), 565–71.

Tan, J., Corciova, S. & Nicholls, D.E. (2019). Going too far? How the public health anti-obesity drives could cause harm by promoting eating disorders. In Cratsley, K. & Radden, J. (eds) *Developments in Neuroethics and Bioethics* (pp. 235–64).

Vadeboncoeur, C., Foster, C. & Townsend, N. (2016). Freshman 15 in England: A longitudinal evaluation of first year university student's weight change. *BMC Obesity*, 3, 1–9.

Vögele, C., Lutz, A. P. C. & Gibson, E. L. (2018). Mood, emotions, and eating disorders. In: Agras, W. S. & Robinson, A. (eds) *The Oxford handbook of eating disorders* (pp. 155–86). Oxford University Press.

Watson, H. J., Yilmaz, Z., Thornton, L. M., et al. (2019). Genome-wide association study identifies eight risk loci and implicates metabo-psychiatric origins for anorexia nervosa. *Nature Genetics*, 51(8), 1207–14.

Alcohol

6

High levels of alcohol intake, and 'binge drinking' in particular, are such a traditional feature of student life that it can feel both churlish and pointless to challenge the situation. Many young British white people start to drink more heavily when they are free of the constraints of life in the family home and when they reach 18 – the age when it becomes legal to purchase alcohol, coinciding with the age of most students when they first arrive at university. I was surprised to find that despite continuing high levels of alcohol consumption in the UK adult population overall, there have been sustained reductions in alcohol consumption over the years from 2005 to 2015 in the student population (Ng Fat et al., 2018). This may be explained, though, at least partly, by the increased numbers of international students from non-drinking cultures. More recently, research on student alcohol use in the wake of the COVID pandemic is still emerging and suggests that male students and staff have increased their alcohol consumption. We do not yet know whether this will be a significant lasting change.

There is now a wider range of recreational drugs to choose from, so that this generation is not obliged to turn to alcohol when they search for mind-altering agents. However, I have separated considerations of recreational substance use into different chapters for alcohol and other drugs (discussed in Chapter 7), because the channels of access are different, subject to different controls, and likely to require different approaches to harm reduction in university communities.

The increased risks of heart and liver disease, cancer and even future dementing illnesses are too far in the future for young students to hold in mind when they face the immediate challenges of their particular developmental stage of life. The consequences of accidents and drunk driving charges are of course important and relevant to students, but they are not sufficiently closely linked to *mental* health to warrant detailed discussion in this book.

The Scale of Alcohol Use in Universities and the Wider UK Community

The stereotypical expectation that students will drink heavily is often framed positively, with negative attitudes towards those who do not. Non-drinkers can be perceived as unsociable, strange or disapproving. Like the young nurses who cared for Jolie in the case study, 79% of students say that drinking and getting drunk is part of university culture, according to a National Union of Students (NUS) report (Alcohol Impact, 2018). The NUS's Alcohol Impact runs a wide-ranging annual survey to uncover student attitudes, behaviours and experiences linked to alcohol consumption, and to track long-term trends in these aspects.

Jolie spent months in a specialist clinic, hoping to recover from anorexia nervosa in time to take up her place at university. Nurses encouraged her to practice coping with university life by going out to eat in cafes, shopping in supermarkets and cooking meals, and several explicitly suggested she should practise drinking alcohol. They told her 'Getting drunk is an important part of your education.' When she protested they told her this was because of her fear of the calorie content of alcoholic drinks.

Data from the annual Health Survey for England from 2005 to 2015 (Ng Fat et al., 2018) found that the proportion of 16- to 24-year-olds who were current non-drinkers increased from 18% in 2005 to 29% in 2015.The increase is mainly due to an increase in those who have never drunk alcohol: from 9% to 17% over the same period. For those who were drinking, there were some improvements, including a fall in drinking above recommended limits from 43% to 28%. Young people in full-time higher education showed consistently lower consumption than those not at school, college or university. However, there is still clear evidence of a student binge-drinking culture in our universities.

The high levels of binge drinking within the student population are the most worrying aspect of the problem, as the age group is not yet likely to show the burden of chronic alcohol dependence. Later in this chapter, some of the consequences of the binge drinking student culture are discussed. One concern is the distortion of the central purpose of university life from being one of scholarship and education to one of intoxication, and the assumption that 'social life' and 'partying' are synonyms for becoming drunk to the point of incapacity.

We may not have to give up alcohol completely. Some cultures and subcultures use alcohol and other substances as 'facilitators' to relaxed, sociable and creative states, and the occasional extreme experience of intoxication can be managed as a sort of 'initiation' into late adolescence. However, the scale of alcohol use in current university culture appears to be occurring at the expense of honouring values dear to modern higher education, including mental well-being, physical health, academic achievement, diversity and respectful sexual relationships.

Findings from the Students and Alcohol National Survey

2% drink most/every day
23% drink 2–3 days a week
20% get drunk on purpose about once a week
21% say they do not drink (never, or have stopped drinking)
60% of those who say it can be difficult not to drink too much (38% overall) say it is because alcohol helps them to relax / socialise
79% agree that drinking and getting drunk is part of university culture.
70% think that students drink alcohol to fit in with their peers
76% say there's an expectation for students to drink to get drunk
Before they started university, 47% thought that students got drunk most of the time.
10% said they were aware of safe or responsible drinking campaigns/activities at their university
Only 1% had taken part in these campaigns/activities.

Alcohol Impact (2018)

Alcohol in the Transition to University

Whilst the subjective experience of reaching extreme intoxication can become an enjoyable leisure activity in itself, the prime value of being a drinker of alcohol is for most students a social one. Alcohol makes students feel that they belong and that provides an enormously reassuring feeling of security. Belonging, attachment and connectedness are fundamentals for most of us and young students face the huge challenge of creating new networks and connections. Not only is alcohol a relaxant, providing self-medication for anxiety, but the ritual of drinking it with others promotes belonging. The very fact that it is a somewhat incapacitating thing to do to oneself builds trust in the vulnerability and gentleness of others in the group. Alcohol brings about enough disinhibition to allow the sharing of personal material that would otherwise only emerge in a trusting relationship. Alcohol can therefore feel like an accelerated route to trusting relationships.

For a majority of UK students, the transition to university at age 18 co-occurs with the attainment of legal drinker status and increased exposure to alcohol consumption, both among peers and in drinking environments. Symbolically and legally, the age of 18 is a proxy for the move from a hierarchy where parents and teachers make and enforce the rules to one where 'peer rules' are most evident and powerful. There is an expectation that alcohol, taken on a communal as well as individual basis, facilitates relief, reassurance, romance and friendship. In this context, it's almost a 'no-brainer' to join the drinkers. Authoritarian prohibitions might only strengthen the sense of solidarity within the student group.

Readers who have already read Chapters 2 and 3 on the transition to university life will remember the prominence of alcohol use in the process of transition and peer group development for new students. It is likely that alcohol has the same role as a social lubricant when students leave halls and take up residence in shared flats and other accommodation. It is worth revisiting and re-emphasising the particular emotional context for these students, or we are doomed to enter into paradoxically well-meaning but self-defeating dynamics.

Brown and Murphy (2020) carefully interviewed 23 first-year students and heard how their pre-arrival concerns over new peer relationships were subsequently reduced by drinking together. This reinforced participant perceptions of alcohol as beneficial for hastening development of social connections, in turn reducing anxiety and supporting successful transition. For non- or low-drinkers in the study, social connectedness without alcohol use was reported as more challenging. Alcohol was perceived as a readily available, effective tool for hastening social connectedness. This made students resistant to alcohol education messages.

Some students had already been online to Facebook groups linking students from the same residences or to chat sites such as 'Student Room', where current and previous students post information on halls, social activities in the area and other aspects of university life. They described planning drinking events, with previous residents suggesting 'big pre-drinks' sessions to meet up and break the ice on arrival. New students felt that online groups like this were helpful in starting to create an image of campus life and also providing opportunities for development of social connections.

Many student groups and societies enact 'initiation rites' for new members, who are required to prove their courage or commitment to the society in a risky or humiliating way. Members may be expected to keep the rites secret. Drinking is usually involved. This so-called hazing has long been a feature of US fraternities and sports societies, and has spread to the UK via movies and social media. It has caused considerable concern. For instance, the rugby union governing body, the Rugby Football Union, warned that initiations at university clubs were putting people off playing rugby (BBC Newsbeat, 2017).

In December 2016, student Ed Farmer died in his first term at Newcastle University after attending an agricultural society initiation where rounds of 100 triple vodkas were ordered. Universities UK launched the new advice for institutions in collaboration with Newcastle University, and several institutions have banned society initiation rites specifically because of the dangers of alcohol poisoning (Busby, 2019).

Students' Attitudes to Theoretical Risk

University authorities and even student unions, the formal voice of the student body, have increasingly taken steps to distance themselves from the alcohol-imbued culture of 'Freshers' Week', but this contrasts heavily with flyers and promotional material available everywhere around campus from local bars and clubs, which focus predominantly on drink promotions. Brown and Murphy's (2020) researchers heard that student and staff expectations, based on social norms, interpersonal messages and experiences, were that, whether or not alcohol is stated explicitly as part of social activity, this is assumed anyway. It was simply presumed by all participants in the research that drinking would be the primary social activity for new arrivals. For parents, university staff or even student unions to challenge this powerful dynamic requires careful strategy and the mobilisation of considerable forces. Simplistic opposition merely demonstrates ignorance and impotence.

Students in the study were asked whether they remembered being signposted to webpages on alcohol safety as part of the university's induction. Content had been written by university staff and included tips for a safe night out, warnings over problems stemming from excess alcohol use and strategies to reduce consumption. Most students did not recall seeing the webpages, so researchers showed them the content and asked for their thoughts. Most of these students then strongly rejected the warnings and consumption-reduction messages and criticised them as paternalistic and unrealistic.

Some of the rituals around alcohol that particularly appeal to students are various drinking games and organised pub crawls. Students have usually been informed and warned in advance about the increased consumption involved and risk of negative outcomes, but young people do not on the whole respond in the same way as older adults to theoretical information about risk.

How Much Is Too Much?

UK Guidance on sensible drinking limits changed in 2016 from 21 units for a man and 14 units for a woman per week to 14 units for both men and women.

It was also advised that people should have at least 2 days off alcohol per week and not consume more than 2–3 units of alcohol on any one occasion.

This advice fails to account for such individual differences as age, gender, body size and co-morbid health concerns. People consuming alcohol within these limits may still exceed driving limits. Many young people appear to drink more heavily without harm.

Recognition of links between alcohol and likely consequences is more important than numbers.

Young adults in their physical prime are expected to embrace high levels of risk in pursuit of worthwhile goals. Historically, society has depended on young people being prepared risk death to engage in battle or to endure childbirth. Even today, many games and sports are associated with high physical risk. Shared risk can be part of the bonding experience of participation, and for high-achieving students the element of competition in sports and games is an important spice. Brown and Murphy (2020) comment 'Social benefits were being prioritised over risks among this cohort at this point in time. . .. Although previous drinking experiences were highly variable, the expectation of the centrality of alcohol to university social activity was universal.'

Some students are more risk averse, but have lived out their childhoods with the experience that caring adults ensure their safety while they enjoy a range of activities. When those around them permit them to participate in activities, they presume someone is looking out for their safety. It is hard to suddenly be responsible for your own risk assessments and monitoring. Luckily, most students have already established a habit of looking out for the safety of peers on nights out and when drinking together, but those who drink alone or who become separated from the group are at greater risk of both acute harms and of drinking beyond group norms.

Alcohol and Student Finance

Chapter 9 makes the argument that financial concerns are one of the important determinants of student mental health and observes that most students are still learning to manage their own budget. They are doing so in the context of commercial interests around them – including those of their university, which depends on their fees, and the interests of local businesses.

We might be dismayed by the amount of money students expect to spend on alcohol, but it can be even more concerning to find that for some, this represents larger amounts of alcohol than expected. Bars and pubs use special offers and inducements to students to drink more. However, a great deal of the alcohol consumed is bought more cheaply in bulk in supermarkets and consumed in homes and halls before going out for the night – a practice called 'pre-loading'.

The NUS reported that 48% of respondents to their survey regularly start drinking either at home or a friend's house before they go out for the night, and 21% said they regularly deliberately get drunk at home before a night out (Alcohol Impact, 2018). Some also deliberately refrain from eating so they can get more drunk. The very common practice of 'pre-loading', may have started as a way to save money on drinks in bars and clubs by drinking shop bought alcohol before going out. For some students it may be a way to deal with social anxiety before leaving home. However, it has now become an expected part of the ritual of a night out as much as a money-saving ploy.

The practice of purchasing drinks in 'rounds' was common, with 17% of respondents reporting they almost always buy alcoholic drinks in this way (Alcohol Impact, 2018). This can be a worry for less-affluent students. It is a more expensive practice because of the social imperative for each group member to 'stand their round', and also leads to more alcohol being consumed. This is another example of how the craving to 'belong' can trump the individual's self-care and longer-term values.

Anecdotally at least, the introduction of minimum unit alcohol pricing in Scotland had little effect on student alcohol use. The target of the intervention was the extremely low-price alcohol that tends to be used by chronically dependent older drinkers. Students say that on the whole they do not use this.

Whilst the direct cost of alcoholic drinks is one factor, the effects of consuming alcohol on other aspects of spending are important too. For instance, students who participate in internet gaming or in online gambling may do so when intoxicated and be more likely to lose control over what they spend. Lynch et al. (2004) found that young gamblers had significantly raised levels of alcohol and drug misuse.

Students who have eating disorders may struggle with alcohol too. The calorie content of alcoholic drinks is one factor that may tend to limit alcohol consumption for some, but some people cut back on nutritious food in order to 'save calories' for drink. The levels of malnutrition will then be higher than a person's weight would suggest. Moreover, the disinhibiting effects of alcohol are likely to trigger out-of-control binging on both food and drink. The vicious binge-purge cycle is further exacerbated.

Commercial Exploitation of the Student Drinking Culture

Orme and Coghill (2014) remark that 'Any regulation of student alcohol use is . . . being attempted within a setting where it contrasts with both informal narratives and economic benefits to business, with campus environments currently limited in the extent to which they are health promoting.' The UK has a considerable investment in the production and sale of alcohol and a whole hospitality industry based around selling alcoholic drinks. Students are seen as likely clients and are, by their own admission, susceptible to advertising and to special offers such as 'happy hours'. In a survey, 21% of students said they take advantage of drink offers such as 'happy hours' and buy larger measures of alcohol because they're on offer (Alcohol Impact, 2018).

> The alcohol industry is a small, but not insignificant, part of the UK economy, contributing £46 billion a year, around 2.5% of total GDP, to national income.
> The most prominent UK study suggests that being a problem drinker is equivalent to the effect of not having a degree on a person's chances of finding work.
>
> Bhattacharya, A. (2017). Splitting the Bill: Alcohol's Impact on the Economy. *Institute for Alcohol Studies: London, UK*

Another example of special offers is the phenomenon of commercially sponsored 'pub crawls' for students. Quigg et al. (2013), studied student drinking patterns and blood alcohol concentration on four commercially organised pub crawls in three different UK cities.

On average, each participant consumed more than 16 alcohol units (more than the recommended limit for a whole week's consumption) over the course of the night. Nearly all had 'preloaded' prior to joining the pub crawl. A fifth had consumed alcohol in the street despite street drinking bans, 14% had hurt themselves (e.g., fallen over), 9% vomited and 7% had been in an argument during the pub crawl. Moreover, 14% of students reported being involved in sexual activity.

The researchers say that organisers had implemented a range of measures to manage and supervise the pub crawls, but that these measures were relatively ineffective. The study authors conclude by suggesting that organisers, local authorities, universities and students bring in measures to make pub crawls safer. It does not appear to have occurred to the researchers to consider a ban on such activities.

A more recent study, conducted in four Swedish university cities, demonstrates that private parties also host hazardous levels of student drinking (Elgàn et al., 2019). 'Preloading' was almost universal, and 86% of women students and 87% of men students reported 'hazardous levels' of alcohol intake. This study concluded that alcohol intoxication and hazardous use among Swedish university students is a concern, and that the university setting is an important arena for implementation of alcohol prevention strategies.

Alcohol and Academic Performance

There is little doubt that alcohol is potentially damaging to brain function over the longer-term, and that heavy alcohol use disrupts academic performance at the levels of interrupting attendance or ability to work. From results of the Harvard School of Public Health College Study of US undergraduate alcohol use, Wechsler et al. (2000) reported that frequent heavy episodic drinkers are much more likely to miss class and get behind in schoolwork. The subtler effects of high or uneven alcohol levels on memory and creativity are less clear, particularly in young adults.

An older study involving 66 US colleges and universities very neatly reported that 'A' students consumed an average of 3.2 drinks per week, while 'B' students consumed 4.6, 'C' students 5.8, and 'D/F' students 8.4 drinks per week (Presley et al., 1996). Such findings suggested a strong, negative correlation between undergraduate alcohol use and academic performance. However, these studies have flaws. Thombs et al. (2009) used more sophisticated analyses of grades, used breathalysers rather than relying only on self-report, and most importantly took account of a range of confounding factors to demonstrate that the link between grades and alcohol consumption is not so straightforward.

Alcohol and Fitness to Practise

In the case of students of the healthcare, teaching and legal professions, there are concerns beyond meeting required educational standards. The graduating student must also be declared a fit person to practise. An active alcohol or drug problem that has come to the attention of the university or college might debar the individual concerned from graduating. The high levels of alcohol use in students (and indeed of practitioners) of the professions and the implications of this are discussed in Chapter 19.

Alcohol and Student Sexual Behaviour

Sexual behaviour in university students is discussed in more detail in Chapter 12. Many of the research findings are likely to be relevant to the wider population of the same age group, rather than being specific to students, however this book tries to focus on work that has specifically examined university populations, including staff as well as students wherever the research allows.

Goldstein et al. (2007) found that amongst female university students – as in the broader population - alcohol use was more likely in new sexual encounters and associated with lower use of contraception or discussion of safe practices. A substantial body of research in several different countries has also found that for students, sexual assault, and also sexual behaviour that is later regretted, is often associated with alcohol and other substance misuse by both parties (e.g., McCauley et al., 2009). Many of the assaults involved are described as 'incapacitated rape' rather than 'forcible rape'.

Testa et al. (2015) explored whether drinking episodes contribute to sexual aggression by first-year US college men and concluded that drinking episodes increased the odds of both aggressive and non-aggressive sex with a new partner. However, the situation was not just a matter of the pharmacological effects of alcohol on sexual aggression. The authors suggest that the situations and environments in which alcohol is consumed can influence sexual behaviour too.

Much of the earlier research in the field came from the United States, but one notable project stems from the UK. Researchers from Liverpool John Moore University's School of Law and the Public Health Institute collaborated on an interdisciplinary programme of research. They explored the experiences and attitudes of students towards alcohol intoxication and non-consensual sexual activity. They also consulted lawyers about legal treatment of intoxicated rape complainants.

They identified a drinking double-standard: whilst women were blamed more for their assault as their level of intoxication increased, increased intoxication in men resulted in a reduction in perception of their responsibility for perpetrating a sexual offence. There was a lack of understanding and confusion amongst students regarding the law of rape and the meaning of consent, especially in cases involving intoxication. Barristers highlighted that alcohol consumption disproportionately impacted on the credibility of the victim at trial, rather than the culpability of the defendant.

As a result of the research, Liverpool city council launched a media campaign aimed at men between 18 and 24 years old, and specifically students as users of the night-time economy. The campaign ran in Liverpool city centre in 2012. Campaign evaluation demonstrated that it had effectively conveyed the message that having sex with someone who is exceptionally intoxicated amounts to rape. Further research and projects based on the original project have focussed on fostering dialogue with young men (Carline et al., 2018).

The Relationship between Alcohol and Mental Ill Health

Jacklyn's parents became worried by her dishevelled appearance and cynical attitude on video calls. They were concerned she was depressed and asked her to refer herself to student counselling.

The counsellor found that Jacklyn had symptoms of marked social anxiety, but quickly picked up on the fact that she was drinking heavily to blot out her anxiety. In fact, she was now drinking instead of going out with friends rather than drinking to relieve fears of going out. This was interfering with her academic work too.

Jacklyn gave permission for her general practitioner to be involved. The problem was still relatively short-lived, and she was able to manage her anxiety with prescribed medication and cognitive behavioural therapy techniques rather than alcohol, and to catch up on her studies.

Despite the focus of the book on mental health, I am not sure that it is particularly helpful in this context to debate whether alcohol misuse constitutes a mental disorder. For some people, such as those who benefit from the work of Alcoholics Anonymous, it is a useful construct to conceptualise destructive alcohol use as an addiction, and to see addiction as a mental disorder. For psychiatrists and other mental health professionals, alcohol misuse can be designated a mental health condition in its own right if certain criteria are met, but this won't usually be the case for young undergraduates. Developing a dependence on an addictive substance or experiencing lasting brain changes generally takes some years.

For this reason, well defined dependence is unusual in young people, particularly those who have succeeded in entering higher education. It is more likely to be observed in older students or members of staff. The immediate problem around alcohol in students is harmful or hazardous episodes of drinking. There is also the risk that such heavy drinking is the precursor of a longer-term pattern, with the consequent risk of dependence.

The two internationally used classifications take slightly different approaches to diagnosis, with the US Diagnostic and Statistical Manual of Mental Disorders, Fifth Edition (DSM-5) system making it more likely that a person could meet diagnostic criteria. The box summarises DSM-5 criteria for alcohol use disorder. According to DSM-5, alcohol use disorder is 'a problematic pattern of alcohol use leading to clinically significant impairment or distress, as manifested by at least two [of the specified criteria], occurring within a 12-month period.'

DSM-5 Alcohol Use Disorder (AUD): 2+ of 11 Problems

1. Alcohol is often taken in larger amounts or over a longer period than intended.
2. There is a persistent desire or unsuccessful efforts to cut down alcohol use.
3. A great deal of time is spent obtaining or taking alcohol or recovering from its effects.
4. Craving, or a strong desire or urge to use alcohol.
5. Recurrent alcohol causes failure to fulfil role obligations at work, school, or home.
6. Continued alcohol use, despite persistent social/ interpersonal problems caused or exacerbated by alcohol.
7. Social, occupational, or recreational activities given up/reduced because of alcohol use.
8. Alcohol use in situations in which it is physically hazardous.
9. Alcohol use continued despite knowing it is causing physical or psychological problems.
10. 'Tolerance' - i.e., need for increased amounts of alcohol to achieve intoxication or desired effect, or diminished effect with use of the same amount.
11. Withdrawal effects – either the characteristic withdrawal syndrome for alcohol, or the need to take more alcohol or a related substance, such as a benzodiazepine, to relieve or avoid alcohol withdrawal symptoms.

It is rare for a student to be diagnosed as having an alcohol use problem in isolation. Far more commonly, the presenting problem will be a disorder such as anxiety, depressive disorder, or even mania and hypomania. Sometimes the drinking to excess can be a symptom of manic disinhibition. More often, alcohol excess in the context of a mental disorder is a result of the person trying to calm down their symptoms of acute anxiety or to temporarily improve their mood.

Interestingly, there is a subtle extra link between mental ill health and alcohol. Kenney et al. (2018) found that college students with anxiety and depressive symptomatology were more susceptible to the perception that their peers drank heavily and approved of heavy drinking. This increased the likelihood that the depressed or anxious students would themselves drink to excess. The researchers suggest we should particularly address such students' views of alcohol, given the known links between perceptions of peer consumption and students' own behaviour.

Alcohol and Student Suicide

Student suicide is addressed in Chapter 17, but it is worth emphasising the association with alcohol in this chapter too. After depression, alcohol use is the commonest modifiable factor in prevention of suicide in the population as a whole. Kalk et al. (2019) describe addressing misuse of alcohol and other substances as 'a missed opportunity in suicide prevention'. It is not only alcohol-dependence that increases risk; acute intoxication is particularly important in younger deaths. The review cites evidence that national suicide rates increase as per capita alcohol consumption increases, and are associated with a culture of drinking to intoxication. The World Health Organization estimates that every fifth suicide would be prevented if alcohol were not consumed in the population. There is evidence that engaging with treatment and staying in contact with support reduces these risks (Kalk et al., 2019).

These findings can be applied to the student age group. In the Stanley et al. (2009) study of 20 young students who died by suicide, five students with a diagnosis of depression were also described by parents or friends as having alcohol problems. Likewise, heavy cannabis use in three cases was associated with both alcohol problems and depression.

A recent study from England used toxicological analysis to examine patterns of alcohol and cocaine use prior to suicide in a large sample of people – not specifically students (Bailey et al., 2021). The authors found that alcohol and cocaine use were both predictors of suicide, and that that people with very high levels of blood alcohol at the time of the suicide were more likely to have used cocaine than those not using alcohol.

These authors all urge us to reconsider the lack of emphasis given to substance use in many national suicide prevention strategies. For example, Talk to Frank (www.talktofrank.com), the public health advice website about substances, does not mention that alcohol or cocaine use is associated with suicide. The otherwise helpful training programmes produced by the Zero Suicide Alliance (www.zerosuicidealliance.com) fail to address substance use and intoxication, and do not acknowledge that conversations with people at high risk of suicide may be hampered by the difficulty in communicating usefully with a person who is drunk or high.

Alcohol and COVID

At the time of writing, emerging evidence suggests that male students, at least, increased their alcohol consumption in response to campus closures and other sequelae of COVID. Lechner et al. (2020) found that students in Ohio used significantly more alcohol in response to lockdown. Increased alcohol consumption was less marked in those reporting better social support. In Eastern Europe, Gavurova et al. (2020) found that it was male students who significantly increased alcohol consumption, whereas the female respondents to their study reported higher stress levels.

In the UK, Evans et al. (2021) found that alcohol use decreased rather than increased in their undergraduate sample, but this sample was made up almost exclusively of female students. Carr et al. (2022) found that UK university staff and postgraduate students were drinking to concerning levels as the community emerged from COVID. Around

20% of their participants were found to reach the cut-off for hazardous drinking, and 30% were drinking more than before the pandemic.

As we emerge from lockdown, it remains to be seen whether patterns of alcohol use return to pre-COVID levels. The situation is further complicated by difficulties in accessing treatment through workforce issues and increased demands on mental health services. Threats of financial and social deprivation from the war in Ukraine and other factors may also promote further 'self-medication' using alcohol.

The Plight of the Non-Drinker

After this litany of the biological, psychological, reputational and societal risks posed by alcohol, it is remarkable to have to ask whether *not* drinking can possibly be bad for you. But this does seem to be the case for many, increasingly vocal, students.

In their study of alcohol use in the transition to university, Brown and Murphy (2020) found that even those who self-defined as non-drinkers anticipated a dominant drink culture. They spoke of having to make special plans in the knowledge that they would be excluded from typical student social activities. Some took on part-time work, others arranged multiple visits from family to keep busy. These new students had to hold themselves aloof from the mainstream experience of transition. This might amount to exclusion from important academic and career networking. It certainly damages the individual's societal integration. It may increasingly be seen as a failure of the university community to incorporate and tolerate diversity.

International students – who provide considerable financial resource for most UK universities – can be among the most vocal critics of UK university alcohol culture. Students, staff and visiting academics from mainland Europe are often surprised by the pattern of binge drinking rather than enjoying regular alcohol consumption with food. Those from the Far East, and especially those from Muslim cultures, can struggle to tolerate what they may see as irreligious or disgusting. Most of all, they experience social exclusion as a result of not participating in the 'drinking cliques'.

Students and staff who may be trying to recover from an alcohol or substance misuse problem will also be disadvantaged, as will people whose mental or physical disorder, or vulnerability to such disorders, makes it dangerous for them to drink. And of course, there are those who make the choice not to drink. As students have remarked, 'there don't seem to be any societies for white non-drinkers' and 'I have to justify my non-drinking to you, but you don't seem to have to justify your drinking to me'.

Dr Fatemeh Nokhbatolfoghahai (personal communication) and colleagues at the University of Glasgow have used focus groups and individual interviews with medical students to explore how alcohol can be a force for exclusion. They recommend that in addition to the existing education about negative health consequences of drinking alcohol, education about the social consequences of drinking culture is warranted. Their work is discussed in Chapter 19 on the mental health of students of the professions. The students they interviewed agreed that events arranged by student societies were alcohol centred: 'In theory, it's just a sports weekend . . . but it's actually a weekend where you get really drunk.'

Another student described behaviour that must surely come under the heading of 'micro-aggression' if not downright bullying: 'Some people . . . have taken my not drinking as a challenge . . . the reason I stopped going to events was because people have tried pushing drinks into my hand.'

Even when not being challenged, or excluded from drinking events, these students did not want to be in the company of drunken people. They said that being sober created a perpetual barrier to conversation when interacting with people under the influence of alcohol.

> Jeremy, a geology student, had insulin dependent diabetes which he struggled to control at times. He found that taking no alcohol at all simplified life and improved his health. His friends at school, who had known him for years had all gone to different universities and he struggled to mix with his hallmates. He had never felt 'different' from other people as a result of diabetes, but he did feel uncomfortably different as a result of not drinking.
>
> On his first field trip, he met up with a group of Chinese students who were horrified by the drunkenness of fellow students. He began to socialise with them, helping them to perfect their English, and being introduced into their culture. As his course progressed, he began to see career opportunities as well as friendships as a result of being adopted into the group, but he confided to his sister that he did wish he also belonged to a friendship group in his own culture. With his Chinese friends he again felt 'different' because of his ethnic origin.

Student societies have traditionally 'incentivised' participation on the basis of providing free alcohol. Those which did not, or which specifically excluded alcohol, were expected to be poorly attended. Currently pizza, including vegetarian and vegan pizza, appears to be a welcome incentive to attend meetings, even if considered a poor second to beer.

Nokhbatolfoghahai's team call for broader-based interventions. They suggest campaigns to build understanding between students of different cultures and proclivities, so that the social exclusionary potential of alcohol is understood by all. This could open new debates on alcohol and social inclusion/exclusion, equality of employment and networking opportunities and the cultural role of intoxication.

Prevention and Treatment of Harmful Alcohol Use in the University

Interventions that tell us to change our health risk behaviour can fail because we simply dismiss the message. It can feel like unwelcome criticism of what we do and who we are, and often feels like 'nagging' rather than support. Leffingwell et al. (2007) found that students who drank alcohol were more critical of a health message about the risks of alcohol and rated the problem as less important than students who did not drink alcohol.

Although alcohol awareness and safe drinking campaigns are commonly undertaken at UK universities, such approaches show little impact on consumption (Larimer, 2007). Moreover, alcohol awareness efforts delivered in drinking settings, such as Student Unions, are often considered incongruent with the perceived purpose of the setting (Brooks, 2011).

In the past century, general practitioners and alcohol misuse experts developed the skills of motivational interviewing (Rollnick & Miller, 1995) to sidestep the oppositional dynamic, the 'resistance' that blocked uptake of health advice.

Key Principles of Motivational Interviewing

Anticipate ambivalence – when thinking about changing drinking behaviour ambivalence is the best you can expect, in fact!
Express empathy – it is too easy to forget what a large ask we are making.

> **Roll with resistance** – it is a particularly good time to express empathy when the individual goes into 'refusal' or 'fight' mode. When we find we are 'locking horns' we need to set aside the need to win and show the individual we are on their side.
>
> **Develop discrepancy** – means helping the person understand that they want things that are mutually incompatible, such as, on one hand, friendship with people who expect them to drink heavily and, on the other hand, the time, money and energy to complete a challenging degree.
>
> **Support self-efficacy** – however strongly motivated an individual, they will need the capability to push through with the task. Getting them to recall times when they have succeeded in a demanding achievement can mobilise strengths and skills – and build strong supportive relationships with helpers and mentors.
>
> (Rollnick & Miller, 1995)

This century has seen great strides in the science of behaviour change, so that there are now other arms in the therapeutic arsenal alongside motivational interviewing. One of these is the technique of 'social norming'. This depends on the idea that heavy drinkers often believe that their peers are drinking the same or more than they are. It also exploits a student's wish to be part of the group. Presented with evidence that they are an outlier compared to the average student, heavier drinkers tend to reduce. Some individuals find it helpful to use the safe drinking guidelines issued by UK Government as 'norms for healthy adult drinkers' but using data from peers has a more immediate and powerful impact.

A study based in Leeds (Bewick et al., 2008) tested out the feasibility and effectiveness of a web-based social norms alcohol intervention. The authors found that 55% of participants were students reporting potentially problematic alcohol consumption. All participants were randomly assigned to receive the intervention or not. Participants in the intervention condition received feedback on their own alcohol consumption and social norms information every time, they visited the website. There was feedback on their level of alcohol consumption, associated health risk, advice about whether consumption should be reduced or maintained, and comments about binge drinking behaviour. Social norms information told them the percentage of students who drank less alcohol than them, taken from Leeds University student survey data.

Disappointingly, there was no significant change in the total number of alcohol units consumed over a week, but there was a significant decrease in units consumed per average occasion – in other words a reduction in 'binges'.

More recent research recognises how important it is not to simply provide information and advice, but to address the mindsets that dismiss health messages scornfully. One study incorporated the theory of planned behaviour into studies like the one just described (Norman et al., 2018). This involves exploratory work to find out the beliefs that are guiding student behaviour and then understand how they can be balanced. Researchers worked collaboratively with students themselves to discuss common assumptions and behaviours and to film short videos of students discussing drinking culture.

In total, 3000 new university students were included in the study (Norman et al., 2018). Participants who received the theory of planned behaviour messages had significantly less favourable cognitions about binge drinking, consumed fewer units of alcohol, engaged in binge drinking less frequently, and had less harmful patterns of alcohol consumption during their first 6 months at university than the control groups. This research is impressive in seeking to understand the students' experience and thinking before trying to impose solutions.

Systemic Approaches to Reduce Harmful Alcohol Use

Alcohol Impact is a harm reduction behaviour change programme, to support students' unions and universities in fostering productive, healthy and inclusive student cultures surrounding drinking. To date, we've reached over 200 000 students, including through the participation of 200 sports clubs. Five thousand students have been actively involved with the programme, and 50 student auditors have received in-depth training. Our annual surveys have been completed by 46 000 students.

We've had great feedback from Alcohol Impact partnerships of students' unions and universities. Since Alcohol Impact began, among the participating institutions, there's been a 50% increase in the number of non-alcoholic events during welcome week; a 40% decrease in students' exclusion from campus venues due to drinking-related incidents; and a 20% reduction in students being rejected from the union bar due to intoxication and aggression.

alcoholimpact.nus.org.uk
www.drugandalcoholimpact.uk/

Beyond the work of individual institutions there are national organisations concerned with student welfare, often run by students themselves or run collaboratively. These have an important online presence, influence with government and university officials, and credibility with students themselves. It is important to 'nudge' conditions so that it is easier for students to live in a sober environment, and it becomes more inconvenient and less glamorous to participate in an unhealthy consumption – this was the line of thinking behind the striking reduction in smoking achieved in the UK by separating smoking from activities such as indoor eating, dancing and meeting.

Alcohol Impact is a programme managed and delivered by the NUS, now incorporated into its Drug and Alcohol Impact website. It is an impressive, whole-institution approach to responsible consumption of alcohol by students. It offers student unions the chance to work in partnership with their parent universities and local communities, to achieve an accreditation mark. This hallmarks that the university has created conditions for a social norm of responsible alcohol consumption. The programme offers a mix of institution-wide behaviour change approaches and interventions.

Dry Campuses in the United States

Some US universities offer 'dry campuses' where staff and students are not allowed to drink alcohol on campus even when they reach the legal drinking age. In the United States this is 21 rather than 18, so the social context is different. The dry campus rules means that no college facilities at all allow drinking, including dining rooms, canteens and university accommodation.

Concerns have been expressed that those students who wish to drink are forced to do so in secrecy and will not get the help they need, or that they will leave the university site to drink in parts of town where alcohol is permitted – perhaps at risk to their own safety. Some 'wet campus' universities nevertheless provide 'dry dorms' and dry fraternities and sororities for those students who wish to join them.

The dry campus policy relieves pressure on underage students who may otherwise be pressured to drink, and appears to successfully avoid problems faced by 'wet' campuses such as drunk driving offences, accidents and injuries, and legal problems. It has also been claimed that students can participate more fully in societies and other university activities without the complication of intoxication. Universities in North Carolina attempted to overcome the problem of students drinking in the local community rather than on campus by developing a 3-year 'campus–community coalition'. This successfully implemented environmental strategies to reduce high-risk drinking and its consequences (Wolfson et al., 2012).

Reflections

The experience of writing this chapter has emphasised how deeply embedded alcohol consumption is in UK life in general and in university life, especially for young students. The chapter has required more cross-referencing to other mental health concerns than any other. Alcohol, because it is an almost universally accepted recreational drug in the UK, plays a prominent role in virtually every other facet of university mental health, physical and mental disorder, accidents, and interpersonal and social trauma. A great proportion of this harm is related to the 'binge drinking' culture rather than necessarily to the overall amount of alcohol consumed, although that is of concern for the longer-term.

Alcohol consumption increases when young people enter university. This provides opportunity and responsibility to examine and address the situation. Whilst heavy-handed condemnation of young people's behaviour is likely to be counterproductive, we need to find creative and collaborative ways to reduce alcohol consumption and develop less harmful patterns of use. If we do not, we will continue to experience high levels of psychosocial damage, mental disorder and increased prevalence of suicide.

Questions to be Explored Further

What are the pros and cons of aspiring to a 'dry campus' vs concentrating on eliminating extreme 'binge' drinking?

How can we heal the social divide between students who use alcohol as an essential part of student life and those who find drunkenness unacceptable?

What are the overlaps and interactions between students' use of alcohol and other recreational drugs?

What changes in academic outcomes and in indices of mental health and disorder might result from a significant reduction in alcohol consumption in universities?

Practice Points

Societal Background

- There are high levels of alcohol in the UK population, with a particularly damaging pattern of drinking in 'binges'. Recent reductions in student alcohol consumption may reflect the larger proportion of female and overseas students now attending, and extreme alcohol use remains embedded in student culture.

- Since COVID and lockdown, male students, postgraduates and academic staff are likely to have increased their alcohol consumption.

Transition to University Life

- The initial transition to university marks a rise in alcohol intake, partly to reduce social anxiety and also to 'belong' to the prevailing culture. Information campaigns and paying lip service to disapproval does not work.
- The student age group tends to be less risk-averse than older groups. It falls to university authorities in partnership with the local community to control high-risk alcohol intake.

Sexual Health and Safety

- The risks of unwanted and unprotected sexual behaviours rise significantly when alcohol is taken. This should be factored into all campaigns around sexual assault and sexual safety on campus. Alcohol should not be seen as a mitigating factor in perpetrating any offence.

Suicide Prevention

- Death by suicide, as well as deliberate self-harming, are associated with alcohol use. Reduction in alcohol use is an important modifiable risk factor in the current need to address suicide rates.

Student Mental Health Services

- Mental disorders are strongly associated in a variety of complex interactions with alcohol use. Abstaining from alcohol may result in striking improvements in mental health as well as academic performance for vulnerable students. Suddenly stopping after heavy drinking may require supervision and sometimes medication to prevent sudden withdrawal syndrome.
- In some cases, heavy alcohol use is associated with other substance misuse disorders, and with gambling and gaming to excess.

Rights of Students and Staff Who Do Not Use Alcohol

- The rights and well-being of non-drinkers need to be supported by the peer community as well as authorities. Projects are needed to develop welcome robust activities and entertainments that are alcohol free.
- It should be treated seriously as an offence to induce or force someone to drink.

University Authorities

- Clear alcohol policies should be in place for both staff and students. Such policies should outline consequences if a student or staff member uses alcohol during the working day, or engages in high-risk alcohol-associated behaviour on university premises. Policies should be linked to clear pathways to counselling and treatment alongside any disciplinary action and monitoring.

References

Alcohol Impact (2018). *Students and Alcohol National Survey: Research into higher education students' relationship with alcohol 2017-18*. NUS.

Bailey, J., Kalk, N. J., Andrews, R., et al. (2021). Alcohol and cocaine use prior to suspected suicide: Insights from toxicology. *Drug and Alcohol Review*, 40(7), 1195-1201.

BBC Newsbeat (2017, 25 October). *Uni rugby initiations 'totally unacceptable' says RFU*. BBC. www.bbc.com/news/newsbeat-41755960

Bewick, B. M., Mulhern, K. B., Barkham, M. & Hill, A. J. (2008). The feasibility and effectiveness of a web-based personalised feedback and social norms alcohol intervention in UK university students: A randomised control trial *Addictive Behaviors*, 33(9), 1192–8.

Bhattacharya, A. (2017). *Splitting the bill: Alcohol's impact on the economy*. London: Institute for Alcohol Studies.

Brooks, O. (2011). 'Guys! Stop Doing It!': Young women's adoption and rejection of safety advice when socializing in bars, pubs and clubs. *The British Journal of Criminology*, 51, 635–51. https://doi.org/10.1093/bjc/azr011

Brown, R. & Murphy, S. (2020). Alcohol and social connectedness for new residential university students: Implications for alcohol harm reduction. *Journal of Further and Higher Education*, 44(2), 216–30. https://doi.org/10.1080/0309877X.2018.1527024

Busby, E. (2019, 23 September) *Universities urged to help prevent deaths from binge-drinking as Freshers' Week begins*. Independent. www.independent.co.uk/news/education/education-news/university-freshers-week-alcohol-deaths-binge-drinking-ed-farmer-health-warning-a9114046.html *accessed 31/10/2021*

Carline, A., Gunby, C. & Taylor, S. (2018). Too drunk to consent? Exploring the contestations and disruptions in male-focused sexual violence prevention interventions. *Social & Legal Studies*, 27(3), 299–322.

Carr, E., Davis, K., Bergin-Cartwright, G., et al. (2022). Mental health among UK university staff and postgraduate students in the early stages of the COVID-19 pandemic. *Occupational & Environmental Medicine*, 79(4), 259–67. https://doi.org/10.1136/oemed-2021-107667

Elgàn, T. H., Durbeej, N. & Gripenberg, J. (2019). Breath alcohol concentration, hazardous drinking and preloading among Swedish university students. *Nordic Studies on Alcohol and Drugs*, 36(5), 430–41. https://doi.org/10.1177/1455072519863545

Evans, S., Alkan, E., Bhangoo, J. K., Tenenbaum, H. & Ng-Knight, T. (2021). Effects of the COVID-19 lockdown on mental health, wellbeing, sleep, and alcohol use in a UK student sample. *Psychiatry Research*, 298, 113819.

Gavurova, B., Ivankova, V. & Rigelsky, M. (2020). Relationships between perceived stress, depression and alcohol use disorders in university students during the COVID-19 pandemic: A socio-economic dimension. *International Journal of Environmental Research and Public Health*, 17(23), 8853.

Goldstein, A. L., Barnett, N. P., Pedlow, C. T. & Murphy, J. G. (2007). Drinking in conjunction with sexual experiences among at-risk college student drinkers. *Journal of Studies on Alcohol and Drugs*, 68(5), 697–705.

Kalk, N. J., Kelleher, M. J., Curtis, V. & Morley, K. I. (2019). Addressing substance misuse: A missed opportunity in suicide prevention. *Addiction*, 114, 387–8. https://doi.org/10.1111/add.14463

Kenney, S. R., DiGuiseppi, G. T., Meisel, M. K., Balestrieri, S. G. & Barnett, N. P. (2018). Poor mental health, peer drinking norms, and alcohol risk in a social network of first-year college students. *Addictive Behaviors*, 84, 151–9. https://doi.org/10.1016/j.addbeh.2018.04.012

Larimer, M. E. & Cronce, J. M. (2007). Identification, prevention, and treatment revisited: Individual-focused college drinking prevention strategies 1999–2006. *Addictive Behaviors*, 32(11), 2439–68.

Lechner, W. V., Laurene, K. R., Patel, S., Anderson, M., Grega, C. & Kenne, D. R. (2020). Changes in alcohol use as a function of psychological distress and social support following COVID-19 related university closings. *Addictive Behaviors*, 110, 106527.

Leffingwell, T. R., Neumann, C. A., Leedy, M. J. & Babitzke, A. C. (2007). Defensively biased responding to risk information among alcohol-using college students. *Addictive Behaviors*, 32(1), 158–65.

Lynch, W. J., Maciejewski, P. K., & Potenza, M. N. (2004). Psychiatric correlates of gambling in adolescents and young adults grouped by age at gambling onset. *Archives of General Psychiatry*, 61(11), 1116–22.

McCauley, L., Ruggiero, K. J., Resnick, H. S., Conoscenti, L. M. & Kilpatrick, D. G. (2009). Forcible, drug-facilitated, and incapacitated rape in relation to substance use problems: Results from a national sample of college women. *Addictive Behaviors*, 34, 458–62.

Ng Fat, L., Shelton, N. & Cable, N. (2018). Investigating the growing trend of non-drinking among young people; analysis of repeated cross-sectional surveys in England 2005–2015. *BMC Public Health*, 18(1), 1–10.

Norman, P., Cameron, D., Epton, T., et al. (2018). A randomised controlled trial of a brief online intervention to reduce alcohol consumption in new university students: Combining self-affirmation, theory of planned behaviour messages, and implementation intentions. *British Journal of Health Psychology*, 23, 108–27. https://doi.org/10.1111/bjhp.12277

Orme, J. & Coghill, N. (2014). Wasted potential: The role of higher education institutions in supporting safe, sensible and social drinking among students. *Health Education Journal*, 73(2), 192–200.

Presley, C. A., Meilman, P. W., Cashin, J. R. & Lyerla, R. (1996). *Alcohol and drugs on American college campuses: Use, consequences, and perceptions of the campus environment: Volume III: 1991–1993.* Carbondale, IL: Southern Illinois University.

Quigg, Z., Hughes, K. & Bellis, M. A. (2013). Student drinking patterns and blood alcohol concentration on commercially organised pub crawls in the UK. *Addictive Behaviors*, 38(12), 2924–9.

Rollnick, S. & Miller, W. R. (1995). What is motivational interviewing? *Behavioural and Cognitive Psychotherapy*, 23(4), 325–34.

Stanley, N., Mallon, S., Bell, J. & Manthorpe, J. (2009). Trapped in transition: Findings from a UK study of student suicide. *British Journal of Guidance & Counselling*, 37(4), 419–33.

Testa, M., Parks, K. A., Hoffman, J. H., Crane, C. A., Leonard, K. E. & Shyhalla, K. (2015). Do drinking episodes contribute to sexual aggression perpetration in college men? *Journal of Studies on Alcohol and Drugs*, 76(4), 507–15.

Thombs, D. L., Olds, R. S., Bondy, S. J., Winchell, J., Baliunas, D. & Rehm, J. (2009). Undergraduate drinking and academic performance: A prospective investigation with objective measures. *Journal of Studies of Alcohol & Drugs*, 70(5), 776–85. https://doi.org/10.15288/jsad.2009.70.776

Wechsler, H., Lee, J. E., Kuo, M. & Lee, H. (2000). College binge drinking in the 1990s: A continuing problem. Results of the Harvard School of Public Health 1999 College Alcohol Study. *Journal of American College Health*, 48(5), 199–210.

Wolfson, M., Champion, H., McCoy, T. P., et al. (2012). Impact of a randomized campus/community trial to prevent high-risk drinking among college students. *Alcoholism: Clinical and Experimental Research*, 36(10), 1767–78.

Substance Misuse

Different Concepts of 'Drug', 'Substance Misuse' and 'Addictions'

The drug culture within universities is somewhat different from, and more intense than, that seen in a similar age group of non-students. It is different again from the particular population of patients with addictions and substance misuse problems seen in most psychiatric clinics. Complex and diverse motivations drive behaviour, and the youth and vulnerability of students on a campus make them ready prey for people wanting to sell drugs, as well as curious and intelligent experimenters in the field of their own brain chemistry. Student union policies do not always match those of the authorities, making it hard to work together. Yet again there is a balance to be struck between the rights, risks and responsibilities involved, and little in the way of easy answers in a field that changes by the year. There are no clear answers. We are even struggling to define the potential problems, and to get a sense of scale. However, there is an all-too-common feeling that nothing can be done, so it is important to outline some options and choices.

We need to find a shared stance somewhere between rigid disapproval and avoidant complacency. Academic research can be helpful (though it is all too scarce) since media articles rely on emotive flavouring to attract attention. It is important that the scientific examination of facts and consequences should include consideration of emotional, behavioural and social as well as physical aspects.

This chapter considers the scale and consequences of student drug use, and the different ways individuals within UK universities interact with mind-altering chemical substances – often thought of as 'drugs'. Other chapters will of course discuss the role of prescribed psychoactive medications (such as so-called antidepressants), which are taken under medical supervision, whilst alcohol is considered in Chapter 6. Within psychiatry, behaviours such as gambling have been classified under the concept of 'addictive behaviours', and certain patterns of online behaviour such as shopping and gaming may also meet criteria for addictive problems. However, substance use or behaviour patterns do not have to meet criteria for 'addiction' in order to harm people.

Substances Commonly Used in Universities

DRUGS TAKEN SPECIFICALLY FOR THE EXPERIENCE THEY OFFER

Hard drugs: drugs that are commonly associated with addictive or dependent use (e.g., heroin, crack cocaine and methamphetamine).

New psychoactive drugs/ legal highs/emerging psychoactive substances/ novel psychoactive substances: narcotic or psychotropic drugs that are not controlled by

United Nations Conventions, but which may pose a public health threat comparable to that posed by controlled drugs. In such an unregulated market, names and chemical composition vary enormously. Some widely available examples include the stimulant mephedrone, and the synthetic cannabinoid 'spice'.

Prescription drugs: medicinal products that, under the UK Medicines Act 1968, are available only on prescription by a certified practitioner. These particularly include sedative and pain-relieving drugs.

Recreational drugs: drugs that are commonly associated with recreational use (e.g., cannabis, ecstasy, LSD and cocaine powder).

DRUGS TAKEN FOR OTHER SPECIFIC PURPOSES – People using these drugs rarely identify as drug users, and prevention and treatment need to address the motives for use.

Cognitive enhancers: usually drugs prescribed for attention deficit hyperactivity disorder or narcolepsy but taken by those without a diagnosis (e.g., methylphenidate and modafinil).

Image- and performance-enhancing drugs: drugs used to lose weight (e.g., laxatives and amphetamines), or to gain weight or increase physical performance (e.g., anabolic steroids).

There is no intention here of limiting the discussion to cases where individual students or staff meet criteria for 'addiction'. Our focus is on drugs that are acquired by the individual for self-medicating or recreational purposes. There is usually a financial cost involved. Acquiring the drugs is often through illegal or semi-legal channels, increasingly online. Quality control is at best uncertain. Long-term physical, especially neurological, risks are concerning. So are drug interactions with prescribed or other drugs or with alcohol. The substances we are discussing here range from 'legal highs' through cannabis – the most common of the substances used by students – to the illegal 'hard drugs' such as heroin, and related chemicals, which of course bring extra risks if injected. Drug use can bring students or staff into a criminal underworld and may leave them with their own criminal record, or with the anxiety of being liable to one if discovered.

As clinicians, parents and directors of studies, we may have passed the age of familiarity with current street slang and attitudes. There are many nicknames given to 'street' drugs in their different forms. The poetic charm of the slang involved, the rituals connected with drug use and the whole online and real-life culture are part of the powerful attraction. For outsiders to the drug culture, it is mystifying, and some of us feel reluctant to confront a problem when we do not 'speak the language'. Professionals in specialist drug clinics probably do need to equip themselves with appropriate vocabulary and awareness of current trends, but there is little point in providing an attempt at a glossary here, as the prevailing names and trends change fast and vary across the country.

Motivations for Drug Use

One stereotype of student drug use is the idea of 'partying', in which young people seek the enjoyment of a chemically altered mind. Disinhibition is welcomed by the user and feared by authorities because of the potential for violence and aggression, including sexual aggression. This is very like the stereotype of the young binge-drinker, with the added thrills and threats of the transgressive nature of drugs. If we adopt this stereotype, the solution may appear to be a 'criminal justice' approach to drugs on campus, focussed on policing and regulation.

In contrast, 'self-medicating' is a term recognising that people can use alcohol and other drugs to relieve painful states of mind, particularly anxiety. This stereotype leads to sympathy for individuals concerned and a wish to provide treatment for underlying distress and disorder.

Students themselves report various reasons for engaging in drug use. Among the 56% of respondents to the National Union of Students (NUS) Students' Drug Survey who reported engaging in drug use, 80% said they used drugs for recreational purposes, 39% used drugs to enhance their social interactions and 31% had done so to help deal with stress (Release & National Union of Students, 2018). Others cited reasons such as improving confidence and enhancing sex.

In practice, it is not always clear, even to the user, where the boundary is crossed between becoming intoxicated for the sheer pleasure of a mind-altered experience, and becoming intoxicated to relieve the experience of social anxiety at a party, for instance. Some substances build up physical or psychological dependence, so that what may have started a pleasure-seeking intoxication turns into a need to avoid the discomfort of withdrawal symptoms. Motivation partly depends on an individual's profile of vulnerability and strengths, but drug use is also highly influenced by the availability of the drug market and socially endorsed peer behaviours. Students' incredibly strong craving for 'belonging' recurs repeatedly in the pages of this book.

Amongst students and other academics, a different sort of self-medication occurs, too. Some substances are taken to improve concentration or stamina or wakefulness. Amphetamines and other drugs that are medically approved to treat attention deficit hyperactivity disorder (ADHD) and narcolepsy may be used by people without these diagnoses to try to improve exam performance or to stay up all night to meet assignment deadlines. People with eating disorders and other body-image disorders often access drugs that are purported to increase metabolism and cause weight loss, whereas athletes and bodybuilders may use potentially dangerous muscle-building substances, as well as strong painkillers to allow continuing exercise despite pain.

Students are of course vulnerable, like all of society, to become accidentally dependent on painkillers, from paracetamol for headaches and period pains, through to strong opiates for joint or other pains. Such problems are unlikely to respond to the sorts of campaigns, preventative projects and treatment services needed to target the acknowledged and substantial problems of culture-led substance misuse in UK universities.

Julia, a young lecturer, had smoked cannabis as an undergraduate, when it was offered socially. She had never bought supplies for herself or others, and merely accepted it as part of hospitality at social gatherings. She prided herself on her open-minded approach to student experimentation and was uncomfortable when older staff members showed serious concern about the student drug culture.

She was approached by a first-year student Anne, who asked her advice about a flatmate's involvement in using, and possibly selling cocaine. Julia felt out of her depth, and was reluctant to speak to her own peer group in case there was a knee jerk disciplinary response. She suggested the counselling service, although she knew Anne was not suffering from a mental disorder. The counsellors acknowledged Anne's realistic concern that her environment was unhealthy for her as a result of someone else's drug use. They redirected her to accommodation services who helped her find another flat.

This chapter does not address the conundrum of whether it is most helpful to consider problematic drug misuse as constituting a mental disorder in itself. Instead, it examines a group of observed behaviours that may arise from a variety of drivers, not all of them mental disorders, and not all from the same sort of mental disorder. Sometimes it is not the drug-using students themselves who present for help, as the story of Anne demonstrates. There can be no easy answers to management of problems that arise. University cultures that vary in their tolerance to drug use and in their implementation of legal and university rules. Staff and fellow students still have to work out how to protect individuals and limit damage as far as possible, whilst pushing for clarity and support from policymakers.

It is a dilemma here, as in so many situations, as to whether young students have the ability to exercise responsible individual choices on every occasion in which they are confronted with them. Schools and families are not particularly successful at protecting today's teenagers against drug use, but such protections as there are fall away suddenly in the transition to university. By this stage most preventative interventions rely heavily on prescribing enhanced individual responsibility rather than on changing the environment, or providing firm interpersonal support to restrain students from using drugs.

Legal Background and How This Relates to the UK University Context

British Law has oscillated between a criminal justice approach and a mental health approach to drug use for more than half a century. Government policies have consistently tended to rates of drug-related crime and drug deaths as the chief outcome measures. These are not necessarily the best measure of drug harm in our universities.

Until the 1960s the medical treatment of dependent drug misusers was a separate provision from the punishment of unregulated use and supply. The 1960s and 1970s saw increased recreational drug use, and the 1964 UK Drugs (Prevention of Misuse) Act introduced criminal penalties for both possession and intent to supply. The Misuse of Drugs Act 1971 introduced a tiered system of drug control, and special restrictions on prescribing controlled drugs. A network of specialist treatment clinics was introduced.

By the late 1980s, the Department of Health felt that HIV posed a greater threat to public health than drug misuse, and shifted to a harm reduction approach with needle exchanges and substitute prescribing. However, by the end of the century there was a move away from health driven policy towards addressing drug-related crime. The premise was that a minority of severe addicts were responsible for the majority of criminality, so the 2002 Drug Interventions Programme provided rapid treatment for offenders.

Over the present century there has been growing critique of maintenance prescribing and harm-reduction strategies, and renewed emphasis on abstinence-based recovery. The 2012 Health and Social Care Act made local authorities responsible for commissioning drug treatment, so resources are not ring fenced from the central UK government. Local authority decisions on treatment are made in the context of competing priorities.

According to a Home Office (2016) report, 18% of young people of age 16–24 had taken an taken an illegal drug or used a substance unlawfully in the past year; 9% in the past month. In the same age group, 5% were defined as frequent drug users (having taken an illegal drug or used a substance unlawfully more than once a month, on average, in the past year). Use of any class A drug was around 10-times higher among people who frequently visited nightclubs, pubs or bars at least four times in the past month.

A great many official documents and guidelines focus their concern on the criminal correlates of substance misuse, and especially on problems of drug supply in prisons and their contribution to criminal behaviour and reoffending. Areas of social deprivation and poor housing are also seen as particularly vulnerable to drug misuse. This narrow focus is even the case in the various guidelines and documents produced by the National Institute for Health and Care Excellence, although this body is part of health services rather than criminal justice or social care.

At face value the preoccupation with drug use in socially deprived settings might not seem applicable to the student population, but particularly at the time of COVID lockdown, many students have complained of poor housing, financial difficulties and being confined to an institution where drug trafficking is rife. And indeed, it does appear that university students, despite the many protective factors available to them, are more vulnerable to misuse of drugs than the same age group outside the university.

Current Situation and Trends of Drug Use in Students

In his very first week of university, Sam was approached outside the library with an offer of 'weed'. He also discovered that many dealers were also advertising on social media – Snapchat, Instagram and WhatsApp. It was as easy as ordering in a pizza, at any time of the day or night. And because of social media and online deliveries continuing throughout lockdown, the drugs economy was able to flourish despite the pandemic.

Over the past decade there has been increased awareness of and attention to drug use in universities. Bennett and Holloway (2014) remarked on the paucity of UK research in the field and complained that 'a review of the literature of campus-based drug prevention found only two examples of programs operating in the UK'. They reported that

> drug misuse on the university campus studied was widespread in terms of the types and patterns of drug misuse. The most troublesome findings concern the high levels of multiple drug use, the use of some of the most dangerous drugs (including crack and powder cocaine and heroin, as well as ketamine), and the list of recorded harms experienced as a result of drug misuse.

Their study demonstrated that university students reported higher rates of use for all 14 drug types than did young people in the general population.

In this sample, the 12-month prevalence rate was around one in five students. One in ten were multiple drug users. Since then, annual prevalence of illicit drug use among students has increased, with about a quarter of university students recently reporting drug use in the current academic year (Bennett & Holloway, 2019). Half obtained drugs solely from friends and associates and one-fifth obtained them solely from external dealers. A quarter used friends and associates as well as external markets. Over a third of the students who used drugs said that they had also supplied drugs. In many cases, 'supplying' drugs amounted in practice to sharing them or giving them away.

Release and National Union of Students (2018) found that 56% of the almost 3000 students surveyed had used drugs at some time, with 39% being current users.

Cannabis was the only drug reported as being taken regularly rather than on 'special occasions'. This suggests that drug use is common but perhaps not as frequent or extreme as we might fear. However, as with alcohol, when there is a growing population of 'moderate' but increasing consumption, the prevalence of severe and even fatal consequences grow too. Of those who used drugs, 14% had come into contact with the criminal justice system as a result of doing so.

Eva Crossan Jury, NUS vice president for Welfare, acknowledges the gravity of the problem. She says 'We are witnessing record-high deaths involving cocaine and MDMA/ecstasy, and it is incumbent on institutions to take steps to protect the health and well-being of students who use drugs', but she believes that a punitive approach may be doing more harm than good. Referring to the NUS report, she says 'The fact that at least 21 students were permanently excluded from their studies for simply possessing a drug, and one in four students caught with drugs for their own personal use were reported to the police, is archaic and harmful.'

When a student is caught in possession of a controlled drug, educational institutions adopt a range of disciplinary outcomes. Release sent freedom of information requests to 151 institutions to analyse drug policies of UK higher education institutions (Release & National Union of Students, 2018).

The most common formal disciplinary procedures for student drug possession were:

- formal warning
- temporary exclusion
- permanent expulsion
- reporting the student to the police
- eviction from student accommodation and
- referral to fitness to practise procedures.

Around half of the institutions identified 'no further action' as a possible outcome, indicating an informal resolution. Only 35% of the students surveyed as part of the same study said they were aware of their university's drug policy (Release & National Union of Students, 2018).

In the 2016–17 academic year, there were at least 2067 recorded incidents of student misconduct for possession of drugs. While many were resolved via a formal warning or another type of sanction, such as a fine, a quarter of these were reported to the police. There were 21 permanent exclusions from higher education for possessing a drug for personal use. The Times reported in 2018 that the number of UK students disciplined for drug use had risen by 42% over the previous 2 years (Gilligan et al., 2018).

Reports of disciplinary action linked to personal possession of drugs suggests attempts to eradicate drug use altogether in universities. At present there is little confidence that it is possible to achieve eradication, even within relatively circumscribed university communities. However, universities do not want to be seen to ignore grave dangers and student drug deaths.

There is a discrepancy between the way society treats the drug alcohol in contrast with other drugs. We do not criminalise alcohol use as such, but do endorse penalties for driving or working when intoxicated. Becoming willingly intoxicated may be seen as part of an irresponsible action rather than as an excuse for it. At present, penalties do focus more on the criminality of supplying illegal substances rather than on personal possession or use, but as we have seen, it can be hard to distinguish between these activities.

Access to Drugs

Researchers from London and Liverpool (Moyle et al., 2019) recently explored the use of social media and 'apps' to supply and access drugs. They conducted an international online survey of over 350 drug users, with average age 18 years. The study was not confined to UK students but is clearly relevant. More than three quarters said they regularly used Snapchat for buying drugs, and a fifth used Instagram. A wide range of substances was available, from cannabis, LSD and ecstasy, to prescription medicines such as opioids, benzodiazepines and 'smart drugs'.

Online drug dealing has been possible for decades, but such trading was limited to the 'dark web' and traded in cryptocurrencies like bitcoin. Its move to modern, pictorial social media sites provides implications of normality, safety and quality. Young people told the researchers that seeing photos and videos of the drugs on offer reassured them that the substances were legitimate. Many believed that the digital communication was all encrypted and therefore protected from law enforcement. However, this is not necessarily the case. It is likely that these deals will leave some sort of online footprint.

The salience of online drug availability and the gradual increase in the proportion of international students studying in UK universities combine, so that substance use in the UK reflects global trends, although the consequences and treatment opportunities will occur in the local context. The high geographical mobility of the student age group may also take them into cultures where attitudes to drug use are extremely different from those on a UK campus. When students and staff travel abroad on university schemes, they need to learn the cultural and legal climate of the other country. Drug laws and customs need to be particularly emphasised.

Harms and Disadvantages of Drug Use in Universities

Whilst the physical health risks of substance misuse are regularly cited as reasons for abstinence, there is little evidence that young students experience a helpful and restraining sense of concern when confronted with 'the facts'. The student age group tends to be physically strong and resilient, and nothing like as risk averse as their seniors.

Young people are not likely to refrain from drug use because of social disapproval by their elders. They are more likely to be motivated by the attitudes of their peers, and more concerned by difficulties in social function or lowered grades, although they may not make the connection between such problems and their drug use. Most of us are skilled in denial when it comes to behaviours that in the short-term feel good and only bring medium- or long-term harm. Drug testing is a controversial practice, but it has the advantage – like the use of breathalysers for alcohol – of linking the substance use immediately with a consequence such as an imposed penalty. Some organisations do carry out drug testing on members of their teams, but it is an unpopular notion with universities.

When Bennett and Holloway (2019) asked the students in their studies about adverse effects, they were mostly concerned by mental ill-effects:

> Cannabis was cited by students as causing: paranoia, panic attacks, anxiety, depression, insomnia, fainting, 'whitey' (feeling faint with whitening of the skin), nausea, flashbacks, psychosis, disorientation, loss of mobility, temporary blindness, lethargy and psychological addiction. The main effects associated with ecstasy use were similar to those described for cannabis and included: paranoia, panic attacks, anxiety, depression, insomnia, hallucinations,

and lethargy. Ketamine was reported as being associated with various harms including: loss of mobility, speech impediment, abdominal cramps, and unconsciousness. Cocaine use was reported as causing: addiction, depression, aggressiveness, memory loss, and vomiting. Mephedrone was associated with panic attacks and parts of the body turning blue.

Potential consequences of the different substances of abuse often show marked individual variations or differ according to the user's developmental stage. It is well-nigh impossible to conduct rigorous controlled scientific studies on humans. Most evidence is observational, relies greatly on self-report, and usually cannot tell whether substances were pure or adulterated.

Substance misuse, whether illicit drugs or alcohol, has particularly dominated thinking in Fitness to Practice concerns around medical, legal and education students. This is considered further in Chapter 19. The General Medical Council and similar codes of practice consider substance misuse to be a mental health concern, but at the same time adopt a disciplinary stance. Universities could host expert debate as to whether it is possible to integrate the two contrasting attitudes and provide examples of approaches that do justice to both viewpoints.

Drug Harms to Mental Health:

- Distress from physical damage, both acute (such as respiratory arrest) and longer-term (e.g., liver damage or blindness).
- Mental damage resulting from chemical effects on the brain and nervous system, acutely (e.g., seizures or psychosis) and longer-term (e.g., depression, memory damage or eventual dementia).
- Cognitive damage, adverse effects on studying and poor grades.
- Results of intoxicated behaviour and withdrawal (e.g., aggression, sexual disinhibition, suicidality and self-harm or becoming the victim of sexual abuse).
- Social and interpersonal damage (e.g., guilt and shame resulting from drug-driven behaviours, loss of focus on friendships when obtaining drugs is prioritised, road traffic accidents or injuries to self or others when intoxicated).
- Financial anxieties (e.g., turning to dealing, the sex industry, gambling and other unhealthy ways to get money for drugs).
- Reputational damage, trouble with the law as a result of drug use or associated criminal behaviour.
- Reputational and cultural damage to the university community (e.g., damage to the mental well-being of all students and staff, including abstainers, affected adversely by the effects of drug culture, especially within student accommodation and on campuses).

Perceived Benefits to the Use of Illegal or Non-Legal Substances in University Life

So far, the risk of damage from substance 'misuse' appears to logically outweigh benefit, perhaps even more than in the case of society's favourite drug, alcohol. Alcohol is at least quality controlled, regulated and available without criminal contact. However, students do not seem to be greatly deterred by the risks, and the institutional environments of campuses and halls, as well as online arrangements, facilitate dealing and use of substances rather more than does the outside community. Some student unions have even facilitated harm-reduction programmes to help students assess the quality and safety of drugs they have acquired, and describe attitudes towards more responsible use of substances that bring them closer to the way alcohol is managed. Members of student groups familiarise themselves with risks and first aid strategies and explicitly look out for each-others' safety.

In a world where medically prescribed drugs are the mainstay of treatment for most physical and mental disorders, and where cosmetic and aesthetic medicine and surgery are openly practised, it is becoming hard to maintain that mind altering chemicals should be reserved austerely for the treatment of intolerable mental pain, and only at the discretion of doctors. Some types of drug fall into the category of neither treatment for a diagnosed disorder, nor drugs of pure 'recreation'. Society has not worked out whether its objections to such use are based on concern for the risks to the person's health and safety, or on concerns that using such 'artificial' means to achieve goals constitutes 'cheating'.

The terms 'smart drugs', 'study drugs' and 'nootropics' refer to prescription drugs used to improve concentration, memory and mental stamina. methylphenidate, levoamphetamine/dextroamphetamine and modafinil are the most common. They are medically prescribed to treat disorders such as narcolepsy and ADHD. They have been commonly used on US campuses for a couple of decades and are increasingly seen here in the UK too. When 1000 University of Cambridge students were surveyed by the student newspaper *Varsity*, in 2009, 10% said they took 'medication without prescription to help work' (Lennard, 2009).

Seven years later, in 2016, the University of Oxford student newspaper *Cherwell* published a survey indicating that 15% of students said they took such drugs without prescription. A recent European study co-authored by Robert Dempsey of Staffordshire University (Helmer et al., 2016), found that the majority of university students believe it is normal to use such drugs to enhance academic performance. Such perceptions may be an exaggeration of the amount of such self-medicating, although the sense that it is so normal may become self-fulfilling in an environment where 'belonging' and matching behaviour to that of others feels more reassuring than cool assessment of risks and benefits.

Many children and young people are already prescribed such drugs as treatment for ADHD, without clear understanding of potential long-term harms and benefits. We are not yet sure whether the improved function conferred by the drugs will translate into healthier brains later in life, or whether the cost of short- to medium-term improvement may be damage to long-term brain health. We might argue that such risks should only be taken by young people who cannot live a reasonable quality of life without them. This does seem to be the prevailing argument from senior researchers and clinicians, and it is supported by UK law, but rarely effectively enforced. Ragan and colleagues argue that we should seriously debate the use of 'cognitive enhancers' not only in the light of the current climate, but because more specifically targeted interventions are already in development. These are not only drugs but gadgets such as electrical stimulators and computer gaming-style exercises (Ragan et al., 2013).

There is a parallel here with the use by athletes of performance-enhancing drugs. For many of us, the concern is overwhelmingly for the welfare of athletes, driven so compulsively to achieve that they willingly sacrifice their health for their sport. It is not illegal, though, to engage in extreme training that causes severe joint damage or injury, and we are only recently starting to recognise the physical and emotional abuse of young people that is sometimes perpetuated in the name of 'coaching'.

However, drug testing is ubiquitous in elite sport and athletics, not perhaps because it is seen as abuse of the body but because it represents 'cheating'. The use of performance-enhancing drugs in student sport and of body-building drugs in student gyms is as concerning as outside the university. Universities, though, have a range of controls and regulatory strategies they can bring to bear, and will increasingly need to do so to protect the reputation of the institution.

This concept of drugs representing a form of cheating also arises in the context of using drugs at exam times. Some UK institutions have considered drug testing to stem the rise of cognitive enhancement drugs being used by young people to improve their academic performance. Occasional use of stimulant drugs at exam times only might be considered to be cheating because it presents a picture of ability that the person cannot regularly replicate. However, some people are prescribed such drugs in all intellectually demanding situations. Many of us rely on large amounts of caffeine to get through a day's work. It is hard to see where boundaries should be drawn.

Long-term use of amphetamine-based and other 'smart drugs' may not be safe, even if medically sourced. Data from large population studies finds chronic use of stimulant drugs is associated with increased risk of Parkinson's disease and dementias in later life, and with increases in road traffic accidents and criminal convictions in the medium-term. The health risks that newer drugs could pose are still unclear, but using them without a prescription is illegal, and can lead to unwanted effects such as increased anxiety and heart rate, and even manic episodes and psychosis in predisposed people.

It is hardly surprising that academic institutions assume that 'education' about such drugs is the answer. Oxford was one of the first universities to introduce workshops about smart drugs. But providing information and education is not as powerful as we would like when the students are still young, vulnerable and desperate to belong to the prevailing norms. Such education and information might even facilitate acquisition of drugs and fire up curiosity.

UK-Wide Interventions to Prevent and Treat Drug Misuse

Much of the official UK guidance on prevention and management of substance misuse, overlooks the student population. I was unable to find any direct reference to university students in the National Institute for Health and Care Excellence guidance, despite its claim that

> This guideline covers targeted interventions to prevent misuse of drugs, including illegal drugs, 'legal highs' and prescription-only medicines. It aims to prevent or delay harmful use of drugs in children, young people and adults who are most likely to start using drugs or who are already experimenting or using drugs occasionally.

In 2017, Public Health England (Burkinshaw, et al., 2017) published a review of the international evidence on what can be expected of the drug treatment and recovery system. They found consistent evidence that providing needle exchanges and/or opioid substitution (prescribing methadone or buprenorphine) reduced HIV and hepatitis rates, and that specialist drug treatment services were associated with crime reduction. The good news was limited though. After 6 months of treatment for illicit opiate use, abstinence rates were substantially lower than those reported in research studies, and drug-related deaths in England were considerably higher than elsewhere in Europe.

Once more, this document failed to address the special case of the student population and emphasises the reduction of drug-related crime rather than the need to protect social and mental health. In theory, students belong to the age group at the highest risk of being both perpetrators of crime and victims of crime, but I have been unable to find statistics or studies that examine university students as perpetrators. Research into student welfare tacitly assumes that crime comes into universities from the outside community. There is an apparent taboo here. As a result, it is difficult to assess whether reduction of drug-associated crime is even a relevant concern in our universities.

Prevention and Treatment of Substance Misuse in UK Universities

Most universities do have a drug policy, stating that the use of drugs is prohibited on campus. This sets up yet another possibility for an adversarial, disciplinary approach. It is widely criticised by students themselves as unhelpful, and is not commonly invoked in the permissive drug culture that appears to have become normalised on university campuses. On the one hand, harsh policies and penalties do not work as well as more lenient but reliably enforced consequences. Disciplinary or police input fails to demonstrate concern for student welfare. On the other hand, failing to address the harms of substance misuse also fails to demonstrate concern either for students who suffer direct drug damage or those who are harmed by the consequences of the drug culture.

It is an enormous challenge to find effective ways to help students adjust their behaviour when they are exposed to multiple powerful influences – opportunities and incentives to use drugs, perceived norms, interaction with others, and their own personality traits. Current evidence from research in schools, colleges and universities suggests that prevention should focus on skills for healthy socialisation, nurturing and safe environments, realistic social norms, social skills, and impulse control strategies. Information provision is necessary but on its own such contributes little to changing behaviour.

Environmental prevention is a powerful tool for changing human behaviour by modifying its regulatory, physical, social and economic context. Social and other environmental cues and social norms, and their perception, are vital drivers of drug use – as of so much else. Changing the physical environment of nightlife in the university and surrounding neighbourhood may be part of the answer. Ironically, many campuses have seen considerable success in eradicating cigarette smoking but continue to witness increasing illegal and non-legal drug use.

In the wider community, both preventative and treatment strategies for addressing substance misuse engage the support of partners or parents in supporting abstinence or reduced consumption (Simon & Burkhart, 2021). Since most students move to live away from home where they have not deep trusting relationships close at hand, there is an obvious gap in potential support.

Universities are reluctant to engage in more rule setting. There are risks that polarised attitudes to drug taking could lead to splits in staff-student relationships. These can damage mutual respect and the growth of maturity. Institutions characteristically reject attitudes that smack of 'paternalism', both out of genuine, liberal respect and also out of horror at the implications of acknowledging higher levels of responsibility for student welfare.

At one extreme, the University of Buckingham controversially introduced contracts for students to sign up to not using drugs, bringing sniffer dogs on campus and even into students' rooms. Others, like Lancaster University, have focussed on 'ensuring the integrity of the examination process' and considered drug testing around exams to discourage 'cheating'.

In contrast, many student unions have offered 'harm reduction' approaches such as provision of kits to test drug purity and advice on first aid for intoxicated fellow students. In 2015, Newcastle University lifted their zero-tolerance ban on campus drugs. Their campus offered a service of testing drugs to identify their nature and purity levels and 'amnesty' from legal action for anyone seeking healthcare input.

In the years that followed, the students' union at The University of Manchester introduced a £2.50 drug testing service and the University of Birmingham provided students with drug education and access to free drug testing kits. The University of Sheffield students' union provides advice on harm reduction, such as how to take safe dosages and how much water to drink. Unions in some institutions collaborate with the charity 'The Loop', which offers drug purity testing at music festivals and other large-scale leisure events.

There would be potential advantages to monitoring the whole range of approaches, at least until such time as research data demonstrates the superiority of one or other in terms of outcomes. In theory, at least, different groups of students would benefit from the different solutions offered. Some might move on from 'harm reduction' to abstinence that would be best supported on a drug free campus or within a drug-free, alcohol-free hall of residence. Performance-enhancing and 'smart drugs' may represent a somewhat different phenomenon, requiring different boundary-setting.

Since the turn of the millennium, traditional fear-based approaches of health promotion have been found to be largely ineffective and have gradually given way to motivation-based approaches and more recently the 'social norms' approach to health promotion (McAlaney et al., 2011). The social norms approach recognises that people tend to overestimate how much their peers take drugs and consume alcohol. These perceptions lead them to consume more than they would if they had more realistic perceptions. In the end there is a self-fulfilling spiral as rates of drug use increase. The media perpetuate these overestimates as they are more 'newsworthy', particularly when accompanied by shocking anecdotes. The aim of the social norms method is to use media campaigns and personal feedback to explicitly correct such misperceptions. The work started in the United States but some studies (e.g., Degenhardt et al., 2018) have generalised the model to European and Australian contexts.

So far, we have struggled, in the UK, to find effective interventions for prevention of substance misuse. Schools and universities most commonly use drug education and awareness approaches. These have fared poorly in evaluations. The 'Study Safely' project for students in London, based on a harm-minimisation approach, produced no significant behavioural change (Polymerou, 2007). A joint initiative between the UK Home Office and the Department of Health provided a pack to inform student welfare officers about drugs, alcohol and sexual health, and how to raise awareness among students. This was similarly ineffective (Polymerou, 2007).

In contrast, an early study of brief face-to-face motivational interviewing (described in Chapter 6) found that students assigned to receive motivational interviewing had lower rates of reported drug consumption at the 3-month follow-up compared with the comparison group (Larimer, 2007).

The MyUSE project (Dick et al., 2020), is currently being trialled. The study design explicitly addresses disappointment with previous interventions and identifies weaknesses that need to be tackled. It acknowledges that student support services are limited in their capacity to deliver face-to-face interventions to large numbers, and proposes the use of digital interventions. However, it plans to improve on mere information-based interventions by adopting effective behaviour-change models.

The ambivalence of drug-using students about help-seeking is acknowledged, as in classic motivational enhancement approaches. This study takes the model further by intensive collaboration with students themselves. Students are not only part of the original design but also involved in repeatedly testing, reviewing and monitoring its effectiveness.

Resources for People Seeking Help with Substance Misuse

FRANK is a government-run support service that provides information about drugs, plus advice for people who use drugs, and their parents or carers.
Call the Frank helpline: 0300 123 66 00
Release www.release.org.uk/offers free, confidential advice on drugs law for people who use drugs, and their families.
Email: ask@release.org.uk or call the helpline: 020 7324 2989.
SMART https://smartcjs.org.uk/ free advice
Email supportservices@smartcjs.org.uk
Addaction – mental health, drug and alcohol charity

Organisations for People Living with a Person Who Uses Drugs:

Adfam has local support groups and information online for families affected by drugs and alcohol.
DrugFAM offers phone and email support to people affected by other people's drug or alcohol misuse.
Email: office@drugfam.co.uk or call the helpline: 0300 888 3853.
Families Anonymous http://famanon.org.uk/ is based on the same principles as Alcoholics Anonymous. It runs local support groups for the family and friends of people with a drug problem.
Email: office@famanon.org.uk or call the helpline: 0207 4984 680.

Practice Points

At a Societal Level

- We still need clarity as to whether society is pursuing eradication of non-medicinal drugs or accepting them into society with safer arrangements for their consumption.
- Lessons can be learned both from the benefits and challenges of the UK smoking 'ban' and from the history of 'prohibition'.
- In the case of alcohol, the 'tip of the iceberg' of problem drinkers grows when the 'iceberg' of all drinkers grows or increases average consumption. This is likely to be

the case for other drugs. Widescale reduction is likely to benefit the most severely affected.

- Drug use prevention, treatment interventions and real life intervention all need more rigorous research to discover what works and what does not.
- Legal, medical and other agencies considering drug use need to appreciate that the student population is a particularly vulnerable group.

At the Level of University Authorities and Policies

- Regulations about drug use should be reviewed regularly. There are different motivations for the different categories of substance use on campus. Each may need its own approach.
- Provide a graded and varied range of options for student drug misuse. Both disciplinary and therapeutic input may be considered, perhaps in parallel. Interventions short of expulsion should be carefully monitored by an appropriate person to whom the student is accountable.
- Drug-related crime, child protection issues and vulnerable adult issues may need to be considered and referred for police and social work input on their own merits.
- Students, academic and non-teaching staff, leaders and management should all have a say in establishing and reviewing policy.
- Universities are ideally placed to conduct research on the potential harms and benefits of drug use and into treatments and interventions. This can unify the university community in a common quest for knowledge and well-being.

School-Leavers, Parents and School Teachers Advising Senior Pupils on Transition to University

- Substance misuse is already widespread in schools and needs to be addressed there.
- the greater freedoms and vulnerabilities of leaving home make university undergraduates particularly vulnerable to starting or increasing substance misuse.
- Students and their supporters can influence the culture by asking in advance about university policies, including those around substance misuse.
- Whilst medication is often prescribed helpfully for children and young people with ADHD, it carries risks, both known and unknown. It should not be too readily prescribed, and should be monitored and reviewed.
- Students who already take prescription medication are at greater risk of drug interactions, of having their medication misused, and of being unable to access early medical review unless this is set up in good time (see Chapters 2 and 3).

Teachers, Tutors, Directors of Studies and Fellow Students

- Try not to glamourise the drug culture, refrain from joking about it and discourage others from doing so too.
- Call out intoxicated behaviour and do not use it as an excuse for behaviour that would not be tolerated in a sober person.
- Encourage discussion and debate rather than merely provision of information.
- Individuals facing drug-related concerns can often access helpful advice from university counselling services and mental health advisors.

- Treatment options range from NHS and private clinics, charitable and third sector resources, and self-help support groups. Staff should prepare a list of useful online resources as a first-aid response for students with concerns, whilst further support is organised.
- Confidential group-based support such as that provided by 12-step groups may provide particular advantages for students living away from home, particularly those who are socially isolated.
- It is important to provide compassionate help for students struggling with substance misuse problems.
- It is dangerous and unhealthy to allow a culture of heavy drug use and associated behaviours in student accommodation and on campus. All members of a university need to actively consider where the line is drawn and who they can consult when there are problems.

References

Bennett, T. H. & Holloway, K. R. (2014). Drug misuse among university students in the UK: Implications for prevention. *Substance Use & Misuse*, 49(4), 448–55. https://doi .org/10.3109/10826084.2013.846378

Bennett, T. H. & Holloway, K. R. (2019). How do students source and supply drugs? Characteristics of the University Illegal Drug Trade. *Substance Use & Misuse*, 54(9), 1530–40. https://doi.org/10.1080/10826084 .2019.1590415

Degenhardt, L., Glantz, M., Bharat, C., et al. (2018). The impact of cohort substance use upon likelihood of transitioning through stages of alcohol and cannabis use and use disorder: Findings from the Australian National Survey on Mental Health and Wellbeing. *Drug & Alcohol Review*, 37(4), 546–56. https://doi.org/10.1111/dar .12679

Dick, S., Vasiliou, V. S., Davoren, M. P., et al. (2020). A digital substance-use harm reduction intervention for students in higher education (MyUSE): Protocol for project development. *JMIR Research Protocols*, 9(8), e17829. https://doi.org/10 .2196/17829

Gilligan, A., Griffiths, S. & Stokel-Walker, C. (2018, 29 April). *Universities failing students on drugs as punishments soar*. The Sunday Times. www.thetimes.co.uk/article/ universities-failing-students-on-drugs-as-punishments-soar-kkxnjm9k7

Helmer, S. M., Pischke, C. R., Vriesacker, B., et al. (2016). Personal and perceived peer use and attitudes towards the use of nonmedical prescription stimulants to improve academic performance among university students in seven European countries. *Drug & Alcohol Dependence*, 168, 128–34.

Home Office (2016). *Drug misuse: Findings from the 2015/16 crime survey for England and Wales*. www.gov.uk/government/ statistics/drug-misuse-findings-from-the-2015-to-2016-csew

Larimer, M. E. & Cronce, J. M. (2007). Identification, prevention, and treatment revisited: Individual-focused college drinking prevention strategies 1999–2006. *Addictive Behaviors*, 32(11), 2439–68.

Lennard, N. (2009, 6 March). *One in Ten Takes Drugs to Study*. Varsity Student Newspaper. www.varsity.co.uk/news/1307

McAlaney, J., Bewick, B. & Hughes, C. (2011). The international development of the 'Social Norms' approach to drug education and prevention. *Drugs: Education, Prevention and Policy*, 18(2), 81–9, https:// doi.org/10.3109/09687631003610977

Moyle, L., Childs, A., Coomber, R. & Barratt, M. J. (2019). #Drugsforsale: An exploration of the use of social media and encrypted messaging apps to supply and access drugs. *International Journal of Drug Policy*, 63, 101–10.

National Institute for Health and Care Excellence (2017). *Drug misuse prevention: Targeted interventions.* National Institute for Health and Care Excellence. www.nice.org.uk/guidance/ng64

Burkinshaw, P., Knight, J., Anders, P., et al. (2017) *An evidence review of the outcomes that can be expected of drug misuse treatment in England.* London: Public Health England. https://assets.publishing.service.gov.uk/government/uploads/system/uploads/attachment_data/file/586111/PHE_Evidence_review_of_drug_treatment_outcomes.pdf

Ragan, C. I., Bard, I. & Singh, I. (2013). What should we do about student use of cognitive enhancers? An analysis of current evidence. *Neuropharmacology*, 64, 588–95.

Polymerou, A. (2007). *Alcohol and drug prevention in colleges and universities: A review of the literature.* Mentor UK.

Release & National Union of Students (2018). *Taking the hit: Student drug use and how institutions respond in the UK.* London: National Union of Students. www.release.org.uk/publications/taking-hit-student-drug-use-and-how-institutions-respond

Simon R. & Burkhart G. (2021). Prevention strategies. In: el-Guebaly N., Carrà G., Galanter M. & Baldacchino A. M. (eds) *Textbook of Addiction Treatment.* Cham: Springer. https://doi.org/10.1007/978-3-030-36391-8_7

Chapter 8

Social (and Anti-social) Media
Are Universities in Competition with an Invisible 'Virtual' Curriculum?

Every chapter in this book acknowledges how in recent decades – and particularly since smartphones came onto the UK market in 2007 – virtually every aspect of our lives, but disproportionately of students' lives, has moved online. The lockdown experience gave extra momentum to finding ways to communicate, administrate, teach and learn online, as well as to buying, selling and spending so much of our leisure there.

At least half the world's population uses social media, and in the West half of all young people spend more than 10 hours a day online. It has become essential for 'keeping up' socially – being informed about the events of our daily lives – as well as politically. We rely on its feedback for our self-esteem, validation, confidence and sense of belonging.

Much of the 'media wisdom' of the past can be directly translated for the digital age. For instance, experts' concerns about how content in media such as Instagram drive body-image obsession were already voiced in the 1970s in reference to glossy magazines and colour television. Beyond the content of what is communicated, though, there is evidence that 'the medium IS the message'. Just as the availability of writing and later of printing had profound changes on human society, virtual realities and virtual communications bring opportunities and risks for the human psyche.

The power of the Internet to seize and keep hold of our attention is not due only to the quality of media content. Articles, apps, adverts, pictures and videos that capture our attention, however briefly, are logged through clicks and scrolls, noticed through 'likes' and other reactions, shared online, and subsequently proliferate. Material that fails to gain attention is quickly drowned out – the survival of material depends entirely on its being attention-grabbing. Technology companies and advertiser have been accused of intentionally capitalising on this potentially addictive aspect of the Internet, at the cost of ethical considerations, in particular society's mental and physical health.

The 'permissive' approach of recent years has exposed dangers inherent in our immersion in online experience. It's no longer acceptable for institutions to leave their most vulnerable members to manage their own survival in the exploitative online environment. Young people have led the way in becoming 'digital natives' and are now maturing into adults who can guide the younger generations. Universities though, are often led and governed by an older generation who are less comfortable with digital media. It is important too, to remember that algorithms govern each individual's experience of being online. For example, a 60-year-old married, Indian, female professor of history is likely to experience a very different online world from that accessed by an 18-year-old, single, white, gay male student of nursing. Moreover, there is growing evidence (Firth et al., 2019) that whereas currently the cognitive stimulus and connectivity offered online is overall beneficial to older adults, effects on the developing brains of children and adolescents may on balance be more detrimental.

Growing Evidence of Harms

A naïve psychiatrist from the last century, time-travelling into today's world would see psychosis all around. People walk about in public apparently talking to themselves. Ideas and messages and voices are delivered directly into their heads, they have lost the structures of eating and sleeping when others around them eat and sleep, and they are sometimes out of touch with what their families and friends would see as 'reality'. We may smile, because we know the 'reasons' behind the illusion, but living online leads us to enact mental states that were traditionally recognised as hallmarks of mental illness. That should at least give us pause.

In fact, if we wanted to invent a device that could generate in ordinary people many of the features of a variety of mental illnesses, social media would fit the bill nicely. In its relentless 24/7 overactivity, inflated sense of possibility and opportunity, encouragement of over-spending and sexual disinhibition, the online environment provides a manic world. This is often followed by exhaustion, despair and amplification of the negative thoughts and images of depression. Elements of both addiction and obsessive–compulsive behaviour are fostered, whilst attention deficit towards the outside world is generated by the compelling nature of the online environment. Twitter breaks down discourse into the smallest possible chunks as if to accommodate the demands of shorter and shorter attention spans. Meanwhile, body-image dysphoria and eating disorders are generated by bombarding us with unrealistic and unrepresentative visual images of bodies, inviting and providing comparisons and scornful judgements. Compassion – for one's self and others – does not come easily to social media.

Students and patients repeatedly tell us that they take great comfort from belonging to groups of like-minded people, who share their painful experiences and sympathise with their ways of coping. This misses the problem that a group which normalises and colludes with dysfunctional ways of coping can be ultimately harmful even whilst bringing comfort. The healthy ideal would be a group which can sympathise with the hardship whilst seeking healthier ways to cope with anguish, and to rejoin the wider community without being isolated by mental pain. Social media and online groups are not able to discriminate between the two different dynamics, and risk trapping people in closed loops, where questioning and dissenting voices are systematically excluded.

Early Concerns

The first smart phones came on the market in 2007, bringing greater availability to the Internet and the added facility of 'apps'. Even before that, in 2005, Dr Gary Cooney and I examined the associations between mental ill health in young people and the time they spent online. We asked three groups of 16–25-year-olds about their online behaviour. One group was made up of senior students from a local high school and college, the second was made up of young people attending a psychiatric day hospital, and the third was a series of those presenting to the accident and emergency department after taking a deliberate overdose or self-harming in other deliberate ways.

The healthiest group – the young students – spent considerably less time online, whilst the most time online was reported by the deliberate self-harm (DSH) patients.

Many of these told us they had used social media as a platform for researching and enacting their DSH, and in some cases that it was people from their online community who then called an ambulance. Our findings were of course more nuanced than this stark summary. One teenager wrote movingly of the support he received over social media after a family bereavement, at a time when he couldn't bring himself to leave the house, but still felt comforted by friends. Another spoke of her horror when seeking help online for her depression, only to be confronted by pictures of self-inflicted wounds, but added that she had then discovered an online support group that helped her.

We were frustrated that at that time our peers seemed reluctant to countenance our concerns and argued strongly that the Internet was a powerful positive force in mental health. Over the following decade however, research demonstrated potential online risks to mental health as well as benefits. We were sufficiently concerned to suggest that it was time to explicitly include an 'internet history' within the standard psychiatric assessment (Cooney & Morris, 2009). We still find it helpful to ask explicit questions about what is happening to a person online. Whilst we now assume that people do live an online life in parallel with their 'real' life, we remain remarkably coy about sharing it with each other or enquiring about specifics. It is accorded almost more privacy than the physical body, which doctors at least expect to examine and scan. Some instinct seems to warn us that people do things online that it would be uncomfortable to discuss.

Growing Evidence of Internet Effects on Young People's Mental Health

A study of US adolescents (Twenge et al., 2017) examined two nationally representative surveys alongside statistics on suicide deaths, and depressive symptoms. Adolescents who spent more time on 'new media including social media and electronic devices such as smartphones' were more likely to report mental health issues, and adolescents who spent more time on non-screen activities (in-person social interaction, sports/exercise, homework, print media, and attending religious services) were less likely. Suicide rates increased between 2010 and 2015, especially among females.

Another US study – likewise based on the self-reports of young people themselves – found that 78% of young people said they check their mobile devices at least hourly and that 50% of teens felt they were 'addicted to them' (Common Sense Media, 2016).

Meanwhile in the UK, the 2017 UK Digital Study reported a marked increase in mental disorders and explicitly associated this with online behaviour. The Royal College of Psychiatrists invited a young woman 'influencer' to address their 2021 Annual Congress, to give an insider view of the experience alongside those of psychiatric researchers and clinicians. Oenone Forbat, who has 135 000 followers on Instagram, told attendees that more than two thirds of these followers find that social media has a net negative effect on their mental health. They cited 'FOMO' (fear of missing out) and making comparisons with other people's lives and appearances as the most powerful factors in driving low mood and anxiety.

Social Media in the Time of COVID

Many academics and clinicians came to endorse the notion that life is healthier the less of it we spend online, and in particular the less of it we spend on social media sites.

However, at that point, the COVID pandemic and its associated series of lockdowns moved many activities online, normalised and familiarised all generations with technology and virtual reality. Amongst those most affected were university students living in halls. During the lockdown imposed by the pandemic they were denied the usual opportunities to socialise, exercise, explore real life sports and hobbies, attend live lectures, concerts, exhibitions and performances or even shop normally. Instead, they were thrown back on the unchosen company of hall-mates, they had to access classes online, and these were often mere recordings rather than interactive 'real-time' screening. Meanwhile, they were particularly vulnerable to the lure of social media.

> Students living in a university residence during COVID were expected to follow lockdown rules strictly, and were subject to consequences if rules were broken. One such consequence was being sent to do an hour's weeding in the gardens. Several students who were assigned this task returned to the gardens on a voluntary basis, and asked permission to do more work there. Eventually this became the basis of a gardening society.
>
> These students were amused to discover later that researchers found gardening to be one of the most mentally healthy activities during lockdown.

An early study from China confirmed our fears as to the results of lockdown social media use on students' mental health (Zhao & Zhou, 2020). In total, 512 Chinese college students participated in this 'snapshot' survey undertaken at the end of March 2020. The students completed measures of social media use, COVID-related stress, negative affect, secondary traumatic stress, depression, and anxiety. As expected, results indicated that greater social media use was associated with worse mental health. More exposure to news via social media was associated with even greater depression for participants who were vulnerable to 'disaster stress'.

As the pandemic has continued, further studies confirm that in all age groups and situations a worldwide 'infodemic' has damaged mental health. Isolation without the Internet may have felt almost intolerable in the past, but part of the cost of this convenience has been the widespread 'infodemic' we now experience. For students new to university accommodation such bombardment added to the torrent of social media feeds, course-related material and Zoom interactions at their fingertips.

The Enemy of Sleep

Activity on social media can be harmful not only in itself, but because it is an obstacle to other activities and behaviours that contribute more positively to our quality of life. Obviously, when we scroll 'mindlessly' we are not getting on with work or study, although taking some time out from effortful work is not necessarily a bad thing. Things are more serious when sedentary online activity replaces the experiences of fresh air, physical activity and socialising. People eat over their phones or laptops rather than in company, or they may not eat at formal times or at tables at all, risking malnutrition and obesity. As well as nutrition and the social benefits of mealtimes, sleep too may be lost the service of social media activity and online gaming.

The international nature of the Internet overrides time zone considerations. Students may have lost their circadian rhythms before they arrive at university. Not all households observe a structured day with regular communal mealtimes, expectations of timely attendance at school and some encouragement to switch lights out early on school nights, but many parents do provide some guidance, structure and example. Students may struggle to replicate these when they leave home. Not all university courses provided the discipline of daily morning lectures and checks on attendance, and for those that did, COVID restrictions took teaching online, so that it was usually available to be accessed at any hour the student might choose.

Much has been made of the sleep-opposing nature of 'blue light' from screens, but in practice the more powerful disruption is that online designers deliberately make sites so powerfully attractive that it is anxiety provoking to switch off. We feel a fear of missing something, whether in terms of achievement, bargains, opportunities, hearing 'news' or gossip, or even the fear of being discussed behind our backs. People describe scrolling through social media sites as 'soothing' because the level of stimulation is fairly undemanding and relieves the anxiety associated with switching off. It nevertheless stands in the way of sleep.

Once sleep is lost, or postponed, the body's circadian rhythms are disturbed, and the brain misses out on the optimal hormonal and chemical environment for digesting and filing the memories of the day. A study of 10 000 teenagers conducted jointly by University College London and Imperial College London confirmed that social media use before bedtime damages the quality of sleep, and having a phone in the bedroom overnight both disrupts sleep rhythms and reduces how long the young person sleeps (Kelly et al., 2018). The study found that more than half the participants slept with their phones in case they should get a call or message during the night. This expectation puts the brain on alert the whole time, rather like the experience of being a junior doctor on call, or a young parent who knows they will be woken in the night to feed a baby. These latter experiences are notorious times of stress and greater vulnerability to mental illness.

Research has borne out repeatedly that sleep deprivation damages mental health and academic and athletic performance. Individuals with a personal or family history of certain mental disorders are especially vulnerable to sleep deprivation, but none of us is immune to the damage.

Memory Issues

For the first time in history, the majority of us have access to almost all existing factual information quite literally at our fingertips. We can all quite easily access material that in the past was scattered in different libraries, and we can do so without the assistance of human librarians. We can then enter into online debates and discussions on an international basis. Depending on our preferred learning styles and available time, we can be taught interactively, sometimes even without fees, by a range of courses and teaching packages, and our learning can be stimulated and tracked in psychologically sophisticated ways. It could be argued that this makes the Internet a highly competitive rival to the institution of the traditional university. Why do students, families and governments continue to fund expensive places on traditional university courses, as well as paying for accommodation away from home? This has become a pressing question in the light of the COVID lockdown experience.

Leaving aside for the moment the question of the optimal time to physically leave home, and related questions of increased social autonomy and responsibility, we are now faced with new concerns about the different ways our brains acquire and assimilate learning in the context of online information repositories. There are implications for everyone, but particularly for children and young people, laying down deep memories that will remain available as reference points and scaffolds for future learning. Some emerging evidence indicates that disengaging from the 'real world' in favour of virtual settings may induce quite profound neurocognitive changes.

For instance, now that we can readily access information online, we are more likely to remember where the facts could be retrieved rather than the facts themselves. Our brains do quickly become reliant on the Internet for information retrieval (Sparrow et al., 2011). This is not the first time in history that our brains have changed with the advent of new technology. When humans first learned to read and write, it became possible to record history, accounts and other knowledge for future reference. It was no longer essential to memorise everything, or to employ specially gifted bards, scholars and other experts. Some academics are similarly optimistic rather than worried by the idea of relying on the Internet for factual memory storage. They believe this may actually free up cognitive resources from the grunt task of rote memorisation so that more ambitious creative thinking becomes possible.

Already, internet resources have facilitated large scale research projects that gather rich data far more conveniently than has ever been possible. Social media makes self-reported measurement and online behaviours deceptively easy to observe, but there are risks that such research will neglect nuances that are harder to capture online.

Attention Deficit by Design

Mobile phones have become the priority for our focus. McCoy (2016) examined students' use of phones and other digital devices in the classroom and found that more than a fifth of them admitted using their devices for activities unrelated to class. This is unsurprising considering that social media are driven by business goals. Algorithms have been designed using use random reinforcement schedules to hold attention, regardless of any collateral damage. Our attention is the most valuable commodity available to the owners of the sites and apps, as it translates into information and into money – the two leading forms of power in the modern world. Sean Parker, a founding president of Facebook described this goal frankly. He said, 'The thought process was: How do we consume as much of your time and conscious attention as possible?' Teachers and lecturers may ask students to switch off their phones during classes, but it may not be so easy for them to comply without practice. Switching off a smart phone can plunge young people into distracting levels of anxiety. Many will merely switch them to silent mode.

Even students who stick to using their phones to research aspects of the topic being studied are stressing their brains with such multi-tasking. Those who engage in frequent and extensive media multi-tasking in their day-to-day lives perform worse in a range of cognitive tasks. Even short-term engagement with an extensively hyperlinked online environment reduces attentional scope for quite some time after coming offline (Ophir et al., 2009).

The Californian company Dopamine Labs vaults its attention-grabbling techniques with pride. It uses 'behavioural economics' to change behaviour. This involves the use of psychological behavioural conditioning, hypothetically mediated by the brains' own dopamine reward pathways. Ramsay Brown, the company's 28-year-old co-founder describes the neurotransmitter dopamine as the 'sex, drugs and rock'n'roll molecule' and claims that it mediates these behavioural techniques. The company is proud of its ability to increase rates of adherence to programmes such as healthier diet, running and other exercise apps, and the learning of languages. Many of us can testify to their effectiveness. We might wonder whether university teachers could follow suit and use the same sorts of reinforcement in their own teaching. Most of us can approve to some extent of pro-educational use of behavioural economics. We worry when the same principles of enhanced adherence are applied to extremes, or to situations of dubious ethical value, such as gambling sites, shopping or political movements.

The term 'internet addiction' was originally coined in the last century but has not been adopted by any of the official, internationally recognised disease classifications. By now most of us would meet criteria, as society relies more and more on the Internet, and we are distressed when deprived of access. People may become compulsively trapped in different aspects of online activity. Problematic internet gaming is certainly well recognised, whilst compulsive gambling is a problem that has been amplified in its online form, just as health anxiety has become almost endemic since the advent of search engines like Google. Dysfunctional accessing of pornography is another phenomenon that has been hugely facilitated by the Internet, but does not depend on it in the sense that it can be termed 'internet addiction'.

When older studies conducted research into 'internet addiction' they were studying the phenomenon of young people with extreme online gaming habits. Zhou et al. (2011) reported that the brains of these young people showed significantly less grey matter, suggesting deficits in the brain's capacity for planning, decision-making, and impulse control. The changes could theoretically have been pre-existing deficits that made them susceptible to compulsive gaming, so the researchers conducted a randomised controlled trial. They found that 6 weeks of engaging in an online role-playing game were followed by significant reductions in grey matter within the orbitofrontal cortex – a brain region implicated in impulse control and decision making. We cannot necessarily say whether these findings are specific to online gaming, or reflect the consequences of other types of internet usage.

From a university viewpoint, it is important to notice that a group with similar demographic to our students is vulnerable to extreme dysfunctional behaviour associated with significant brain changes.

Drug Dealing on Apps and Social Media

Drug addiction and dependence, as well as culturally tolerated recreational drug use, have long been facilitated online. In the past, though, this involved accessing the 'dark web', and perhaps paying in crypto currencies. Only a minority of students would access this. More recently though, drugs of all sorts have been available not merely online but via attractive social media sites and apps, which resemble those students would use to buy fashion, electronics, groceries, books and holidays. They accept payment through credit cards and PayPal. The pictorial social media sites provide implications of normality, safety and quality. Just before the pandemic, researchers from London and Liverpool (Moyle, 2019) explored the use of social media and 'apps' to supply and access drugs. More than three quarters of their respondents regularly used Snapchat for buying drugs, a fifth used Instagram. The students were able to purchase a wide range of substances from cannabis, LSD and ecstasy, to prescription medicines such as opioids, benzodiazepines and 'smart drugs'. Many students wrongly assumed that the digital communication was all encrypted and therefore protected from law enforcement, whereas in fact it is likely that their deals will leave some sort of online footprint. Student drug use is discussed in more detail in Chapter 7.

Making purchases of drugs or any substance or service, entering into online gambling, or becoming involved in online investing and crypto currencies, all carry a heightened risk of a student's getting into financial difficulties. Financial distress is itself a powerful driver of mental ill health, and is discussed in more detail in Chapter 9.

Obsessive Compulsive Engagement with Online Sites

Obsessive–compulsive disorder (OCD) puts the patient in a state of constant doubt and fear. The fear – for instance a fear of contamination or other catastrophic harm to the self or others – causes avoidance and anxiety-relieving behaviours, such as cleaning, checking or seeking reassurance from others. The doubt means that any relief is short-lived, so that checking and other behaviours have to be repeated at ever shorter intervals.

Conscientious people tend have a degree of such behaviours, and many academics and professionals are strongly obsessional and perfectionistic. Like other mental conditions, OCD has advantages if it is not so intense as to be dysfunctional. Digital devices have certainly tuned into our obsessional nature, and their use can tip previously well-functioning people into frank disorder.

Smartphones have normalised widespread habitual 'checking' behaviours, characterised by quick but frequent inspections of the device for incoming information from news, social media, or personal contacts. These habits are thought to be the result of behavioural reinforcement from 'information rewards'. Effectively we are conditioned to keep checking, and even to increase checking.

On top of this habitual checking – almost a behavioural tic – many of us experience a compulsive need to immediately 'google' when we do not have information to hand. This is particularly the case when the information is about personal health and physical symptoms. The plethora of available sites, often conflicting in their advice, brings both immediate relief and increased doubt, and can powerfully increase health preoccupation and anxiety by mechanisms that were unavailable in the past, even to medics, healthcare workers and librarians. Beyond search engines, people may also turn to social media for reassurance, and are likely to join groups of similarly worried people. In the past it was medical students who notoriously believed they were suffering from whatever disease they were studying that week and became trapped in a vicious circle of focus on illness that robs a person of perspective. The focus on the feared catastrophe distracts them from getting on with healthy life tasks, and may ironically mask the presence of other risks that need to be addressed. One example is where people become so afraid of 'unhealthy' food that they restrict their diet to the point of malnutrition.

Students may be particularly at risk of obsessive health checking online when they first face the onset of physical symptoms as an independently living adult. Without parents to turn to, they use the Internet. The new challenge of working out what is pathological and what is within the normal range can lead some students to engage in obsessive online checking and even the purchase of unnecessary or harmful products. Testing kits, cures and remedies are a lucrative online business.

We should encourage students with health anxiety to understand that the behaviour is not a solution but a problem in its own right, and suggest they seek medical advice both about the physical symptoms and on the appropriate sources of information and support. They should share with their doctor the fact that they have a problem with obsessional health anxiety so that this too can be managed within the doctor–patient relationship.

Body Image Obsessions and Eating Disorders

Every year since 2009, Girlguiding has been polling more than a thousand girls up to age 21 for their Girls' Attitudes Survey. In 2021, 71% of their respondents said they experienced online harms, above all body confidence issues (Girlguiding, 2021).

The biggest worry was comparisons with other girls' bodies, especially how they looked in photographs and the number of 'likes' their photographs received. Psychologists believe that it has always been normal human social behaviour to make 'upward social comparisons'. This cognitive process can be hijacked, though, by the environment manufactured on social media, which showcases only the highly edited successes of people whose images have usually been digital manipulated for maximum physical attractiveness. Such drastically high levels for comparison would rarely be encountered in everyday life and would be balanced by encounters with ordinary and less attractive bodies. The more visually dominated social media such as Instagram and Snapchat are particularly powerful in leading to poor body image and negative self-concept.

Young women are particularly likely to conflate body image and self-worth. Followers of the influencer Oenone Forbat tell her that an insidious 'diet culture' permeates most media platforms, putting pressure on young women to lose weight. Pressures and advice can arrive unasked for within the social media site, then if someone starts actively looking online for ways to lose weight, they open floodgates to the torrent of advice from the diet and gym industries, personal monitoring gadgets, quack remedies, dangerous weight loss drugs, pro-anorexic advice and 'tips' and bizarre concepts like 'thinspiration' 'fitspiration'. 'thigh gaps' and the rest. Even the opposing jargon and images of the 'body positive' movement maintain the focus on bodily appearance, even if they glorify more diverse body shapes, abilities and colours.

Depressingly, research confirms that adolescents (particularly females), who spent more time on social media and smartphones have a greater prevalence of mental health problems, including depression, than those who spent more time on 'non-screen' activities. Those who spent more than 5 hours per day online had a 66% increased risk of suicide-related outcomes compared with those who spent only 1 hour or less (Twenge et al., 2017).

What can we do about this? In the past patients with severe eating disorders experienced considerable relief when their mobile phones were taken away on admission to hospital. Once mobile phones were again permitted in hospital wards, and became seen as a human right, we continued to ask some patients to surrender their devices for most of the day, with prescribed times for communication with family and friends. We also set up groups and one-to-one sessions for explicit discussion of how the phones were 'feeding' the disorder. Patients were encouraged to uninstall those apps and sites that increased the body checking and measurement, weight tracking, calorie counting, exercise monitoring and competitive comparisons with fellow patients. It was painful for them to do this, and they repeatedly relapsed into old habits, but when they could persist, it was remarkably effective in getting rid of the dictatorial anorexic thoughts. For young people who are vulnerable to an eating disorder, it is a good principle to minimise online time as much as possible and disable monitoring apps.

Socialising Online

It was striking from the Girlguiding surveys that whilst the girls themselves believed the biggest online harm was to their body confidence, their parents were largely unaware of this concern but feared their daughters being 'groomed' by sexually predatory older men. Indeed, more than 60% children admitted they had met in real life with someone they had initially met online without their parents knowing. Once young adults are away from home it becomes even easier to outwit parental protections. Any increase in their maturity may leave them still vulnerable to sexual exploitation.

In a remarkably short time, the proportion of social interaction that take place online within social networking sites has grown dramatically. Our connection with these sites is also meshed with the offline world. The etiquette of sexual behaviour in the modern university, and its relationship to mental health, is considered further in Chapter 12. Students typically see the goals of university life as not only achieving a course of study, a degree qualification and enhanced entry into the world of work, but also as forging life friendships and finding sexual partners. Like the rest of society, they go online to find friends and partners, and like us all they become somewhat confused by whether the same codes of behaviour cover what is posted online and what happens offline.

Social media posting shares with the world of television, film and music videos the phenomenon of presenting fantasies, fictions and narratives that would not be acceptable in 'real life'. However, it is only in social media and individual messaging on media platforms that the spectator can move into the role of participant. It appears to be tacitly accepted that young people exchange intimate pictures and engage in 'sexting', but there is little discussion of what constitutes indecency, where the boundaries of privacy lie, what constitutes trust, and whether it is even helpful in every case to try to separate out who is the 'abuser' and who is 'the abused'. The stereotype of a young woman student preyed upon by an older male abuser does of course exist, but there are also many cases where a sexually abusive culture is generated within an online group.

Firth et al. (2019) summarise the literature as showing that our brains process online and offline social networks in surprisingly similar ways, but comments that online social media is bending some of the rules – potentially at the expense of users. For instance, whereas real-world acceptance and rejection is often ambiguous and open to self-interpretation, social media platforms directly quantify our social success (or failure), by providing clear metrics in the form of "friends", "followers", and "likes" (or the potentially painful loss/absence of these). Given the addictive nature of this immediate, self-defining feedback, social media companies may even capitalise upon this to maximally engage users.'

Reputation and Shame

Shame is an experience that has potent links with anxiety, depression, OCD, trauma, eating disorders and the whole stigma of mental illness. Shame and fear of being shamed affect healthy people too, but the chronic experience of oneself or one's family or group as inherently bad and undesirable is damaging to healthy function.

> Javier, a young man with remarkable knowledge of the political situation, and a flair for communication, was already making a name for himself in campaigning for his local political party. He was delighted when a party official asked him to consider standing for parliament, but declined. No one of my generation, he said, will survive long as a politician. There is always too much in your past on social media that your enemies can use against you.

As children develop, the notion of a personal reputation that is respected by others grows too, together with fears of reputational damage. We have some sort of sense that each of us has a 'record' with medical, educational and civic authorities. By the time students reach university they are keen to actively protect that 'record'. These days, their social media footprint stands alongside official records, as a more or less ineradicable script of less formal behaviour and remarks. Not all students had the forethought or the parental protections to ensure maximum privacy settings. Messages, photographs and video recordings can be broadcast without the originators' or participants' permission. We do not so far have a recognised process by which someone can formally disown previous views they expressed or cancel aspects of their former behaviour.

In parallel with the endurance of evidence, there has sprung up a culture of directing condemnation and hatred towards a person rather than maintaining respect for the individual whilst opposing particular opinions or arguments. This stifles and impoverishes the quality of debate, as well as threatening human well-being.

As young students reach adulthood, they are more likely to be held personally to account for their online behaviour. Professional training now routinely incorporates advice about appropriate online behaviour for members of the professions, but students do not always understand how far different platforms link up or how much of their personal data and digital footprint can be traced back to them.

> Jeanne, a student teacher, booked herself into the university counselling service complaining of severe anxiety and panic attacks. It was only after 3 sessions that the therapist asked her 'What's going on for you online?' She told her counsellor that she was a sex worker. She had no regrets about doing this, loved being able to earn large sums for one evening's work, and was confident she was looking after her physical health and personal safety.
>
> She was increasingly anxious about potential damage to her reputation. She was terrified that her parents and family would find out and that it would prevent her from working as a teacher. She had used the Internet as part of her work, and was afraid the material could be traced, particularly if clients decided for whatever reason to breach her privacy.

Online Bullying

In my youth there was a fair chance that home was haven for those bullied at school, whilst children with an unhappy home life could regard school as a sanctuary. These days those involved carry the bullying around in their own mobile phones 24 hours a day, and fear to switch off even in bed. Cyber bullying is not always as clear cut as bullies on one side and victim on the other, although that can be the case. More often a dynamic is generated where individuals participate in unhealthy communications – competitive, cancelling, taking and giving offence, posting unwisely when intoxicated, over-aroused or disinhibited, saying things for effect rather than out of conviction and then shamed or condemned by the ineradicable nature of postings. People unwisely or innocently give their trust and then experience public online betrayal.

By the time they start university about half of all adolescents say they have bullied online, and a similar proportion admit they have engaged in cyberbullying (Peebles, 2014). It is unlikely that such behaviour stops when young people leave school or turn 18. Both bully and victim are negatively affected. The bullying may include publicly jeering at individuals or at their partners or families, making racist, gender-based or appearance-based comments, excluding them from groups, and public shaming by images as in 'revenge porn' and 'fat shaming'.

At a National Union of Students 'round table' in 2017 students described the unrelenting and addictive nature of social media, which they accessed on multiple devices. Students described being exposed to 'around-the-clock' harassment, bullying and trolling, including racism and Islamophobia. Social media exacerbated students' need to feel validated by others, and some believed it had increased the risks of hate crime, sexual violence and abusive relationships.

While extensive research had already examined cyber-bullying in school settings, Mishna et al. (2018) were among the first to formally report a high rate of cyberbullying in a university. Their exploratory study of 1350 Canadian students found 25% of respondents had a private video or photo shared without their permission and 28% were sent angry, vulgar, or intimating messages. Perpetrators were most likely to be a friend (50%), another student (20%) or an intimate partner (18%), and 20% of those who had experienced cyber bullying reported stress and anxiety.

At least one study has linked this sort of bullying online to DSH (Heerde & Hemphill, 2019). Social media and internet sites have contributed to the normalisation of DSH, and even of suicide, as if it were a logical, appropriate response to distress rather than a tragic but dysfunctional coping mechanism. There are sites and groups online, with an international reach, that imply DSH may be even desirable, so that it becomes competitive.

Students are on the whole more open minded than many of their elders in accepting mental illness without stigma. This can be a healthy attitude, but there is a real risk that social media could treat mental illness as 'cool'. Young people may then be encouraged to relate to each other in terms of their weaknesses more than their strengths. Exposure to DSH by others is known to increase the likelihood that others will behave in the same way, and photographs or videos are a particularly powerful form of exposure.

Analysis of children in the Avon Longitudinal Study of Parents and Children cohort (Mars et al., 2014) found that DSH starts around puberty, especially in girls, and is associated with increased risk of suicide and of depression and anxiety in the later teens and early twenties. There is a problem in assessing and managing DSH symptoms as teenagers turn 18. Schools and child and adolescent mental health services tend to see DSH behaviour as a focus for treatment in its own right, or to see it as part of a disorder of anxiety, depression or trauma. Adult services, though, are more likely to see DSH as a hallmark of a personality disorder, and seldom regard this as amenable to treatment. Fortunately, many people experience a maturing process that leaves them able to cope without DSH, but this maturing process could be blocked by continuing to access online groups and sites that actively or implicitly promote DSH.

Social Media and Suicide

When Molly Russell took her life in 2017 at the age of only 14, her family found graphic posts about suicide and self-harm on her Instagram account. Her family mobilised public demand for regulation of the Internet and a formal duty of care by tech companies. The Online Harms Bill is currently going through Parliament. The tragedy is all the more poignant because such a very young, vulnerable schoolgirl was harmed, but it would be a mistake to focus legislation too much on protection of children, when students do not suddenly become streetwise as they turn 18, and in fact experience a temporary increase in vulnerability and deterioration in mental health when they start university. The links between social media use and death by suicide are discussed further in Chapter 17.

We need to campaign for nuanced and effective regulation, which offers realistic protection to all vulnerable people, not only those who happen to be under 18 years old. At the same time, reviews and debates around the effects of such regulation on freedom of expression need to continue. Broad public regulation needs to be supplemented by local, institutional regulation and by personal self-regulation by individual students and scholars. There is a well-evidenced international youth awareness of mental health (YAM) programme, which can demonstrate reduced suicidal attempts and ideation as well as reduced rates of depression in participants. However so far it is only delivered in schools. Those fortunate enough to have accessed YAM might benefit from a 'refresher' course as they start university life, whilst for those who have not had the opportunity to participate in YAM, we need a version of the intervention that is specially modified for the university student setting. This would require trials to ensure that such a modification is effective. It is a particularly attractive feature of the programme that it improves other aspects of mental health as well as reducing suicidal ideation.

Doing More to Mitigate the Effects of Social Media on Mental Health in Universities

The experience of moving more of our lives online during lockdowns has made our virtual experiences more salient than before in all of our consciousness. There has been much more debate and acknowledgement of concern about social media and its effects on mental health, in families, in public, on radio and television, and of course online. University research departments have contributed evidence to inform these debates. In university governing bodies, though, the emphasis has been on protecting corporate reputations, with a disciplinarian perspective on using the Internet.

Most universities' websites acknowledge the existence of social media, but more in terms of reputational damage to the university rather than as a threat to the community's mental health. For instance, this is the statement from one establishment, though in practice similar wording can be found on most UK university websites:

> Inappropriate use of social media can be damaging to the reputation of the university as well as have a negative impact on students, staff and the wider community, so we have put together these guidelines to help you avoid this.

Advice is couched very much in terms of a list of 'don'ts'. It implies an individualistic approach to 'misconduct' rather than a thoughtful consideration of the broader effects of overreliance on virtual media for the mental health of whole communities and social groups. There are limits to what individuals can do by themselves. We might undertake a periodic 'digital detox', learn how to set up our own safeguarding filters and 'curate' our own feeds. This involves regularly and systematically deleting, blocking and 'unfollowing', so that for instance images of thin white young women do not automatically pop up all the time. It is hard though to change our relationship with social media without considerable negotiation with others.

In concert, families, friendship groups, classes and potentially whole institutions, could do much more. Some actions might include decisions about favouring certain less exploitative platforms over others, respecting 'device-free' hours or days, and agreeing to switch mobile phones off during mealtimes, bedtimes and class times.

There are organisations that facilitate this sort of planning. In February 2018, the US Center for Humane Technology launched a film, website and campaign, 'The Truth About Tech', to raise awareness of dangers of spending too much time on smart phones and tablets. The Center's founders formerly worked in big tech companies such as Google, Facebook and Twitter, so they are credible and persuasive. Enlightenment about the goals and mechanisms of Big Tech leads many of us to resolve to reduce time online. In practice, our initial individual enthusiasm wears thin. This movement, though, perpetuates the debate and offers resources for teachers, families and young people to stimulate action at all levels of society to create an online environment that is beneficial to core human values without relentlessly favouring money-making at whatever cost.

Virtual Mental Health Consultations and Therapy

As our colleagues predicted earlier this century, the Internet does have the potential to facilitate large scale, convenient, flexible and life-changing contributions to psychiatric and psychological treatment. There is great faith placed in the power of technology to rescue our young people from health problems. A recent Lancet review of young people's health acknowledged that 'Non-communicable diseases of adolescents including mental and substance use disorders, and chronic physical illnesses are becoming the dominant health problems of this age group' and said 'information and broadband technologies present an exceptional opportunity for building capacity within sectors and coordinating actions between them' (Patton et al., 2016). The paper provides very little discussion, though, of the harms attributable to adolescent use of the very technology it proposes as their saviour, claiming that 'the development of the new media has been so rapid that research efforts to understand their effects have failed to keep pace with their growing influence.'

Two years on from the start of lockdowns, clinicians and patients are making mostly positive observations about online interventions, although in the initial crisis, there was frustration around delays, regulatory obstacles and widespread reluctance to trust treatment to the small screen. Student counselling and psychotherapy services were effectively closed to many for a distressingly long time.

This is in contrast with optimistic predictions in research literature and even in research trials of technology-based psychological interventions. We have lagged in harnessing, in an ethical and transparent manner, those behavioural strategies used by the industry, using natural language processing, sentiment analyses and machine learning. Yet these elements could theoretically help patients and their carers to identify increased risk for suicide or relapse, for instance.

Ironically, the detailed data held on us as individuals by big tech companies is not mirrored by the detail found in our medical records. Yet meticulous online databases could provide students – geographically mobile, and across different care systems – with personalised health profiles. These could combine research evidence with the patient's personal physiology and experience to suggest the best available interventions. Virtual platforms might then be used to monitor – if not always to deliver – those interventions. We could help students look at the analyses of their own online behaviour (as well as other behaviours) in the light of their own reports of mood, anxiety and other symptoms. They could then observe how their behaviour was impacting their feelings, and the feedback would guide and reinforce their efforts in therapy.

Powerful techniques are now used in online behavioural psychology in social media and apps, and they are harming the mental health of our students. These same techniques, though, could be regulated, monitored and harnessed in the service of positive mental health. At the same time, strong evidence suggests that offline experiences are generally a healthier and richer option. This is likely to be true in the delivery of counselling and psychotherapy too.

> I saw Jinty online for a psychiatric assessment. She was anxious, slightly depressed, and provided a history of an eating disorder in her early teens, which she told me had completely resolved. She was studying for 14 hours a day and was academically successful. She volunteered at a charity shop at weekends, and sang in a rock choir. After three appointments I was at a loss as to how she could be experiencing the levels of anguish she described. Objectively I could find no formal psychiatric illness. Reluctantly we agreed on a trial of antidepressant medication. She came to the clinic in person to have her blood pressure checked and to collect a prescription.
>
> Even in masks and at a safe social distance, I realised within minutes that Jinty was very high on the autistic spectrum. A range of sensory cues only added up now that I could see Jinty in movement, interacting socially with a receptionist, walking from waiting room to office, selecting a seat, responding to the unexpected, rather than delivering her prepared account in front of a screen. There may be other senses – smell, body vibration, touch, personal space, rhythm of response in speech – that are muted or muffled in online communication.

The Internet can offer useful material, including mental health resources, but we need to ensure this is available to students when they need it and not lost like a needle in the haystack of information. Students may struggle to know what is safe and effective. They may come up with the impression that they will need to pay for private counselling, or may complete exercises on apps designed for people with entirely different needs. For example, anorexic patients often follow weight losing and physical exercise apps, whilst people with OCD find themselves trapped in relaxation or meditation rituals that are counterproductive for them though helpful to others. At present there is still too much outdated 'information' describing self-help peer groups and initiatives that no longer happen, perhaps because the energetic students who ran them have moved on. University intranets have a useful role in selecting up to date and helpful information, and may in future be able to provide each student with a personal 'dashboard' tailor-made in anticipating their needs.

Practice Points

At the Societal Level

- We are only just waking up to the relentless commercial interests driving our online interactions. Society needs to protect young brains in particular from exploitation and harm.
- Awareness and understanding are a crucial first step but not enough.
- Legal and institutional regulation is essential but may not occur without grass roots campaigning.
- There is still a generation gap in terms of expertise, being 'media smart'.

Schools and Families

- The school and family setting usually provides some protection and online safety education.
- This needs to be reinforced and revisited during the transition to university.
- Schools could have a useful role in sharing and developing evidence-based online education that could be adopted and adapted by university staff and unions.

At the Level of University Authorities and Policies

- Student use of social media is not only a potential threat to the reputation of the individual and the university but is currently damaging student well-being and academic performance.
- University websites and intranets can be valuable repositories of respected health information, signposting and self-help resources, but these need to be kept up to date.

Teachers, Tutors, Directors of Studies and Fellow Students

- Online teaching works best when it is part of a structured timetable, delivered and accessed in 'real time' when possible. Interaction with teachers and fellow students is a hallmark of a healthy university experience. Try to avoid online 'multitasking' by putting phones away during classes.
- The university community is healthier when outdoor, physically active, and real life social interactive experiences are prioritised.
- When you are concerned about someone's mental health or well-being, it is helpful to include a questions such as 'What's going on for you online?'
- Counsellors and other clinicians can usefully employ online therapy delivery to bridge gaps when students are away from the campus.

References

Common Sense Media (2016). *Dealing with devices: The parent-teen dynamic.* www.commonsensemedia.org/technology-addiction-concern-controversy-and-finding-balance-infographic

Cooney, G. M. & Morris, J. (2009). Time to start taking an internet history? *The British Journal of Psychiatry*, 194(2), 185.

Firth, J., Torous, J., Stubbs, B., et al. (2019). The "online brain": How the Internet may be changing our cognition. *World*

Psychiatry, 18(2), 119–29. https://doi.org/10.1002/wps.20617

Girlguiding (2021). *Girls attitudes survey.* www.girlguiding.org.uk/globalassets/docs-and-resources/research-and-campaigns/girls-attitudes-survey-2021-report.pdf

Heerde, J. A. & Hemphill, S. A. (2019). Are bullying perpetration and victimization associated with adolescent deliberate self-harm? A meta-analysis. *Archives of Suicide Research*, 23(3), 353–81.

Kelly, Y., Zilanawala, A., Booker, C. & Sacker, A. (2018). Social media use and adolescent mental health: Findings from the UK Millennium Cohort Study. *EClinicalMedicine*, 6, 59–68.

Mars, B., Heron, J., Crane, C., et al. (2014). Clinical and social outcomes of adolescent self harm: Population based birth cohort study. *BMJ*, 349, g5954.

McCoy, B. (2016). Digital distractions in the classroom: Student classroom use of digital devices for non-class related purposes. *Journal of Media Education*, 7(1), 5–32.

Mishna, F., Regehr, C., Lacombe-Duncan, A., et al. (2018). Social media, cyber-aggression, and student mental health on a university campus. *Journal of Mental Health*, 27(3), 222–9. https://doi.org/10.1080/09638237.2018.1437607

Moyle, L., Childs, A., Coomber, R. & Barratt, M. J. (2019). #Drugsforsale: An exploration of the use of social media and encrypted messaging apps to supply and access drugs, *International Journal of Drug Policy*, 63, 101–10.

Ophir, E., Nass, C. & Wagner, A. D. (2009). Cognitive control in media multitaskers. *Proceedings of the National Academy of Sciences*, 106(37), 15583–7.

Patton, G. C., Sawyer, S., Santelli, J. S., et al (2016) Our future: A Lancet commission on adolescent health and wellbeing *The Lancet.* 387(24), 23–78.

Peebles, E. (2014). Cyberbullying: Hiding behind the screen. *Paediatrics & Child Health*, 19(10), 527–8. https://doi.org/10.1093/pch/19.10.527

Sparrow, B., Liu, J. & Wegner, D. M. (2011). Google effects on memory: Cognitive consequences of having information at our fingertips. *Science*, 333, 776.

Twenge, J. M., Joiner, T. E., Rogers, M. L. & Martin, G. N. (2017). Increases in depressive symptoms, suicide-related outcomes, and suicide rates among U.S. adolescents after 2010 and links to increased new media screen time. *Clinical Psychological Science*, 6(1), 3–17. https://doi.org/10.1177/2167702617723376

Zhou, Y., Lin, F., Du, Y., et al. (2011). Gray matter abnormalities in Internet addiction: A voxel-based morphometry study. *European Journal of Radiology*, 79(1), 92–5.

Zhao, N. & Zhou, G. (2020). Social media use and mental health during the COVID-19 pandemic: Moderator role of disaster stressor and mediator role of negative affect. *Applied Psychology: Health & Well-Being*, 12, 1019–38. https://doi.org/10.1111/aphw.12226

Finance and Mental Health

A considerable body of evidence demonstrates that for people in general, financial stress is associated with worse physical, psychological and social well-being. The mechanisms may be direct – as consequences of poor nutrition or housing – or indirect – arising from the social implications of having little money. The converse is also true: poor health is likely to lead to impaired financial management.

On the shoulders of that body of literature demonstrating the psychosocial stresses and increased levels of mental illness associated with financial hardship in the community, research has turned more specifically to student debt. In 2008, Nelson et al. (2008) reported that students with high credit card debts were not only more likely to feel stressed but also to engage in more physical altercations, binge drinking, substance misuse and to be overweight. There are vicious cycles at work. 'Stress proliferation' occurs, with each stressor increasing the development of others.

As with so much research into mental health and student life, most studies come from the United States. In that higher education system students have long been expected to finance their own studies. State grants have been a particularly British phenomenon, and the upheavals of the shift to student loans are still felt. Some research has specifically focused on UK students. One meta-analysis found that 41.7% of those with a mental health disorder reported being in debt, compared with only 17.5% without (Richardson, 2013). Looking at it the other way round, 15.5% of students who had debts had a mental health disorder – almost double the 8.9% of those not in debt. The authors found a statistically significant relationship between debt and depression, suicide completion or attempt, problem drinking, drug dependence, neurotic disorders and psychotic disorders. Later, Richardson (2015) showed that financial difficulties in students increased the risk of students developing an eating disorder. Students experience vicious spirals as mental disorder and financial concerns interact over their university career.

Recent studies acknowledge the complexity of the situation. There is no linear relationship between actual size of debt, or financial poverty, and subsequent mental health consequences. Evidence suggests that the relationship between finances and mental health may be attributed to amount of stress about debt rather than actual debt (Richardson et al., 2017). Ross et al. (2006) found that Aberdeen medical students' healthy functioning is related to their perceptions of their own levels of debt rather than level of debt per se: 'Students who worry about money have higher debts and perform less well than their peers in degree examinations … and may have mental health problems.' Obviously this does not sanction leaving students in financial hardship, but does suggest that financial confidence and the ability to manage and tolerate inevitable debt are important factors in remaining mentally healthy at university.

Roberts et al. (2000) established that students 'who had considered abandoning study for financial reasons had poorer mental health, social functioning, vitality and physical health and were also heavier smokers'. Among students who were parents of young children 79% reported difficulty paying family bills. These authors were among the first to demonstrate that financial stress can bring UK students into contact with a criminal world. They found that 'being in debt was associated with knowing people involved in prostitution, crime or drug dealing to help support themselves financially'.

More recent research prefers to use validated measures of mental health problems rather than relying on self-report, and uses longitudinal designs to track the development over time of student confidence or distress in managing financial matters. Richardson et al.'s (2017) longitudinal study of UK first year students from a range of universities corroborated previous self-report studies that greater subjective stress about debt exacerbated anxiety, depression, stress, as well as global mental health over time. The literature suggests that the financial concerns are usually the primary factor in leading to poor student mental health, rather than poor mental health problems leading to financial deterioration. However, worsening mental health, alcohol and substance misuse amplify financial chaos, setting up those vicious spirals. Over the course of a year

> Greater financial difficulties predicted greater depression and stress cross-sectionally, and also predicted poorer anxiety, global mental health and alcohol dependence over time. Depression worsened over time for those who had considered abandoning studies or not coming to university for financial reasons, and there were effects for how students viewed their student loan. Anxiety and alcohol dependence also predicted worsening financial situation suggesting a bi-directional relationship. (Richardson et al., 2017)

Financial Changes in the Circumstances of UK Students

In the 1950s most UK local education authorities paid student tuition fees and provided grants to support students' living costs. The 1962 Education Act made it obligatory for local education authorities to do so. By the early 1980s there was still a minimum grant for all, but any extra depended on declared parental income, with no legal obligation on parents to make up the sum. The Student Loans Company was founded in 1990 to provide low interest loans to students to help make up living costs. The 1998 Teaching Higher Education Act introduced a student contribution of £1000 a year towards tuition costs. Maintenance grants were replaced by repayable student loans, and student contribution to tuition fees has gradually increased. Since 2016, postgraduate students are also entitled to student loans. Devolved governments in Scotland and Wales opted to pay for student tuition, but maintenance grants are largely replaced by loans across the UK.

Students may also take out private loans. Sometimes a university acts as a financial intermediary to 'certify' the loans; others are 'direct to consumer'. Such 'direct to consumer' loans involve an 'origination fee' and high and variable interest rates rather than the fixed rates of government loans. Where the student or their family has an excellent credit rating, the repayment terms are significantly better than where credit is poor. Students from poor backgrounds suffer disproportionately from the all-too-common delays in accessing government loans, and poorer universities may be less able to draw on their own wealth to provide bursaries and scholarships for students in need.

Meeting the Extra Costs of a Mental Disorder at University: DSA

Disabled Students' Allowances (DSAs) are Government funded allowances designed to ensure that students who have a longer-term health condition or 'disability' are not disadvantaged in accessing their university studies. When a student discloses their mental health disability to the university, this generally sets off the process of inviting them to apply for a DSA, but a student who later decides to request help or develops their disorder later on, may of course apply.

> The following website provides an estimate of whether the student is likely to be eligible for DSA
>
> www.surveymonkey.co.uk/r/HE-support-checker
>
> Guidance on the application process is available at
> https://diversityandability.com/dsa-find-your-way/

A DSA is not a loan and is not financially means tested. The amount received depends on individual needs. Students with longer-term mental health conditions as well as those with physical disabilities are eligible for DSAs. A formal specific psychiatric diagnosis is not required, but the student must provide evidence of meeting criteria for the mental health condition, such as a letter from a GP or psychiatrist. Dual or multiple diagnoses, including for instance autism, attention deficit hyperactivity disorder, visual or hearing impairments, dyslexia or epilepsy, are taken into account in deciding the level of allowance needed.

Graduate students as well as undergraduates are eligible, provided that their course is longer than 12 months. Distance learning courses are included. Whilst international students may not be formally eligible, some universities can help them to access equivalent funding. It is important for students to understand that there may be different funding streams they can be supported to access, and that they are not expected to undertake the application process unaided. It is an important part of the role of university mental health professionals to help steer students through the complicated pathways to help as well as delivering some of that help on campus.

For many students with mental health problems, the greatest benefit to receiving a DSA is being able to access one-to-one support from a specialist mental health mentor. This important role is mentioned in several chapters of this book and is described further in Chapter 18. Counselling and some other university services often have long waiting lists and limited, fairly short duration of contact with those services. Specialist mental health mentoring, on the other hand, provides regular, flexible long-term input from a qualified mental health professional, and usually from the same individual for the length of the university course.

Finance after Graduation

Many graduates describe loan repayment problems. It is not the Student Loans Company but the tax man who calculates and collects repayments. When overpayment has occurred, the money should be returned with interest, but bureaucratic delays are reported. The system is complex, with terms repeatedly changing depending on when the loan was taken out, and for some individuals the complications of having to repay several different loans. It is demanding of time and expertise for a young person to manage debts and responsibilities at the start of their working life, when few individuals can afford the services of a financial advisor.

> As a graduate who still has outstanding student debt, I find the name 'loan' or 'debt' problematic. Friends have experienced mental and financial anguish trying to repay the 'debt' early. If they had stuck to the standard repayments until retirement (when the remainder is written off) they would likely never have to repay the full amount.
>
> Changing the name to 'graduate tax' might not change the financial reality of regular payments, but I wonder if it could be psychologically beneficial.

In the United States, Walsemann et al. (2015) analysed 13 years of data from nearly 9000 adults, and found student loan debt was correlated with lower levels of psychological well-being for 25- to 31-year-olds, even after accounting for income, family wealth, occupation, and the level of education attained. Walsemann commented that 'people seem to be putting off marriage or home ownership, choosing jobs in high-paying instead of meaningful careers.' Financial obstacles to childbearing might be particularly daunting for women graduates facing the significant decline in fertility over the period of repaying debts.

Financial Situation of Staff and Mental Well-Being

It is far harder to find research on the relationship between the financial situation of university academic and support staff and their mental health. The focus of media and research publications is on relationships between pay and 'satisfaction', rather than mental health. At the time of writing (October 2022) university staff are considering industrial action because levels of pay are currently lower in real terms than in previous decades, and because the pay rises offered are below inflation rates.

This threat of action may be a healthy sign of anger at reduction in status, and a signal that staff are demanding greater appreciation. It does not necessarily reflect mental ill health, although Chapter 13 certainly finds much to be concerned about in the mental well-being of university staff. An individual's pay by itself does not tell us the whole story about the financial health of the staff member. Those with pre-existing debts and many outgoings and responsibilities will of course have more precarious finances than those who belong to two-income families or have other sources of wealth. This may partly explain the finding from two decades ago that UK female academics are more satisfied with their pay when compared with their male colleagues (Oshagbemi, 2000).

As yet, there is no evidence to predict the effects of growing pay dissatisfaction and industrial action on the mental health of either staff or the wider climate in the university. The disruption to student teaching, and the public declaration of conflict between staff and management within a university community is unlikely to be benign.

The Commodification of Higher Education

The end of the UK's state grant system in favour of a loan system has done much to make a higher education a commodity. A dynamic of financial imagery has built up around this – with metaphors such as 'investment', 'human capital', 'value for money', 'entitlement' and 'market' dominating academia. Members of academia who remember the previous system often comment on this.

One experienced counsellor observes that universities 'went from feeling like state institutions, like schools and the NHS, to being commercial institutions.' Students and perhaps their parents, she says, are now clients who purchase academic products rather than apprentice academics. Whilst this model may seem 'more American', she feels that it is different. For the UK this is a profound change in UK attitudes, rather than simply the ways things have always been.

This senior counsellor observes at one extreme those students completely funded by rich parents or independent incomes who are 'entitled' and 'just living the lovely life' and so perhaps 'more forgiving of the university'. At the other extreme are the students who rely on loans and part time jobs who may be 'hard working but anxious, demanding and resentful'. Such dynamics split the student community and appear to place some students in opposition to the authorities.

The financial metaphor enters into the system of marks and degree grades, all plugging into a world where self-worth is too commonly expressed in numbers – marks, grades, income, age, body weight and numbers of 'likes'. Whilst non-selective education at primary and even secondary level has been advocated for many years, 'league tables' persist, and high levels of competition characterise the university environment, from student competition to enter 'top' institutions to competition within and between universities for research funding and high scores on the Research Excellence Framework. Competition is often invoked as a healthy drive, particularly in capitalist narratives. However, psychological evidence suggests that high levels of competitiveness are particularly detrimental to women, and may be counterproductive overall in terms of achievement as well as damaging to mental health.

The Wealth of the Institution

Just as the financial and mental distress of even a minority of students or staff members affects the well-being of a broader university community, so the financial situation and management of an institution will affect the ethos and well-being of all members.

A well-maintained and comfortable university environment has direct academic benefits. Provision of excellent libraries, laboratories and lecture halls affects mental well-being. Subsidising good accommodation and food, sports facilities, common rooms, counselling services and medical facilities might also directly affect mental health – with academic spinoff. Most important is the resource available to attract and retain excellent staff, so that students receive – and give – the satisfaction of small group teaching, one-to-one attention, and healthy adult attachments.

It is obvious that universities require money, and their options for acquiring it, together with the terms on which they can spend it, are limited by the political climate. It is salutary to examine advertising matter. Whilst most public institutions advertise for staff, there is a contrast between the ways they advertise for 'clients'. Thus, private hospitals publish lavish advertising features aimed at potential patients, whereas the NHS certainly does not advertise for patients. Primary and secondary schools in the UK state system rarely aim advertising material at pupils or parents, whereas private schools offer Open Days and expensively produced publicity. The Times Higher Education (THE) periodical carries increasing amounts of advertising material for universities, often in pull-out supplements. These are mostly for non-European institutions, but UK universities also advertise, both internationally and at home. The UCAS website, for instance, states that

> Marketing is a crucial part of recruitment for both universities and colleges, while an increasing number of businesses are keen to reach the lucrative student demographic.
> That's where we can help. Through our subsidiary UCAS Media, we're able to offer our members and commercial partners a suite of marketing and creative services designed to reach every student audience – via social media, email marketing, print media, online advertising and much more.

Evidence for the risks and benefits for students of being characterised as part of a 'lucrative demographic' is currently lacking.

Edward Lucas (2019), in an essay for The Times, writes that

> western cultural institutions are encouraged to be entrepreneurial – competing for customers, sponsors and partners – at home and overseas. Little stops them doing deals with authoritarian states.

He lists China, Saudi, Russia, Iran and Turkey as examples of states donating money as a means to influence course content and research, as well as *'spying on troublesome students'*. Lucas welcomes the recent report by Universities UK (2020) on the risks of foreign collaboration. This acknowledges that risks to universities are not limited to the theft of intellectual property and data, or the security of university campuses.

'There are also threats to the values that have underpinned the success of the higher education sector: academic freedom, freedom of speech and institutional autonomy.... self-censorship and an environment that appears closed in terms of transparency and accountability to staff.' Lucas describes how 'Chinese students shun course modules that include sensitive material, or write their assignments in a way that will not get them into trouble at home.'

There are particular dilemmas for students, researchers and other staff wanting to speak out against the situation, in that doing so may irretrievably damage international career prospects. Administrators may be most concerned to bring in more money from foreign students so as to rise up league tables. Other students simply want to get on with getting their degrees with minimal trouble, and feel that defending national culture and intellectual freedom is not their business. While we work towards culture change, counsellors and other mentors need to be aware of the increased vigilance and fears – including fears for family members – that some international students may experience. The mental well-being of members of a university is ultimately linked to the financial contracts into which the institution enters.

Freshers' Finances and the Thirst for Belonging

Most students arrive at university with the financial confidence or anxiety inherent in their background. This often reflects the financial situation and attitudes of their families, and perhaps – in a more complicated way – of their school background. Being the first in a family to attend university, and having to take up paid work while studying due to financial pressures have both been identified as risk factors for poor mental health among students (Student Minds, 2019). Meanwhile, some religions and cultures teach attitudes to money and particularly to 'usury' that make a loan system very uncomfortable.

'First generation' students and those from Black and minority ethnic backgrounds often experience the attitude that 'investing' a large amount of money in higher education is not a safe thing to do and neither they nor their family may be familiar with the way in which student financing works in the UK. Mere provision of information is unlikely to provide reassurance. Prospective students also need opportunities to discuss and digest the issues with trusted peers, with parents and teachers too. It might be helpful to set up meetings between university finance staff and parents and school staff in areas where few pupils attend university. This could reassure the adults around the normality of incurring managed debt, whilst guiding them on the safest ways for their children and pupils to do so. Even parents who are not in a position to financially support their adult children can contribute by helping them manage and understand their finances. Those who fear or disapprove of debt, or who distance themselves from the financial issues involved can increase student anxiety around money, regardless of the precise financial situation.

> J was the oldest son in a large, loving and ambitious Asian family. Everyone worked long hours in the family business to ensure he could attend a prestigious university, but it was understood that he would study law, medicine or business, in order to repay the family investment by financing the fees and living costs of his younger siblings. He would joke that his youngest sister should pay him back by financing early retirement for him, but in practice both knew that she would be expected to 'pay' by caring for their parents in old age.
>
> Whilst the siblings had less disposable income than many of their peers, they felt secure in the arrangements that were 'masterminded' by the extended family.

Once at university, the actual financial situation is modified by young students' inexperience in managing their own finance, by their personality, peer expectations, and the demands and opportunities of the institution to which they belong. Some will still have parental wealth to fall back on. Others may not, for reasons of harsh reality or else pride. Opportunities to earn extra income from a part time job may relieve financial pressures, but may also contribute to overall fatigue and stress.

Reid et al. (2020) have attempted to tease out exactly how financial worries result in poorer grades. Controlling for background variables, they showed that financial concern was mediated by changes in 'stress' and 'sense of belonging' at university. The crucial role of healthy 'attachments' in making learning possible is well-known in schools but not always made explicit in adult education. However, the sense of belonging has long driven lucrative alumni loyalties to old schools and universities. For many students and staff, this sense of belonging is not important not only a route to high grades and financial donations, but is the most rewarding aspect of university life. Conversely, the sense of being poor when other students are rich can be part of 'imposter syndrome'.

> I was sold a dream of upward mobility. But from cash to culture, it's clear my working-class background still counts against me. . . . . .my first year has exposed the significant wealth disparities between me and other students. . . .My privileged counterparts will be able to explore opportunities in the form of unpaid internships; I need a career path that provides monetary stability. . .One [friend] told me how she dreamed of pursuing a career in acting, but soon realised that the financial insecurity of that industry means

that it won't be an option...I've learned that our class shapes our economic, cultural and social capital, and much of our potential, from birth. This is something a Cambridge degree cannot erase.

Daniella Adeluwoye www.theguardian.com/commentisfree/2019/sep/23/cambridge-university-upward-mobility-working-class-background

Maladaptive Financial Coping Strategies

A few students find themselves trapped in disastrous financial predicaments. For these students, extreme financial stresses can be part of a picture of extreme mental distress that requires psychological as well as practical management. Some students fall victim to damaging strategies that may have appeared at first to provide financial solutions, but end up compounding the financial situation and bringing devastating troubles on top.

Some students become sex workers to make money for their studies. This is often portrayed in media as a choice by which glamorous young women exploit their youth and beauty for a luxurious life with rich older men. The reality is often very different. Vulnerable students can be sexually exploited by powerful individuals who take most of their earnings and intimidate them. Students working as drug dealers may also be vulnerable to both disease and exploitation by criminal networks, and the two spheres are of course linked. Student sexual behaviour is discussed further in Chapter 12, and drug use in Chapter 7. These practices impact on mental health of the individuals obtaining their income this way. They also affect the reputation and mental health climate of the universities in which they operate.

Gambling and Gaming

Gambling and gaming can affect mental health both when they constitute an addictive mental disorder in themselves, and indirectly through the financial consequences and the effects of these on stress and relationships. There is evidence that pathological gambling is associated with increased risk of having a criminal record too, generally to obtain funds to continue gambling (Blaszczynski & Silove, 1996).

Gambling – and its younger relative gaming – is an almost universally observed human phenomenon. It is not a simple money-making or money-losing criminal phenomenon, but in its extreme is a recognised psychiatric disorder, related to other addictions, and characterised by a quest for the excitement or 'buzz' that it generates. Gaming is a popular pastime among university students, particularly male students, and is not necessarily undertaken for the purpose of making money, although developments in technology are creating more potential overlaps between gaming and gambling. One cliché of the 'typical male student' is of one who lives in squalor, scruffily dressed, burdened with debts but still managing to drink and party. This cliché can be a cover for more serious underlying issues such as problem gambling, financial difficulties, substance misuse problems and mood disorders.

Often, treatment is not sought until a major crisis occurs either financially, personally, in terms of criminal conviction or at work. However, 90% of those affected have started excessive gambling in their teens and experienced insidious damage before the crisis. Average age of starting to gamble is the early teens, so students affected with a gambling problem are likely to already be well-established in the habit. For many students, gaming as well as explicit gambling may represent an attractive way to make money as well as constituting a way to get a 'high' rather like a stimulant drug.

Experts describe how the initial 'winning phase' of gambling moves into a losing phase characterised by 'chasing losses', and borrowing on credit cards, or from friends, using loan sharks and pawn brokers to continue to finance the habit. By this stage, the aim is no longer to make money or even pay off debts but to maintain the gambling experience and continue to feel the 'high'. The activity now serves to distract the person from their worries, which are ubiquitous. Finally, in the 'desperation phase' there is intense mental disorder and social alienation. Other addictive behaviours often accompany this self-destructive picture. Lynch et al. (2004) found that young gamblers had significantly raised levels of alcohol and drug misuse.

The Young Gamers and Gamblers Education Trust (YGAM) (2019) has published research into how gaming and gambling affect student life. YGAM's survey identifies that 47% of students have gambled in the last 12 months. Of these, 16% can be identified as moderate risk or problem gamblers. Students said that they gambled to try to ease and improve their finances whilst at university. Of those who gambled, 59% said they were always worrying about their financial situation while 16% had gambled more than they could afford. The research found that gambling affects students' academic prowess and mental health as well as finance.

On the basis of their research, YGAM calls for limits on advertising around both gaming and gambling. They also recommend a ban on credit card use to place stakes either in person or online, as student problem gamblers were far more likely to use their credit cards 'most days'. They also report that in their experience, a peer-to-peer model of support works effectively to engage students to address gambling problems.

Financial Literacy: An Underestimated Aspect of Mental Resilience

Chisholm-Burns et al. (2017) examined stress levels in a group of American Pharmacy students and found, similar to the findings of Ross in the UK, that it was 'fear of debt' rather than actual levels of debt that increased stress levels. Conversely, those students who described higher levels of 'contemplation and knowledge' about financial matters enjoyed lower stress and experienced greater confidence that they would manage to keep debt low and pay it off rapidly. Indeed, such students tended to keep their debts lower, contributing to a virtuous cycle of high competence leading to high confidence and lower stress. Novilitis et al. (2006) also found that increased financial knowledge did indeed result in less student debt. This implies obvious ways to improve student mental health by educating them from the start – or even before their university careers – on personal financial management.

There is a huge risk of further overloading the fraught 'Freshers' week' timetable, where high arousal levels in new undergraduates make it impossible to lay down much lasting learning. One suggestion would be to offer group-based financial discussions both in school 6th forms and during a pre-term university induction course. Further facilities might include 'drop in' financial counselling to students throughout the academic year, outreach to university societies and organisations, and further professionally organised workshops on future financial planning around the transition period of graduation from university.

A group of university staff and students suggested to me that just as students are currently invited to declare medical and mental health conditions on acceptance of a university place, so they might also be invited to declare financial vulnerability and have the right to financial mentoring. Applicants could be shown how to complete a financial balance sheet, which could be used by them before any disclosure to assess whether or not they would benefit from such mentoring.

> Ben was the only pupil from his school to attend university. He was thrilled to meet people who shared his interests but embarrassed to find how much more money the others had. He avoided socialising for fear of having to get in expensive 'rounds'. One of his hall mates offered to sell him all the course set books second hand, but he had no idea whether she was taking advantage of his gullibility. He decided to do without books altogether and study in the library. His extreme parsimony blighted much of his time in university, until a girlfriend he met in his final year, who came from a similar background, helped him put his concerns into perspective and to seek help for an obsessional condition.

Teaching financial skills can improve both financial and social well-being and play a role in preventing mental disorder, substance misuse and criminal involvement. At the same time, students should have any untreated mental disorders addressed to provide the mental 'space' to acquire and exercise finance management skills. The learning of problem-solving skills and putting them into use requires a sufficiently confident and relaxed attitude. This means that financial counsellors should be alert to the presence of a treatable mental disorder so that the student can use financial skills better, whilst mental health professionals need to bear in mind the potential for financial support and training as part of both cause and effect of a mental illness. In addition to the financial disarray that occurs when individuals become depressed and low in energy, people with manic or hypomanic episodes may experience episodes of disastrous disinhibited spending, and those with obsessive disorders may simply be unable to take the risk of spending sensibly.

Opportunities to openly discuss money matters with peers and facilitating experts can be liberating, particularly to British people who have followed an implicit code that it is 'not done' to discuss money. It is probably necessary, though, to ensure that less well-off students and people from minority cultures can meet with others in a comparable financial situation, as the presence of rich students in such groups could lead to embarrassment and stigma.

Finance workshops for students can include useful discussions on essential and non-essential financial outlay, and cheaper choices. Significant savings can be made by eating in university canteens or cooking in halls rather than ordering take-aways or eating out. Alcoholic drinks are expensive – as is water when bought bottled rather than taken free from taps! The disinhibiting effects of alcohol also make further spending more likely.

There are options for considerable savings by doing without personal grooming expenses from hairdressers, beauty clinics and tattoo artists. Sharing or recycling clothes using charity shops and thrift stores often also appeals to students' ecological aspirations. Even highly intelligent young people may have overlooked the disadvantages to credit card debts, and may need help to consider how to prioritise different sorts of debt.

Building Financial Well-Being at the University Level

Many universities and colleges attempt to provide 'cost containment' whereby tuition fees and accommodation are price-capped for the duration of the course to allow students to budget in advance. The provision of hardship funds, and bursaries for financially stressed and underprivileged students varies according to the wealth of different universities. Bursaries are still offered to nursing and other healthcare students across the UK, because of the perceived need to recruit into these professions. 'Shortage' healthcare specialisms, such as learning disability, command extra funding on top of the standard bursary.

Another potential source of funding for students is scholarships. These carry double connotations, both as prizes for excellence and as one of the routes for a poor student to gain an education. In most cases, though, the monetary value of scholarships has not kept pace with inflation and represents only a small financial benefit. It might be argued that scholarships are a sign that the academic entrance bar is set higher for poor people, and that bursaries are a way that poor students are pressured to opt for unpopular career choices.

Jack was the first member of his family to attend university and was strongly encouraged by his enthusiastic family. He hoped to win a scholarship that would offset the high costs of studying medicine in London, but failed to manage this. His family between them mobilised all possible resource, even including re-mortgaging the family home. They expected J to match their sacrifice by taking on work as a nursing assistant on top of his studies.

This work was exhausting, and he did not maintain his position as an academic high-flyer at this stage, but found the skills he gained contributed to high marks and clinical confidence later in his course. Weekend shifts limited the amount of expensive socialising he could do, but he enjoyed the company at work, and also experienced far less financial stress than many peers who were – on paper – wealthier.

Many institutions have funds, raised by alumni and other donors, specifically to support students who are in financial need. Such funds can be usefully linked to financial counselling facilities. Universities may also have a 'bank' of work placements – in libraries, campus shops or university offices – available for students who are working their way through college. Those students might be encouraged to study less than full time, although the risks and benefits of juggling paid work and study depend greatly on an individual's energies and the demands of their course.

With a high proportion of the population now expecting to attend university, reverting to the old system of maintenance grants for all may be impractical, but at a national and even international level there are calls to revisit the funding of higher education to improve the health, happiness, academic prowess and productivity of the world's graduate workforce.

Practice Points

Societal Awareness

- In higher education finance and mental health are closely linked, albeit in a complex way.
- The relatively recent 'commodification' of higher education in the UK has consequences for the overall mental well-being of university communities, including cultural risks and benefits of seeking finance and competing for fees. Society may wish to review options for funding higher education.

University Financial Services

- Students arrive at university with differing levels of financial concern and confidence. Many go on to graduate with increased financial stresses.

University Mental Health Services

- Debt and financial concern are associated with poorer mental health and academic under-performance at university and lower levels of well-being after graduation. It is always worth asking sensitively about finance and debt when a student is troubled.
- Established mental disorders in turn feed into vicious spirals of decline and must be treated alongside the provision of financial counselling.
- The combination of financial stress with maladaptive coping strategies such as gambling, sex working and drug dealing can lead students into association with a criminal culture, which is destructive for the individuals and their communities. Again, awareness and sensitive questioning of troubled students can reveal opportunities for help.
- Students may be more likely to seek timely support to solve financial difficulties if they perceive financial advisors as sympathetic and supportive rather than angry and blaming.
- Financial literacy is important and can be explicitly taught and supported, with benefits for mental health. Targeted workshops before starting university and during graduation might be supplemented by drop-in clinics.

References

Blaszczynski, A. & Silove, D. (1996). Pathological gambling: Forensic issues. *Australian & New Zealand Journal of Psychiatry*, 30(3):358–69. https://doi.org/10.3109/00048679609065000

Chisholm-Burns, M. A., Spivey, C. A., Jaeger, M. C. & Williams, J. (2017). Associations between pharmacy students' attitudes toward debt, stress, and student loans. *American Journal of Pharmaceutical Education*, 81(7), 5918. https://doi.org/10.5688/ajpe8175918

Lucas, E. (2019, 17 October) *Weekend Essay: Our universities have sacrificed academic liberty for Chinese cash*. The Times.

Lynch, W. J., Maciejewski, P. K. & Potenza, M. N. (2004). Psychiatric correlates of gambling in adolescents and young adults grouped by age at gambling onset. *Archives of General Psychiatry*, 61(11), 1116–22. https://doi.org/10.1001/archpsyc.61.11.1116

Nelson, M. C., Lust, K., Story, M. & Ehlinger, E. (2008). Credit card debt, stress and key health risk behaviours among college students. *American Journal of Health Promotion*, 22(6), 400–7.

Novilitis, J. M., Merwin, M. M., Osberg, T. M., Rochling, P. V., Young, P. & Kamas, M. M. (2006). Personality factors, money attitudes, financial knowledge, and credit-card debt in college students. *Journal of Applied Social Psychology*, 36(6), 1395–413.

Oshagbemi, T. (2000). Correlates of pay satisfaction in higher education. *International Journal of Educational Management*, 14(1), 31–39.

Reid, M., Jessop, D. C. & Miles, E. (2020). Explaining the negative impact of financial concern on undergraduates' academic outcomes: Evidence for stress and belonging as mediators, *Journal of Further and Higher Education*, 44(9), 1157–87. https://doi.org/10.1080/0309877X.2019.1664732

Richardson, T., Elliott, P. & Roberts, R. (2013). The relationship between personal unsecured debt and mental and physical health: A systematic review and meta-analysis. *Clinical Psychology Review*, 33(8), 1148–62. https://doi.org/10.1016/j.cpr.2013.08.009

Richardson, T., Elliott, P., Waller, G. & Bell, L. (2015). Longitudinal relationships between financial difficulties and eating attitudes in undergraduate students. *International Journal of Eating Disorders*, 48(5), 517–21.

Richardson, T., Elliott, P., Roberts, R. & Jansen, M. (2017). A longitudinal study of financial difficulties and mental health in a national sample of British undergraduate students. *Community Mental Health Journal*, 53, 344–52. https://doi.org/10.1007/s10597-016-0052-0

Roberts, R., Golding, J., Towell, T., et al. (2000). Mental and physical health in students: The role of economic circumstances. *British Journal of Health Psychology*, 5, 289–97.

Ross, S., Cleland, J. & Macleod, M.J. (2006). Stress, debt and undergraduate medical student performance. *Medical Education*, 40, 584–9. https://doi.org/10.1111/j.1365-2929.2006.02448.x

Universities UK (2020). *Managing risks in internationalisation: Security related issues.* www.universitiesuk.ac.uk/policy-and-analysis/reports/Pages/managing-risks-in-internationalisation.aspx

Walsemann, K. M., Gee, G. C. & Gentile, D. (2015). Sick of our loans: Student borrowing and the mental health of young adults in the United States. *Social Science & Medicine*, 124, 85–93. https://doi.org/10.1016/j.socscimed.2014.11.027

Young Gamers and Gamblers Education Trust (2019) *How gaming & gambling affect student life.* www.ygam.org/wp-content/uploads/2020/07/FINAL-research_full_report-PRINT-READY-5.pdf

Neurodiversity

The Autistic Spectrum and Attention Deficit Hyperactivity Disorder

10

Conditions such as autism spectrum disorder (ASD) and attention deficit hyperactivity disorder (ADHD) are mentioned but not primarily addressed in Chapters 14–16. People may not struggle so much with the symptoms of these conditions as with the clashes that occur when their ways of experiencing the world are not in keeping with societies' expectations and codes. Such people are known to be particularly vulnerable to mental ill health and mental illnesses. It can be controversial as to how far the vulnerability is intrinsic to the neurological basis of the conditions and how far it reflects having to march to other people's drums.

Even as I use that metaphor, it occurs to me that it might not be readily accessible to some readers with autistic traits. I suspect that entire books are written without consideration for understanding by people at different ends of the neurodiverse spectrum, and this may bring about the sort of stresses we all feel when studying texts that we effectively have to 'translate'.

Like many colleagues, I tend to use the example of left handedness to discuss the nature of neurodiversity. Left handedness can of course be one sign of a serious disorder of the brain, but that is not usually the case. Yet left-handers often feel disabled by having to adapt to a largely right-handed world. Sometimes, the difference is an advantage – for instance in fencing and tennis matches. In the past, adults would force left-handed children to use their right hand instead, and this often caused distress, sometimes extreme disturbance. People with ASD can similarly become anxious, depressed and even suicidal if obliged to simply mimic the behaviours of non-autistic individuals and suppress their authentic selves. This is described as 'camouflaging' or 'masking'.

Some Terms and Abbreviations	
ADHD	attention deficit hyperactivity disorder. Attention deficit disorder (ADD), a previous term, is still sometimes used for adults when the hyperactivity is reduced
ASD	autism spectrum disorder
Aspie	a person with Asperger's syndrome, the former term for high-functioning autism (usually used in a positive way by the people with the condition of themselves)
Camouflaging or masking	taking pains to act like a person without ASD, and to supress ASD behaviour and speech
DSA	disabled students' allowances
ND	neurodiverse person – generally refers to someone with ASD or ADHD

Neurodiversity	the diversity of all people's mental styles but usually used to indicate ASD or ADHD
NT	neurotypical person – someone who does not have ASD or ADHD
Stimming	self-stimulating behaviour such as rubbing hands over a furry object or engaging in repetitive gestures (or words) that may look like nervous habits but can be pleasurable as well as self-soothing
Twice-exceptionality (2e)	refers to gifted students who have some form of disability, usually ASD or ADHD.

Some people challenge the 'medical disorder' model. They suggest that people do not become disabled simply as a result of having impairments to body or mind. Instead, the disability arises when societal barriers interact with individual differences, so that some individuals are unable to benefit from systems that only cater to the dominant culture.

However, some parents of autistic children and parent-led organisations, as well as some autism researchers and some autistic people themselves, have in turn protested that high-functioning activists present an unrealistic picture of how very disabling autism can be. They do not want to deflect attention and resources away from the struggles of more severely affected individuals and their families. They worry that certain features of autism should be addressed and treated rather than accepted.

The term 'neurodiversity' can be used to span both medical and social models, recognising that both inherent vulnerabilities and societal obstacles can be damaging for people with these conditions. This is the broad sense in which I will use the term in this book. I use the expressions 'autism spectrum *disorder*' and 'attention deficit hyperactivity *disorder*' and their abbreviations ASD and ADHD rather than such terms as 'autistic spectrum *condition*', because the research evidence and political discussion mostly uses those terms. I have also used the expression 'diagnosis' not only to describe the process of diagnosing mental disorders in people with ASD, but also to describe the identification of ASD itself. This is again, mainly a matter of common usage, although 'identification' might be a less medical word to use. One advantage of the word 'disorder' and even more so the word 'diagnosis' is that it does imply that doctors and other mental health professionals have a responsibility to provide a service. It is hard to imagine how the conditions could be reliably identified and formulated without a professional training in mental health and further specialist expertise.

The expression 'people with autism' has been criticised as wrongly and pejoratively separating a condition that is intrinsic to the person. After years of learning to speak about 'people with anorexia' or 'people with schizophrenia' rather than 'anorexic patients' or 'schizophrenics', we are being challenged to think of people with ASD as 'autistic people'.

In recent years, the UK Government has increasingly recognised that ASD brings significant unmet social and healthcare needs. This recognition led to the Autism Act 2009; the first disability-specific legislation passed in the UK. The Autism Act required the Secretary of State to produce statutory guidance for local authorities and health bodies to meet the needs of adults with ASD.

Neurotypical syndrome is a neurobiological disorder characterised by preoccupation with social concerns, delusions of superiority and obsession with conformity. There is no known cure.

Laura Tisoncik, 1998, quoted in Silberman's 'Neurotribes'

It has to be acknowledged that there are considerable problems with the idea of a binary neurodiverse/neurotypical divide. It's hard to imagine a gold standard set of criteria for being 'neurotypical' (although autistic wits have suggested a definition), or a way to define the cut-off. Many of us would not meet criteria for an ASD or ADHD diagnosis but recognise many of their traits in ourselves. It was interesting to read National Institute for Health and Care Excellence (NICE) (2012) guidelines recommending that clinicians should clearly introduce themselves, clarify their role and speak respectfully to people with ASD, as well as ensuring that the environment be calming and predictable. Most of us would benefit considerably from the same respect.

Whilst ASD has been at the centre of concerns for students with neurodiversity, the neurodiversity paradigm has extended to include ADHD, which is still usually spoken of as a disorder, although is increasingly embraced as part of a personality profile. ASD and ADHD are often found in the same individual, as are a range of other conditions such as dyslexia, dyspraxia, and dyscalculia. On the whole, our universities make excellent provision for these latter conditions, regarding them as the domain of educational psychologists and specialist teachers. There has been work suggesting that Tourette syndrome and perhaps even some variants of obsessive–compulsive disorder may be related to ASD and ADHD. This chapter, though, will confine itself to consideration of ASD and ADHD.

When we discuss neurodiversity, it is worth helping the individual to find a conceptualisation of their condition that leads to positive outcomes for their situation, rather than getting too caught up in our own views. One study (Griffin & Pollak, 2009) interviewed a range of students whose 'neurodiverse' conditions included autism, dyslexia, developmental coordination disorder, ADHD, and stroke. All the students described uniformly difficult schooling careers involving exclusion, abuse, and bullying. However, those who tended to see themselves as 'different', with a range of unusual strengths and weaknesses, had higher academic self-esteem, confidence in their abilities and career ambitions, than students who saw themselves as having a 'disadvantageous medical condition', who were more focussed on achieving disabled students' allowance (DSA) and compensation for their condition. Many of the students reported gaining the sense of themselves as 'different' rather than 'defective' through contact with neurodiversity advocates in online support groups.

Autism Spectrum Disorder

I can deal with change a lot better now than I could in the past, but things still catch me off guard sometimes. Moving house every year, new lecturers every term, and so many other parts of 'normal' uni life can pose a difficulty for people with autism. I have to actively spend time preparing myself before a change and adjusting afterwards.

Some of the situations I find most difficult are ones where I don't have time to prepare. For example, when one of my lectures changed location midway through term. As soon as that happened – despite attending consistently to that point – I stopped going to the lecture. I didn't know why, but I felt completely unable to attend; it was like I had a mental block. My brain couldn't adjust to having the same unit but in a different place without any warning. Reflecting on this has helped me recognise it and helps stop it happening in the future. However, it would be useful for universities to understand the potential unintended consequences of what must seem like 'small' changes to most people.

Elizabeth Blackwell Institute for Health Research (2020)

On ASD, the 11th edition of the International Classification of Diseases and Related Health Problems (World Health Organization, 2022) provides this summary:

> Autism spectrum disorder is characterized by persistent deficits in the ability to initiate and to sustain reciprocal social interaction and social communication, and by a range of restricted, repetitive, and inflexible patterns of behaviour and interests.

The essential features of ASD are communication difficulties, unusual interests, and repetitive or 'stereotyped' behaviours. Regularity, sameness and repetition can be positive sources of pleasure as well as being soothing. Autistic people usually find it hard to tolerate changes in routine, will sometimes become very anxious around social interactions and often do not use conventional body language or communicate by varying their tone of voice.

Students and staff with ASD can have significant cognitive strengths. These can include extraordinary capacity for memorisation and unusual attention to detail. Enormous amounts of information may be learned about restricted topics. Some individuals exhibit enhanced visuo-spatial skills such as drawing or ability to play a piece of music after hearing it only once. Many academic pursuits benefit from such attributes and when the individual is fulfilled in a course well-matched to their interests, this goes a long way to reducing stress.

One study carried out at the University of Cambridge, asked students to complete a scale known as the Autism Spectrum Quotient. Scores in students overall were similar to a control group. Students who were studying sciences and mathematics scored higher than social sciences and humanities students, with mathematicians scoring highest of all. (Brugha et al., 2011). This illustrates the sorts of speciality where the brains of people with ASD have made particular contributions, but we should not play too much into stereotypes and push people into these subject choices.

There are lots of great things about being autistic. I'm really passionate about the things that matter to me, I love learning new things, and when I'm allowed to be myself, I'm apparently very funny (if people's reactions to the things I say are to be believed!). But more than anything, I'm a very accepting person. I know what it feels like to be different and to be excluded, so I try my hardest to show people they can be themselves around me.

Autism is my way of being. I don't know how to experience the world without autism, and so much of my energy goes into navigating a neurotypical world. When I was diagnosed, the psychologist compared being autistic to being left-handed. There isn't anything inherently wrong with it, but the world just isn't set out to be accessible to us. I work around it for the most part; I've spent 20 years of my life learning to pass as neurotypical, and I'm very good at coping now, but there are still times when it can make things more difficult.

Elizabeth Blackwell Institute for Health Research (2020)

Asperger's Syndrome

Asperger syndrome, also known as Asperger's, was the name of a neurodevelopmental disorder that is no longer recognised as a diagnosis in itself. It was a term to describe ASD without intellectual deficits and is sometimes called 'high-functioning autism'. Most students with an ASD are likely to have been in this category. Both international diagnostic classifications have merged it into (ASD). The syndrome was named after the Austrian paediatrician Hans Asperger, who, in 1944, described children in his care who struggled to form friendships, did not understand others' gestures or feelings, engaged in one-sided conversations about their favourite interests, and were clumsy.

The term 'Asperger's', and its affectionate diminutive 'Aspie', used to describe people who identified as having the condition, were catchphrase headlines in the massive increase in ASD awareness, particularly for cognitively able autistic individuals, that has taken place over the past three decades. There is still a great deal of useful online material using the expression. It is hard to think of a convenient replacement, but continuing to use the term would be a controversial option because of the discovery that Prof. Asperger may have collaborated with Nazi death camps in World War II.

Prevalence of ASD in Society and in Universities

Around one in 100 people in the UK would qualify for a diagnosis of ASD (Brugha et al., 2011). Rates of diagnosis are rising, though it is not clear whether this is a result of increased ascertainment or a true increase in prevalence. In the UK the number of autistic students at university increased from 1.8% in 2004 to 2.4% of the student population in 2008 (Macleod & Green, 2009). These numbers are expected to have increased even further since these data became available partly due to investment in equality and diversity programmes and widening participation agendas.

Gurbuz et al. (2019) present the alarming statistic that 'less than 40% of autistic students successfully complete their studies (VanBergeijk et al., 2008; Newman et al., 2011)'. However, their sources are from US studies and are over a decade old, so we may hope that this is not the case in the UK in the 2020s.

Male students and staff are between 4- and 9-times as likely to be diagnosed with ASD as their female counterparts. This is partly because females are more likely to use 'camouflaging' or 'masking'. These terms refer to the ways in which autistic individuals act like their neurotypical peers. It may also be the case that professionals expect ASD to be a more likely diagnosis in boys and men, and possibly the preponderance of male subjects in research has shaped the very definitions of ASD to describe how it presents in males. My experience of working in eating disorders services taught me that many young women with anorexia nervosa had undiagnosed ASD at the root of their condition, and this, strikingly, is a disorder diagnosed predominantly in women. Many of my patients had fathers and brothers with ASD, suggesting that the genetically inherited cognitive style of these families is common to both ASD and anorexia.

Assessments and Support in Universities

In the past, ASD diagnosis was usually made in child and adolescent mental health services (CAMHS). Some students will arrive at university having be diagnosed in the traditional way. A comprehensive assessment involves a specially trained multidisciplinary team that observes child and family across multiple settings, and includes assessment for cognition, psychomotor function, verbal and nonverbal strengths and weaknesses, style of learning, and skills for independent living.

Many children with ASD are initially diagnosed as having ADHD. Others may never be offered the intensive diagnostic procedure, or they or their families may decline. It is not unusual for students who did not meet criteria for ASD in CAMHS, particularly girls, to be later found to have ASD on further clinical investigation

Adult diagnosis requires painstaking clinical examination and thorough medical history gained from both the individual and other people who know the person, focusing on childhood behaviour patterns. There is no widely accepted equivalent of the formally rated interviews used to diagnose children, but there are questionnaires that can guide clinical discussion and alert us to symptoms and features we may not have thought to enquire about. Parents, especially mothers, can provide invaluable information in finding out whether the current picture is a reflection of longstanding patterns or the result of a current disorder such as anxiety or depression.

We may not consider autism as a mental health condition in itself, but mental health problems are among the most common and serious challenges experienced by people high on the spectrum. Almost 80% autistic adults experience a mental health problem. They often complain that they are unable to access community mental health support on the mistaken basis that there are separate specialist services for autistic adults (Lever & Geurts, 2016). Autistic people have reported being 'punted' between different settings; often from mental health services that are not confident in 'dealing with autism' to learning disability services, which can be poorly integrated with mental health services.

This can obviously be a particular issue for adults who do not have an intellectual disability. Untreated mental disorders may escalate until emergency inpatient care is required. Alongside the difficulty in accessing routine services, up to 10% of adults in inpatient mental health settings are autistic, although only 1% of the UK population has ASD (Tromans et al., 2018).

The increased awareness of and provision for intellectually able people with ASD in universities may be going some way to bridging the gap in services and possibly providing training and awareness to non-university settings. Students with ASD can present to student support services with a range of problems. The leading symptoms include depression, suicidality, anxiety and obsessive–compulsive features. The condition may also come to attention as a result of behaviour that is disruptive or socially inappropriate.

Diagnostic assessment is available from different sources in different parts of the UK. It may be provided by NHS mental health services, the National Autistic Society, or university disability services. Each university should clarify a properly resourced pathway that does not involve long waiting lists.

Diagnosis benefits students or members of staff in several ways. It provides a framework for the individual and their peers to understand the nature of this condition. It gives students access to DSA funding that can pay for the support of a specialist mentor. There is also opportunity to plan appropriate modifications to parts of the course.

Assessment for comorbid disorders is a crucial part of a comprehensive ASD assessment. These can have a greater effect on a person's outcome and functioning than the core symptoms. Sometimes it is extremely difficult to differentiate between a lasting feature of autism and a temporary difference resulting from a different, treatable mental condition.

For instance, I have had the experience that depression, anxiety and the 'starvation syndrome' of anorexia nervosa can all mimic features of ASD. In those cases, the symptoms are reversed by recovery from the disorder. For instance, reduced social motivation or difficulties in social situations can turn out to be the results of a treatable social phobia. Compulsive behaviours in obsessive–compulsive disorder can appear similar in presentation to restrictive and repetitive behaviours observed in ASD, and indeed recent evidence has suggested some neurobiological overlap. Social disinterest and atypical social communication may be classic symptoms of depression. On the one hand, this means we have to be tentative in suggesting an ASD diagnosis in the presence of other conditions. On the other hand, even when such conditions are treated, many individuals will still need support and management for underlying ASD.

Vulnerability to Mental Health Disorders

It can be difficult to identify mood disorder in some people with ASD. As discussed, some of the features of the condition include differences in social verbal communication and less use of body language and facial expression. A substantial proportion of autistic people, including those with high intelligence also have alexithymia. This term is derived from Greek words meaning literally 'no words for emotion' but it is used in psychology to denote more than the lack of words. People with alexithymia have great difficulty getting in touch with and identifying their feelings in the first place, even when those feelings cause them to suffer. Alexithymia describes a phenomenon, it does not constitute a diagnosis in itself, and therapy can often help people learn to overcome it in part.

Since alexithymia and social communication differences may cause delays in getting help and treatment, it is helpful for other people to take responsibility for noticing changes in the person's functioning or behaviour. These can include changes in sleep, concentration or increased social withdrawal, for instance. It is common experience that people with ASD are better at completing forms than reporting feelings to other people, so self-report scales should be made available where possible.

Hollocks et al. (2019) conducted a systematic review and meta-analysis of anxiety and depression in adults with ASD. At any one time 27% had anxiety disorders, and 23% depressive disorders. Over their lifetime the estimates were that 42% would have an anxiety diagnosis and 37% a diagnosed depressive disorder. Unfortunately, the use of questionnaires, the presence of intellectual disorders and the age range of subjects, made the authors wary of concluding they had discovered accurate estimates. When considering the student population, we can be even less confident. However, the massive interest in ASD at every level of society and the fact that universities are so well placed to design, conduct and recruit for studies in this field, should yield better information before too long.

ASD and Depression

Depressive disorder may be the most frequently diagnosed single comorbid psychiatric illness in ASD (Ghaziuddin et al., 2002), and of course often co-occurs with anxiety disorders (See Chapter 16 for further detail on the nature of depression and anxiety disorders). A review of depression in ASD two decades ago (Ghaziuddin et al., 2002) points out that unusual slowness of speech, walking or other physical movements are useful indicators that a person with ASD may be depressed.

Irritable and oppositional behaviour may also be symptoms. Those who know and understand the student's particular fanatical interests may notice changes in these, sometimes even a complete loss of the usual preoccupations. The associated anxiety may bring about increases in obsessional or self-soothing behaviours too.

There are a couple of modifiable reasons why people with ASD might be more prone to depression. Teenagers with ASD and other neurodevelopmental disorders are far less likely to exercise or play team sports than their peers, and sedentary behaviour is linked to a higher likelihood of being depressed. One small review (Lang et al., 2010) found that, remarkably, for children and young adults with ASD, physical activity and aerobic exercise interventions were not only mood enhancing but showed significant reductions in odd movements, aggression, and off-task behaviour as well as improvements in academic engagement and appropriate motor behaviour.

Joni was a gifted maths student who had been diagnosed as having ASD when at school. She often felt lonely and misunderstood and constantly believed people were laughing at her. Starting university was a positive experience. 'People get me at last' she told her parents. She involved herself with the autistic community online and sometimes at real life meetings and became militant about neurodiversity. She refused to apply for DSA as a matter of principle as she believed she was 'otherwise abled'.

She was dreadfully upset by the ending of her first romantic relationship and plunged into depression. Her doctor advised her to reconsider applying for DSA as this would provide for her to have longer-term mentoring for all her mental health needs.

Joni was matched with Mary, a mentor who specialised in the needs of people with ASD. They met for exactly 1 hour every Wednesday in term time. It was always the same mentor, in the same, peaceful room in the Chaplaincy Centre. Sometimes they ended up in logical debates where Joni was always determined to win the argument. Mary would gently draw her attention to this pattern and after a while Joni was able to notice it too, and to laugh together about it.

Joni described Mary as someone who could explain the neurotypical world to her and sometimes vice versa. She said it was like having an interpreter. Both women insisted that the work was not therapy, although it did support Joni to survive the way she felt when her boyfriend left her. She would sometimes refer to Mary as a 'friend' but usually corrected herself.

When Joni graduated, with spectacular grades, her parents suggested she nominate her mentor for an award, but she felt this would be inappropriate as Mary had told her she was 'simply doing her job'. She was accepted to undertake a PhD at a particularly prestigious university and asked her parents to help her find a new mentor there.

Another issue that faces students with ASD is isolation and loneliness. Social difficulties and need for solitude do not mean the individual does not crave the feeling of belonging, the affection of other people and the chance to be playful. Many of the interventions that have been found to prevent or relieve mental disorder in people with ASD have caring relationships at their heart. Even treatments such as physical exercise, prescribing anti-depressant medication and delivery of cognitive behavioural therapy rely on their being led by a trusted, caring figure.

Students with ASD might feel themselves initially courted but then rejected by evolving social groups at university because of problems with social skills and social understanding. Some universities in the United States and UK use 'buddy schemes' in which another student will act as a buddy to the student with ASD, perhaps living for a reduced rent with the student with ASD, making sure they are understood, sometimes socialising or attending activities together, and planning calendars and study timetables together. There can be a risk that the person with ASD becomes too attached and becomes a burden to the fellow student, or that the person with ASD is devastated when the buddy moves on. It's essential that buddies belong to an official peer group providing supervision and support. If possible, there should be teams of buddies so that transitions or buddies' time off are cushioned.

ASD and Anxiety Disorders

People with ASD experience high levels of diagnosable anxiety disorders, including specific phobias, agoraphobia, generalised anxiety disorder, social phobia and obsessive–compulsive disorder. Even those without a diagnosis speak of high baseline levels of anxiety. One explained, 'If the average person has a baseline anxiety level of 1 or 2 on a 10-point scale, my baseline is generally a 6.'

Further anxiety may stem from preoccupation over possible violations of routines and rituals, from being placed in a situation without a clear schedule or expectations, from stress about exams or presentations or from concern with failing in social or sexual encounters.

Zukerman et al.'s (2022) study, discussed later in this chapter, compared psychiatric symptoms in students with and without autism. As expected, the students with ASD had significantly higher levels of anxiety and depression. After a year, it was levels of anxiety disorder symptoms that predicted how much progress the students had made in adapting to university life. This suggests that focussing efforts on reducing anxiety levels, or helping students gradually become more resilient to anxiety, might be powerful in improving their quality of life.

ASD and Eating Disorders

Judith studied linguistics but was rarely seen in lectures or classes. She found her hall of residence to be too loud and messy and frequently retreated back to her family home at weekends. She spent most of her time in the library studying or sitting in the library café with mugs of black coffee and an open book. She was an emaciated figure, always dressed in many layers of black clothes even in summer.

She presented immaculate coursework, so it was a surprise when suddenly she stopped returning assignments. She was found almost moribund in her bedroom and spent months in hospital. She was diagnosed with anorexia nervosa, depressive disorder and probable ASD.

She was obliged to gain weight, and as she became better nourished, clinicians were amazed and delighted to observe that her depression lifted and a much more sociable, humorous personality emerged. The strange rituals and exclusions that were so noticeable at the dining table melted away too and she began to eat like a healthy person.

Her mother said she was finally seeing Judith's personality as it had been when she was a child. She was terrified that Judith would revert to restricting her eating and they would 'lose her again'.

Chapter 5 is devoted to the consideration of eating, weight and body image concerns in universities. There has been considerable interest in links between ASD and anorexia nervosa, which warrants consideration here. It is also important to note that many people with ASD have certain rules and rituals about eating behaviour that may result in their losing or gaining large amounts of weight and/or suffering from nutritional deficiencies, as well as causing social inconvenience and embarrassment. Clinicians tend to call these 'feeding disorders.' Somewhat confusingly, we reserve the term 'eating disorders' for where there is an obsessive drive to lose weight, because of body image concerns. People with 'eating disorders' are also likely to use overexercising, purging and other ways to lose weight, besides restricting their diet.

In 1983, Professor Chris Gillberg (1983) wrote a short letter to the British Journal of Psychiatry from the University of Gothenburg. He described three boys with 'infantile autism' who had female cousins with anorexia nervosa and asked, 'Is there a possibility that a common biochemical disturbance may interact with other factors (brain damage, starvation, cultural factors) to cause autism in young boys and anorexia nervosa in pre-pubertal girls?'

Since then, growing research has attempted to elucidate the nature of the relationship between the two disorders, focusing on both elevated presence of ASD in anorexia nervosa and shared underlying difficulties in cognitive, social and emotional functioning. One particularly interesting consideration is the difficulty with 'interoception' that is seen in both conditions. In other words, people struggle to perceive what is going on inside their body – they almost literally lack 'gut feeling' and do not notice or misinter-pret feelings of emptiness or fullness, for instance.

The apparent association has been fruitful in many fields of research and practice, calling into question traditional diagnostic boundaries, highlighting the underdiagnosis of ASD in females, and of anorexia nervosa in males, generating new treatments that take account of the best ways to work alongside people with ASD to support people with anorexia, and collaborating with people with lived experience of each or both of the conditions to demand that impoverished or non-existent services be improved.

However, some of the leading experts in the field have examined the evidence and urge caution on conflating the roots of anorexia nervosa and ASD. Westwood and Tchanturia (2017) summarised current understanding. They point out that studies are somewhat unsatisfactory in using differing assessment tools and inconsistent recruitment approaches from patient groups. It is clear that virtually all the studies consistently report higher than expected ASD symptoms amongst people with anorexia nervosa. What cannot be shown from present research is whether these symptoms represent an underlying common neurodevelopmental disorder or whether they are mere similarities in cognitive and socioemotional functioning, which may be seen in other psychiatric diagnoses.

Whilst we await further research, it's helpful to be aware of both the likely increase of eating and feeding disorders in people with ASD of both genders. We should also use ASD-friendly approaches to people with eating and feeding disorders as they may have an undiagnosed ASD condition.

ASD and Suicide

Anecdotal reports that autistic people are more likely to die by suicide have been validated by a large and well-constructed study based on Danish data. Researchers (Kõlves et al., 2021) used the Danish a nationwide database to analyse data of more than 6 million people ages 10 and older living in Denmark from 1995 to 2016. More than 35 000 people had a diagnosis of ASD. The key finding was that people with ASD had a more than three-fold higher rate of both 'suicide attempt' and death by suicide than people not diagnosed with ASD.

Among autistic people who attempted suicide or died by suicide, 90% had a co-occurring mental health condition. The researchers also found that high-functioning autistic people were at higher risk of suicide and speculated that this may be because as they were less likely to be closely monitored and supported. Recently, a study suggested that a high proportion of people who died by suicide had shown many autistic traits and could have been suffering from undiagnosed autism (Cassidy et al., 2022).

Social and Sexual Issues

Students with ASD find themselves at university with an additional "hidden curriculum" of social rules that people expect each other to just know without being taught. Sexual behaviour in society has traditionally relied for decades, even centuries, on implied rather than explicit communication and – obviously – on body language. This can be a nightmare for individuals who require much more explicit, specific and literal information, and for whom experience of body language is more an expression of their need for self-soothing ('stimming') than a subtle communication of desire or approach. On top of these problems, student sexual etiquette in the 21st century is a minefield of assumptions and conflicting codes (see Chapter 12), although the etiquette of requesting and confirming explicit consent to sexual behaviour is being introduced and taught in university campaigns.

Students with ASD often appear naïve. They may be told by their peers as a joke to say something or do something that is sexually inappropriate, and they may be at risk of being taken serious advantage of sexually. The mental health consequences include anxiety, and of course traumatic stress responses.

Students on the autism spectrum must often be explicitly taught what is appropriate to say to a person he or she may find attractive (or indeed to someone they do not). These students may have had sex education at high school but now need reminder discussions appropriate to their developmental level. This includes how to protect themselves from disease and unwanted pregnancy. There are also more complex discussions to be had about maintaining longer-term couple relationships beyond the first few dates, and about ending relationships and surviving rejection.

There are a range of books and online resources that explicitly explain scenarios not only for the student with ASD but also for someone dating a person with ASD, and many very witty and engaging personal accounts of sex and romance on forums and blogs. These are all too often transient or quickly out of date. This book prefers to offer direction to formal organisations that have the resource to keep them updated and that are subjected to scrutiny and constructive criticism by membership and reputable funders. At the time of writing, the UK National Autistic Society focuses mostly on sex education for parents and children, but the US Organization for Autism Research provides a freely available multimedia series of modules on sexual behaviour for people over age 15 (researchautism.org).

Interventions to Support Students with ASD

Given the vulnerability of people with ASD to mental illness and other psychosocial problems, preventative measures are particularly important and worthwhile.

Environmental Modification

Most of the NICE (2018) guideline recommendations for supporting people with ASD in NHS settings have equal validity in university environments. Whenever there are opportunities for new building, or redecoration of old facilities, involving students and staff with ASD is good practice. It is worth remembering that an individual's specialist equipment and support needs expenses can be claimed from the DSA.

The key principles in planning a mentally healthy built environment for people with ASD are

- Reducing sensory overstimulation and
- Improving predictability

Sensory issues can be addressed by using low-arousal colours like cream on walls and furnishings, avoiding detailed and prominent patterning, reducing noisy, harsh or echoing acoustics with screens, carpets or special baffles, and taking care that smells, however delicious, from kitchens and canteens do not leak into learning spaces. Fluorescent lighting should be reduced or shaded as much as possible, and glare from sunny windows shielded with blinds. Unlike schools, universities do not oblige students to wear uniform so students are blessedly liberated from itchy fabrics or tight school ties, and they will be encouraged rather than discouraged from using their own personal adjustments such as dark glasses, baseball caps and ear defenders to mitigate sensory overload. Some students find that they are still distracted and distressed by the noise and movement of others around them and will often benefit from an individual room for examinations, and a small side room where lectures can be live streamed to them.

Predictability can be increased with appropriate signage – but not to the extent of having crowded, jarring notices and posters everywhere. Continuity of staffing in libraries, receptionists, residence staff and servers in food outlets, is much appreciated. Being readily identifiable because of a dress code or coloured lanyards and badges is important but does not preclude the need for people to introduce themselves and their roles explicitly until these are clearly known and remembered. In this way staff build up trust and a sense of security. They can act as calming influences and as human signposting. Training both academic and non-academic staff to use language and behaviour that is helpful to the ASD community results is appreciated by the whole community.

Private sector accommodation can prove more restful than halls of residence, which tend to be noisy.

Teaching, Mentoring and Buddying Support

Again, the key task is to help the person manage change and over-stimulation. University and college can be much less predictable than high school. Clashing course commitments can cause anxiety in many students, especially those whose anxiety levels are already high. Planning ahead, providing the student with their schedule of classes and assignments at the beginning of each semester offers helpful predictability.

Many students with ASD say they are 'visual learners' and benefit from maps, diagrams and being shown rather than told what to do. In the same way, written and printed timetables that provide an overview are more memorable and soothing than relying on sporadic electronic prompts.

Although ASD often co-occurs with ADHD and specific learning disabilities, in practice social-emotional misunderstandings or confusions and sensory overload are the most likely problems to crop up in the classroom. A good place to start is by ensuring that the location of the learning experience is calm. The appearance of the room matters, but perhaps even more crucial is to make sure there are no distracting or frightening noises. A large echoing lecture hall can be transformed by carpets, soft furnishings, allocated seating and peaceful student behaviour.

Difficulty with social relationships does not mean that the student with ASD always does better with solitary learning. They often prefer to learn with authoritative adults in one-to-one settings, or in settings where interaction is not expected such as lectures, although the environment of a large lecture hall may be intolerable as we have said. They may be able to cope with and even enjoy peer group interaction if it is well-structured and task oriented.

Because students with ASD struggle to decipher social cues, teachers find it best to maintain a calm tone of voice, particularly when providing feedback. Increased excitement or volume in the tone of voice may be misinterpreted and eclipse the meaning of the words. The use of explicit, concrete language is good teaching practice at the undergraduate level in any case, but especially helpful to students with ASD.

Students with ASD tend to develop passions (even fixations) on specific topics, objects, or interests. Their knowledge of these narrowly focused areas of expertise can be impressive and demonstrate the level of mastery a student is capable of. Teachers can capitalise on that motivation by relating new skills to the topic of fascination.

It is always worth having an agreed crisis plan in case the student feels overwhelmed. This often involves taking a break and going outside for a while. Better still, learning should be broken up into routines with frequent predictable breaks so that the person with ASD can recharge.

> The most important piece of practical help I have received at uni is around exams. I can now be assessed through coursework rather than exams. I find coursework much less anxiety provoking, and it allows me to achieve in ways exams never could. This has made more of a difference than I can explain and allows me to demonstrate my knowledge in a much more accurate way.
>
> Another thing that has helped has been to have content broken down into smaller sections. This is particularly valuable when I am feeling overwhelmed. Taking the time to sit with me and help me untangle everything has been invaluable, and I am incredibly grateful to the staff members who give their time to help me when I need it.
>
> On the topic of staff, knowing there are people I can go to when I'm having a panic attack or feeling overwhelmed, and who can help me calm down, has been incredibly helpful. The staff in my department have been amazing, not only with helping me in the moment, but also in helping me learn to manage my anxieties. Regular contact with my personal tutor has made a world of difference, as has having 'safe' people.
>
> Finally, having advance notice about anything out of the ordinary is incredibly helpful. By allowing me the extra time to process things before they happen, I am able to cope with them a lot better. This can range from things such as having a different lecturer, a different location, or what the content of the lecture will be.
>
> Elizabeth Blackwell Institute for Health Research (2020)

Intensive Support Projects for Students with ASD

One recent US study evaluated a multi-facetted university programme for autistic students (Zukerman et al., 2022). As part of their participation, autistic students lived in an on-campus residence with a peer-mentor without autism who was instructed to promote positive social interaction, and also frequently attended social events with other students with ASD and peer-mentors. They drew on evidence that social anxiety is a strong predictor of failure to thrive, and studies that demonstrated benefits of peer mentor ('buddy') interventions, to measure benefits over a year of the programme.

The researchers hypothesised that such levels of exposure to dyadic and group social interaction would lead to improved adaptive behaviour and reduced levels of psychiatric symptoms by the end of the year. All students with ASD who had been offered the programme over the 14 years of its existence had accepted so they believed it would be unethical to have a control group who were deprived of the programme. They set up a form of control group in terms of a group of students without ASD, some with social anxiety and some without. Neither of these groups had access to the programme so the comparison was less than ideal.

By the end of the year, the students with ASD had statistically significant reduction in depressive symptom reductions. The other two groups of students did not, so this is suggestive of benefits from the programme. It might be possible to repeat the experiment at a university that has not already embedded such a programme, so that adding in more intense support could be compared with a more realistic control group. Meanwhile, it would be fascinating to hear more about the experience of the peer mentors themselves, in terms of their motivation for participating, the benefits and difficulties they experienced and useful advice for others taking up the role.

It was impressive to see that the mentors were given considerable support and supervision. If the scheme were to be rolled out in the UK, issues of payment, insurance and training would be particularly important. These mentors received a residence stipend, attended two-hour group meetings with program coordinators two to three times each semester to discuss autism, expectations/instructions (e.g., setting boundaries with mentees, communication techniques) and university procedures (e.g., exams, academic accommodations, program policies).

ASD and COVID

The health and safety measures put in place to mitigate the impacts of COVID have proved particularly disruptive for some autistic individuals. The social withdrawal involved may have been almost a plus in some cases, but the unpredictable frequent changes to regulations was highly distressing. Facial recognition in masks and other PPE became even more challenging for people with ASD who struggle with facial recognition and with interpreting facial expression.

Some people with ASD developed an intensive preoccupation with the infection. This could have driven some of the innovative work against the pandemic. Others suffered from obsessive health anxiety. Emerging from lockdown restrictions has involved further uncertainty, change and disruption, and for those who still fear infection it may be hard to venture back into company.

Physical distancing, restrictions on activities, new telework arrangements, and the shift to virtual learning can cause significant disruptions to precious daily routines, and some students found themselves trapped either in halls or in their parents' homes, which could become overcrowded or noisy. Anecdotally, some people with ASD told us they welcomed solitary home working at first and only later discovered how isolated and lonely they had become.

Early research on young people with ASD as we emerge form lockdown suggested that overall, they engaged less in physical activity and more in screen time. Both are behaviours that increase risk of depression.

Resources for Autism

The National Autistic Society autism.org.uk

Organization for Autistic Research https://researchautism.org/

Silberman, S. (2017). *Neurotribes: The legacy of autism and how to think smarter about people who think differently.* Atlantic Books.

Hendrickx, S. (2015). *Women and girls with autism spectrum disorder: Understanding life experiences from early childhood to old age.* Jessica Kingsley Publishers.

McKibbin, K. (2015). *Life on the autism spectrum-a guide for girls and women.* Jessica Kingsley Publishers – follows the story of Alison, a girl diagnosed with Asperger Syndrome, through both childhood and adulthood.

Attention Deficit Hyperactivity Disorder

ADHD is the other main neurodevelopmental condition recognised in major diagnostic classifications. People with ADHD experience troublesome levels in inattention, of hyperactivity and impulsivity across all the different contexts of their lives. In some cases, the person behaves in ways that might be normal for a much younger child. The past two decades have brought a fundamental shift in understanding the essence, of the disorder so that it no longer seen as a matter of problem behaviour, but as a result of different kind of brain function.

The term ADHD was not in common use until the 1980s, but British psychologist Cyril Burt (1937) described a category of the "excitable and unrepressed child" in his book on the "backward child" in 1937. In the same year, Charles Bradley (1937) published a paper describing the effects of psychostimulant medication in school students with various behaviour disorders. He writes

> The psychological reactions of 30 behavior problem children who received Benzedrine sulfate for one week were observed. There was a spectacular improvement in school performance in half of the children. A large proportion of the patients became emotionally subdued without, however, losing interest in their surroundings. A variety of other definite behavior changes were also noted.

We now see ADHD as a common mental health disorder that begins in childhood. We now recognise that it frequently persists into adulthood. The diagnostic criteria were originally developed for children, and childhood hyperactive behaviours tend to subside with age or may be replaced by an inner restlessness, which is difficult to quantify. However, characteristics such as inattentiveness, organisational problems and impulsivity often persist. In the past adults with ADHD may have relied on finding places in society where these symptoms could be accommodated. Some, as they grew older managed to figure out ways to cope with their condition. Others did not cope and failed to thrive after leaving school.

ADHD commonly co-occurs with other specific learning disabilities, neurodevelopmental conditions (such as ASD, dyslexia and dyspraxia), mental health conditions, and physical health problems. The diagnosis usually arises when the child or young person is obliged to try to fit into social structures that demand much more self-regulation, sustained attention and control for longer periods than they can they manage. Attendance at nursery or school is the usual prompt for diagnosis, although the characteristics have been present in the child from the start of their life.

Like ASD, ADHD appears to be one end of a spectrum across the population. There is no clear cut-off for diagnosing the condition, any more than we can state a precise height at which we describe someone as 'tall'. This of course leads to controversy as to whether a treatable disorder actually exists. There is growing criticism of the tendency to 'medicalise' normal experience. In the case of ADHD there is concern that pharmaceutical companies stand to make profit from prescribing of the condition and so may influence increased diagnosis. In such a situation, clinicians have no simple 'cut off' point, but need to assess in each individual whether having a diagnosis and potentially treatment is more likely to be helpful or harmful to the student's flourishing, both now and in the future.

Both cognitive and emotional problems are well documented in ADHD. It is often associated with difficulties in working memory, in response inhibition (so that students blurt out comments without having time to consider them), and in organisation. Like the symptoms of inattention, difficulties in these areas may become more apparent as the demands of school, work and university increase (Brown, 2009).

Alongside the intellectual problems, ADHD is often associated with problems in emotion regulation, mood, and irritability, which cause disabling interpersonal problems, including difficulties getting on with parents, teachers, doctors and other authority figures – the very people needed to help with assessment and support.

In contrast with those high-functioning individuals with ASD, who would not want to be relieved of their condition and see it as a fundamental and even welcome part of their personality, people with ADHD are more likely to want to be relieved of their symptoms, although there are advantages. For instance, ADHS can confer the ability to maintain an unusually prolonged and intense level of attention for tasks the person finds interesting or rewarding; this is known as hyperfocus.

The Particular Relevance of ADHD for Students

Even getting to university can be challenging in the context of ADHD, although sympathetic parents and teachers, and often the benefits of medication, can provide support. These are withdrawn when a student leaves home, school and the CAMHS environment. University then demands self-directed study, attending classes in different places at different times, note-taking, time management of course work and submission, and on top of these, taking charge of all the ordinary arrangements of life. We do not yet have a comprehensive review of the impact of ADHD on the educational outcomes of university students in the UK or even the rest of Europe. A comprehensive review of the (mostly North American) literature about university students with ADHD was conducted by Sedgwick (2018).

The review found that on the whole these students showed poorer performance in time-limited exams and overall academic achievement. They tended to get lower classes of degree. Students with ADHD also reported lower levels of social adjustment, social skills, and self-esteem in relationships. Some research found that ADHD put students at increased risk of overuse of the internet and social media, and they were considerably more likely than peers to misuse tobacco, alcohol and other licit or illicit substances.

The review found that students could offset their struggles to some extent by positive mental attitudes and engagement in physical exercise, and intellectually gifted students, especially female students, used their intelligence to cope despite the obstacles. These are the so-called twice-exceptional or 2e students who are gifted but have some form of disability, usually ASD, ADHD, dyslexia or dyspraxia. The concept is still a controversial one and not recognised in the Diagnostic and Statistical Manual of Mental Disorders or the International Classification of Diseases and Related Health Problems. It is the case, though that students who get good grades but still report ADHD symptoms are most at risk of not getting diagnosed and treated.

Just before the COVID pandemic, the UK Adult ADHD Network convened a meeting of practitioners and experts from England, Wales, and Scotland, to discuss issues that university students with ADHD can experience or present with during their programme of studies and how best to address them. They published a helpful and hopefully influential report on the collective analysis, evaluation, and opinions of the expert panel and published literature about the impact of ADHD on university students (Sedgwick-Müller et al., 2022).

Jeremy was a gifted classical violinist and folk fiddler, from a large family of artists and musicians. He could turn his hand to almost any instrument. His music teachers at a large comprehensive school had appreciated his talents and treated him as part of the 'music department family'. His forgetfulness and disorganisation were tolerated as part of his personality. Even his heavy smoking was overlooked, and peers looked after him out of appreciation for his gifts and sweetness of temperament.

When he moved away to a Conservatoire where he knew few people, he found it impossible to find his way on time to classes in different buildings, he fell out with flatmates because of the noise of his practising, and he began to drink heavily. He dropped out before the end of the first term and returned home, very depressed.

He was referred to a psychiatrist who identified probable ADHD alongside his depressive symptoms. Treatment was successful, though partly because he was now back with a group of people who supported and appreciated him. He signed up for a less prestigious course, but was able to part-fund his studies with what he earned from local 'gigs' and other part time work in the music world.

Prevalence

The reported worldwide prevalence of ADHD in adults is 2%–3%. A UK study suggested 7% students self-reported above-threshold symptoms of ADHD. The prevalence of ADHD was reported to be around 5% in the United States and 8% in a Chinese student cohort (Sedgwick-Müller et al., 2022). The very term 'disorder' means that a person's symptoms are bad enough to cause problems in daily living. It is not surprising that the prevalence of 'disorder' is higher in university life, because symptoms that prove disabling in an academic context may not count as disabling in life outside a university.

On the other hand, the rates of ADHD, including undiagnosed ADHD, are very high in people attending mental health services. Eberhard et al. (2022) studied young people in the student age range (18–25 years) who were first-time attenders at a Stockholm psychiatry clinic. Careful in-depth assessments revealed that 63% of these young people met criteria for either ADHD or ASD or both. Most of the patients, particularly the young women, had not been diagnosed in childhood. For instance, 48% of the female clinic patients met criteria for ADHD, though only 12% of them had been given this diagnosis in childhood. Amongst children diagnosed with ADHD there is famously a high proportion of boys, but the ratio in this clinic was even higher. Their findings underscore the importance of screening for ASD and ADHD in adult psychiatric services regardless of referral reason, so that treatments can take account of all aspects of the individual's mental profile.

Assessment in Universities

In the past there was some stigma about an ADHD diagnosis. Parents often worried that it reflected on their ability to properly 'control' their child. Other children might tease the child for 'being special needs'. Teachers would suspect it was a euphemistic excuse for naughtiness or just another disruptive threat to an orderly classroom, general practitioners (GPs) and even some psychiatrists insisting that no such condition existed. It was pointed out that the apparent 'epidemic' seen in the United States might be amplified by the opportunities of pharmaceutical companies to sell medication.

These days, whilst we are of course concerned to avoid 'over medicalising' the normal difficulties of everyday life, and rightly wary of flooding a community with drugs that have potential street value and unknown long-term effects, most professionals accept that there is indeed a treatable condition, known as ADHD. We realise now that people do not necessarily 'grow out' of the condition as they reach adulthood, and many adults are now keen to have their struggles validated by having a diagnosis. Because the condition tends to run in families, parents often identify their own ADHD when their children are diagnosed.

Self-diagnosis, using online resources, has become extremely common, but finding a recognised NHS or even private clinic to conduct a thorough assessment is exceedingly hard. I am often contacted by desperate friends and colleagues asking to be signposted to services either for themselves or their student children. Meanwhile, in my clinics, I commonly meet people – especially young women in the perinatal clinic – who have been referred for symptoms of depression, anxiety or eating disorders, but who use the referral opportunity to tell me about their belief they may have ADHD and ask whether I can officially confirm this. Often they are right, and approaching parenthood is an appropriate time to receive support and treatment. Sometimes, though, it emerges that their symptoms are better explained by a diagnosis of ASD, or even by diagnosing both conditions together. Whole families can benefit from an accurate diagnosis and plan.

One problem for students with ADHD is that it is commonly classified in educational settings as a specific learning difficulty, rather than as a mental health condition (see www.hesa.ac.uk/collection/c17051/a/disable). It is still classified as a 'disability' under the Equality Act 2010, which gives universities the responsibility to make reasonable adjustments to remove systemic barriers and provide extra support for disabled students, to enable them to engage fully in their programmes of study and to benefit from university life in general. There are also disadvantages to this, though.

Data collected about students with ADHD is gathered all together with that collected about students with the other specific learning difficulties, such as dyslexia for instance.

This means that we do not have the extremely useful figures on numbers of students with ADHD in each institution, or any details on their progress in comparison with that of students with other conditions.

The other big disadvantage is that within the NHS, ADHD is, in contrast, regarded as a mental health disorder, and one that may require the prescribing of a controlled drug (the psychostimulant medications are Class B and Section 2 drugs). Under NICE (2018) guidelines, diagnosis is a specialist-only diagnosis, with GPs providing support to specialist services through shared care protocols. Adults who turn to private services for a diagnosis may face having to continue to pay for private prescriptions, as GPs do not usually recognise such diagnostic pathways in their protocols. This can be the case when parents have paid for a private assessment for their student child.

Substantial costs, both financial and otherwise can arise from delayed treatment. Students who have already invested in large student loans and started courses with enthusiasm really struggle with the typical 1–2-year delay on NHS waiting lists. Under-performance at university can have a long-term negative impact on someone's career and drop-out can be a real risk. For these students, the misuse of caffeine products or non-prescribed stimulants may become attractive options for self-medication.

The UK Adult ADHD Network recommend that students with possible ADHD should therefore be fast-tracked for an initial assessment by NHS services, but in many areas such services are so far very sparse, and it is not only students for whom long waits can be disastrous. Young working adults with demanding jobs and families to care for might be even further disadvantaged if the student population were prioritised in principle.

Universities might alleviate the problem somewhat by collaborating with NHS clinicians to design a formal training in assessment and monitoring of ADHD in adults. This might be acquired by mental health professionals both within and outside universities, and accredited so that GPs could negotiate protocols with these trained professionals, calling in the expertise of identified Psychiatrists only when needed.

Vulnerability to Other Mental Health Conditions

ADHD is associated with other neurodevelopmental and mental disorders as well as some non-psychiatric disorders, which can cause additional impairment, especially in modern society.

In a study by Anastopoulos et al. (2018) in a sample of university students with ADHD, 55% had at least one comorbid mental illness and 32% had two or more, most commonly depressive and anxiety disorders. A paper published in the same year looking at the Swedish general adult population with ADHD found very similar figures (Chen et al., 2018). In a Swedish population database study, 50% women and 35% men with ADHD had depression or anxiety disorders. 30% women and 40% men with ADHD had substance misuse disorders.

Treating ADHD may be a way of reducing the burden of risks to both mental and physical health that result from 'self-medication' and impulsive behaviours. These involve smoking, alcohol and other substance misuse, risk taking, accidents, and the stresses that arise when people become overwhelmed and cannot organise their lives, as well as the distress when interpersonal and academic goals are lost. Once such disorders have occurred, it is important but not sufficient to treat the ADHD. The secondary disorder must be treated in its own right.

ADHD and Eating Disorders

Here we will focus on eating disorders in the context of ADHD; eating disorders are discussed more broadly in Chapter 5. Swedish database material (Yao et al., 2019) has shown that there is an increased risk of all types of eating disorders in people with ADHD but that from a genetic point of view, ADHD is more closely associated with the eating disorders bulimia nervosa and binge eating disorder (BED) than with anorexia nervosa.

The similarities between BED and ADHD are particularly interesting. The commonest of the main eating disorders, BED is a psychiatric disorder characterised by loss of control leading to frequent, compulsive episodes of excessive eating (binges). The diagnostic criterion of 'a sense of lack of control of eating during the episode', implies that BED is a classical impulse control disorder. There is an emerging body of clinical evidence to show that a loss of impulse control in BED is a causal factor in bingeing on palatable foods. Heal and Smith (2022) found evidence supporting the hypothesis that BED is an impulse control disorder with similarities to ADHD, including responsiveness to stimulant drugs. In the case of BED, the drug lisdexamfetamine has been approved to treat BED in the United States but not in the UK.

People who have BED are more likely to be overweight or obese, so it would be interesting to see whether people diagnosed with both disorders are less likely to be overweight and to show BED symptoms when treated for ADHD. It is commonly observed in children who take stimulant drugs to treat their ADHD that they lose appetite somewhat and become underweight. Indeed, parents are encouraged to give 'drug holidays' outside school term time to avoid growth being affected.

ADHD and Suicide

Balazs and Kereszteny (2017) conducted a systematic review of the evidence and confirmed previous suspicions that ADHD confers an increased risk of 'suicidality' in both sexes and in all age groups. As in the case of ASD, the risk is mediated by the increased occurrence of comorbid mental disorders in people with ADHD. It was interesting that in both forms of neurodiversity, females were almost as likely as males to die by suicide compared with the predominantly male deaths in the 'neurotypical' population.

On the basis of these findings, the authors urge clinicians to screen patients attending mental health clinics for suicidal ideas. In fact, psychiatrists and other mental health staff are emphatically taught to make this a regular part of enquiries with all patients. Sadly, it is not always possible to know how a patient who is sober and hopeful in an afternoon clinic might feel later that night, perhaps after 'partying', and in the case of people with ADHD, the impulsivity that characterises the condition can make risk assessment even harder.

Management of ADHD

Educational Support

In addition to treatment for the disorder, many students with ADHD require adjustments to the University structures. Because of distractibility and poor 'working memory' they may take more time to digest complex concepts and organise their work on the page. In examinations they can benefit from extra writing time, a quiet room at from others to reduce distractions, with an invigilator who is familiar with ADHD. They benefit from being given breaks rather than having to sit for long stretches. Outside examinations academic coaching and mentoring can assist with planning ahead and organisational skills and prevent the student falling behind. Procrastination, misjudgement of how long tasks take, and forgetfulness, are all common features of the condition, so that agreed flexibility in deadlines may be necessary. Sometimes, a good solution is for the student to study on a part time schedule rather than complete the degree in the usual 3 or 4 years. Sadly, this may be unacceptable because of wanting to keep up with a peer group.

Physical Exercise

The physical benefits of moderate to vigorous physical activity are well known, and the antidepressant effect is such that NICE guidelines recommend exercise as a first line treatment. Sedgwick-Müller (2022) summarises evidence that aerobic physical activity can improve attention and other cognitive functioning in older adults and improve attention deficits and other ADHD symptoms in children over and above the benefits of methylphenidate treatment.

Medication

Pharmacological treatment with stimulants (methylphenidate or lisdexamfetamine) is recommended as the first line treatment for adults with ADHD by NICE (2018) 'if their symptoms are still causing significant impairment in at least one domain after environmental modifications'.

The stimulant medications, related to amphetamines, include methylphenidate (sold under brands such as Ritalin, Concerta and Equasym), dexamphetamine (Dexadrine) and lisdexamfetamine (Elvanse). They work quickly, but the effect wears off quickly too. Slow-release preparations mean the student can usually take tablets just once a day. The dose will usually be more than that prescribed for children, so students already diagnosed may need adjustments to the dose to remain effective. Many students prefer the flexible use of prescribed stimulant medication with optimum doses during times of essay writing and exam preparation, and no medication between terms and on days without academic work. This is a pattern of use often recommended to children, so they may already have established this pattern.

Jenna was diagnosed with ADHD as a teenager and managed successfully, using physical exercise as a strategy to help cope. At university she was delighted to have a mental health mentor, who prompted her to stay organised, not only with her studies, but also when her financial situation became chaotic.

As exams approached, she found herself spending more time in the library and less in the gym. She also began to struggle with binge eating, which had been a previous problem despite cognitive behavioural therapy at age 16. She decided to accept the option of taking Ritalin, despite her family's misgivings.

There was no miracle in terms of studying, but she did find herself bingeing less and was delighted to tell her mentor that she had not scraped her car since starting the medication. The mentor was not aware that she was driving and was concerned to hear that Jenna had had several accidents at the wheel, though luckily these had been fairly minor.

If stimulants cannot be tolerated or are ineffective, atomoxetine (Strattera) is a 'non-stimulant' medication. This takes longer – perhaps several weeks – to become effective, compared with stimulant medications.

Medication does not cure the condition any more than painkillers cure arthritis. Benefits are lost if the medication is stopped. Pharmacological treatment of ADHD appears to protect against substance use disorders in people with ADHD. However, it is reasonable to be cautious about risks of 'sharing' or even selling medication as 'smart drugs' to peers.

One systematic review of 176 studies about the long-term educational outcomes of untreated versus treated ADHD found that students who were treated for their ADHD had better academic outcomes than students with untreated ADHD (Arnold et al., 2015). Those who were treated with both medication and psychosocial treatments did better than those who had either of these alone. However, we still need to better understand how university students with ADHD adjust to life at university, the academic challenges they face, and how these are managed or overcome.

Resources for ADHD

www.rcpsych.ac.uk/mental-health/problems-disorders/adhd-in-adults – Information package as part of the Royal College of Psychiatrists' information series for patients, carers, family and friends
https://ivypanda.com/blog/adhd-definitive-guide/ – US website with useful hints on managing studies and other aspects of life at university
adhduk.co.uk– UK-based and, unlike much of the ADHD material that focusses on children, this has much on adult and student ADHD.

Practice Points

At a Societal Level

- We should all, whatever our role, increase awareness that students with ADHD and particularly ASD are particularly vulnerable to developing mental health disorders, which appear to increase the prevalence of suicide in this group of people. The neurodevelopmental condition acts as an amplifier to the mental illness in causing suicide.
- Despite growing interest in both ASD and ADHD in young adults, many people who could benefit from diagnosis have not received it. These people are even more vulnerable as they are not provided with the support available to students with neurodiversity.

At the Level of University Authorities and Policies

- Universities should recognise neurodiversity as conferring risk for mental health conditions and suicide. Evidence-based support and monitoring can reduce the risk of these occurring and can also reduce dropout and improve academic and psychosocial outcomes for these students.
- Staff training in recognition and management of neurodiverse conditions should be delivered at levels appropriate to staff roles.
- ADHD waiting lists at NHS clinics are too long. University mental health staff may be able to create recognised training programmes and negotiate agreements about diagnosis and prescribing with local GPs.

Mental Health Clinicians

- Professionals need to be aware of underdiagnosis of both ASD and ADHD in girls and probably in ethnic and other minority groups.
- Creative solutions are needed so that students do not wait for years on waiting lists.

Teachers, Parents, Tutors, Directors of Studies and Fellow Students

- Lay people who take on caring or 'buddying' roles for people with neurodiversity need to be well-supported within a helping community rather than expected to shoulder responsibility alone.

References

Anastopoulos, A. D., DuPaul, G. D., Weyandt, L. L., et al. (2018). Rates and patterns of comorbidity among first-year college students with ADHD. *Journal of Clinical Child & Adolescent Psychology*, 47(2), 236–47.

Arnold, L. E., Hodgkins, P., Kahle, J., Madhoo, M. & Kewley, G. (2015). Long-term outcomes of ADHD: Academic achievement and performance. *Journal of Attention Disorders*, 24(1), 73–85.

Balazs, J. & Kereszteny, A. (2017). Attention-deficit/hyperactivity disorder and suicide: A systematic review. *World Journal of Psychiatry*, 7(1), 44–59. https://doi.org/10.5498/wjp.v7.i1.44

Bradley, C. (1937). The behavior of children receiving benzedrine. *American Journal of Psychiatry*, 94(3), 577–85.

Brown, T. E., Reichel, P. C. & Quinlan, D. M. (2009). Executive function impairments in high IQ adults with ADHD. *Journal of Attention Disorders*, 13(2), 161–7.

Brugha, T, McManus, S., Bankart, J., et al. (2011). Epidemiology of autism spectrum disorders in adults in the community in England. *Archives of General Psychiatry*, 68(5), 459–65.

Burt, C. (1937). *The backward child*. London: University of London Press.

Cassidy, S., Au-Yeung, S., Robertson, A., et al. (2022). Autism and autistic traits in those who died by suicide in England. *The British Journal of Psychiatry*, 221(5), 683–91. https://doi.org/10.1192/bjp.2022.21

Chen, Q., Hartman, C. A., Haavik, J., et al. (2018). Common psychiatric and metabolic comorbidity of adult attention-deficit/hyperactivity disorder: A population-based cross-sectional study. *PLoS ONE*, 13(9), e0204516.

Eberhard, D., Billstedt, E. & Gillberg, C. (2022). Neurodevelopmental disorders and comorbidity in young adults attending a psychiatric outpatient clinic. *Psychiatry Research*, 313, 114638.

Elizabeth Blackwell Institute for Health Research (2020, 9 December). *Autism at university – being an autistic student*. University of Bristol.

Ghaziuddin, M., Ghaziuddin, N. & Greden, J. (2002). Depression in persons with autism: Implications for research and clinical care. *Journal of Autism Developmental Disorders*, 32, 299–306. https://doi.org/10.1023/A:1016330802348

Gillberg, C. (1983). Are autism and anorexia nervosa related? *The British Journal of Psychiatry*, 142(4), 428.

Griffin, E. & Pollak, D. (2009). Student experiences of neurodiversity in higher education: Insights from the BRAINHE project. *Dyslexia*, 15(1), 23–41.

Gurbuz, E., Hanley, M. & Riby, D. M. (2019). University students with autism: The social and academic experiences of university in the UK. *Journal of Autism and Developmental Disorders*, 49(2), 617–31.

Heal, D. J. & Smith, S. L. (2022). Prospects for new drugs to treat binge-eating disorder: Insights from psychopathology and neuropharmacology. *Journal of Psychopharmacology*, 36(6), 680–703.

Hollocks, M. J., Lerh, J. W., Magiati, I., Meiser-Stedman, R. & Brugha, T. S. (2019). Anxiety and depression in adults with autism spectrum disorder: A systematic review and meta-analysis. *Psychological Medicine*, 49(4), 559–72.

Kiani, R., Alexander, R. & Brugha, T. (2018). The prevalence of autism spectrum disorders in adult psychiatric inpatients: A systematic review. *Clinical Practice and Epidemiology in Mental Health: CP & EMH*, 14, 177.

Kõlves, K., Fitzgerald, C., Nordentoft, M., Wood, S. J. & Erlangsen, A. (2021). Assessment of suicidal behaviors among individuals with autism spectrum disorder in Denmark. *JAMA Network Open*, 4(1), e2033565. https://doi.org/10.1001/jamanetworkopen.2020.33565

Lang, R., Koegel, L. K., Ashbaugh, K., et al. (2010). Physical exercise and individuals with autism spectrum disorders: A systematic review. *Research in Autism Spectrum Disorders*, 4(4), 565–76.

Lever, A. & Geurts, H. (2016). Psychiatric co-occurring symptoms and disorders in young, middle-aged, and older adults with autism spectrum disorder. *Journal of Autism and Developmental Disorders*, 46(6), 1916–30.

MacLeod, A. & Green, S. (2009). Beyond the books: Case study of a collaborative and holistic support model for university students with Asperger syndrome. *Studies in Higher Education*, 34(6), 631–46.

National Institute for Health and Care Excellence (2012). *Autism spectrum disorder in adults: Diagnosis and management.* www.nice.org.uk/Guidance/CG142

National Institute for Health and Care Excellence (2018). *Attention deficit hyperactivity disorder: Diagnosis and management.* http://nice.org.uk/guidance/ng87

Newman, L., Wagner, M., Huang, T., et al. (2011). *Secondary school programs and performance of students with disabilities: A special topic report of findings from the National Longitudinal Transition Study-2 (NLTS2). NCSER 2012-3000.* National Center for Special Education Research.

Sedgwick, J. A. (2018 University students with attention deficit hyperactivity disorder (ADHD): A literature review. *Irish Journal of Psychological Medicine*, 35(3), 221–35.

Sedgwick Müller, J. A., Müller-Sedgwick, U., Adamou, M., et al. (2022). University students with attention deficit hyperactivity disorder (ADHD): A consensus statement from the UK Adult ADHD Network (UKAAN). *BMC Psychiatry*, 22, 292. https://doi.org/10.1186/s12888-022-03898-z

Tromans, S., Chester, V., Kiani, R., Alexander, R. & Brugha, T. (2018). The prevalence of autism spectrum disorders in adult psychiatric inpatients: A systematic review. *Clinical Practice & Epidemiology in Mental Health: CP & EMH*, 14, 177.

VanBergeijk, E., Klin, A. & Volkmar, F. (2008). Supporting more able students on the autism spectrum: College and beyond. *Journal of Autism and Developmental Disorders*, 38, 1359–70. https://doi.org/10.1007/s10803-007-0524-8

Westwood, H. & Tchanturia, K. (2017). Autism spectrum disorder in anorexia nervosa: An updated literature review. *Current Psychiatry Reports*, 19(7), 1–10.

World Health Organization (2022). *ICD-11: International classification of diseases (11th revision).* https://icd.who.int/

Yao, S., Kuja-Halkola, R., Martin, J., et al. (2019). Associations between attention-deficit/hyperactivity disorder and various eating disorders: A Swedish nationwide population study using multiple genetically informative approaches. *Biological Psychiatry*, 86(8), 577–86.

Zukerman, G., Yahav, G. & Ben-Itzchak, E. (2022). Adaptive behavior and psychiatric symptoms in university students with ASD: One-year longitudinal study. *Psychiatry Research*, 315, 114701.

11 Ethnically Diverse University Communities

Challenges for Students and Staff from Black, Asian and Other Minority Ethnic Backgrounds

Zara was academically bright and a strong athlete. She went to a run-down school in an area of Birmingham where Black families were in the majority. She thrived at her first university, an institution in Inner London with a racially diverse student population, and an equally diverse community outside.

She won a prestigious graduate scholarship to the University of Cambridge and found herself 'suddenly in this bizarre little town in East Anglia'. She felt that people did not really 'get' her sense of humour, the all-white porters in the lodge were less friendly to her than to white students, and she was homesick for the first time in her life.

White readers of this book might benefit, as I did, from some background reading. Reni Eddo-Lodge's (2017) *Why I'm no longer talking to white people about race* helped explain what Black individuals feel when asked to speak for their entire culture, and left me with some insight into what it feels like to be discounted. Robin DiAngelo's (2018) *White Fragility* provided a role model in terms of a white woman wrestling with the ethical imperative to give back power and privilege. Articles in the British Medical Journal such as those by Nazroo et al. (2022) provided a medical and mental health perspective. Such 'homework' is a helpful preparation for hearing from people who know first hand about structural as well as personal racism. Some reading of history, research and popular paperbacks can then alert us to items in the media and in day-to-day life, that flesh out theory and highlight the concerning legacy of racism.

Black activist staff and students told me they were weary of feeling duty-bound to campaign on racial issues whilst white peers could simply get on with their studies. Black academics spoke of being labelled troublemakers, and seen as aggressive or 'entitled' if they spoke about racial issues. Such activists may have to sideline their own well-being to fight for racial justice. They have less time and energy for personal relationships, for academic work and in some cases for navigating their first time living away from home. The extra stress – plus the racist incidents that inspire and accompany the work – can cause students to fall behind in their studies or experience mental disorders. The weariness expressed sounded close to depression, when people said, 'It seems like you white people are only just waking up to things we've been trying to say forever!'

Dr Jason Arday of Cambridge University points out that few Afro-Caribbean students get as far as PhDs, but if they do, their topic is disproportionately likely to be research on Black, Asian and minority ethnic (BAME) people in universities! Academics should be free to research any topic, in the knowledge that BAME issues will be addressed by the whole community. I had initially assumed that it would be disrespectful to 'trespass' into the territory of BAME understanding but now realise that it is disrespectful to be a bystander whilst people fight their own battles for justice.

Searching for words that don't give offence has often been difficult too. My 'white fragility' seeks the 'correct' expressions as a defence against blame, but obviously the real need is to find ways to talk without blocking further communication. We can't afford to be cavalier about using offensive terms, obviously. It's more important to try to find ways to repair the hurt to others rather to be defensive about our own embarrassment. Learning what terms cause hurt was particularly revealing. Attempts to be inclusive often mean tagging the words 'and other' to any descriptor or acronym, yet it is precisely this experience of being considered 'other' that lies at the heart of the damage.

The Range and Scale of Ethnic Diversity in UK Universities

This chapter's focus is on people in UK universities who either consider themselves or are considered by others to be of minority racial origin. I reluctantly use the term 'BAME' to encompass this range. The focus is not on international students, although there is some overlap. Among home UK students more than half are 'BAME', with a high proportion of 'Black' people who grew up in the UK, often in minority ethnic communities who may speak English as a first language. In contrast, most UK international students are Chinese, and for them, like many other international students, use of language is a primary concern. Of course there is overlap. Many staff and students juggle several interacting challenges to their mental well-being.

Identifying people – and oneself – as belonging to a racial group not considered mainstream, is often about appearances. Skin colour is an obvious hallmark, and one less in the individual's power than costume or behaviour. A mixed-race Black student told me 'My mother is Jewish and proud of it, but sometimes she chooses not to wear her Star of David emblem when she goes out. I have to wear my black face every time I leave the house, and I have to be in a state of constant alertness to deal with the reactions it will draw.' A young Pakistani woman spoke of her guilt at pretending to be Italian to avoid prejudice. One exception was the tiny Gypsy, Traveller and Roma community whose student representatives spoke about racial disadvantage without any visible badge of minority ethnic status.

Ellie Mulcahy of the Gypsy, Traveller and Roma (GTR) communities speaks of the problems of receiving hate crime and racism without 'being Black'. A third of UK people surveyed admitted to holding prejudice again GTR groups and half hold an 'unfavourable view' of them.

These groups have the worst educational outcomes in the UK using any outcome measure, and are poorest represented in student and staff groups. They experience material poverty, cultural isolation and transition stress from many moves, and are victims of prejudice and discrimination. Like some other BAME groups, they fear inclusion will bring cultural dilution and are even afraid to identify as GTR because of the fear of stigma, so research is difficult.

They do in fact want educational opportunities but fear the process. They have massive fears of the debt involved and there are few role models of members of their community going to university.

Khunti et al. (2020) argue against the use of terms such as 'BAME', emphasising that 'There will never be a perfect term to encompass ethnic diversity, but researchers should avoid reinforcing perceptions of homogeneity where none exists, or excluding groups that do not fit within BAME terminology. Even "ethnic minority groups" is an imperfect collective term, and researchers should be prepared to break it down further to ensure that their findings benefit those who need them most.' Gee Yen Shin (2020) responds that 'the only commonality is that they are not white'. Sadly, this is the very commonality I have to address here. Cultural detail between and within different groups is important, but perhaps the priority is to oppose racism in UK universities – or any communities. The theme of this chapter is how treating people as 'non-white' in UK universities is bad for mental health.

Part of the solution can be to respect, explore and nurture diverse cultures within our society. An indispensable first step is for white people to acknowledge and equitably share our unfair privileges and dismantle racially constructed hierarchies of power.

'Racism' and How It Matters

The Synergi Collaborative Centre (2016) defines racism as

> Prejudice, discrimination, or antagonism directed against someone of a different race based on the belief that one's own race is superior. The belief that all members of each race possess characteristics, abilities, or qualities specific to that race, especially as to distinguish it as inferior or superior to another race or races.

Synergi goes on to show that racism is not limited to the individuals' active demonstration of such beliefs:

> Institutional racism is defined as the collective failure of an organisation to provide appropriate and professional services to people because of their colour, culture or ethnic origin. it can occur without any awareness of it happening.

The very concept of 'race' is a slippery one. The notion is taken for granted but hard to define biologically. For instance, anatomists can identify physical traits that show how a person is related to a broader population group but cannot generally identify precise 'racial' boundaries between those groups. As communities we continue to engage in self-defined ethnic and racial group identities. This is a way for groups of people to assert their rights, protect property and culture, provide social support and a sense of belonging. Racism and attacks on other groups can be symptoms of competition for scarce resources. In the present context, these resources may include places at desirable universities, jobs and promotions, accommodation and research grants.

Race and Ethnicity Interact with Other Disabling Factors at University

The concept of 'intersectionality' describes how aspects of a person's social and political identities combine to create different modes of discrimination and privilege. Examples include gender, wealth, caste, sex, class, sexuality, religion, physical disability, and physical attractiveness, interacting with each other and with race. Non-white students are more likely to be 'first gen' – the first generation in their families to receive higher education. Intersectionality operates like compound interest on disadvantage.

Discrimination can drive inequalities and lead to health problems that in turn worsen inequalities and social exclusion, and amplify cycles of deprivation. These structural and institutional dimensions are especially pertinent to the context of student mental health.

Education is often seen as a potential way out of deprivation, but for non-white people this is limited. Research shows that ethnic minority people with degrees are less likely than white graduates to secure employment, and their lifetime earnings are less than those of the white majority population.

Structural and Institutional Racism

Racism occurs as a whole thread through communities as well as existing at the one-to-one interpersonal level. It has been classified along the dimensions of structural, interpersonal and institutional racism, which overlap and are interdependent (Nazroo et al., 2020). Structural racism involves processes and procedures, rather than specific intentions, and involves cultural and ideological matters as well as material commodities and physical actions. Within institutions such as universities both structural and interpersonal racism interpenetrate and support one another rather than being distinct phenomena.

Racism on UK University Campuses

University leaders have made some progress in setting and meeting diversity and inclusion goals to hire and promote more Black faculty members, administrators and professional staff and to improve the lives of BAME students, particularly since the Black Lives Matter movement. We could be tempted into complacency by universities' own professions of anti-racism. Such proclamations are essential for a good international reputation. Often, Black staff and students complain that there is too much 'virtue signalling' and defensiveness, with avoidance of blame rather than genuinely seeking the benefits of a confidently diverse community.

Throughout the UK education system substantial gaps in attainment remain between ethnic minority and white pupils. Overall, travellers and Black Caribbean pupils have the lowest attainment, and rates of permanent exclusion at about three times those for all pupils. These figures make it unsurprising that just 6% of Black school leavers attended a Russell Group university, compared with 12% of mixed or Asian school leavers and 11% of white school leavers. Dumangane (2016) explores obstacles such as a lack of Black teachers and academics as role models, Black men being labelled as 'trouble' or 'low achievers' by teachers in secondary school; and assumptions made about their capabilities due to their ethnicity.

Since 2008, the entire UK population has seen an increase in the proportion with a degree-level qualification, with much higher relative increase for non-white people. Indeed, by 2011 people from most ethnic minority groups were more likely than white British people to have degree-level qualifications and less likely to have no qualifications (Lymperopoulou & Parame shwaran, 2015). However, while around three-quarters of white students achieve a good degree, this is true for fewer than half of their Black peers, even when they enter university with the same qualifications. And of all categories, Black students are most likely to drop out after their first year of study.

Among university academic staff, BAME people report being judged and treated negatively in relation to their experience and expertise and, like their colleagues working in other sectors, they remain poorly represented at the highest levels. In 2018, BAME people made up only 2% of UK academic staff and just 0.7% of professors. After graduation, analysis of official statistics by the TUC shows that BAME workers with degrees are more than twice as likely to be unemployed than white graduates. These numbers point to poor chances of achievement. What the numbers cannot show us is the detail of the incidents and attitudes that damage the potential for achievement.

> As a Scottish Black woman married to a white American man, I am under no delusions. This brutality against Black people has been present ever since the transatlantic slave trade . . .
> When I became a professor in 2015, I was invited to a lunch to welcome new professors. . . . I happened to be the first of the new professors to arrive . . .
> A professor . . . who had graduated . . . at a similar time as me, greeted me as I walked in saying 'Hi Helen. What are you doing here? I mean . . . what are you being promoted to?' . . . His own sense of white privilege, of being entitled to sit at the professorial table, made it impossible for him to see me in that role.
> I had been shocked to discover, when appointed, (2015) that I was only the 18th Black female professor in the UK – out of over 20 000 professors in total. . . . it's crucial we all realise that the transatlantic slave trade is not really history . . . We are, all of us, living in the long tail of that skewed distribution the low expectations of Black people, worldwide, and the brutality against them, are modern versions of the slave owner's chains and the overseer's whip.
>
> Minnis, H. (2020, 9 June). The Herald.

At present, there are short-term disincentives to ethnic diversity for universities seeking commercial and 'league table' success. Professor Kehinde Andrews of Birmingham City University asserts that whilst universities cherish a liberal, left-wing reputation, they are inherently deeply conservative, and that 'universities are still allergic to hiring Black people'. Universities with lots of Black British-born students tend to be low in league tables and have low graduate employment rates.

This sort of statistical overview clearly does not describe the quality of the atmosphere and attitudes students and staff experience in their daily lives, but does suggest that there are larger structural forces involved. We are not only discussing episodes of racial harassment from one student to another. Attempts to 'weed out the bad apples' are unlikely to solve the larger problems. Adding of 'Black texts' to a reading list achieve at best symbolic, at worst merely cosmetic improvement.

This chapter focusses on how the experiences of BAME students and staff relate to mental health and mental illness. It is also important to consider whether access to mainstream mental health resources is subject to the same barriers and obstacles for BAME people as those that diminish their full participation in higher education. The improvement of mental health for this group might have welcome consequences for the educational experience and academic achievement not only of minority groups but also the whole university population.

Racism and Mental Health in UK Universities

The place of racism as a cause of mental illness, or factor that leads to poor health, is still contested. However, a large and growing body of robust evidence demonstrates that racism leads to mental illnesses. Samples such as the UK Household Longitudinal Study have demonstrated the prevalence of racism in twenty-first-century Britain and its negative associations with greater psychological distress (poorer mental functioning), poorer physical functioning and lower life satisfaction over 2-year follow-up, adjusting for baseline scores (Hackett et al., 2020)

Racism acts as a physiological stressor, both in its more overt forms and as so-called micro-aggressions involving casual disparagement, perhaps even being feared, avoided or overlooked. These subtle influences can result in pessimism, and difficulties adjusting and recovering from trauma, and psychosis, depression and substance misuse are more likely in those exposed to racism.

Physical violence obviously leads to injury and often post-traumatic stress, while verbally hurtful comments about appearance or hostility towards a specific race threaten identity and status in the individual and their close groups. Earlier chapters of this book have emphasised the developmental importance for undergraduate students of building identity as individuals and members of communities. Threats and disruptions to the sense of the belonging self are all the more damaging at the threshold of maturity. Racially motivated behaviour functions as an attack on a person's very identity as a member of a category or group. Even when an individual is not personally attacked but observes racism towards others, it is still experienced as a threat (Nazroo et al., 2020)

For me it is Totally about Belonging!

I feel I don't belong here. Imposter syndrome is very common, particularly among first year students, especially if you're a woman, and it is definitely stronger in BAME students. I wonder if a better induction programme would have helped.

You see, the university isn't built for us, in fact it is built to keep us out. The classes taught are very white. Of course, it is expected that you adapt to the culture of a place you have chosen to come to, but when is 'adapting to the culture' oppressive and like returning to colonisation? What are the pros and cons of choosing to wear your national dress on formal occasions instead of gowns?

I do wish the university would stop thinking it's their job to build our resilience. We had to be expert in that to even get here. All Black parents give their children 'the talk' when we're young. Couldn't it be the uni's job to provide a space where we don't have to be resilient all the time, and it feels more like home, you know, where the portraits and monuments are not all white men and women or else photos of noble half-naked Black people or starving babies.

S, in workshop discussion

Fear of being victim to assault and racism is itself harmful, and undermines resilience, hope and motivation. People of visible migrant or ethnic minority heritage, who see themselves as targets of negative attitudes, live with the chronic stressor of fear. This generates irritability and pessimism for the whole group.

It is known that a mother's anxiety can affect the development of her unborn child. Generations of racism and associated deprivations mean that potentially, BAME students are more likely than others to have been stressed from early life, and certainly long before arriving at university. This has not simply resulted in yet another group of people damaged by chronic stress. Boyce and Ellis (Boyce & Ellis, 2005), proponents of the adaptive calibration model of stress point out that

> our developmental systems have been shaped by natural selection to respond adaptively to a range of different contexts. When people encounter stressful environments, this does not so much disturb their development as direct or regulate it toward strategies that are adaptive under stressful conditions; conversely, when people encounter well-resourced and supportive environments, it directs or regulates development toward strategies that are adaptive in that context.

They suggest that not only would this lead to people with adverse backgrounds being more responsive to further trauma, but they would also show the greatest propensity to benefit from positive environments. Other research is confirming that the association between adversity and mental ill health is extremely complex.

Much of the literature on mechanisms for racism comes from the US but can be applied cautiously to the UK context, particularly when the subjects of the studies are university students. Williams et al. (2018) minutely examined the relationships between self-reported frequency of experiences of micro-aggressions and anxiety, stress & trauma symptoms in 177 students. The study took account of both gender and 'negative affectivity' – the mindset which might cast a negative slant on all interactions – these African American students experienced clinically measurable symptoms as a result of racial mistreatment.

A systematic review of (mostly American) studies examined the cumulative effects of racism in adolescents of age 11–18 (Cave et al., 2020). There were significant associations between accumulated racism and later mental health outcomes and health-harming behaviours such as substance misuse. The health effects of racism varied depending on the age at which the exposure to racism occurred. This emphasises that students will likely have already accumulated damage from exposure to racism by the time they attend university, and highlights the developmental sensitivity of the experiences.

It is now possible to explore the potential neurobiological pathways by which discrimination affects brain and emotional health. Like other forms of social stress, the experience of racism has been shown to raise levels of the 'stress hormone' cortisol. Indeed, the pathways involving our hypothalamus, pituitary and adrenal glands appear to become unable to normalise levels in the context of chronic perceived threat (Berger & Sarnyai, 2015). Work on a campus in Texas (Cheadle et al., 2020) involved 100 students wearing sensors and providing daily survey data to link racism-related experiences, negative emotions, and skin conductance (which reflects emotional arousal). Racism-related experiences were associated with both increased negative emotion and heightened skin conductance.

In the UK, qualitative research methodology was used to examine the accounts of 32 BAME students at a London University to explore the social experience of racism (Arday, 2018). Themes that emerged included lack of belonging, isolation, and marginalization, and in particular barriers to accessing culturally appropriate mental health services.

Ethnicity and the Nature of Mental Illness

A huge longitudinal study of 40 000 UK households found that once we take account of racial discrimination and other socioeconomic factors, there is there is little difference between people's vulnerability to mental disorder (Wallace et al., 2016). The authors found that cumulative exposure to racial discrimination has negative long-term effects on the mental health of ethnic minority people. In other words, the higher rates of mental illness in minority populations are likely to be the result of racism, not of any inherent vulnerability in particular ethnic groups.

Within all cultural groups, regardless of racial or ethnic identities, the presentation of psychiatric disorders will be characterised by reference to the range of what is regarded as 'normal' in terms of attitudes and beliefs in that culture. Phenomena such as delusions and obsessions are likely to vary according to the environment – for instance ideas of possession by the devil were more common in the UK a century ago, whilst being sent cryptic messages by a television newsreader occurred frequently when I was a junior doctor. Both then and now, some societies do not accept the concept of 'mental illness' and individuals from such societies are more likely to deny symptoms such as depression or to present it in the form of physical symptoms such as very real pain or bodily weakness.

If we are not culturally sensitive to different presentations of mental distress in different cultures, we will miss opportunities to provide support and treatment. It is also important to question the impression that the nature of mental illness among ethnic minority people is necessarily more florid and more violent. There are higher psychiatric admission and detention rates among ethnic minority groups, especially Black male patients. Ethnic minority people are also more likely to be subjected to forcible treatment, seclusion and restraint (Synergi Collaborative Centre, 2018). This may be related to these people having received less management of their condition at the level of general practitioner (GP) care, and more access through forensic services and the criminal justice system. One plausible suggestion has been that BAME groups avoid services unless or until their disorders have become too florid to ignore. They may fear racism from institutions invested with authority and power, and have bad experiences of treatment personally or have heard such accounts in the community. It may also be that services make it difficult for BAME people to access, or are unable to understand their symptoms when they do present.

Obstacles to Appropriate Mental Health Services for BAME Students and Staff

Even in an anti-racist university environment, mental disorders will inevitably occur, and require treatment. It is a frightening experience to become aware that we are developing a mental illness, or that this is happening to a close friend or family member. Most of us are reasonably confident to approach services to help us with a physical illness, but this is less often the case for mental illness. University students, as a young and educated group, tend to experience less stigma than average in admitting to mental illness, but continue – as this book asserts – to experience obstacles to accessing help. For BAME students there is the potential for extra stigma. When we already carry one label of 'otherness' which has to be compensated for, we resist any further potential label of 'defectiveness'. Mental health professionals are known to expect greater disturbance in BAME patients, making them potentially less welcoming; other members of BAME communities are more likely to report bad experiences of care and less likely to urge their peers to access to services. All this undermines help-seeking and support.

People's personal fears of racism are not always taken seriously or are denied – even if they have experienced racism. The experience of not being heard, or being mistrusted, or being treated with hostility, are commonly expressed by Black services users, and reveal implicit power dynamics that act as a context for inequalities. In the US, it is likely that Black students are unable to afford the higher quality medical care available to richer white students, but in the UK our national health service (NHS) should theoretically offer equal healthcare to all.

Students need to be introduced to mental health care systems long before they become too ill to evaluate them properly. They require clinicians who are not only culturally sensitive and aware, but also expert in different responses to prescribed medications. It is unrealistic to demand that we always match patients with individual clinicians of the same race – let alone the same race, gender and age group. It may help, though, when students can see that clinical teams are ethnically diverse, with representation from people they can identify with, and a spread of roles, so that some of the professors and consultants are Black as well as a proportion of lower paid staff being white people.

It is also worth remembering that BAME communities, even more than white students, tend to prefer less formal sources of emotional support before resorting to psychiatric services. These range from family and friends, religious advisors, church members, the use of prayer, pharmacists, 'alternative' medications and substances offered by fellow students. They may also prefer help from their GP to the stigma of attending a mental health clinic (Barksdale & Molock, 2009). When the issues are of trust and privacy it can be counter-productive to automatically connect these options to NHS mental health services. All the same, confidential links can be made, and permission to consider onward referrals often becomes possible in the context of well-developed trusting relationships.

Mental Health and Academic Achievement in BAME Students

It is inappropriate to use academic achievement as a single index of for mental health, but it is theoretically likely that a racist culture damages learning capacity in victims and witnesses. The links between good mental health and higher academic achievement are important, too, in motivating university authorities to bring about change towards a more diversity-friendly environment .

We have already seen that Black students tend to have lower degree marks than their white counterparts, and this is also the case for students with a mental illness. Figures from the UK Office for Students (2019) show that in 2017–18, three-quarters of students with a mental health condition graduated with a first or a 2:1, but only half of Black students with a mental health condition did so. There are also differences in the extent to which a mental illness blocks progress. Only 77% of Black students with mental illness continued with their degree into the second year, compared with 87% of all students with mental illness.

Mental well-being and success in academia are different issues, but there are important links. Educational psychologists have long been aware of these, at least since Vygotsky's (1978) sociocultural theory. This asserts that the process of learning occurs in an interpersonal context, scaffolded by the support not only of teachers but also of parents, caregivers, peers and the wider culture.

Neil, a charismatic and hard-working Black student, consistently failed to get the high marks he wanted, although he was by no means failing. Professor P remarked in retrospect that had Neil been white he would have taken him to task for failing to back up his pronouncements with solid evidence. Neil urged his own views and opinions without enough academic rigour. The professor was afraid that any criticism would be construed as racism. As a result, the student was deprived of robust challenges that might have transformed his approach to work.

Professor P wished there had been a forum for academic staff to confidentially discuss dilemmas of this kind, where he could have been supported to address the issue with Neil in a positive manner. As it was, he felt that the only way to highlight the problem beyond the individual level would be if a student was seriously failing, or if he needed to pursue disciplinary action.

The interpersonal atmosphere acts to modulate levels of arousal. It provides stimulation and encouragement where necessary, or soothing and calm if there is too much arousal. Psychotherapists have always sought ways to bring about the most effective arousal levels in their patients to foster change and maturity, and a similar effect seems to be needed in the classroom or study. In contrast, acute or chronic stress is a handicap to learning. This makes evolutionary sense; our brains have to deal with threat by not becoming too immersed in mental states, or relaxing into play. At any moment a burst of adrenaline may be needed to trigger fight or flight from danger. The more chronic and severe the threat, the more easily startled the body becomes. Attention is always divided and academic learning is difficult. However, too little stimulation results in poor learning too.

Racial attacks, whether direct or witnessed, and cumulative micro-aggressions, act like any chronic threat as a handicap to optimal brain function, akin to the effects of post-traumatic stress disorder. At a chemical level such stress compromises well-being and tips people into frank mental illness more easily. Paradoxically, one form of white 'fragility' may operate to deprive BAME students of full participation in the University experience, if teachers and peers avoid robust engagement with them for fear of being accused of racism.

Improving Experiences of Ethnic Diversity in Our Universities

It is essential to start from an acknowledgement of systemic and interpersonal racism in UK institutions, but this does have to be followed by action to start the process of reparation, including attention to mental health inequalities. A recent paper published in the British Medical Journal makes three key recommendations: giving back property taken by 'brutal dispossession' by colonial powers, the laying aside of 'white fragility' so that white people's discomfort no longer blocks progress and the following of ethnic people's leaders' own recommendations (Smylie et al., 2022).

An End to Complacency

One recent text (Pilkington, 2020) summarises accumulating research as showing that '[Black and minority ethnic] staff and students continue to experience considerable disadvantage ... universities typically see themselves as liberal and believe existing policies ensure fairness; they thus ignore adverse outcomes and do not see combating racial inequalities as a priority.'

Reference to 'universities' generally means university authorities, which, as we have seen, are overwhelmingly white organisations. For the time being, then, it is crucial that white people in power make themselves allies to healthy ethnic diversity, opening minds to awareness of white privilege and phenomena such as micro-aggressions. Such a stance can be profoundly uncomfortable, but sophisticated intellectual institutions can embrace the discomfort with justifiable pride.

The University of Glasgow had always prided itself on its eighteenth and nineteenth century abolitionist stance and providing higher education for James McCune Smith, who was born into slavery and then became the first African American in the world to be awarded a medical degree. In 2016, however, the university commissioned a study into its relationship with slavery as well as with abolition, and examined some 'less palatable' aspects of how it benefited from the slave trade. These revelations led to a call for 'reparative justice' in today's university setting, including working with the University of the West Indies.

Reforming Complaints Procedures

The principles and processes of awareness, active quest for evidence and invoking the principles of 'reparative justice' can be effective at many different levels within a university setting. Bureaucratic complaints procedures are widely criticised by students, who find them counter-productive and re-traumatising, and even offensive in demanding that victims have to take responsibility for change.

In October 2018, Ella McPherson and Monica Figueros launched a digital reporting platform *The Whistle*, to collect testimonies and eye-witness accounts of racism. Their aim is to sidestep legalistic, oppositional dynamics around individual 'complaints' in favour of gathering a description of the whole climate of what is dished out and what is experienced. Postings attract immediate comment and support when racism occurs. Over time a picture emerges of a whole climate or attitudes and dynamics, which planners can use to inform constructive responses.

Meanwhile, Liyana Kayali describes Sussex University's *Restore Respect* project, which manages complaints about racism using principles of restorative justice. The project uses trained facilitators who hold a series of careful preparatory meetings with each side before setting up an encounter. Students feel that such procedures are more accessible and less likely to result in trauma and distress than cumbersome all-or-nothing disciplinary approaches. This approach can also embrace issues of identity and intersectionality without having to rigidly 'tick boxes' proving racism.

Legal Structures

Despite pejorative implications of invoking the law, with its dichotomous views of 'perpetrator' and 'victim', our evolving legal systems have much to offer to transforming diversity. All UK jurisdictions are signed up to protect globally agreed human rights, and have enshrined these protections in law. These include the 1997 Protection from Harassment Act and the 2010 Equalities Act, which makes it a legal obligation for public institutions to manage racism. Laws like this can become mere empty promises from the Government unless we use them to bring organisations to account. Barrister Georgina Calvert-Lee, at McAllister Olivarius, recommends that we 'use the legal stick when the carrot does not work'. She helpfully dispels some common misperceptions about the law. For instance, the legal definition of 'harassment' DOES in fact take into account the feelings experience by the harassed person, even if the perpetrator did not intend to elicit those feelings.

She also explains that whilst internal university complaints procedures might be expected to be a 'softer' approach than invoking the law, such procedures are in practice formal disciplinary processes against the 'accused'. The student bringing the complaint is generally not allowed to access evidence, attend hearing, make submissions, bring along a legal representative, see full outcome details or appeal against decisions. The focus appears to be on whether or not to punish the alleged perpetrator, rather than on providing justice to the complainant. A formal legal approach might offer greater transparency for the student or staff member bringing the complaint.

Co-production of Policy with BAME Staff and Students

It has been demonstrably beneficial to BAME students to provide advocacy, BAME representatives in Unions and other additional supports through faculty and peer mentorship. Such initiatives appear to improve retention and graduation rates. An interesting variant is 'reverse mentoring' in which a BAME student leads in teaching a senior white member of the university about their cultural needs. Outside dyadic work, planning bodies need to include a significant proportion of BAME individuals rather than the all-too-common appointment of single representatives. This is not only tokenistic but isolating and pressurising for the individual, whose well-being is all too likely to suffer.

Black students told me that BAME cultures are often characteristically 'collectivist'. 'This can sometimes feel a bit stifling, but everyone feels backed up', said one young person. Given the chance, students instinctively replicate these communities at university – they seek each other out, create pockets of community, BAME societies and Facebook groups. They protect each other in real life and on social media, 'making circles against bullies'. It is challenging to get the best balance between fostering these nurturing groups and encouraging new, diverse 'tribes' that do not require shared ethnic identity as the basis for trust.

Training for Staff and Students

Most universities do provide staff training in ethnic awareness, but are criticised for simply providing it to 'tick boxes'. It may be too generic to enact significant change. Some institutions have adopted 'unconscious bias training' (UBT). The UK Equality and Human Rights Commission recently reviewed UBT, concluding that eliminate unconscious bias and risks 'backfiring effects'. It appears that where UBT participants are exposed to biases that appear fixed or unchangeable they may conclude that efforts to change are pointless (Civil Service HR, 2020). Moreover, they criticise the provision of single session mandatory training without regular top up.

Dom Jackson Cole, of SOAS University of London proposes a two-part staff training course done on a departmental basis. The first part would involve identifying and acknowledging racial biases, the need to decolonise curriculum and prepare appropriate responses to perceived racism. A second workshop would involve action – a detailed mapping and redesign initiative with implementation goals that can be held to account. This would ensure that training is not an isolated exercise but is used to help drive broader university initiatives.

I would add to this suggestion the proposal that not only academic but also domestic and administrative staff should be included in such training, and that 'cultural competency programmes' should be provided to every new student at whatever stage. Training projects should routinely include consideration of the whole spectrum of student well-being from promoting positive diversity to highlighting pathways to treatment for mentally ill BAME staff and students.

Black Universities?

It can feel repugnant for those of us in the UK to envisage an institution where the students are by definition all from BAME backgrounds. This may sound like apartheid. However, not all UK schools are co-educational, and some are dedicated to the education of specific minority groups, for instance Catholic or Jewish schools. In higher education, Newnham College is an all-women's College within the University of Cambridge, accepting application from any individual who self-identifies as a woman. The UK, then, does accept some provision of protected educational settings for minority groups who choose them.

In the US 85% Black students attend predominantly white institutions, but research suggests there are distinct advantages for those who attend historically Black colleges and universities. Black students at historically Black colleges and universities had more positive self-image, stronger sense of racial pride, better academic performance, greater social involvement, and higher occupational aspirations whilst those enrolled in predominantly white institutions experienced more feelings of isolation, alienation, and low social support. (Darrell et al., 2016).

In contrast, the UK does not have historically Black universities but rather experiences the phenomenon that newer universities, particularly those in London, attract more BAME students. BAME students made up 51% of all UK students in London, compared with 21% of UK students at all other higher education providers outside of London. I have not found evidence as to whether BAME students are more likely to thrive at these London universities compared with their counterparts at universities elsewhere.

Better BAME representation across the whole of academia, and particularly at senior levels could do much in terms of recognising and enacting healthy ethnic diversity. Social debate continues about getting the balance right between the advantages and disadvantages of protected but less diverse environments. In the meantime, BAME students may wish to consider the ethnic mix and reputation of universities to which they consider applying, and their families and advisors may also wish to be explicit in acknowledging the dilemmas involved in such choices.

Culturally Appropriate Services, BAME Counsellors and Mental Health Clinicians

Mental health service providers both on campus and in the wider community have been working alongside BAME students and staff to redesign service delivery and publicity. Whilst students are expected to be fluent in English, communications about services and campaigns can feel friendlier and more accessible when translated into different languages for international students, or presented in culturally accessible ways, such as cartoons, story-telling and word of mouth. Senior lecturer Judith Francois of Kingston University set up an innovative approach, using storytelling and pictorial resources created by artists to explore cultural understanding and well-being with undergraduate and postgraduate students. Counsellors and clinicians might offer visits and discussions to university societies, sports centres and chaplaincies where BAME students hang out, rather than rely on laminated notices in toilets to direct students to help.

Where it is not always possible to offer students a counsellor of their own ethnic group, it should always be common experience to have people of colour working as clinicians, and for all of them to be regularly trained in cultural considerations, even when they cannot personally share the student's background and life experiences. The more ethnically diverse the staff mix, the more likely individual staff members are to understand each other's culture and challenges, so that clients have the transformative experience of being effectively helped by a person whose physical appearance is different from that of their own ethnic group.

For those students who strongly prefer to consult with a BAME counsellor, it may be possible for them to access someone working in a different institution using telemedicine – even the offer of such choices can make strides in building trust between a troubled student and their treatment team.

White therapists and clinicians often describe feeling embarrassed about raising race and culture in the context of discussion mental health. This could lead to avoidance of important issues. Questions do not need to be heavy handed. Helen Minnis, Professor of Psychiatry at Glasgow University, recommends asking a simple question such as 'is there anything about your culture or religion that might be relevant here? She warns clinicians against the habit of relying on 'the feeling in the room', as this can be a short cut to our own unconscious racism. She argues that 'our most powerful tool, replacing stigma in our diagnostic toolbox, is respectful curiosity'.

The Equality Challenge Unit's Race Equality Charter

Advance HE is an institution operating in more than 100 universities across the world and is already known for its Athena Swan Charter (Bhopal & Henderson, 2019), which allows universities to hallmark themselves as leaders in gender equality. Its race equality charter has been designed to improve the representation, retention and experiences of BAME students and staff. Since 2015, it has offered bronze and silver race equality charter awards for good practice in ethnic diversity. Universities are given up to 3 years to collect data, set up a self-assessment team, identify obstacles and strengths, and develop and audit goals. Only 70% of submissions are successful at first application as there is an exacting set of standards. Advance HE reports that for many universities, simply discussing racial inequalities is a major step; developing effective actions will take more time, commitment and understanding. Whilst the primary focus is social justice rather than mental health, the framework is a good discipline for improving mental well-being and including mental health care in its scope.

The Glass Half Full

It is important and impressive to find that BAME students, though by no means a homogenous group, can boast several areas of unusually strong mental health, despite the climate in which they have to function. For instance, suicide rates are lower in Black students (Gunnell et al., 2019) and they are less likely to drink alcohol (Siebert et al., 2003) or to experience eating disorders (Eisenberg et al., 2011) compared with white students. They report higher levels of spirituality, which is associated with better mental health in student populations(Luna & MacMillan, 2015).

American research has called for an approach that examines positive aspects of BAME mental health whilst not denying formidable racialised stressors and attainment disparities. Dawnsha Mushonga claims that in terms of mental health in Black US college students 'the glass is half full' (Mushonga, 2021). It is all too easy to focus on the deficits and handicaps that BAME students and staff experience and to overlook their resilience and expertise in managing their challenges.

Practice Points

Governments and Broader Communities

- Despite repeated 'wake up calls' such as the Black Lives Matter movement, there is still a long way to go in terms of reparation to non-white communities for past white privilege. This is important for the well-being of present and future community well-being and mental health.

University Governors and Managers

- There needs to be an end to the complacency that liberal university culture has superseded racism.
- Better nurturing of ethnic diversity in university communities can be associated with improved academic achievement.
- Universities should actively seek to appoint more BAME staff.
- Disciplinary procedures need to offer greater openness to those who make complaints of racism (and of other forms of discrimination and harassment).
- Institutions should sign up to Advance HE's race equality charter.

All University Staff

- Staff groups should assertively welcome and support BAME staff to be appointed and in seeking research grants and publications.
- Senior staff should consider engaging in 'reverse buddying' with BAME juniors and students, to expand understanding of issues.

White University Staff and Students

- There is a need to overcome discomfort and defensiveness about our own racism to prevent this 'white fragility' from blocking progress.
- Respectful curiosity is a healthy alternative to avoidance and defensiveness.
- One-off mandatory trainings require revisiting and regular updating. Certain approaches to training are not evidence-based to result in effective change, so these should be monitored.

Mental Health Practitioners within the University and in the NHS

- More BAME practitioners improve the ethnic diversity of the clinical group, whether or not BAME students and staff opt to meet with a clinician of non-white ethnicity.

- Where clients do feel safer with a non-white clinician, telemedicine and links with other agencies can make this possible.
- Work is needed with GPs to provide enhanced culturally sensitive treatment at the primary care level to prevent escalation of mental illness.
- BAME students need extra support to return to their studies after a mental illness as they are at greater risk than their white counterparts of dropping out.

Families and Parents

- Families from all ethnic backgrounds should take account of a university's reputation for diversity.
- It is helpful to ask whether the institution has signed up to the race equality charter.

Students from BAME Backgrounds

- The UK does not have predominantly Black universities, but there are student societies and informal groups which allow experience of one's own culture and the sense of secure belonging this can provide.
- Individuals should not feel obliged to sacrifice their educational experience to focus on issues of racism and discrimination.

I would like to express my appreciation of conversations about this chapter with Helen Minnis, Professor of Child and Adolescent Psychiatry at the University of Glasgow, Shubulade Smith CBE, Consultant psychiatrist at the South London and Maudsley NHS Foundation Trust (SLaM), senior lecturer at King's College, London and Clinical Director at the NCCMH (National Collaborating Centre for Mental Health) and forensic services, SLaM, Cindy Chew, Consultant Radiologist, NHS Greater Glasgow and Clyde, Honorary Clinical Associate Professor, University of Glasgow. and Dawn Edge, Professor of Mental Health & Inclusivity, University of Manchester.

I am also grateful to colleagues, students, staff and contacts from a range of ethnically diverse background. students and staff for their thoughtful and helpful contributions to this particular chapter.

References

Arday, J. (2018). Understanding mental health: What are the issues for black and ethnic minority students at university? *Social Sciences*, 7(10), 196.

Barksdale, C. L. & Molock, S. D. (2009). Perceived norms and mental health help seeking among African American college students. *The Journal of Behavioral Health Services & Research*, 36(3), 285–99.

Berger, M. & Sarnyai, Z. (2015). "More than skin deep": Stress neurobiology and mental health consequences of racial discrimination. *Stress*, 18(1), 1–10. https://doi.org/10.3109/10253890.2014.989204

Bhopal, K. & Henderson, H. (2019). *Advancing equality in higher education: An exploratory study of the Athena SWAN and Race equality charters*. British Academy/Leverhulme Research Report.

Boyce, W. T. & Ellis, B. J. (2005). Biological sensitivity to context: I. An evolutionary-developmental theory of the origins and functions of stress reactivity. *Development and Psychopathology*, 17(2), 271–301.

Cave, L., Cooper, M. N., Zubrick, S. R. & Shepherd, C. C. J. (2020). Racial discrimination and child and adolescent health in longitudinal studies: A systematic review. *Social Science & Medicine*, 27(250),

112864. https://doi.org/10.1016/j.socscimed.2020.112864

Cheadle, J. E., Goosby, B. J., Jochman, J. C., Tomaso, C. C., Kozikowski Yancey, C. B. & Nelson, T. D. (2020). Race and ethnic variation in college students' allostatic regulation of racism-related stress. *Proceedings of the National Academy of Sciences*, 117(49), 31053–62. https://doi.org/10.1073/pnas.1922025117

Civil Service HR (2020) *Unconscious bias and diversity training – what the evidence says*. UK Government. www.gov.uk/government/publications/unconscious-bias-and-diversity-training-what-the-evidence-says

Darrell, L., Littlefield, M. & Washington, E. M. (2016). Safe spaces, nurturing places. *Journal of Social Work Education*, 52(1), 43–9.

DiAngelo, R. J. (2018). *White fragility: Why it's so hard for white people to talk about racism*. Boston: Beacon Press.

Dumangane, C. (2016). *Exploring the narratives of the few: British African Caribbean male graduates of elite universities in England and Wales* (Doctoral dissertation, Cardiff University).

Eddo-Lodge, R. (2017). *Why I'm no longer talking to white people about race*. London; New York, NY: Bloomsbury Circus, an imprint of Bloomsbury Publishing Plc.

Eisenberg, D., Nicklett, E. J., Roeder, K. & Kirz, N. E. (2011). Eating disorder symptoms among college students: Prevalence, persistence, correlates, and treatment-seeking. *Journal of American College Health*, 59(8), 700–7.

Gunnell, D., Caul, S., Appleby, L., John, A. & Hawton, K. (2019). The incidence of suicide in University students in England and Wales 2000/2001–2016/2017: Record linkage study. *Journal of Affective Disorders*, 261(2020), 113–20. https://doi.org/10.1016/j.jad.2019.09.079

Hackett, R. A., Ronaldson, A., Bhui, K., Steptoe, A. & Jackson, S. E. (2020). Racial discrimination and health: A prospective study of ethnic minorities in the United Kingdom. *BMC Public Health*, 20(1), 1652. https://doi.org/10.1186/s12889-020-09792-1

Khunti, K., Routen, A., Pareek, M., Treweek, S. & Platt, L. (2020). The language of ethnicity. *BMJ*, 371, m4493. https://doi.org/10.1136/bmj.m4493

Luna, N., & MacMillan, T. (2015). The relationship between spirituality and depressive symptom severity, psychosocial functioning impairment, and quality of life: Examining the impact of age, gender, and ethnic differences. *Mental Health, Religion & Culture*, 18(6), 513–25.

Lymperopoulou, K. and Parame shwaran, M. (2015) Is there an ethnic group educational gap. In Jivraj, S. & Simpson, L. (eds) *Ethnic Identity and Inequalities in Britain* (pp. 118–98). Bristol: Policy Press.

Mulcahy, E. & Angus, A. (2021). Gypsy, Roma and Traveller young people. In: Menzies, L. & Baars, S. (eds) *Young people on the margins* (pp. 94–123). Routledge. https://doi.org/10.4324/9780429433139-5

Mushonga, D. R. (2021). The glass is half full: The need to promote positive mental health in Black college students. *Journal of College Student Psychotherapy*, 35(4), 313–26. https://doi.org/10.1080/87568225.2020.1727804

Nazroo, J. Y., Bhui, K. S. & Rhodes, J. (2020). Where next for understanding race/ethnic inequalities in severe mental illness? Structural, interpersonal and institutional racism. *Sociology of Health & Illness*, 42(2), 262–76.

Nazroo, J. (2022). Tackling racism: moving beyond rhetoric to turn theory into practice. *BMJ*, 378.

Office for Students (2019). *Mental health: are all students being properly supported?* www.officeforstudents.org.uk/publications/mental-health-are-all-students-being-properly-supported/

Pilkington, A. (2020) Promoting Race Equality and Supporting Ethnic Diversity in the Academy: The UK Experience Over Two Decades. In: Crimmins G. (ed) *Strategies for Supporting Inclusion and Diversity in the Academy*. Cham: Palgrave Macmillan. https://doi.org/10.1007/978-3-030-43593-6_2

Shin, G. Y. (2020). The language of ethnicity: blunt, contrived terms should be abandoned. *BMJ*, 371, m4935. https://doi .org/10.1136/bmj.m4935

Siebert, D. C., Wilke, D. J., Delva, J., Smith, M. P. & Howell, R. L. (2003). Differences in African American and White college students' drinking behaviors: Consequences, harm reduction strategies, and health information sources. *Journal of American College Health*, 51(3), 123–9.

Smylie, J., Harris, R., Paine, S. J., Velásquez, I. A. & Lovett, R. (2022). Beyond shame, sorrow, and apologies—action to address indigenous health inequities. *BMJ*, 378, o1688.

The Synergi Collaborative Centre (2018). *The impact of racism on mental health.* https:// legacy.synergicollaborativecentre.co.uk/wp-content/uploads/2017/11/The-impact-of-racism-on-mental-health-briefing-paper-1.pdf

Vygotsky, L. S. (1978). *Mind in society: the development of higher psychological processes.* Cambridge, MA: Harvard University Press.

Wallace, S., Nazroo, J. & Bécares, L. (2016). Cumulative effect of racial discrimination on the mental health of ethnic minorities in the United Kingdom. *American Journal of Public Health*, 106(7), 1294–300. https://doi .org/10.2105/AJPH.2016.303121

Williams, M. T., Kanter, J. W. & Ching, T. H. W. (2018). Anxiety, Stress, and Trauma Symptoms in African Americans: Negative Affectivity Does Not Explain the Relationship between Microaggressions and Psychopathology. *Journal of Racial & Ethnic Health Disparities*, 5(5), 919–27. https://doi.org/10.1007/s40615-017-0440-3

Sexual Behaviour and Gender Identity in Universities

> Sexual health is fundamental to the overall health and well-being of individuals, couples and families, and to the social and economic development of communities and countries. Sexual health, when viewed affirmatively, requires a positive and respectful approach to sexuality and sexual relationships, as well as the possibility of having pleasurable and safe sexual experiences, free of coercion, discrimination and violence. The ability of men and women to achieve sexual health and well-being depends on their:
>
> - access to comprehensive, good-quality information about sex and sexuality
> - knowledge about the risks they may face and their vulnerability to adverse consequences of unprotected sexual activity
> - ability to access sexual health care
> - living in an environment that affirms and promotes sexual health.
>
> Sexual health–related issues are wide-ranging, and encompass sexual orientation and gender identity, sexual expression, relationships and pleasure. They also include negative consequences or conditions.
>
> World Health Organization www.who.int/health-topics/sexual-health

Our universities provide young people with an interpersonal laboratory and with the time and freedom to experiment with relationships. They learn to manage respect, caring, comfort, conflict, rejection, loss and asymmetries in interpersonal power. This chapter considers ways in which sexual behaviour offers interpersonal power and responsibility for members of the university community, how it interacts with other aspects of human development and background culture, and in doing so affects – and is affected by – mental health.

We start with some discussion of current norms, then consider whether there are clear relationships between sexual behaviour and mental health. Universities host a climate of great diversity in terms of sexual orientation, gender identity diversity and fluidity. These issues combine with other aspects of intersectionality to amplify experiences of distress and mental ill health in universities. (Intersectionality is the description given to the experience of simultaneously belonging to different, often stigmatised, social groups – ethnic, cultural, religious, gender or sexual.)

In acknowledging all these issues, this book seeks to hold a focus on mental and emotional health. It is easier to quantify and medically treat physical risks and consequences of sexual behaviour compared with mental ones. Seen dispassionately, sexually transmitted diseases, and unwanted pregnancies are amenable to pharmacological and surgical solutions. In a climate of controversy about sexual morality, it is not surprising that we might try to avoid raising topics that open us up to accusations of being judgmental. This risks overlooking the huge need for emotionally and interpersonally informed discussions about sexual matters.

The chapter also examines prevention and management of sexual assault and abuse. Sexual abuse is such an important cause of psychological trauma that it dominates concerns about the psychological aspects of sexual behaviour. Perhaps we risk overlooking both positive and negative emotional dimensions of less-extreme sexual behaviour. These include romantic communication and miscommunication, rejection and loss, and the context of diverse cultural, religious and moral codes. Preparation for writing this chapter has left me impressed by some similarities in institutional and educational attitudes to alcohol and to sexual behaviour. The 'party line' is to issue warnings and condemnations regarding physical, and to a lesser extent mental health, harms, but meanwhile the assumption is that students will engage in excessive behaviour that cannot be controlled from outside.

Individual students have told me that before coming to university, school sex education focussed almost entirely on physical aspects of sex, warnings of diseases and emphasis on avoiding discrimination of the lesbian, gay, bisexual, transgender, queer and other minority gender groups (LGBTQ+) community. Even the basic contraceptive information that was provided left out discussions of the emotional context in which this would be managed. The ubiquitous feelings of embarrassment and shame in the classroom were ignored and suppressed rather than acknowledged and explored. Some of those in the classroom were seriously worried by what they heard and for a while avoided sexual matters, but most responded with mockery and bravado.

The Current Climate of Sexual Behaviour in Universities

There is a stereotype that students have a lot of reckless sex during their first week at uni. While many home students do not engage in this behaviour you may see or hear things during Freshers' Week that you find shocking or don't agree with. For example, your uni will likely be giving out free condoms. They may also have literature about contraception and sexual health or even at-home STI testing kits...Freshers' Week is intense for a lot of reasons, but you will find that everything settles down after the first week.

British attitudes towards sex may seem casual to you. In the UK is common to have sex before marriage, sleep with a bunch of different people, have one-night stands, kiss in public, live with your partner but never marry them, and do all sorts of other things which you may find a little scandalous.

Having sex with a Brit does not automatically mean that you are dating them. 'Hook-up culture' – having casual sex with someone and never getting into a relationship with them – is common. Some people just aren't interested in dating, so make sure you know what you want before sleeping with someone . . .

Great British Mag. British students and sex: everything you need to know.
https://greatbritishmag.co.uk/student-guide/british-students-attitudes-towards-sex/

There does not appear to be any universally accepted code of what constitutes normal sexual behaviour for the student age group, but there is evidence (Stinson, 2010) that 'hooking up', or casual, short-term uncommitted sexual encounters, has become an increasingly common form of sexual relationship for university students, at least in the Western world. This has generated alarm at 'moral decline in our culture, a reflection of our hypersexualised media, and a promotion of sexual irresponsibility' (Stinson, 2010). However, 'hooking up' does not indicate a lifelong avoidance of more enduring sexual relationships. Casual relationships are characteristic of a normal but fairly transient developmental stage. Later on in university life the experimentation phase of 'hooking up' gives way to more settled, longer monogamous relationships (Stinson, 2010, Netting & Reynolds, 2018).

A striking Canadian study involved surveying students every 10 years since 1980 (Netting & Reynolds, 2018). Between 1980 and 1990, it became socially acceptable for people expressing mutual love to have sex even if not married. There was a fall in 'virginity rate' among female students, and an increase in male students entering monogamous romantic relationships. The research identified three distinct sexual sub-cultures: monogamists (about 55%), abstainers (30%), and multi-partnered 'experimenters' (20% men 14% women). The experimenters reported concurrent partners, most of them casual. These were distinct subgroups rather than a continuous range of behaviours. The authors suggest that sex education programmes may need to target different habits and attitudes for each. For instance, the authors report that in response to the HIV epidemic, abstainers exaggerated the dangers they faced, monogamists over-relied on fidelity as a protection from infection, whilst 'experimenters' increased their use of condoms.

Sexual activity has many aspects. It is a provider of sensations, like a recreational drug, and also a cementer of lasting relationships – perhaps more like wine with dinner. Problems of course arise when different aspects become confused or when participants have different expectations of what is being communicated. Diverse cultural and ethnic assumptions are embedded in the psychosocial and emotional meaning of sexual behaviour. There are commendable efforts to clarify the meaning and validity of consent to sexual activity, but this goes only so far. It is not the same as giving consent to a surgical procedure, although there are parallels – in both scenarios, consent can be distorted if it is demanded without time to consider, and in a distracting or pressured environment. Intoxication affects the ability to consent, and the validity of consent is greater when the relationship with the person seeking consent is one of well-founded trust.

'Casual' and Committed Sexual Relationships at University

Given that universities are places where on the whole a wide range of sexual behaviour is tolerated, it may be less likely that mental health will suffer purely as a result of stigma or discrimination against practices outside mainstream heterosexual culture. Nevertheless, Wade (2017) describes 'hook-up' relationships as highly likely to be associated with alcohol use, depression and emotional distress, problems with attachment and family stress.

In contrast, some students report finding casual sex to be a gratifying, stress-relieving experience that increases a sense of belonging to the university community. We shouldn't underestimate the stresses and distresses of committed, longer-term relationships either. The quest for a potential life partner and trying out of couple relationships is challenging. It is far from simple to try to yoke together the needs and behaviours of two different, developing personalities.

Sexual relationships are most comfortably tried out and survived in the context of stable non-sexual relationships. Friends old and new, and family members, can provide stability, continuity and a different kind of intimacy. However, new students leave this secure base when they leave for university. There may be damage to ordinary friendships when one friend enters a sexual relationship. Competition, jealousy and rejection can occur in non-sexual friendships as well as sexual relationships and of course the two spheres can overlap. Students can be distracted from studying when a sexual relationship is intense. They may struggle to attend the same course or live in the same accommodation as an ex after a break-up.

These normal but painful experiences are particularly difficult for students who live with higher-than-average levels of anxiety. Anxiety disorders are discussed in more detail in Chapter 16. It is worth emphasising that students with autistic spectrum conditions have the double vulnerabilities of communication differences and high levels of anxiety, making sexual interactions potentially confusing and fraught for these students.

Unsurprisingly, researchers have found that students who have committed relationships during their student years' experience fewer mental health problems than those who do not (Braithwaite et al., 2010). It is hard to say which is cause and which is effect. Stable relationships may minimise mental disorders by providing comfort and security during a turbulent and emotionally challenging stage of development. Alternatively, students with fewer mental health problems may be more likely to achieve committed relationships. It may also be the case that though settling early into a stable relationship reduces uncertainty and anxiety, it could also insulate the couple from experimentation towards ultimately more fulfilling relationships.

Some students and staff conduct stable 'long distance relationships' with partners they have already met at home or more recently during travels or online. These relationships used to be considered particularly stressful, but studies suggest that that those in such relationships do not experience significantly lower levels of satisfaction. The couples report enjoyable activities such as 'hanging out on FaceTime', doing homework collaboratively, discussing serious relationship issues, and participating in cybersex (Dargie et al., 2015).

Relationship and Sex Education in UK Schools and Beyond

Students arrive at university having already received formal relationship and sex education (RSE) at school, and influenced by the explicit and implied attitudes from home and peers, the pressures of media, and a varying range of personal experience. In terms of formal education, recent reports and media campaigns have found this to be out of touch with the reality of young people's lives, leaving the pressures they face unaddressed (Ofsted, 2021, Gana & Hunt, 2022).

In 2012, UK activist Laura Bates set up the Everyday Sexism website, which became an international movement and prompted the National Union of Students (NUS) research into 'lad culture' in schools, streets, workplaces and universities. Phipps and Young (2015) found that for female students 'lad culture' dominated the social and sexual spheres of university life in problematic ways. This 'lad culture' amongst young people does not arrive anew at university, but is already seen in schools.

In 2020, in the context of the MeToo movement in the United States, Soma Sara started the Instagram page Everyone's Invited for people to share experiences of gender-based violence at school and university. The UK Government responded with an urgent review of sexual abuse in schools by Ofsted (2021). By the time of the government report, the site had received over 54 000 anonymous testimonies of gender-based aggression including verbal harassment, sexual abuse, exploitation and rape. Respondents often said they had taken their allegations to someone in a position of trust, only to be suppressed, dismissed or ignored.

The initial focus of Everyone's Invited was on schools, but within a week, more than 1000 testimonies of sexual harassment, abuse, misogyny and assault were shared by students at more than 80 UK universities. Unlike schools, universities are legally regarded as independent organisations. This means the Department for Education is unable to intervene directly, but it can issue regulatory guidance, which asks that they make a 'visible commitment' to tackling sexual misconduct.

Key Findings from Ofsted (2021)

- Issues around sexual abuse and harassment are so widespread that they need addressing for all children and young people
- For some, sexual abuse and harassment is so commonplace, that they see no point in reporting it
- Children and young people were rarely positive about the RSE they had received
- Lack of awareness among teachers that abuse is happening. Children say teachers 'do not know the reality' of their lives
- Online sexual abuse is prevalent, group chats are a problem
- Boys are less aware of the problems than girls
- Young people are learning more from pornography than RSE
- Sexualised & homophobic language is common
- Nearly 90% of girls, and nearly 50% of boys, said being sent explicit pictures or unwanted videos happens a lot or sometimes
- 92% of girls and 74% of boys said sexist name-calling happens a lot or sometimes
- 54% of those age 16 and above and 40% of those age 13 to 15 said unwanted touching occurred a lot or sometimes.

In fact, both schools and universities have long been aware of the high prevalence of sexual harassment in their institutions. The NUS survey (Smith, 2010) found that one in seven female students had been victims of serious sexual assault or serious physical violence at university, and 68% had been a victim of sexual harassment. Research by Girlguiding (2014) found that 59% of UK girls and young women of age 13 to 21 years had faced some form of sexual harassment at school or university in the previous year. In 2016, Universities UK's (2016) Changing the Culture report found that support for students was patchy, and there was a need for institutions to embed a zero-tolerance attitude to sexual violence into their policies and create better reporting systems.

In response to these shocking disclosures, students, parents, campaigners, and activists have once again called for better and more comprehensive RSE, and for other measures to address the situation. New and more effective school RSE programmes might be created using the evidence provided by Everyone's Invited and in collaboration with school and university students themselves. This could ensure that relevant and appropriate issues are addressed.

However, a whole new dimension appears to be needed to promote a safe and respectful climate within educational institutions (and of course beyond). This involves exploring the emotional and interpersonal dimensions of sexual behaviour and no longer avoiding the controversial and conflicting belief systems that young people and their families will bring to such discussions.

One example of this is the recent concern about the prevalence of anal sex in young people, which is now experienced by over 28% of 16- to 24-year-olds (Gana & Hunt, 2022). Up to 25% of young women with experience of anal sex report they have been pressured into it at least once. The NHS patient information on anal sex considers only sexually transmitted diseases, making no mention of anal trauma or incontinence, or the psychological aftermath of the coercion young women report. Failure to address important issues 'may not be just avoidance or stigma … there is genuine concern that the message may be seen as judgmental or even misconstrued as homophobic'. The authors believe that better education would allow those who genuinely want anal sex to protect themselves more effectively, whilst those who agree reluctantly to meet perceived media or peer expectations or to please partners, could be helped to feel better empowered to say no (Gana & Hunt, 2022).

Studies from the United States (e.g., Santelli et al., 2018) showed that school-based sex education, including skills-based training in refusing unwanted sex, was an independent protective factor for preventing sexual assault at university. Abstinence-only instruction was not. In interviews, students reported variable experiences with sex education before college; many reported it was awkward and poorly delivered.

Those authors suggest that 'sexual assault prevention needs to begin earlier', but do not consider it is the whole answer (Santelli et al., 2018). They add that 'successful prevention before college should complement prevention efforts once students enter college'. Such prevention might perhaps be modelled on a Canadian programme aimed at women students. It focussed on protective measures such as reducing alcohol intake and considering personal safety and self-care. This was shown to reduce the likelihood that women would be victims of serious sexual assault over subsequent years (Senn et al., 2015).

'Sexual assault prevention' is a useful measurable proxy for a healthy sexual climate. It feels disappointing as an aspiration for a university as a whole. I would suspect in any case, that defensive strategies against assault can only be successful in the context of a society that learns how to express and regulate sexual drives, and discuss their emotional, physical, practical and interpersonal consequences.

There is a welcome movement to bring back the factual aspects of sex education within moral attitudes to relationships. This doesn't mean applying rigid religious or cultural rules, but rather holding a stance of proper concern for everyone's well-being. In the United States, Sharon Lamb and colleagues have pioneered and researched the Sexual Ethics for a Caring Society programme for schools (Lamb et al., 2021). University society benefits when schools have promoted an ethical culture, but it is not enough. Some universities now make it mandatory to attend workshops on consent, usually during Welcome Week. These workshops might be expanded and offered again later in the university course.

There is a risk though that students will simply take on a legalistic message that getting consent is necessary to avoid getting into trouble. We need to understand why consent is important in how we relate to one-another, and to treat each other in a caring and just way. We also need to reopen discussions about the various meanings of sexual behaviour within society, so that it is more than an appetite to be assuaged in a matter-of-fact way. Mental and emotional dangers need consideration as well as the perils of sexual violence, infections and unwanted pregnancy. For the sake of friendly relationships amongst and within different genders, we need to move beyond stereotypes of male rapists and female victims.

Universities do not have the inbuilt expectation of delivering obligatory sex education in a didactic fashion, but they might run courses (both optional and for credits) on matters such as sexual ethics and behaviour, and extend campaigns and research projects beyond prevention of gender-based violence, important though that will always be.

Sex and Social Media

The effects on student mental health of social media and other online, particularly phone-based, communications, are discussed further in Chapter 8. Electronic communication goes beyond other forms of communication by facilitating immediate and huge scale contact with strangers in a paradoxically secret space. Until the widespread use of the internet, most communication was between people who already had some sort of attachment to each other, and group dynamics were smaller. Intimate, late-night communications, perhaps when intoxicated, have always occurred but used not to be amplified across the whole world. There are now situations where a young person in their own residence can be exposed to abuse and threats online that friends or relatives in the same room are unaware of. There is a complex entanglement of experiences of digital and physical gendered violence. Students have described how online threats and insults and so-called 'revenge porn' make them frightened in real life.

Papadopoulos (2010) conducted a review on behalf of the UK Government on the 'sexualisation of young people', which largely confirmed 'the popular perception that young people (and in particular young women and girls) are increasingly being pressured into appearing sexually available'. She felt that the internalisation of media images was powerful in bringing about this culture.

Another change for this generation of students is the ubiquitous use of 'dating apps' to negotiate both traditional dating and casual sexual contacts. Without explaining how it may be that this change threatens well-being, Sawyer et al. (2018) found that young people who used dating apps had higher rates of 'sexual risk behaviours', including sex after using drugs or alcohol. They were twice as likely to have had unprotected sex in the past 3 months, and dating app use predicted the number of lifetime sexual partners. A more recent study (Mori, 2020) confirmed these findings and added that there were significant associations between 'sexting' and symptoms of anxiety and depression, and substance use.

Sexual activity appears to be physically and mentally healthier if contacts are negotiated in real life rather than electronically. This fact raises concerns in the context of the reduced availability of real-life contact during COVID, and the corresponding increase of electronic communication both during lockdown and to some extent subsequently. During COVID, reports from across the world identified a 'shadow pandemic' of gender-based violence (Simonovic, 2020). Increased screen time intensifies risks of gender and sexual violence including online sexual harassment and image based sexual abuse.

Since web-based communication is now a fact of modern life, young people will certainly seek sex and relationship education online. Educationalists and interested collaborators are working to develop and research responsible online packages of sex and relationship education. The best current evidence comes from interventions that involve in person group discussions, though, even if these are based on online presentations.

Students – and all of us – would benefit too from an online climate that allowed responsible discussion of sexual relationships, rather than an automatic entrance into a locker-room atmosphere of pornography and 'lad culture'. There are a number of responsible and helpful online parenting forums. It would be helpful if the same standards of constructive respect could be more readily accessed by young people embarking on sexual relationships.

Student Sex Workers

Roberts et al. (2007) hypothesised that changes in the funding of higher education in the UK were behind the phenomenon of some students entering the sex industry 'in order to make ends meet'. Their sample of undergraduates in the south of England found that poor psychological well-being, drinking problems and difficult financial circumstances were associated with sex work, and although no direct evidence was found linking this to an earlier history of sexual abuse, there was an indirect relationship through the impact of abuse on mental health.

More recent research found that almost 5% of students in the United Kingdom are involved in sex work (Sagar et al., 2015). Students' biggest concern was keeping their work secret. The surveyed universities avoided the topic of student sex work presumably due to fear of reputational damage. 'Pro-feminist' attitudes were associated with seeing sex work as exploitation and oppression of women. Staff knowledge on the legalities of sex work and on appropriate referral pathways was 'inadequate'. The authors argue 'that steps need to be undertaken to make the higher education environment inclusive for all students, including those who work in the sex industry'. This is a contrasting perspective from that of Roberts et al. (2007), in that rather than seeing the situation as one of impoverished students driven to sex work, it conceptualises the issue in terms of enabling young people who choose to engage in sex work to access a university education.

Research based in Berlin, surveyed students in the sex industry and also questioned other students about their attitudes to student sex workers (Ernst et al., 2021). All assumed that the main problem student sex workers have to face would be 'mental distress'. Surprisingly, the authors found no differences in mental health and self-esteem between women who engaged in sex work and age-matched women who did not.

The most frequent service students provided was found to be 'prostitution in the narrow sense' but the student sex workers also provided escort services, striptease, webcam services or erotic massages, or worked as a porn actor. No difference in happiness could be found between sex workers offering sexual intercourse and those not offering it. The students said that their motivation for engaging in sex work included 'fun, financial problems, adventure, higher income, self-affirmation, curiosity and flexible working hours' (Ernst, 2021).

A recent UK study (Palomeque Recio, 2022) investigated 'sugar dating' in universities. This focused on the transactional relationship between a younger woman (sugar baby) and an older affluent man (sugar daddy). Their interviewees described 'having bills to pay' as a critical factor, despite having acquired a student loan, as well as 'the expectation of "fun", the acquisition of symbolic capital, and the forecast of enjoying a superior lifestyle'. The authors suggest that 'the economic context of female students in the UK should be investigated to offer economic alternatives to gendered sexual activities such as sugar dating' but do not make it clear whether this recommendation is based on moral or feminist views, as they do not describe the mental health of their subjects, but, like previous researchers, assume that the women are driven by financial pressures rather than having other choices to meet their expenses.

Sex, Students and Substance Use

Alcohol use is itself associated with damage to mental health in a university context, and its interaction with sexual behaviour is highly likely to amplify the potential mental ill health problems resulting from either behaviour taken singly. The general mental health associations of alcohol use in students are considered in Chapter 6. In this section we focus on the additional mental health consequences of alcohol related sexual disinhibition.

A substantial body of research in several different countries has also found that for students, sexual assault, and also sexual behaviour that is later regretted, is often associated with alcohol and other substance misuse by both parties Many of the assaults involved are described as 'incapacitated rape' rather than 'forcible rape'. Lorenz and Ullman (2016) reviewed research on alcohol and sexual assault, finding that about half of sexual assaults involve victims consuming alcohol before the assault. The victims of such assaults are most likely to be student-aged white women, who have consumed alcohol voluntarily. The authors acknowledge that other factors contribute to risks for and recovery from alcohol-involved assaults and emphasise that sexual violence is never the victim's fault. Meanwhile alcohol use also plays an important role in perpetration risk, and in this case cannot be said to excuse an assault.

Alcohol may confer risk of assault through its physiological effects by altering perception, reducing speed of reactions and impairing decision-making abilities for both perpetrator and victim. These changes can lead to misinterpretation of cues, ineffective communication, inability to resist, and difficulty perceiving and responding to threat. Lorenz and Ullman (2016) characterise the typical results as an intoxicated man misinterpreting friendly cues from a woman as a sign of desire for sexual activity while the intoxicated woman discounts fears of negative sexual consequences. Perhaps in acknowledgement of the role of alcohol-induced miscommunication, or out of shame, or because their assailants were friends or acquaintances, many victims do not label their unwanted sexual experiences as a crime, particularly on college campuses.

Clearly, managing the problem of alcohol-related assaults will involve changes in attitudes, policies and information campaigns. At the same time, it has been shown that interventions to help young women students to reduce their alcohol consumption can decrease their risk of being a victim of 'incapacitated' sexual violence (Clinton-Sherrod et al., 2011).

Victims are not the only topic of research into alcohol-related violence. Research conducted in Liverpool (Liverpool John Moores University, 2014) focussed on reducing alcohol-related aggression in young men. The authors identified a drinking double-standard: whilst women were blamed more for their assault as their level of intoxication increased, increased intoxication in men resulted in a reduction of their perceived responsibility for perpetrating a sexual offence. Barristers highlighted that alcohol consumption disproportionately impacted on the credibility of the victim at trial, rather than the culpability of the defendant. As a result of the research, Liverpool City Council launched a media campaign aimed at young men, especially students as users of the night-time economy. Campaign evaluation demonstrated that it had effectively conveyed the message that having sex with someone who is exceptionally intoxicated amounts to rape.

Sexual Orientation and Gender Identity in the Student Age Group

It is an important paradox that while same-sex orientations and gender identity differences do not in themselves constitute a mental disorder, they do expose those with gender 'non-conformity' to a range of mental health stressors and treatment obstacles. Mental health needs of this population may differ from those of students with more mainstream gender and sexuality. LGBTQ+ students may have had to invest time and emotional energy in working out non-conforming gender and sexual identities. These preoccupations may have occupied time and energy in adolescent years that others used to master other maturational skills. An Australian study of 16- to 29-year-olds, not all students, found LGBTQ+ people were more likely to describe having experience of substance misuse, young age at first sex, multiple sexual partners, and lower ratings of their own mental health than their matched heterosexual peers (Bowring et al., 2015).

The 'minority stress model' has been invoked in a great deal of recent works to explain how members of sexual minority groups experience mental distress and ill health. It describes clashes between minority and dominant values and resultant conflict within the social environment (Meyer, 2003).

Universities may be amongst the most tolerant and welcoming environments for people who are LBGTQ+. Many boast societies dedicated to the interest of sexual and gender minorities. Students who kept their sexual or gender identities secret whilst living at home often choose to 'come out' when at university, and others feel safe to experiment with fluid identities and behaviours. Even so, students who are not cis-gender and heterosexual have higher risks of mental illness, and lower levels of happiness, at least partly mediated by feeling that they belong less to the community, and are more unsafe (Wilson & Liss, 2022).

There are higher levels of attempted suicide in LGTBQ+ young people, higher numbers of deaths by suicide, and differences in triggers and methods of suicidal self-harm methods (Ream, 2019). This suggests that specific interventions, rather than general preventative measures, need to be developed. Countries that acknowledge same-sex marriages, and environments with inclusive anti-bullying policies, have been found to experience lower rates of LBGTQ+ 'suicidal behaviour', but as yet, interventions have not demonstrated reduction in deaths (Ream, 2019).

Transgender Students and Staff

The transition to university life, often a difficult stressor for cis-gender young people, may be welcomed with open arms by those who were unable to trust family, friends or school staff with their sexual orientation. Transgender youth in addition, may only now, at the age of legal majority, be entitled to certain medical or surgical interventions. For a young student it is not simply a case of 'being' part of a minority sexual or gendered community, but of 'becoming' that individual. Negotiating the new identity can exert a huge extra demand on time, organisational skills and emotional energy. Not all students will be ready to 'come out' or transition at the same stage of the process. Potential partners may also be living at different stages. It poses a great burden to have to keep secret the identity of an intimate partner. This seems especially common when a UK-born student is dating an international student whose culture frowns on sexual minorities.

Up to 1.3% of young people identify as transgender. These people have roughly twice the rates of mental illnesses such as depression, suicidal behaviour, self-harm and eating disorders (Connolly, 2016). The same study found that gender-affirming medical therapy and supported social transition correlated with improved psychological functioning.

Until 2010, and possibly more recently, psychiatric diagnoses included 'gender identity disorder'. The change to 'gender identity dysphoria' acknowledges that being in a physical body that is not expressive of the gender one feels can give rise to severe distress. In 2010, the World Professional Association for Transgender Health (Bouman et al., 2010) asserted that

> the expression of gender characteristics, including identities, that are not stereotypically associated with one's assigned sex at birth is a common and culturally diverse human phenomenon [that] should not be judged as inherently pathological or negative.

Political attitudes to transgender rights and issues are currently controversial, with efforts to liberalise legislation receiving high profile opposition, and the Tavistock transgender clinic recently closing out of concerns that it pressured very young people into gender change they were not ready to assume. Few of us have the expertise to judge the reversibility or longer-term effects of treatments, and the discomfort and confusion we may feel about such issues may be experienced by young transgender people as rejection of their identities or personalities, rather than as concern to avoid harm. Unintended stigma is thus added to the open and hostile discrimination seen in the general community, even though it may be less prevalent on campus.

Before considering our role in supporting LGBTQ+ colleagues and students, staff and clinicians alike may have to take thoughtful account of their own identity and their religious and cultural beliefs. Students often complain that their counsellors give the impression that their LGBTQ+ issues are themselves the root of the pathology. However, being in a minority group brings particular risks to mental health and often requires means of prevention and treatment that specifically respect this.

Students coming to terms with sexual orientation, gender identity, or both, may benefit from the support of a therapeutic relationship, even if they do not meet diagnostic criteria for a mental illness, and despite wanting to avoid implications that their sexuality and gender are pathological. Most student counselling services now use a very brief therapy model, which is inadequate for the longer-term work these students need. Exceptions should be made to allow for longer therapeutic contact.

Consequences of Childhood Sexual Abuse for Student Mental Health

Childhood sexual abuse is now well-known to predispose victims to mental disorders. These can take a range of features, and will also often present with post-traumatic symptoms. Single or acutely clustered trauma tends to produce a clear picture of post-traumatic stress disorder (PTSD) with flashbacks, nightmares, avoidance and hypervigilance, chronic repeated abuse often produces a more complex picture with substance misuse, deliberate self-harm and eating disorder symptoms as common features. It is very important though, not to assume that everyone who experiences self-harm, substance misuse or eating disorder symptoms will necessarily have a history of sexual abuse.

The UK Office for National Statistics (2016) crime survey found 11% of women of age 16 to 59 gave a history of sexual abuse in childhood compared with 3% of men; 3% of women and 1% of men had experienced sexual assault by rape or penetration (including attempts) during childhood.

Young women are the group at highest risk of screening positive for PTSD. In an online survey of more than 5000 US undergraduate students (Young, 2007) over 40% of females and 30% of males reported a history of sexual abuse. Higher levels of psychiatric symptoms were reported by both male and female students who had been abused. The researchers found that experience of physically forced sexual assault before starting university was associated with nearly seven-times the risk of forcible sexual assault as a student. It has been suggested that people with PTSD may be at higher risk or further assault because of their use of alcohol and drugs as ways to alleviate their distress.

It is likely that many young women and some men are arriving at university already burdened with significant histories of sexual trauma. Further sexual trauma whilst at university is particularly likely to affect this section of the student community. It is hard to imagine prospective students being asked to disclose previous sexual abuse at the time of university entry, so that efforts to reach out to offer special protection and support have to rely on students assertively seeking this for themselves.

Work with young children who have been sexually abused generally involves interventions with them and their non-abusing parents to re-establish sexual codes and healthy norms. Students arriving at university may not all have received such interventions and may benefit from a reorientation to healthy sexual etiquette within an individual or group therapy programme. Universal compulsory consent workshops must be sensitively led if they are not to retraumatise some students.

Gender-Based Aggression, Assault and Abuse in University Life

A UK national online survey by the NUS, attracted over 2000 responses, describing women students' experiences of harassment, stalking, violence and sexual assault (Smith, 2010). Findings, published in the Hidden Marks report, were that 68% respondents had experienced some kind of verbal or non-verbal sexual harassment. This kind of behaviour – which includes groping, flashing and unwanted sexual comments – had become almost 'everyday' for some women students.

Respondents reported consequences of violence, stalking and sexual assault on their health, experience of learning, confidence and relationships, mental health. One in four victims of serious sexual assault stated that their studies had been affected by the incident, and 13% had considered leaving their course.

One in four female respondents experienced some form of sexual assault at university and one in seven experienced a serious physical or sexual assault. The majority of perpetrators of stalking, sexual assault and physical violence were male fellow students, already known to the victim. The stereotype of a scary stranger emerging from the bushes on a dark night and committing rape is not a likely scenario. Most assaults are by acquaintances in social settings such as student halls or at parties. The prevalence of 'incapacitated sexual assault' is more than twice as common as physically forced sexual assault (Krebs et al., 2009).

The NUS survey (Smith, 2010) found that even those who had been 'seriously' assaulted were unlikely to have reported this to the university or police. The most common reasons given were either that the assault did not seem 'serious enough' or that the victim felt ashamed or embarrassed: 43% thought they would be blamed for what had happened, and a third thought they would not be believed. More than 40% victims of serious sexual assault had told nobody about what had happened to them.

There may have been some truth in their negative expectations. A much more recent study (Shannon, 2022) found that 'institutions worked to protect the perpetrators who were deemed more valuable than the survivor. In some cases, this was because of the 'role the assailant occupied or their potential to make an impact in their field'.

> Jocelyn appeared to be a rather confident, even brash, first year student, who made no secret of her partying, and preference for casual 'no-strings' relationships.
>
> Halfway through the year she referred herself to the counselling service and explained tearfully that she had been forced to have sex by a fellow student in halls. She told the counsellor it reminded her of an incident when she was a 13-year-old schoolgirl. A boy at a party had thrown himself on top of her in a bedroom until they were interrupted in the bedroom by classmates. Jocelyn had pretended to her friends she had wanted to have sex and had been trying to keep up the bravado ever since.
>
> She was afraid that if she reported the recent sexual assault, she herself would be blamed, and she would get into trouble if it came to light that she had used cocaine. She was experiencing flashbacks to the episode that happened 6 years earlier and had become tearful and unable to work.

In 2010, the Hidden Marks report concluded 'that institutions and students' unions should adopt a 'zero tolerance' approach to non-verbal and verbal sexual harassment' and that 'institutions, in partnership with students' unions, should develop a comprehensive policy that would set out the measures they will undertake to tackle violence against women students' (Smith, 2010). Over a decade later, this is still an unfulfilled need. We could be more inclusive too in our aspirations, in the light of what is known now about the experiences of people of all genders, not only women.

In the United States, a large-scale survey of 27 higher education institutions found that over 20% of all final-year undergraduates had experienced sexual violence while studying. This number rose to 33% for final year female students and to 39% for transgender, genderqueer, or questioning students (Cantor et al., 2015).

It's crucial to recognise that staff as well as students can be victims of gender-based violence, as well as be perpetrators (Castelao-Huerta, 2022). It is not always certain whether power differentials mean that students' claims will be prioritised over those of staff or the other way round, but bearing in mind Shannon's (2022) findings, it is important to ensure that investigation of allegations of gender-based violence – or indeed other forms of assault – be carried out independently, so that individuals' desirability to the university does not impede justice.

A change in the climate of gender-based respect is vital for everyone's well-being. It goes beyond prevention of serious assault, vital though that is. Fear and threat can cause chronic damage, and make it harder for young people to learn academic, social and interpersonal skills with curiosity and pleasure. So far, efforts to prevent gender-based violence in universities do not appear to have reduced the overall problem. Inconsistent outcomes are reported for a variety of interventions such as consent workshops, self-defence trainings, and bystander training.

It can be difficult to evaluate whether interventions result in overall improvements in the safety of the sexual environment for students. Projects obviously start on a small scale and may be too small to convincingly demonstrate significant changes. The Canadian programme mentioned earlier (Senn et al., 2015) was shown to reduce the likelihood that women would be victims of serious sexual assault over subsequent years. This is laudable, but relies on potential victims taking steps to protect themselves without further input to improve the context in which they have to keep themselves safe.

In parallel with continued efforts to change the culture, counsellors and other clinicians will need to provide treatment for those affected. Management of an acute sexual trauma involves support around decisions such as who to tell, whether to report to authorities, and how to cope with investigations and trials, as well as the direct effects of the trauma. In theory the management of acute PTSD is different from that of chronic trauma, but as we have seen, many student victims of sexual trauma will turn out to have past histories of previous trauma, which often will have been inadequately addressed at the time. The principles of early management – sometimes called 'psychological first aid' – involves re-establishing a sense of security and stability. People are encouraged to pay attention to healthy routines of eating, sleeping, taking physical exercise and socialising with the people they feel safest with, and resisting maladaptive coping strategies such as alcohol, drugs, or risk-taking behaviours.

None of these healthy routines may come easily into a student lifestyle, and for students with supportive families, a return home is an obvious benefit. The main drawback to this is that it involves avoidance of the university environment. The mind will connect the place where the assault happened with danger, and avoidance will make that connection stronger, so that it becomes even harder to return. It is helpful if the counsellor can continue to offer support by video or telephone links and encourage a return to studies in a graded way if avoidance becomes an obstacle. Obviously, avoidance of genuine danger is healthy, but trauma can also cause unhelpful obsessive avoidance of places or people psychologically but not realistically associated with the event.

Mental Health Conditions and Sexual Behaviour

New Zealand's Dunedin Study found 'a clear association between risky sexual behaviour and common psychiatric disorders' in their 18-year-old participants (Ramrakha et al., 2000). They were surprised to find that even depression, the commonest diagnosis, was associated with increased rates of risky sex, sexually transmitted diseases, and early sexual experience. As so often, the research could not assess how far the mental condition caused the risky sexual experiences and how far it was a response to such experiences.

Students with bipolar disorder are often vibrant and high achieving members of a university community, but are also very vulnerable and at higher risk of suicide. They can experience contrasting sexual disturbances depending on the phase of illness that is affecting them. If they go 'high' they can become disinhibited, with an increased incidence of risky sexual behaviours. By contrast, in depressive episodes, they can feel loss of desire and high levels of shame. Students with bipolar disorder are already at higher risk of suicide, and there is evidence that for people with bipolar disorder, sexual problems are significantly associated with suicide plans or a feeling that life is not worth living (Dell'Osso et al., 2009).

The message for our university communities is twofold. Firstly, students who engage in 'risky' sex may need attention to mental ill health. Sexual health campaigns should include this, and sexual health clinics and general practitioners (GPs) should consider appropriate management and onward referral for students who present with medical sexual concerns. Secondly, students already known to have mental health conditions benefit from specific attention to their sexual well-being. For instance, the National Institute for Health and Care Excellence (NICE) recommends that everyone working with autistic adults 'should be sensitive to issues of ... personal and sexual and relationships. In particular, ... problems in social interaction and communication may lead to the autistic person misunderstanding another person's behaviour or to their possible exploitation by others' (NICE, 2012).

Students who experience mental illness are likely to find that both their condition, and often the medication prescribed to treat it, may impair sexual function and reduce sexual satisfaction. The student age group is particularly likely to be concerned about sexual expression and performance, but doctors and counsellors may overlook the importance of asking about this or find it embarrassing. Without discussion, students may not associate their sexual symptoms with their disorder. Some may believe they indicate a change in sexual orientation or gender identity. Some worry that they are burdened with a separate condition on top of their mental illness. Others are ready to attribute sexual dysfunction to their medication without giving this a chance to become effective.

When medication does cause sexual problems – as psychotropic medications quite often do – the student may simply discontinue their treatment rather than discuss alternative drugs, dose changes or additions to the regime. Young people may also stop taking medication if they begin to gain weight, as this is nowadays such a blow to bodily confidence. Psychiatrists have a range of prescribing options that can minimise weight gain, improve global self-confidence, protect sexual function and still keep mental illness at bay. A helpful review (Montejo et al., 2018) guides clinicians to prescribing strategies that maximise good sexual function for people requiring treatment for a range of mental illness.

Students are not always so aware of other features of mental illness that are obstacles to engaging in sexual and indeed other relationships. These might include lack of eye contact when depressed or in the presence of autistic conditions, compulsive behaviours such as counting or muttering, psychotic experiences such as hearing voices, or the avoidance of social situations in eating disorders because of fear of having to eat. Some mental disorders lead to decreased self-care and hygiene, which makes the patient less attractive to potential partners.

Sexual relationships can also be affected by an individual's experience of stigma, both from other people and the internalised self-stigma many experience. The stigma and the reduction in social functioning that come with mental illness can make it easier for affected students to engage in casual sex rather than pursue romantic relationships that might demand intimacy and disclosure of mental illness. Fear of rejection can be particularly strong for someone already struggling with mental and emotional health.

In some cultures, people – especially women – are frankly deemed less 'marriageable' if they have a mental illness, whilst even enlightened societies can experience unspoken fears and prejudices about such illnesses. This be an obstacle to students from some cultures seeking help as they fear consequences of a formal diagnosis.

Mental illness, then is bad news for healthy sexual experience, and some pharmacological treatments can at least temporarily worsen rather than improve sexual function. Sexual interest and desire can be affected as well as the mechanics of intercourse and orgasm. Stopping medication will rarely improve matters, as the student then relapses into the sexual as well as other consequences of untreated mental illness. Yet when treatment is adjusted and perhaps augmented with appropriate psychological therapies, healthy sexual participation can contribute powerfully to recovery.

Practice Points

University Staff and Students

- UK university life lends itself to experimentation and freedom in terms of sexual behaviour, and orientation as well as gender identity. This can be alarming for members of other cultures.
- The LGBTQ+ community is at higher risk of mental ill health.
- Students with autism spectrum disorder may need extra support to negotiate the role of sex in their development.
- Casual sexual encounters ('hooking up') is particularly common the early terms, but those who settle into more monogamous 'dating' seem to enjoy advantage for mental health and well-being.
- Social media, though highly influential, often provides misleading sex education. High reliance on 'apps' and websites for building relationships is associated with poorer levels of mental health than in-person dating.
- High levels of alcohol consumption and use of other drugs are strongly associated with both perpetrating gender-based violence and becoming a victim.

Parents and Families

- The experience of sexual liberation for some students then poses problems for trust and communication with the family of origin.

Schools

- School pupils report that their RSE classes are poorly delivered and show inadequate awareness of the context to their sexual concerns.
- Certain aspects of sex education in schools can protect students from gender-based violence throughout their university career and beyond.
- There is a need to focus on ethical and relational concerns as well as on the mechanics and physical risks of sex.

University Authorities

- Permissive attitudes to excessive alcohol consumption can increase prevalence of gender-based violence in universities.
- It is unjust to protect perpetrators of sexual violence and harassment out of fear of reputational damage.
- Independent investigators may be needed to prevent inappropriate protection of perpetrators who are perceived as having more power and value to the university, than their victims.

Clinicians: GPs, Psychiatrists, Counsellors and Therapists

- A significant minority of students will have histories of previous sexual trauma and abuse, which may still be unaddressed.
- Mental illness – even common 'depression' – is associated with less healthy sexual experiences. The sexual dimension of life is so particularly important to the student age group that this should be part of any assessment and treatment plan.
- All prescribed medication should take sexual activity into account.

References

Bowring, A. L., Vella, A. M., Degenhardt, L., Hellard, M. & Lim, M. S. (2015). Sexual identity, same-sex partners and risk behaviour among a community-based sample of young people in Australia. *International Journal of Drug Policy*, 26(2), 153–61.

Braithwaite, S., Delevi, R. & Fincham, F. (2010). Romantic relationships and the physical and mental health of college students. *Personal Relationships*, 17(1), 1–12.

Bouman, W. P., Bauer, G. R., Richards, C. & Coleman, E. (2010). World Professional Association for Transgender Health consensus statement on considerations of the role of distress (Criterion D) in the DSM diagnosis of gender identity disorder. *International Journal of Transgenderism*, 12(2), 100–106.

Cantor, D., Fisher, B., Chibnall, S. H., et al. (2015). *Report on the AAU campus climate survey on sexual assault and sexual misconduct*. Westat. www.aau.edu/sites/default/files/%40%20Files/Climate%20Survey/AAU_Campus_Climate_Survey_12_14_15.pdf

Castelao-Huerta, I. (2022). The discreet habits of subtle violence: An approach to the experiences of women full professors in neoliberal times. *Gender and Education*, 34(2), 216–30.

Clinton-Sherrod, M., Morgan-Lopez, A. A., Brown, J. M., McMillen, B. A. & Cowell, A. (2011). Incapacitated sexual violence involving alcohol among college women: The impact of a brief drinking intervention. *Violence Against Women*, 17(1), 135–54.

Connolly, M. D., Zervos, M. J., Barone II, C. J., Johnson, C. C. & Joseph, C. L. (2016). The mental health of transgender youth: Advances in understanding. *Journal of Adolescent Health*, 59(5), 489–95.

Dargie, E., Blair, K. L., Goldfinger, C. & Pukhall, C. F. (2015). Go long! Predictors of positive relationship outcomes in long distance dating relationships. *Journal of Sex & Marital Therapy*, 41(2), 181–202.

Dell'Osso, L., Carmassi, C., Carlini, M., et al. (2009). Sexual dysfunctions and suicidality in patients with bipolar disorder and unipolar depression. *The Journal of Sexual Medicine*, 6(11), 3063–70.

Ernst, F., Romanczuk-Seiferth, N., Köhler, S., Amelung, T. & Betzler, F. (2021). Students in the sex industry: Motivations, feelings, risks, and judgments. *Frontiers in Psychology*, 12, 586235.

Gana, T. & Hunt, L. M. (2022). Young women and anal sex. *BMJ*, 378, o1975.

Girlguiding (2014). *Girls attitudes survey*. www .girlguiding.org.uk/globalassets/docs-and-resources/research-and-campaigns/girls-attitudes-survey-2014.pdf

Krebs, C. P., Lindquist, C. H., Warner, T. D., Fisher, B. S, & Martin, S. L. (2009). College women's experiences with physically forced, alcohol-or other drug-enabled, and drug-facilitated sexual assault before and since entering college. *Journal of American College Health*, 57(6), 639–49.

Lamb, S., Gable, S. & de Ruyter, D. (2021). Mutuality in Sexual Relationships: A Standard of Ethical Sex?. *Ethical Theory and Moral Practice*, 24(1), 271–84.

Liverpool John Moores University (2014). *Developing a Sexual Consent Campaign to Raise Awareness and Educate Young Men on Sexual Activity, Consent, Intoxication and the Law of Rape*. (2014 Research Excellence Framework Impact Case Study). https://impact.ref.ac.uk/casestudies/CaseStudy.aspx?Id=30013

Lorenz, K. & Ullman, S. E. (2016). Alcohol and sexual assault victimization: Research findings and future directions. *Aggression and Violent Behavior*, 31, 82–94.

Meyer, I. H. (2003). Prejudice, social stress, and mental health in lesbian, gay, and bisexual populations: Conceptual issues and research evidence. *Psychological Bulletin*, 129(5), 674–97.

Montejo, A. L., Montejo, L. & Baldwin, D. S. (2018). The impact of severe mental disorders and psychotropic medications on sexual health and its implications for clinical management. *World Psychiatry*, 17 (1), 3–11.

Mori, C., Temple, J. R., Browne, D. & Madigan, S. (2019). Association of sexting with sexual behaviors and mental health among adolescents: A systematic review and meta-analysis. *JAMA Pediatrics*, 173(8), 770–9.

National Institute for Health and Care Excellence (2012). *Autism spectrum disorder in adults: Diagnosis and management*. www .nice.org.uk/Guidance/CG142

Netting, N. S. & Reynolds, M. K. (2018). Thirty years of sexual behaviour at a Canadian university: Romantic relationships, hooking up, and sexual choices. *The Canadian Journal of Human Sexuality*, 27(1), 55–68.

Office for National Statistics (2016) *Abuse during childhood: Findings from the Crime Survey for England and Wales, year ending March 2016*. www.ons.gov.uk/peoplepopulationandcommunity/crime andjustice/articles/abuseduringchildhood/findingsfromtheyearendingmarch2016 crimesurveyforenglandandwales

Ofsted (2021). *Review of sexual abuse in schools and colleges*. www.gov.uk/government/publications/review-of-sexual-abuse-in-schools-and-colleges/review-of-sexual-abuse-in-schools-and-colleges

Papadopoulos, L. (2010). *Sexualisation of young people review*. Home Office.

Phipps, A. & Young, I. (2015). 'Lad culture' in higher education: Agency in the sexualization debates. *Sexualities*, 18(4), 459–79.

Ramrakha, S., Caspi, A., Dickson, N., Moffitt, T. E. & Paul, C. (2000). Psychiatric disorders and risky sexual behaviour in young adulthood: Cross sectional study in birth cohort. *BMJ*, 321(7256), 263–6.

Ream, G. L. (2019). What's unique about lesbian, gay, bisexual, and transgender (LGBT) youth and young adult suicides? Findings from the National Violent Death Reporting System. *Journal of Adolescent Health*, 64(5), 602–607.

Roberts, R., Bergström, S. & La Rooy, D. (2007). Sex work and students: An exploratory study. *Journal of Further and Higher Education*, 31(4), 323–34.

Sagar, T., Jones, D., Symons, K., Bowring, J. & Roberts, R. (2015). Student participation in the sex industry: Higher education responses and staff experiences and perceptions. *Journal of Higher Education Policy and Management*, 37(4), 400–412.

Santelli, J. S., Grilo, S. A., Choo, T. H., et al. (2018). Does sex education before college protect students from sexual assault in college? *PLoS ONE*, 13(11), e0205951.

Sawyer, A. N., Smith, E. R. & Benotsch, E. G. (2018). Dating application use and sexual risk behavior among young adults. *Sexuality Research and Social Policy*, 15(2), 183–91.

Senn, C. Y., Eliasziw, M., Barata, P. C., et al. (2015). Efficacy of a sexual assault resistance program for university women. *New England Journal of Medicine*, 372(24), 2326–35.

Shannon, E. R. (2022). Safeguarding and agency: methodological tensions in conducting research with survivors of sexual violence in universities. *Social Sciences*, 11(8), 350.

Simonovic, D. (2020) *Violence against women, its causes and consequences regarding COVID-19 and the increase of domestic violence against women. Submission to the UN special rapporteur.* Human Rights Watch. www.hrw.org/news/2020/07/03/submission-un-special-rapporteur-violence-against-women-its-causes-and-consequences

Smith, G. (2010). *Hidden marks: A study of women students' experiences of harassment, stalking, violence and sexual assault.* National Union of Students. https://itstopsnow.org/sites/default/files/2018-02/Hidden Marks-A study of women students' experiences of harassment, stalking, violence & sexual assault (NUS).pdf

Stinson, R. D. (2010). Hooking up in young adulthood: A review of factors influencing the sexual behavior of college students. *Journal of College Student Psychotherapy*, 24:2, 98–115.

Universities UK (2016). *Changing the culture: Report of the Universities UK taskforce examining violence against women, harassment and hate crime affecting university students.* www.universitiesuk.ac.uk/sites/default/files/field/downloads/2021-07/changing-the-culture.pdf

Wade, L. (2017). *American hookup: The new culture of sex on campus.* New York, WW Norton & Co.

Wilson, L. C. & Liss, M. (2022). Safety and belonging as explanations for mental health disparities among sexual minority college students. *Psychology of Sexual Orientation and Gender Diversity*, 9(1), 110–19.

Young, M. S., Harford, K. L., Kinder, B. & Savell, J. K. (2007). The relationship between childhood sexual abuse and adult mental health among undergraduates: Victim gender doesn't matter. *Journal of Interpersonal Violence*, 22 (10), 1315–31.

The Mental Health of Teaching and Academic Staff

The original title for this book was 'University Mental Health'. Publishers preferred 'Improving Student Mental Health', but during the course of writing it, I found the importance of a whole-university approach emerged repeatedly. The welfare of staff as well as students is integral to the flourishing of the whole institution. Modern universities need a variety of staff groups including ancillary, administrative and pastoral staff, managers, leaders and non-executive decision-makers, and of course academic and teaching staff. We have thus returned to a version of my original title.

Universities were first set up almost a thousand years ago as communities of academics. The term 'university' comes from the term 'universitas magistrorum et scholarium', meaning the 'entirety', or perhaps 'community', of teachers and students. They were very much based on the relationship of a master and his students (always male), usually clustered in certain subject areas, rather like today's departments and faculties. In the Middle Ages, teachers and students formed corporate bodies – like the trade guilds – to protect their group interests.

It was the scholarship, the teacher–student relationships and the community around this shared value that constituted a university, and for some of us still does. The academics, researchers and teachers are the precious essence of modern universities. Without them there is no university in the real sense of the word. In the twenty-first century, though, academics and teachers as well as their students, find themselves working in a very different sort of 'university'. Two different models of university life emerge in conversations within and outside universities.

One is the common assumption that universities are 'tertiary education' centres, where students automatically progress after high schools, to be recipients of more teaching, albeit at a higher level than before, to sit harder examinations and only then emerge into the adult world with a degree qualification. According to this implicit model, students are still vulnerable adolescents. They are still being educated by others in large groups, in contrast with the old model of younger and older adults working more like master and apprentice with both contributing to the work.

An alternative model is the often-embittered complaint that we have all but turned universities into 'degree factories'. Some people do not complain, of course, but regard a commercial model of education as perfectly valid. This sees students – or their families and national governments – as consumers purchasing educational courses and the qualifications that hallmark them and making demands on the service they have paid for. In this model, universities are the purveyors of education, and academics are hired hands set to work on the conveyor belt to produce teaching or research, which is then sold to the public by the middlemen.

As both these implicit models mix, attitudes to students have changed too. In their grandparents' time students would work towards their degrees while they were still under age 21 and therefore 'children' to whom the university had responsibilities 'in loco parentis'. In contrast, there is now an uncomfortable dynamic that sees staff as having duty of care towards these young adults, whilst also insisting on their adult rights. Individual members of both academic and pastoral staff can feel responsible for the well-being of the students they teach, and also overwhelmed by the impossible scale of that task. Often, they do not feel adequately backed up by university authorities in terms of resources to refer troubled students.

This perceived lack of support can impact on the well-being and mental health of university staff, who may already be managing diagnosed or diagnosable mental disorders of their own, in a post-COVID climate of reduced availability of services in the community.

The main focus of this chapter is the mental health of academic staff, but with recognition that non-academic staff and particularly mental health support staff have their own, frequently different needs. The needs of postgraduate students, who are also frequently employed on a casual basis as university staff, are also considered.

Some of the same principles apply to the many non-academic staff – administrative staff, residence and accommodation staff, librarians, security and domestic staff – who make essential contributions and are organically part of university life. In some research these staff members are studied as 'controls' for the health of academic staff, and usually found to have better mental health, or at least higher levels of well-being (e.g., Fontinha et al., 2019). Unfortunately, I have not found any information on how their mental health is supported.

Mrs Johnson, a well-known chef, suggested to her husband that he might like to invite some of his final year students for dinner at their home. She had fond memories of parties in her professor's house when the two of them had been students at the university where they met.

Dr Johnson was horrified by the idea. He told his wife that he tried to hold his students at arms' length. He felt that any contact with them would potentially expose him to accusations of sexual abuse or of handling their mental health wrongly. This had never happened to him, but he had heard colleagues' stories.

There were times when he felt concerns about students and sometimes suspected that questions about academic aspects of the course might be 'covers' for expressing loneliness or depression. However, he had not attended the optional mental health training the university offered, preferring to focus on research aspects of his work and keeping the teaching within tight boundaries.

What Is Known About the Mental Health of Academic and Teaching Staff

Significant numbers of university staff appear to have poor mental health, with high levels of clinical distress. There has been a significant increase in the numbers of staff accessing support, though with significant variation between universities. University staff are now reporting higher levels of stress and burnout than the general population and low levels of well-being (Shaw, 2014). This does not mean that they are necessarily diagnosed with treatable mental illnesses, although obviously such stresses can precipitate depression and anxiety disorders in those of us who are constitutionally vulnerable. In staff already managing a mental health condition, there may not be a healthy ambient environment for remaining well or recovering from episodes of illness.

One senior, male academic told me

> There is an expectation, implicit in the Research Excellence Framework, quality assurance and appraisal system, that academic staff should be excellent at everything – research, teaching and administration – in order to be considered worthy. When this is combined with expectations from home to be excellent homemakers/parents/carers and with a healthy work–life balance, there is intense stress.

We do not have to rely – as is so often the case – on studies from the United States, as several recent papers have examined well-being in UK academics. Fontinha et al. (2019) found that academic staff report a poorer quality of life than non-academics within UK higher education institutions. One important factor in this was the higher number of extra hours worked per week, which adversely affects work–life balance. Interestingly, those academics who worked up to 10 extra hours were actually more satisfied with their career and believed they had more control at work than those who either did not work extra hours at all or who worked for more than 10 extra hours weekly.

Another study comparing academic staff with non-academic staff in UK universities (Johnson, 2019), whilst agreeing that academics reported higher levels of work overload, and poorer work–life balance, also reported better physical health, better job conditions and work relationships, and less concern about pay and benefits in comparison with non-academic employees. This suggests that the two groups of staff have different needs and concerns. However, such studies do not tell us how working in a university compares with comparable work outside a university setting.

One of the most coruscating criticisms of conditions for academic staff comes from the report Pressure Vessels (Morrish, 2019), whose author describes an escalation of poor mental health among university staff. The report finds a 70% increase in referrals to counselling and a 60% increase in referrals to occupation health for female staff. Morrish (2019) suggests that 'pressure on staff to enhance the student experience has resulted in work-related stress', which negatively impacts upon staff productivity, impacting upon the support they can offer to students and leading inevitably to 'the wasteful loss to the sector of able and experienced personnel'.

Finally, that same year in 2019, a qualitative study was conducted by the group responsible for the university Mental Health Charter. Brewster et al. (2022) conducted six focus group discussions of professional and academic staff. They discussed training in mental health, available support for their own mental health, positive and negative influences on mental health and well-being in their work life, and the relationship between staff and student well-being. Their conclusions – in contrast with some of the other studies – were that the mental health of students does not have to be at the expense of staff well-being, but that there is an 'intrinsic interconnection between staff and student well-being'.

Their report cites the evidence that academic staff in the UK work an average of 51 hours per week, undertake more unpaid work and experience higher work-related stress than the majority of other occupational professional groups and the general population. The research was conducted before the pandemic, but in writing up, post-COVID, the authors hypothesise that 'these pressures may well have been exacerbated as a result of COVID and the 'online pivot' within higher education'.

In 2020, in the unique COVID pandemic and associated lockdown restrictions, a research group at a London university (Carr et al., 2022) conducted an investigation into the mental health of 9800 staff members and 2500 postgraduate students. Although the survey was completed online, this was not just a 'convenience sample' of self-selected respondents, but involved samples specifically invited by email. The survey drew on detailed administrative information about the target population to determine the representativeness of respondents. Researchers were thus able to consider factors previously associated with poor mental health, such as age, gender and ethnicity, as well as factors introduced or amplified by the pandemic and lockdown.

Nearly one in three staff and one in ten postgraduate students had children living at home. Around one in ten respondents reported other caregiving roles besides childcare (Carr et al., 2022). It is already known that carers are more likely to experience symptoms of mental ill health, and this is of course more likely to be part of life for mature students, postgraduates and members of staff than for undergraduates. Provision of childcare and support of other caring responsibilities may do much to improve staff well-being.

Carr et al. (2022) found no evidence of direct associations between remote working and reports of depression or anxiety. However, most of the usual risk factors were amplified by the COVID situation. Staff on fixed-term or casual contracts were more likely to report anxiety symptoms, compared with those on open-ended contracts. Staff who needed, but could not access, healthcare were more likely to show symptoms of depression and anxiety. Reporting a long-term health condition was associated with probable depression and anxiety, and staff members who had to shield or self-isolate were twice as likely to show anxiety.

Around 20% of staff members and 30% of postgraduate research students met thresholds for probable depression or anxiety on the questionnaires. This doubled to around 40% among younger respondents. Other factors associated with probable depression and anxiety included female gender, belonging to an ethnic minority group, caregiving responsibilities and shielding or isolating. Around 20% of respondents were found to reach the cut-off for hazardous drinking on the Alcohol Use Disorders Identification Test, and 30% were drinking more than before the pandemic. The authors found these to be worrying levels of symptoms of depression, anxiety and alcohol use disorder, but admitted that it was hard to be sure of the extent to which elevated mental distress was attributable to the pandemic.

Increasing Threats to the Mental Well-Being of University Staff

It emerges from a reading of the research that while increases in hours worked and consequences for work–life balance are significant, one of the salient complaints is the nature of the extra work. Staff are not complaining about extra time spent on research or teaching, but on the growing bureaucracy required to complete regulatory requirements, metrics, audits and sector reviews such as the Teaching Excellence Framework and the Research Excellence Framework. Academic and teaching staff have to participate, often reluctantly, in the surveillance and monitoring of their own and sometimes colleagues' performance, setting objectives and targets, participating in metrics measures and completing audit exercises. Morrish (2019) describes 'a culture of workplace surveillance'. This engenders feelings that academics are not trusted to have their own sense of responsibility. Similar complaints are heard from staff in the National Health Service (NHS), and from primary and secondary schoolteachers and warrant broader research into interventions to modify the situation in the interests of staff well-being.

Threats to University Staff Mental Health

Short-term contracts
More than 10 extra hours worked each week
Time spent completing metrics, audits and sector reviews
Unsympathetic direct line manager
Overwhelming number of electronic platforms and messages
Overwhelming numbers of extra students added to teaching load
Obligation to support student mental health without adequate training, support or protection from liability
Failure to recognise pastoral care in workload, either in terms of time, prestige and pay
Culture of student well-being taking priority over staff well-being.

Performance management in universities is too often linked to short-term outcomes and expectations, which are seen as unrealistic for many. Participants in these exercises complain that the administrative tasks and monitoring are not helpfully linked to raising standards but are 'setting people up to fail.' Ironically, this is the reverse of good teaching psychology.

The dynamic of threat and of competition rather than collaboration with peers that these exercises foster is unlikely to promote mental health. Staff, like students, rightly seek a sense of belonging and acceptance, and as culture-carriers for universities, can do much to create that atmosphere on campus. However, many academics are employed on a succession of precarious fixed-term contracts, which do not allow for career planning and advancement. More than a third say they experience poor mental health because of worries about their employment status (Morrish, 2019). They are thus unlikely to develop a sense of loyalty and attachment to their institution, or to radiate a sense of positivity and hope.

The sense of belonging to a supportive group can mitigate this distress greatly. Brewster et al. (2022) reports that 'having a supportive team and a good direct line manager has been shown to be important for good well-being, in both the literature and feedback from staff participants in the Mental Health Charter consultation'. This is potentially precarious, though. When key members of staff leave, the benefits are lost unless the ethos of the small groups is part of the whole university culture. One respondent in the Mental Health Charter consultation described how 'when people are struggling with their workload, the answer to that is "Improve your time management."'

Staff as well as students struggle with healthy management of life online (see Chapter 8). Electronic communication contributes to the sense of loss of control and of feeling overwhelmed. Since COVID and the emergence of Teams, Zoom and other communication platforms, online communication has become de rigueur. It encroaches on and potentially invades the privacy of home life and disturbs work–life balance. This problem is by no means confined to university staff and is a phenomenon that society has yet to address satisfactorily.

University staff can feel 'under fire' from increasing demands from audit and monitoring exercises, from increasing electronic communications and also from being asked to teach and support increasing numbers of students without benefit of extra colleagues to share the workload. The solution of teaching in ever larger lecture theatres or over electronic platforms fails to account for the important interactive elements of both teaching and pastoral support. Staff have rightly identified that widening access brings disproportionate demands on pastoral care. One academic spoke of the increased recruitment of international students and proposals for introducing accelerated degrees as 'all a matter of more and faster'. Some report a culture of the well-being of students taking priority over that of staff.

Meeting the increased need to support student mental health requires extra trained staff, both academic and support staff, together with appropriate and effective training, supervision and institutional protection from undue liability. To add insult to injury, academic staff who participate compassionately in student support are often expected to do so without any extra prestige, recognition or pay. It has been suggested that awards to staff voted for by students are a good way of highlighting those that go the extra mile. However, such 'extra miles' should not have to be a competitive prize-winning option, but a properly recompensed part of work with students.

> Dr Jackson, a senior lecturer in politics, introduced a young male student to the counselling service and ruefully pointed out to her colleagues in the student support team that nearly all the student counsellors and mentors were female. One of them responded that at least they were seen as professionals in mental health and paid the same as their male counterparts, whereas Dr Jackson, so far as they could see, was doing all her mental health work on a voluntary basis on top of her academic workload and it was taken for granted that she was just 'being motherly to the students'.
>
> This was a wakeup call. She was enraged to think that this might be the case and raised the issue at annual appraisal. It was satisfying that the work was now formally acknowledged in her workload, and resource was allocated to sending her on special training for the role. However, she was angry that she had to raise the issue herself after several years as a lecturer and was aware that the solution was an individual patch rather than recognition of a systemic need for the role.

The RAND review (Guthrie et al., 2017) examined the mental health of 'researchers'. This is not exactly the same as university academic staff: it includes postgraduate students and reads with the presumption that researchers are engaged in research into the sciences rather than the arts. This study revealed that spending a larger percentage of one's time on research was associated with reduced stress, and that research-only staff reported lower levels of work–life conflict and had better well-being than predominantly teaching staff.

The authors speculate that this may be to some extent confounded by other characteristics of the researchers, for instance they may be more senior. It seems reasonable to consider, however, that university academic staff, unlike schoolteachers, do not come into teaching through a training in education but are expected to add teaching to their primary interest in their academic subject. They may not consider it their primary purpose at work, nor feel confident in their teaching abilities. Moreover, the potential for attracting congratulation (and promotion) rather than complaint may be greater in research than in teaching.

This research also points out that research on emotionally challenging topics such as trauma, abuse or war can put staff well-being at risk. It recommends that staff should receive greater support to mitigate the negative impacts of this work. My experience has been that ethics committees are usually highly sensitive to such issues and tend to insist that provision is made to address potential psychological harms. The well-being of teachers and trainers in such fields requires equal consideration.

Job stress and poor workplace well-being can contribute to reduced productivity – both through absence and through 'presenteeism', where researchers attend work and are less productive. The report translates this into financial terms by quoting an estimate from Shutler-Jones (2017) that the costs to the UK higher education sector could be more than 5% of the sector's total annual income. It may seem crass to imagine we can translate human suffering into purely financial terms, but this may be one of the most powerful ways to negotiate improvements.

The Prevalence of Mental Health Disorders in Academics

While there has been huge interest in stress and poor levels of mental well-being in university staff, recent figures on diagnosable mental illness are harder to find.

A review across different occupational groups (Goodwin et al., 2013) suggested that academics are among the occupational groups with the highest levels of 'common mental disorders'. The review estimated the prevalence of common mental disorders among academics and teachers at 37% – almost double that of the general population (19%). However, the prevalence of psychological disorders was higher in primary and secondary teachers compared to higher education teachers.

A survey conducted in 2014 by The Guardian newspaper (Shaw, 2014) specifically targeted academic staff who had experienced mental health problems and provides data on the relative frequency of different conditions within the sample. Not all the 'conditions' reported correspond with formal diagnoses, and the caveat applies that this is a self-selected sample of respondents. Depression, panic attacks and eating disorders were the most frequently reported conditions, experienced by 75%, 42% and 15% of the sample, respectively.

The RAND review (Guthrie et al., 2017) found that only 6% academic staff disclosed a mental health condition to their university despite the 37% prevalence of mental illness. They make the reasonable point that 'it was unclear whether stress was a result of working conditions in the research environment, or whether research settings attracted particular types of individuals'.

Other chapters in this book observe how a personality profile that includes a vulnerability to certain mental health conditions may also bring abilities and attributes that make such people particularly valuable to the academic community. When this is acknowledged, the appropriate response may not be to blame environmental and interpersonal conditions for all pathology but to accept that there will be some intercurrent disorders needing treatment, albeit in the most supportive possible contexts. Staff who are courageous enough to 'disclose' a mental health condition can anonymously demonstrate the normality of such disorders and the need for proper adjustments to be made to workload and contracts.

Relative Prevalence of Different Mental Health Conditions in Academics Who Report Mental Health Problems

Depression 75%
Panic attacks 42%
Eating disorder 15%
Self-harm 11%

Obsessive compulsive disorder 11%
Alcoholism 11%
Post-traumatic stress disorder 9%
Other mental health problem 7%
Bipolar disorder 4%
Drug addiction 2%
Schizophrenia less than 1%

(Shaw, 2014)

Services to Treat and Manage Mental Disorders in University Staff

As of the summer of 2022, my exploration of a broad range of university websites leaves me impressed by the provision made by universities for providing counselling support to university staff. It is easy to access helpful information simply by putting 'staff counselling at the university of wherever' into any search engine. Websites are then clear, detailed and explicit about choices on offer, how to self-refer or access referral, and boundaries of confidentiality. Most of the larger institutions provide a range of choices for academic, teaching and ancillary staff with mental health problems or conditions.

Virtually all institutions have a contract with a private provider to provide confidential counselling or psychological therapy. These involve individual appointments with a therapist as well as subscriptions paid for by the institution to web-based packages, such as SilverCloud or Togetherall. Larger universities also offer their own staff counselling services, with online or face-to-face options that are not at the same venue as student counselling sessions. Occupational Health is another important and related resource. It is not itself a provider of mental health treatment, but a way to have mental health needs validated and the necessary support negotiated in the staff member's working life.

Obviously, members of staff are more likely than students to have an established relationship with a local general practitioner, through which referrals to specialist NHS psychiatry and psychology services can be arranged. What surprises me is how rarely university staff seem aware of the apparent wealth of support provided by universities for their staff, especially in the realm of psychological support, for which there are long NHS waiting lists. It may be lost in the barrage of information on staff intranets, or possibly the impression given by websites is not an accurate representation of the reality. Quite likely, considering conversations I have had and seen reported in the literature, staff are unconvinced by assurances of confidentiality, unaware that being known to Occupational Health is more likely to be protective than threatening, and wary of allowing their own vulnerability to be managed within the university. Brewster et al. (2022) quote a staff member as saying

> If I say I'm not managing things, then are you going to be promoted, because obviously you don't have any resilience, and it gets so much more stressful. So, I think there is probably a culture of internalising, so you just keep quiet and carry on.

It will take time, training and positive experiences to change views such as this.

We need also to be aware that even in the most enlightened and rational culture, when a person falls prey to a disorder of the mind, they may regress to more primitive thinking patterns. When a person is anxious and depressed, they may see the world through 'negative spectacles'. It is not enough at such times for there to be useful information on web pages. The individual needs help from trusted others. Just as students may need prompting from peers, teachers and pastoral staff, to access help and accept treatment, so may staff, however mature and senior. The absent-minded professors of a century ago were usually supported by a wife or housekeeper. Today's teachers and academics may need to rely on colleagues to nudge them to find help. Such colleagues – and even students – need the institution to have supportive rather than disciplinary pathways in place to facilitate this.

Professor Jones had a bipolar disorder, which he had declared to the occupational health department on taking up his Chair. The disorder had not been an obstacle to a highly successful career in modern languages. He was a popular and charismatic teacher. However, he decided with his psychiatrist's agreement, to change to a different medication to avoid certain adverse side effects. He then slowly developed an upswing in mood. One Monday morning he announced that he would give his lecture at double speed to allow everyone to leave early for lunch, and proceeded to do so, adding in several puns and jokes, which made him laugh more than his audience.

A pair of mature students who knew him well agreed that he might not be well and decided to take their concerns to one of the other lecturers on the course. This colleague spoke with management and Professor Jones was immediately suspended from teaching and informed that 'two female students had made a complaint against him'. The situation became distressing for all concerned, although the professor's partner ensured that he was seen speedily at the hospital and spent a week on the ward there.

It was later agreed that had he been a student rather than staff, there would have been compassionate provision to support him, but staff were not expected to be vulnerable. The incident led to the setting up of pathways to support staff with mental illness without having to use a disciplinary route.

Prof Jones considered taking legal action against his employers for failure in their duty of care and for damage to his reputation but was persuaded that this would ultimately do more damage to his academic career.

In Brewster's (2022) study, policies on staff absence were raised in several groups, with the potential for absences to lead to formal interventions and even dismissal. Another group's discussion centred on the benefits of being able to take days off for well-being purposes, but the difficulties of doing so in practice because of demands on staff time. The problem of how to treat a person's mental condition as an illness requiring treatment and support rather than as bad behaviour to be punished also arises in the context of 'fitness to practice' and the structures around mental disorders in members of the professions such as medicine, law and teaching (see Chapter 19).

The Role of Academic and Teaching Staff in Supporting the Mental Health of Students

Most parents of students and many academics have asked what exactly is meant by 'duty of care' to the students in a university, and how this differs from being 'in loco parentis'. Universities deal almost exclusively with young adults. The tiny minority of students under the legal age of majority are subject to special protections and regulations, but even these students will rarely if ever be under the age of 16. As a result, universities are not called upon to offer levels of protection and care that could be reasonably expected of a parent. The specialist lawyer, Sian Jones-Davies (2019) writes

> In broad terms, institutions owe a general legal duty of care to students to deliver their services (such as teaching and pastoral support) to the standard of the reasonably competent higher education institution and to act reasonably to protect the health, safety and welfare of their students.

This means that in fact, universities as a whole are creating the standards by which they will be judged. It may be that the Mental Health Charter could be used as a benchmark for expectations of 'reasonable' practice, although it seeks to institute excellent rather than merely 'reasonable' practice. Universities across the UK create a sort of general 'norm' whereby some sort of pastoral care is expected of all, but some universities offer more than the minimum. Beyond the general 'duty of care' principle, there is also the matter of contractual obligation, particularly now that universities are seen as delivering an advertised service, according to a commercial model. Paradoxically, promising more than a minimum level of pastoral care opens a university up to more complaints and legal challenges if it is in breach of what is promised.

Obviously, different members of staff will reasonably be expected to have different skills in terms of pastoral support, and academics, library staff and cleaning staff would not be expected to have the levels of pastoral care expertise found in members of the university counselling staff. For the institution to fulfil its overall duty of care though, it is reasonable to expect communication and awareness so that students can be directed to the resources and support they need and staff themselves can receive guidance.

Research by Hughes et al. (2018) speaks of 'the unavoidable role academics are now playing in responding to student mental health'. The research already cited suggests it is not always a comfortable or welcome aspect of the job and it may be that the efforts of some to attempt to avoid, perversely make the culture worse.

Alan Percy, Head of Counselling at the University of Oxford, says staff are not unsympathetic or judgmental so much as afraid of what they might uncover. Their understandable fear that they couldn't handle severe acute mental illness can spread to a sense that even common-sense support and management is dangerous, and they must protect themselves from doing something wrong. In contrast, most students and staff would be able to handle physical problems from a running a burned finger under a cold tap to dialling 999 if someone collapses in a corridor. Of course, we have all been repeatedly drilled in emergency contact numbers, notices in corridors carry details of the nearest official First Aider, and in the longer term the student or colleague with a physical illness has capacity to manage their illness and make decisions. None of these things are necessarily true when the illness or disorder is one of the mind.

Some respondents to the Hughes et al. (2018) study felt they were not always backed up by student mental health services when they asked for support in a crisis. They felt their judgment was undermined. They often felt they were 'left holding the baby' when students were waiting on long waiting lists for formal support either with university or NHS services. Academics described worries about students keeping them awake at night and impacting on their home life. They became exhausted, anxious and even depressed. They often felt that they were not equipped or supported to respond to student mental health problems or how to support students generally. As a result, they were drawing entirely from their own experience or personal support networks. Newly appointed academics were particularly vulnerable, particularly international appointees from different cultures and health systems.

Joyce was a likeable but disorganised second-year English student. She was a lively participant in small group seminars run by Carol, a PhD student. Joyce made several casual but concerning references in the seminars to her own self harming behaviour and low mood. One afternoon when others had left, Carol asked Joyce about her mental health. The answer was 'I often get close to topping myself, don't you?' A few days later, she came to class clearly intoxicated and distressed, so Carol took her aside and suggested she could make her an appointment with Student Support Services. To her surprise, Joyce became angry and forbade her to do so, telling her it would be a serious breach of her confidentiality. She said that so long as she could speak to Carol, she would be safe.

Carol's own PhD supervisor was on sick leave, and she mentioned to her partner, without naming Joyce, that she was seriously concerned about a student and had no one to turn to. He suggested that since she had been able to speak to him without breaching confidentiality, she might be able to contact a mental health advisor to do the same thing. It was a relief to speak with an expert and to have limits of confidentiality and responsibility discussed and clarified.

On balance, she felt she was sufficiently concerned to insist that Joyce seek help for herself, and this did happen. The relationship between Carol and her student became much more distant, but at the end of the semester Joyce sent an email thanking her for taking her mental health seriously.

Some academics have been advised by lawyers that they would be held liable if there were a disastrous outcome for a student who was being supported by an unqualified director of studies rather than by a properly trained mental health professional. Whilst I would expect a good defence lawyer to be able to reassign responsibility in a just way, I would also advise any staff in this situation to protect themselves by documenting formally where they have been obliged to support a student because of the absence of other immediate appropriate treatment. I am aware, though, that this adds to bureaucratic burden in a situation that should not arise in the first place.

Training in Mental Health for University Staff

The focus groups described by Brewster et al. (2022) and Hughes et al. (2018) found that the idea of training was surprisingly contentious. It is understandable that finding time to engage is difficult unless the training were to be mandated as part of agreed workload. For instance, mandatory training could be provided regularly, alongside Fire safety and other necessary training, in a 1- or 2-day block before the start of academic semester, preferably with paid expenses. But some staff were afraid that attending additional training could increase their responsibilities in this area. Others suggested that the training they had received had not been helpful as it was not designed for their role.

One academic complained that

> The thing is with mental health training is it's not for you, it's for you to help the student, that's the institutional message.

Another experienced academic told me

> There was such an explosion of training 'opportunities' and requirements in the past few years that they significantly eroded time for either research or development/preparation/delivery of new teaching.

If mental health training is to authentically engage academic and teaching staff it is essential that it states explicitly, and enacts convincingly, the attitude that the focus is on the mental health of all members of university whatever their seniority, and that the well-being of staff and colleagues is crucial. Self-care and mutual care for colleagues is to be part of the training.

Much of the benefit of mental health training is about forging constructive relationships with support services as well as learning specific information and skills for supporting students and colleagues in distress. When staff from university mental health services deliver the training interactively and show themselves to be approachable and respectful, potentially oppositional relationships between academics and mental health staff can be reconstructed and a sense of confidence in reliable support restored.

Another key anxiety that must be addressed if learning is to take place in such training workshops is the question of liability. Concepts such as 'duty of care' are rarely adequately described or understood, for instance. Academics are often unclear about who holds responsibility for the well-being of a student, whether responsibility sits with the academic, departments or wider university, or in some cases, with the student's parents or family. It has to be acknowledged that academic and pastoral responsibilities cannot be easily separated as academic problems often have a non-academic cause.

Structural boundary descriptions are unlikely to solve the problem. Students turn to approachable academics for support regardless of how the role is described to them. In some instances, academics believe confusion and blurred boundaries are deliberately maintained at an institutional level to encourage them to taken on extra but inappropriate tasks, including assessing student need and triaging.

In order to acknowledge the nuances and uncertainties of such concerns, trainers could use case studies to focus discussion. Sometimes it's particularly informative to work together through situations described by the staff. Trainers should be prepared to take questions, suggestions and requests for clarification to university authorities, unions and legal teams after the training session. This would allow participants to contribute to improvements in the university's services and policies at the point of receiving training.

There are already several well-regarded training resources, including online versions, that cover 'Mental Health first aid' principles and who to call in a crisis, and management of suicide risk. These benefit from being viewed in a group with discussion, and particularly benefit from having local contacts and arrangements highlighted, as each institution has different arrangements and different contact details. Out-of-hours arrangements are particularly important to know. These specifics are among the most useful 'tools' participants take away from the training.

If there is time and interest in the training, information could be provided on mental health conditions likely to require specific adjustments to student life, together with discussion of non-acute help such as advice lines for staff and resources for people who are still on waiting lists or being treated but causing concern.

Stand-alone training, however good, is not enough. Such workshops need to be just one opportunity for academic and specialist mental health staff to work together. NHS staff and other frontline professionals who respond to people in distress usually work within a clear framework of responsibility and comprehensive support, including supervision. Regular confidential supervision groups and 'hotline' advice should be set up for university staff to support their pastoral care. Many staff involved will be part timers or have regular commitments, so a choice of different times may be necessary. Likewise, new staff may arrive long before the next mental health training is available, so that brief 'induction' packs need to be available too, particularly for staff on 'casual' contracts.

Essentials of Mental Health Training for Academic and Teaching Staff

Emphasis on mental health for all staff as well as for students

Information on resources for staff mental health

Clarification of legal responsibilities and boundaries

'Mental health first aid' principles and who to call in a crisis, including out of hours

Coping with suicide risk in students or staff

Information on mental health conditions likely to require specific adjustments in the university

Advice lines and resources for students or colleagues still on waiting lists or being treated but causing concern

Regular and drop-in supervision groups where academic staff and mental health advisors can discuss together both specific and general mental health concerns about students, confidentially

Repeat information on appropriate resources for staff mental health needs.

Academics across a number of institutions admitted with disarming honesty that while they think information and guidance on how to manage specific situations exists, they do not always know where to find it (Hughes et al., 2018). It is more effective when it is easy to ask for help and advice from individuals with appropriate experience. A number of academics felt they would benefit from an opportunity to access supervision for their role, in relation to student distress.

Whilst the research workshops revealed a lack of consensus as to whether training should be compulsory and universal, I would argue that such training does need to be a mandatory part of all staff induction and continuing professional development. It must acknowledge the inevitable overlap of academic and mental health concerns in their own and their colleagues' lives as well as those of their students.

Such training by no means equips academics to be therapists. Those who do chose to take on a more time-consuming pastoral support role should be acknowledged and fully supported within managed pastoral care teams. Those members of staff who do not feel confident in face-to-face support of distressed students can still contribute by supporting the status and rights of those colleagues who do, respecting the expertise and value of this aspect of university life. They may also provide salutary correctives when they observe colleagues becoming over-enmeshed in students' personal problems. One experienced academic told me that

> problems have arisen where staff think they can cope with students who have serious difficulties then find themselves drawn in too much and start to struggle themselves. It is vital to provide some kind of staff support system to minimise this.

If training is not made compulsory, research tells us, 'It is always the same people' who attended training, rather than being representative of the wider academic and professional staff community (Brewster et al., 2022). Student-facing teaching roles in which staff work with small groups of students or one-to-one are often taken by 'casualised' staff, such as PhD students, part-timers and early career researchers. Even if training is available widely within an institution, these staff may be missed out. Such staff members are likely to identify student issues because of the regular contact involved in their role. It is particularly important to provide both a digest of training within a brief induction for these staff and also the opportunity to be paid to attend formal training as soon as possible.

University Counsellors and Mental Health Staff

> Sometimes you'll have people in hospital with psychosis, there will be a couple of suicidal students you are chasing and you still have got four appointments each day and it feels rushing actually, because you've got no lunch and you're juggling seven or eight complex cases in your mind at once, and you can't go home until you know this person is safe, that person is safe.
>
> *University counsellor, cited in Brewster (2022)*

Research by Hughes et al. (2018) has described a 'problematic' relationship between academics and student support services, with academic staff describing a service that felt detached and completely unfamiliar. I have heard teaching staff say that they deliberately avoided communication with counselling staff and assumed that this was mutual in order to assure the students of confidentially. In contrast, student support staff have felt too overwhelmed by increased and growing caseloads to find time to reach out to academic and teaching staff, often commenting that they were obliged to take on work that would be more appropriately managed within NHS services if those were adequately staffed. This is a distortion of the role they were employed for, which is to support the academic community and relive academics of pastoral roles that go beyond their expertise and capacity.

The different mental health services catering for the needs of university staff and students are discussed further in Chapter 18. The mental health supports funded by universities themselves are particularly important resources, though, as they were set up specifically to relieve teaching staff of the task of managing student mental ill health. Their expertise involves both delivering direct service and also case-managing the support the student needs, including medical, psychological, financial and academic needs. Academics who do manage to build strong working relationships with counselling and other student support services emphasise the high value of these links.

After 2 months in the local eating disorders ward, Jackie was ready to return to university. Two weeks before she left hospital, her consultant invited the university's mental health advisor to a discharge planning meeting, attended also by her parents who travelled up specially, and the outpatient therapist who would take over her care.

Ms Zhang, the mental health advisor, offered to link with different offices at the university to propose various kinds of support. She contacted the accommodation office to arrange a warm room in halls near to Jackie's course lectures, and found a group of 'buddy' students to take turns to accompany her to meals.

Ms Zhang made contact with Jackie's director of studies so that she was not penalised when she missed classes to attend hospital appointments. Work would be copied and made available to her. With Jackie's agreement, she would attend the next review meeting, so that

Jackie's new therapist could receive feedback on progress with university life and ask for further adjustments to her university life if needed. Meanwhile she would support Jackie to apply for a mental health mentor, who could then take over the support and communication.

Jackie's director of studies had found her illness stressful for the whole department, as the young woman had come close to death, but refused treatment until almost the end. The academics had felt overwhelmed by the situation and unaware of how much pastoral support was in fact available from the university.

Just as teaching and academic staff need specific support for their own mental health if they are to support their students, so it is crucial for this to also be the case for the staff at university counselling and support services. They will be obliged by their professional bodies to access supervision and continuing professional development, but in terms of where they access any required treatment for their own mental health conditions, arrangements need to be carefully considered, as mental health professionals in any locality tend to know each other and feel uncomfortable about sharing symptoms and difficulties despite confidentiality.

The Interaction between the Mental Health of University Staff and That of Their Students

Staff and student well-being are inextricably linked, in both university and school settings. The situation at present may be exacerbated by the obstacles and difficulties staff perceive in providing support for their students' mental health, and by the very notion that the two issues are separate. I know from my psychotherapy practice that the quality of the therapist-patient relationship has more influence on outcomes than the precise model of therapy offered. In the same way, the personal relationships between students and their teachers have the potential to improve both academic outcomes and mental health. Educational psychologists have studied this phenomenon more in school-children than in adults, but recent research repeatedly confirms that meaningful relationships between students and teachers in higher education brings similar benefits. (Hagenauer et al., 2023).

In 2014 Hagenauer and Volet (2014) observed that the teacher–student relationship at university was 'an important yet under-researched field'. They cited research demonstrating that in schoolchildren secure attachments and high-quality relationships have an impact on motivation, social competence, academic outcomes, reduction in dropout and well-being in general. Those who benefit most from such high-quality relationships are usually the most vulnerable and disturbed children. A counter argument is that adults have to develop the resilience at some point to stand on their own two feet. Ecclestone and Hayes (2009) criticised the 'dangerous rise of therapeutic education' for undermining that resilience and building an expectation of vulnerability that then becomes a self-fulfilling prophecy.

In higher education, teacher-student relationships are formed between adults, albeit in a hierarchy where the roles are not equal. Teaching settings tend to be more fragmented, with less frequent interactions between teachers and students. Teaching is just one scholarly activity expected of university educators, so that frequency of contact with undergraduates may be fairly low.

Academics teaching in Australian universities highlighted that more frequent contact and in smaller groups facilitates more satisfying student-teacher relationships

(Hagenauer et al., 2023). Such teaching has characterised the teaching offered by Oxbridge colleges and other high-prestige universities for many years and may be an important ingredient in high standards as well as in well-being. Prevalent student–staff ratios, combined with high research expectations, currently preclude this.

Tellingly, research on this topic is more likely to focus on the effects on the students than on the teachers. Even those researchers who highlight the value of the relationship for high-quality teaching and learning, tend to conclude with a call for teachers to enhance their interpersonal skills rather than considering how to explore and foster such relationships on both sides. In a recent study, Hagenauer et al. (2023) interviewed experienced university teachers in two Australian universities to explore the relationship from the teacher perspective. The academics stressed how each relationship is characterised by mutuality. Higher education teachers often 'flatten the hierarchy', applying student-centred approaches, prioritising students' ideas and opinions Students, in turn, have to take on a higher responsibility for their studies.

The balance between 'closeness' and appropriate boundaries was complex. Teachers had to judge the cultural expectations, age, maturity, gender and personality of each student. then set boundaries to protect staff whilst offering the right degree of professional and interpersonal approachability. One academic spoke of trusting students with their mobile phone number, whilst others said that was 'a total no-no'. Such discussions could form a useful part of staff mental health training.

Lay-Hwa Boden (2013) examined the benefits of close and supportive relationships for first-year students. Positive teacher-student relationships enhance students' confidence, lessen the transition shock and reduce the risk of detachment from the university. In her research close relationships involved some appropriate mutual personal disclosure (remembering names, acknowledging holiday plans and birthdays), not treating students as numbers, listening to students' concerns, building rapport with them and answering their emails.

The Australian staff (Hagenauer et al., 2023), whilst agreeing with the importance of interpersonal enjoyment of the teaching relationship, put more emphasis on the importance of professional boundaries. These staff agreed on the importance of caring behaviour, when students are struggling, being willing to listen to students' academic problems and fears and contacting absent students. Still, the teachers frequently highlighted that their care must have limits. They considered that it was important to reliably and promptly answering calls and emails, but also cautioned students not to be over-reliant and expect answers at any time. According to many of the university teachers, too much closeness can become uncomfortable, and it was deemed improper or even dangerous (e.g., becoming connected on social media).

There is so far very little work on how digitalised learning environments affect teacher-student relationships. My own experience with medical students has been that they have craved live interpersonal contact and sought out opportunities to link up with staff online to compensate for the isolation and loneliness of lockdown. Meanwhile university teachers – like schoolteachers – have struggled so much to deliver the professional content of their teaching in electronic form that these demands have often distracted them from developing relationships with their students as they would have liked.

I would very much endorse the call for more attention to be paid to the relation between the teacher-student relationship and teachers' occupational well-being and engagement in teaching.

Positive Mental Health amongst University Academics and Teachers

Not all university staff have poor mental health, thank goodness. In the many decades of a potential academic career, however, the majority of people can expect to meet criteria for a diagnosable mental illness and some point (Caspi et al., 2020), and will experience stress and distress falling short of illness criteria. Universities can be places in which staff are able to pursue meaningful work, in a supported and stimulating environment, that benefits their well-being. Rates of suicide for those working in a higher education institution, are lower than the national average, in contrast with primary schoolteachers, where it is almost twice the national average.

University staff benefit from that sense of belonging, which is so important to the mental health of adults as well as young students. When university teachers in the Brewster et al. (2022) study were asked about factors contributing positively to their well-being, they spoke of 'making a difference' through the provision of teaching and pastoral support to students as significant in their overall role satisfaction, fulfilment, and well-being. Some remarked

> my favourite day of the year is graduation, because I go to graduation and it's like, I'm looking at my children ... They've actually learned something. They've achieved something.
>
> I still feel incredibly privileged to be doing a job I love. And the difference I can see in a student coming to see me, who might be thinking about dropping out, really struggling, and then seeing an improvement.

My own experience of teaching students and trainees in several disciplines has been mostly one of delight. For those of us who relish the learning experience, teaching lively students not only obliges us to increase and reinforce our own learning, but also challenges and changes our old assumptions and areas of ignorance. The sheer playfulness of teaching at an advanced level is very good for mind and spirits.

Practice Points

At the Institutional Level

- Formal university policies should ensure academic and teaching staff do not have disproportionate responsibility for student well-being and clarify that staff well-being is an integral part of duty of care.
- Indemnity should be assured for staff doing their best and following principles of the institution's mental health training.
- Structures are needed to allow staff mental illness to be flagged up in a compassionate and supportive rather than using disciplinary pathways.
- There should be a regularly reviewed mandatory annual mental health training for all teaching and academic staff, with pay for part time staff. Feedback from such training should continue to inform university mental health policy.
- Major surveillance exercises and other sources of administrative overload should be reviewed as a priority, and at least paid as overtime rather than being automatically seen as part of the professional contract.
- Institutions should acknowledge the inevitable pressures of balancing pastoral support with the other expectations of academic roles. They need to be rewarded financially and in terms of status and recognition.

- More commitment is needed to provide for sustainable careers and pathways from graduation and postdoctoral research to tenured lectureship.
- It is estimated that 5% income is lost to the sector through staff ill health. Investment of even a part of this sum in increasing staffing and improving staff job security and conditions might reap returns.

Line Managers, Appraisers and Working Culture

- Line managers can do much to foster a work environment in which respectful conversations about mental health are possible. The culture of 'more and faster' should be resisted in favour of high-quality consolidation.
- Staff should be able to identify mental health problems, without fear of judgement or negative consequences for their career.
- Attitudes to mental illness and need for sick leave need to be more considered, with care taken that sick leave that cannot be covered is not left to the convalescent staff member to catch up on return to work.
- Appraisers and job planners should fully engage with university policies on rewarding pastoral support financially and in terms of status and recognition.
- Pastoral care of and by part time, temporary and casualised staff, including postgraduate students, should be particularly considered rather than assuming full time semester-long availability of all staff.

Student Support and University Mental Health Staff

- Student support and university mental health staff are best placed to design and deliver mandatory mental health training for all staff. This should prioritise mental well-being of staff themselves and make good links and networks between academic and support staff.
- In addition to ensure regular communication and improved understanding between academics and Student Services, universities there should be increased opportunities for structured engagement, regular contact and shared sense of purpose.
- Academic and teaching staff could be offered a mental health advice hotline manned or on call 24 hours a day, so that academic staff can access advice on mental health concerns about their students' or colleague's mental health. Regular drop-in confidential group supervision slots should be available to staff supporting students who have mental health needs.

Academic and Teaching Staff

- Are far less likely than students to 'disclose' a diagnosable mental condition to their university. Having the courage to do so would highlight need and demand for better consideration of a whole-university approach to taking health needs into account.
- Would be well advised to seek contact with occupation health rather than waiting passively for a crisis referral. The occupation health office can validate staff legal and contractual rights to have mental health needs supported.

- Benefit from nurturing professional relationships with individual members of student counsellors and other support staff.

Students, Schools and Families

- Should prepare for and acknowledging the greater maturity required in the adult student-teacher relationship and the reciprocity of adult relationships.
- Whilst pastoral care is part of the student/teacher relationship, and teaching and academic staff can be expected to keep matters confidential, it should be expected that serious concerns about mental health will be discussed in a confidential setting with counselling and other student support staff.

References

Brewster, L., Jones, E., Priestley, M., Wilbraham, S. J., Spanner, L. & Hughes, G. (2022). 'Look after the staff and they would look after the students' cultures of wellbeing and mental health in the university setting. *Journal of Further and Higher Education*, 46 (4), 548–60.

Carr, E., Davis, K., Bergin-Cartwright, G., et al. (2022). Mental health among UK university staff and postgraduate students in the early stages of the COVID-19 pandemic. *Occupational and Environmental Medicine*, 79(4), 259–67.

Caspi, A., Houts, R. M., Ambler, A., et al. (2020). Longitudinal assessment of mental health disorders and comorbidities across 4 decades among participants in the Dunedin birth cohort study. *JAMA Network Open*. 3(4), e203221. http://doi .org/10.1001/jamanetworkopen.2020.3221

Ecclestone, K. & Hayes, D. (2009). *The dangerous rise of therapeutic education*. Routledge.

Fontinha, R., Easton, S. & Van Laar, D. (2019). Overtime and quality of working life in academics and non-academic: The role of perceived work-life balance. *International Journal of Stress Management*, 26(2), 173.

Goodwin, L., Ben-Zion, I., Fear, N. T., Hotopf, M., Stansfeld, S. A. & Wessely, S. (2013). Are reports of psychological stress higher in occupational studies? A systematic review across occupational and population-based studies. *PLoS ONE*, 8(11), e78693.

Guthrie, S., Lichten, C. A., Van Belle, J., Ball, S., Knack, A. & Hofman, J. (2017). *Understanding mental health in the research environment: A rapid evidence assessment*. Santa Monica, CA: RAND Corporation. www.rand.org/pubs/research_reports/ RR2022.html

Hagenauer, G. & Volet, S. E. (2014). Teacher–student relationship at university: An important yet under-researched field. Oxford Review of Education, 40(3), 370–88. 10.1080/03054985.2014.921613

Hagenauer, G., Muehlbacher, F. & Ivanova, M. (2023). 'It's where learning and teaching begins-is this relationship': Insights on the teacher–student relationship at university from the teachers' perspective. *Higher Education*, 85, 819–35.

Hughes, G., Panjwani, M., Tulcidas, P. & Byrom, N. (2018). *Student mental health: The role and experiences of academics*. Student Minds. www.studentminds.org.uk/ uploads/3/7/8/4/3784584/180129_student_ mental_health__the_role_and_experience_ of_academics__student_minds_pdf.pdf

Jones-Davies, S. (2019). The legal position: obligations and limits. In Barden, N. & Caleb, R. (eds) *Student mental health and wellbeing in higher education: A practical guide* (pp. 18–39).

Lay-Hwa Boden, J. (2013). What's in a relationship? Affective commitment, bonding and the tertiary first year experience: A student and faculty perspective. *Asia Pacific Journal of Marketing and Logistics*, 25(3), 428–51.

Morrish, L. (2019). *Pressure vessels: The epidemic of poor mental health among higher education staff*. Oxford: Higher Education Policy Institute.

Shaw, C. (2014, 8 May). *Overworked and isolated: Work pressure fuels mental illness in academia*. The Guardian. www.theguardian.com/higher-education-network/blog/2014/may/08/work-pressure-fuels-academic-mental-illness-guardian-study-health

Shutler-Jones, K. (2011). *Improving performance through wellbeing and engagement: Essential tools for a changing HE landscape*. Wellbeing. http://affinityhealthhub.co.uk/d/attachments/44-shutler-jones-2011-1526946099.pdf

An Overview of Mental Disorders in Students and Staff

PERSONALITY DISORDERS

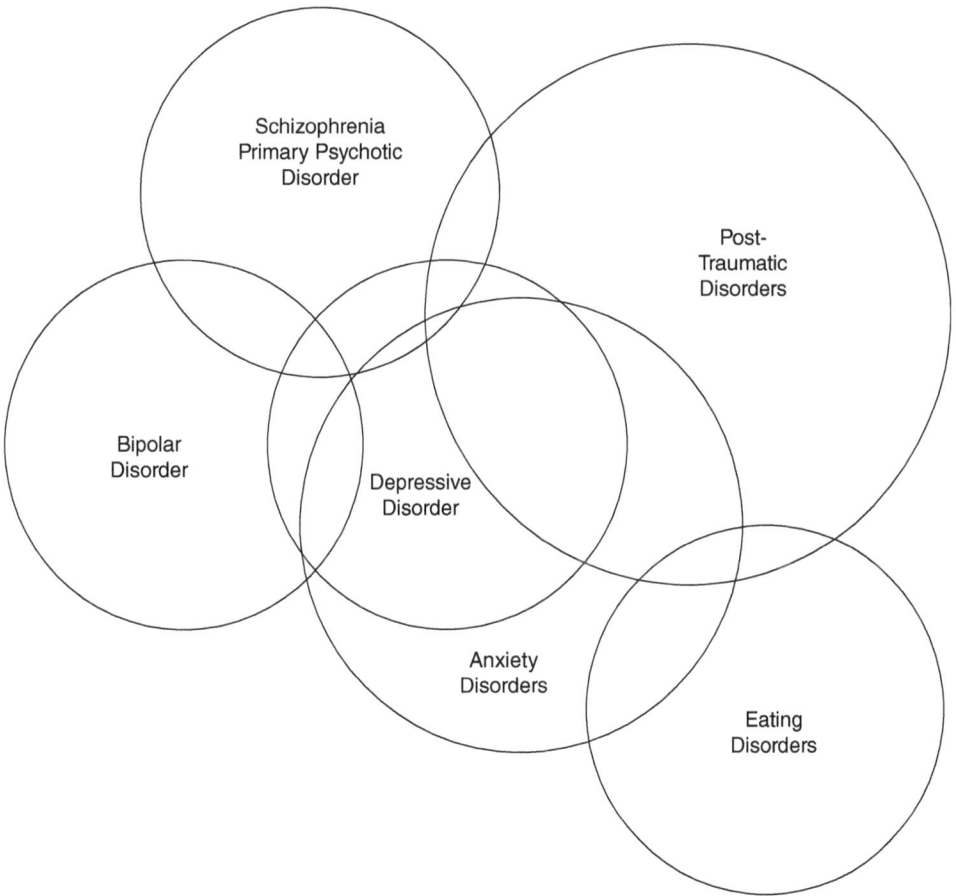

AUTISTIC SPECTRUM + NEURO DEVELOPMENTAL

Figure 14.1 Overview of mental disorders and their interrelatedness

This chapter does not provide details of symptoms and treatments of mental illnesses in any expectation that directors of studies, tutors, non-academic staff, parents and fellow students should expect to diagnose or manage a student's or colleague's disorder. That would be inappropriate and potentially dangerous. All the same, some intelligent awareness is important so that we don't engage in the superstitious avoidance that isolates and deprives people with mental illness. Sometimes mental health professionals will call on members of the university community to be part of the care around a patient. It is important to acknowledge that there are mental illnesses that cannot be safely managed purely by kindness, talking with peers or even counselling. At every level of contact with students who have mental health difficulties we need to know how to involve more specialist input.

For those readers who have or are in the process of exploring a diagnosis of their own mental difficulties, I hope the accounts provided here help make sense of the experience, and explain the uncertainties and obstacles to offering simple answers. The same factors that make it hard to reach clearcut diagnoses when patients are so young, are the very factors that allow for optimism and good prognosis. It has long been known, and more recently demonstrated by research, that some of the very characteristics that make a person more vulnerable to mental illness can also underlie considerable creative strengths. For instance, Power et al. (2015) found that 'polygenic risk scores for schizophrenia and bipolar disorder predict creativity'.

The UK has a strong anti-psychiatry movement. Psychiatrists have been accused of 'medicalising' mental ill-health. Where psychiatry – or any medical discipline – is a business, closely linked to the pharmaceutical industry, there may be a temptation to try to explain all distress and discomfort with a diagnosis, and to sell medication at a profit. In the UK, though, my overwhelmed national health service (NHS) colleagues genuinely resist inappropriate diagnosis and prescribing. We certainly do see cases where mental illness is driven or exacerbated by lifestyle problems. Part of our work involves advocating that people pay attention to routines, sleep, good diet, exposure to nature and daylight, moderate physical activity, lower intakes of alcohol and other substances, and good interpersonal relationships.

At the same time, we believe that there ARE mental illnesses, disorders of the mind. These form our core caseload, alongside those cases where mental 'ill-health' has increased to the level of meeting diagnostic criteria for a named 'disorder'. It is important to acknowledge both sorts of disorder.

Jill had worked as an English lecturer for decades without promotion. As a single mother with no help in the home and no family locally, she had little time for her own writing and research but took on huge amounts of teaching. She found her work increasingly exhausting and unappreciated. After participating in industrial action, which failed to achieve any changes in pay or conditions, she asked her general practitioner (GP) to sign her off with 'stress' for a week. She had fallen behind in marking and preparation and was unable to sleep. She regularly skipped meals and noticed her concentration and memory had dipped. Her doctor found that her symptoms met criteria for a depressive disorder and offered medication, but Jill resisted this 'label'. She said she had been damaged by overwork rather than an illness and needed rest not medicine.

This book as a whole examines the whole issue of mental health in our UK universities, as well as its relationship to 'physical' health and to social well-being or adversity.

In the realms of both physical and mental health, we can often hypothesise a spectrum in which 'illness' and 'disorder' occur when there is a lack of healthy function and an increase in unhealthy function. There are also conditions where there is a very clear difference from normal function or from the person's own usual behaviour and experience. Chapters 15 and 16 describe some of the main psychiatric disorders. They are not absolute bars to a university course or career, but may interrupt or even sabotage it, particularly if they are not identified or acknowledged and if appropriate support and adjustments are not in place. Chapter 18 considers the services available to members of a university to support their recovery and management of a mental health condition.

Jean, like her father and older sister, had bipolar disorder. She was diagnosed at age 17, when she became over-elated and disinhibited on a school residential trip. She was drinking alcohol, which was uncharacteristic, and responded to teachers with irritation and then physical aggression. She was admitted to a local hospital and then transferred to a ward in her home area. She took a year away from education to recover and start on the same medication that had helped her relatives maintain stability in their high-achieving lives. She was reluctant to accept any 'label' but believed that since she had been detained in hospital on a compulsory basis under the Mental Health Act, this would be 'on record', so she declared it to her prospective university and was offered mental health mentorship and other 'disability support'.

By the end of her first year at university she had settled in well socially and academically, despite failing to attend any of the mentoring appointments arranged for her. She continued to take her medication, prescribed by the new GP practice. Her parents had 'nagged' her to sign up with the practice nearest the university and they regularly checked on her by phone.

The high-risk period for onset of schizophrenia, bipolar disorder, as well as common mental disorders such as anxiety and depression is in late adolescence and early adulthood, coinciding with entering higher education. Some students are affected by long-term conditions with onset in mid-adolescence, such as anorexia nervosa. Others might be staring to develop features, which later attract diagnoses of addictions. Hence university students span an age range in which a wide spectrum of mental illness is seen. In the United States it has been estimated that mental disorders account for nearly a half of the disease burden for young adults (World Health Organization, 2008).

What Do We Mean by 'Mental Illness' or 'Mental Disorder'?

The language we use is constantly shifting. Some terms include 'mental illness', 'mental health problems', 'mental health difficulties', 'mental ill health', 'psychological problems', 'emotional disorders' and 'mental health issues'. This is not so much a matter of trying to be scientifically accurate as to avoid giving offence to people with stigmatised conditions. Perhaps it also reflects our primitive fear of mental illness, so that we avoid even naming them – the 'Voldemort' phenomenon. Recently, several people have told me that they have 'mental health', without appearing to notice the contradiction.

I have provided a personal glossary of terms I may use in this chapter. Most mental health colleagues would understand my use of them, though some would disagree as to the most helpful vocabulary to in different settings. The main value judgment I feel in the use of any of these terms is that I regard 'mental health' as referring to a positive and desirable state of being, whilst I use 'mental illness' to refer to a state of being that is by definition an obstacle to the best quality of life. Another feature of my own use of words is that I find it helpful to hypothesise that mental experience reflects brain function (and in some cases brain structure). I am comfortable with a medical model of mental illness, using that term 'medical' in its best, most holistic sense.

Mental health	Literally, this should refer to good mental health, just as 'health' implies that a person is enjoying good physical health. It has become common practice to avoid terms such as 'mental illness' and 'mental disorder' and particularly the word 'psychiatric'. If this is a well-intentioned effort to avoid giving offence then this sadly implies that having a mental illness is an offensive matter, and to my mind plays into stigma. Alternatively, there may be a reluctance to give a name to feared conditions – there was similar avoidance of the word 'cancer' in the days when all cancer was believed to be incurable
Mental illness, mental disorder, psychiatric illness, disorder	I use these terms more or less interchangeably in the book, and see the same sort of usage by other authors. Some people prefer the term 'mental condition', though this might be thought to also refer to a condition of wellness. Another alternative is 'mental ill-health', although this avoids suggesting the actual presence of a diagnosable illness.
Diagnosis	The name given to an illness or disorder, suggesting that conditions attracting this label share causation and are likely to respond to treatment provided for others with the same condition.
Formulation	A description of how a person came to have a particular diagnosis, or combination of diagnoses. It summarises the predisposing, precipitating and perpetuating factors, to allow tailor made management. Physical, psychological and social factors are all considered.
Acute/chronic	An 'acute' illness is relatively short-lived, although since mind and brain take longer to heal than other parts of the body, an 'acute' episode may take many months. There is a start and finish to an acute illness, with healthy function between episodes. 'Chronic' illness implies that the disorder is long term or even permanent.
Mental disability	Long-term dysfunction from either a chronic illness or a permanent underlying vulnerability to repeated episodes of illness can result in a disability. Some mental illnesses are formally granted the status of a 'disability' in the eyes of authorities such as university entrance, benefits agencies and occupational health.

Symptoms, signs, features	Observed or measured features of any illness form the basis for reaching a diagnosis. Symptoms are those features experienced and described by the patient, whilst signs are the features other people observe.
Patient	I use this term to describe a person receiving assessment or treatment for an illness. Research suggests that they themselves, like most clinicians, prefer the word to such alternatives as 'client' 'service user' and 'sufferer'.
Psychotic/non-psychotic	A 'psychotic' experience is one which is not commensurate with objective reality (although philosophers may question what that in fact means!). Some disorders, such as schizophrenia, are characterised by psychotic experiences, whilst others, such as depressive or anxiety disorders, may never involve experiences of psychotic intensity.
Personality disorders	A particularly complex concept implying a long-term ingrained propensity to certain reactions, experiences, relationship patterns and behavioural responses, which may predispose to or co-exist with other mental illnesses.

Some mental conditions, if not lifelong, are at least 'undergraduate-long'. Bipolar affective disorder (formerly known as 'manic depressive disorder') is generally recognised to be a lifelong vulnerability, which declares itself in acute episodes. The person may experience healthy high quality of life in between these episodes. Obsessive–compulsive disorder can follow the same sort of pattern, with acute episodes and remissions, but can also take a more lasting form, particularly if untreated.

Pros and Cons of Diagnosing a Mental Disorder

Diagnosis is essential to good medicine. Diagnosis implies that we understand the causes and likely consequences of a condition. It focusses research on the hunt for treatments – not only drug treatments but psychotherapies too – and allows people with the diagnosis to make sense of what is happening to them and learn from the experience of their fellow patients. An accurate diagnosis can also act as a warning that people in that diagnostic group might be harmed by treatments that can help those with similar symptoms but a different diagnosis. For instance, if two students show the very same symptoms of depression, but one of them has a diagnosis of bipolar disorder, then this second student should not be prescribed the same 'antidepressant' drugs, because of a risk of triggering a manic episode.

Juno was a high achiever at school but struggled with life in student halls. She often failed to give in assignments on time, and became anxious and unhappy. She was unable to face taking the antidepressants her GP prescribed then came to the accident and emergency department having swallowed a whole boxful, washed down with vodka. She attended the psychiatric outpatient clinic regularly over the course of her second year. Her psychiatrist reached a diagnosis of obsessive–compulsive disorder, and she joined a long waiting list before accessing psychological therapy. She was reluctant to take any medication out of concern it could 'contaminate' her brain, and she continued to struggle with symptoms.

However, she told her psychiatrist she was profoundly grateful to him for providing a diagnosis that made sense to her, and that she could use as an explanation in speaking with other people. She hoped that in time she might even consider medication as she increasingly came to trust her doctors.

There are still doubts as to the precision of our current diagnoses in some areas of medicine, but the quest to identify and refine them is part of progress. Many areas of psychiatric diagnosis remain uncertain. Research progresses so fast that every few years classifications have to be revised, but each time this occurs, older research is to some extent invalidated for people diagnosed under the new understanding. In some parts of the world health insurance only covers treatment when formal diagnostic criteria are met, so that internationally recognised diagnostic categories are extremely powerful. In the UK, the wish to practice 'evidence-based medicine' has led to greater use of international classification systems, but we also enjoy greater flexibility to assign a 'clinical diagnosis'. A patient's symptoms may not completely match formal criteria, but are close enough to the spirit of the diagnosis for the professional to have faith in the benefits of similar approaches and treatments.

There are two main classification systems for mental disorders. One is the World Health Organization's. International Classification of Diseases (ICD) now in its 11th edition. It includes both physical and mental disorders, and is the preferred system in the UK for collecting data. Individual patients are not usually informed of the exact section and subsection under which their disorder has been categorised. Meanwhile, the American Psychiatric Association has its own Diagnostic and Statistical Manual (DSM) now in its 5th edition. It has a highly respected tradition of use in defining research participants. There are certain differences between the two systems, which provide for debate and challenge but are not really helpful to individual patients.

In practice, like all doctors, psychiatrists understand an illness by looking at the overall picture the patient shares with them, and considering this in the context of their clinical experience and familiarity with research studies. They have to hold in mind ambiguous alternatives and tolerate uncertainty whilst providing patients and families with as much clarity as possible.

ICD-11 is replacing ICD-10 in the UK as from 2022. It allows for greater diagnostic flexibility, reflecting good clinical practice and the exercise of clinical judgment rather than symptom counts or rigid duration of symptoms. ICD-11 also has the advantage of adopting a 'lifespan-approach'. Thus, mental disorders that primarily occur in childhood and adolescence are not grouped separately as in the past. Moreover, ICD-11 provides guidance for classification adjustments to specific cultural contexts. These advances make the new diagnostic system more helpful to the university student population.

A 'hair-splitting' approach to diagnosis is not helpful. There is a risk that overstretched services might use failure to meet full formal diagnostic criteria to exclude people who could benefit from treatment. Another risk is that 'checklists' of symptoms encourage people with mild expressions of these symptoms to jump to the conclusion that they may have a disorder when the threshold for severity is not there. Most of us who have been medical students have had the experience of diagnosing ourselves repeatedly with the topic of the week's lectures.

University academics typically deal with life by giving names to ideas and phenomena and debating them, renaming as necessary, and shaping and advancing each other's notions and attitudes. There is obviously a huge advantage in being able to use well-considered diagnostic categories to understand our fellow scholars' experiences of distress and disability. Diagnosis and discussion are essential for psychoeducation in the student population, and a recent study by Cadge et al. (2019) illustrates both advantages and disadvantages to the use of diagnosis in severe menta illness, in this case schizophrenia.

These students – all UK home students from different ethnic backgrounds held a general misconception that schizophrenia caused multiple personalities, with more Indian students perceiving upbringing as a causal factor in the development of the illness and more Pakistani students perceiving possession by a spirit as a cause. Most students perceived schizophrenia as stigmatising with perceptions of the disease as shocking and a weakness, impacting on image and status. Further, even in this highly educated cohort most students perceived schizophrenia as dangerous, with associations of violence and unpredictability, despite the fact most people with schizophrenia are not violent or dangerous. The belief schizophrenia does not exist or is 'all in your head' was also expressed. For me, one telling point is that the very word 'schizophrenia' shocked participants, with one student commenting on the fact they were taken aback when told the interview would be about schizophrenia (Cadge et al., 2019).

Over my psychiatric career I have watched successive attempts to soften the shock of diagnostic labels and their implications. Sometimes this is a laudable effort to avoid stigma, sometimes a less laudable effort to minimise the challenge that lies ahead of the individual or family to whom we are breaking the news, and to make it easier for ourselves as doctors. We also need terms that respect the condition whilst allowing time – even years – for the precise diagnosis to become apparent. ICD-11 offers the alternative expression 'Primary Psychotic Disorder' in place of 'Schizophrenia'. This may allow people to shrug off the baggage of false assumptions and myths associated with the word, and still achieve some clarity in terms of what they are dealing with. I suspect that the best way to 'rehabilitate' some of our terminology will be the provision of more effective treatments. In my childhood, people avoided the word 'cancer', preferring terms like 'tumour' 'SOL (space-occupying lesion)' and 'the big C'. Frank use of the word 'cancer' has become much easier when there is hope of treatment and even cure.

Developmental Considerations

If the reader is already irritated by so much that is unclear and ambiguous in this description of mental illness, I'm afraid my further remarks on brain development will only add to the frustration. Parents, teachers, and professionals working with adolescents are uncomfortably aware how young people's behaviour becomes unpredictable and unstable as their bodies grow and change. Different individuals master the range of intellectual, interpersonal and social skills at different rates both in terms of their own profile of growth and in comparison with peers. It is a turbulent time, reflecting enormous growth and then 'pruning' of brain tissue. Hormones of puberty influence brain shape and directly modify behaviour too, and the whole thing is shaped by interactions with the nutritional, physical and social environment. Pioneering brain scanning studies (Giedd, 2008) have demonstrated that the adolescent brain continues to change and develop well beyond the end of growth in height, particularly in young men. This means that students will be experiencing dynamic brain changes stimulated by their own physiological development alongside the mental growth stimulated by the intellectual and social challenges of university life.

It is difficult to assess and diagnose a disorder in a 'moving target'. We are keen to make early diagnoses of treatable conditions because of evidence that the longer our brains have to live with the damage of a disorder, the more ingrained it can become. On the other hand, we do not want to interfere with the striking but normal oscillations of a brain that is settling down to a healthy balance. We sometimes physically over-protect young people, but in other contexts allow them to risk physical injury in the interests of challenging themselves to greater growth and achievement. We are only starting to consider how much psychosocial and emotional risk young people need to thrive. We cannot wrap students in cotton wool, but perhaps we are not really wrapping them in enough insulation at present and have a duty to provide psychologically healthier structures. For instance, there is debate about the extent to which coaches should risk the physical – and mental – well-being of young athletes.

What This Chapter Does Not Address

Some significant mental conditions are merely mentioned here, and dealt with in other, more focussed chapters. The so-called eating disorders and other body-image disorders, for instance, are discussed in Chapter 5. Alcohol use and misuse is addressed in Chapter 6, and other recreational and 'smart' drugs are covered in Chapter 7. This is because understanding them is part of a broader spectrum of psychosocial climate, and because for young students, such behaviour can lead to mental and social problems without reaching levels regarded as constituting an illness.

In contrast, issues of gender and sexuality, are concerns that campaigners have fought to have recognised as part of the range of healthy humanity, rather than disorders. People in these and other minority groups can be more vulnerable to developing mental illnesses as a result of the stigma and exclusion they often experience. It's a common complaint of people in LGBTQ+ groups, though, that professionals too often focus on the fact of their gender or sexuality rather than on the nature of their symptoms of depression or distress.

For the same reason, the book carries a separate chapter on mental health aspects of neurodiversity. Campaigners for these groups too have insisted on the different but valid differences in their thinking styles and abilities as part of the healthy range rather than as disorders or disabilities in themselves. I agree with this stance, whilst sympathising with the extra mental and emotional stresses that come from living with a significant difference in a culture set up for mainstream majorities.

Deliberate self-harm and suicide are not in themselves diagnosable disorders, though they are often manifestations of mental illnesses.

Is Mental Illness Preventable?

The founders of our cherished NHS predicted that providing excellent care and public health measures would almost eradicate illness. It is now recognised that there are limits to what preventative measures can achieve. Few people would claim that rheumatoid arthritis, ulcerative colitis, or type 1 diabetes can be prevented by lifestyle interventions, for instance. Most people would accept that there is still little that can be done to prevent many cancers and some heart disease. No-one is surprised when healthy young people become acutely physically ill, and yet mental illness has a much higher prevalence than physical illness in the young.

On the other hand, there is still a widespread assumption in modern society that all mental illness represents an unacceptable failure of 'mental health' in some way. There is another myth that mental illness springs purely from social adversity, so that avoiding childhood trauma, encouraging openness and talking about feelings could virtually eliminate 'mental breakdown'.

At the other extreme, an older or more traditional attitude sees mental illness as a potentially lifelong disability in certain people, whilst the rest of us are not subject to symptoms. This view expects the mentally ill to refrain from full participation in public life, unless they can be 'fixed'. They would not be expected to attend university, for instance.

Finally, there is still a persistent attitude in some cultures and subcultures that there is no such thing as mental illness. Either supernatural or metaphysical notions of good and evil, or of morality may be invoked, or else the psychiatric profession is accused of generating the very symptoms they aspire to treat. Many of us think that we do not hold any of these beliefs and yet still behave as if there is something shameful or morality weak in experiencing mental illness.

As psychiatrists, most of us believe that even in the most ideal social environments, some people will be vulnerable to developing a mental disorder. They are not only affected by the external environment, but also by the internal biochemistry of the brain. This is often inherited down many generations, and so determined both before and after birth. Current thinking would regard those of us who are vulnerable as still having much to give to and receive from a university education. The possibility of doing so, though, depends on the right treatment being made available in a matter of fact and respectful manner.

Most of the chapters in this book examine the whole range of UK university mental health and considers systemic interventions rather than specifics of highly specific treatments for the worst affected individuals. The next few chapters in contrast, acknowledge that a significant minority of students and staff benefit from recognition and evidence-based treatment of a treatable mental illness.

Is Attending University Bad for Your Mental Health?

I have been asked whether the very existence of a book with a title like this one presumes that going to university increased the risk of mental illness. It does not intend to strike fear into students, staff or parents as they consider investing in a university education for their children. There is even evidence that students enjoy better mental and physical health than their non-student peers, though they may have pre-existing advantages that influence both mental health and likelihood of going to university. It is likely that those living in a family home, attending a relatively small educational institution such as a school, enjoy considerable protection from mental and physical health threats. On the other hand most steps towards maturity involve exposing ourselves to greater risks.

Civilisation involves cushioning those risks to some extent for the maturing individual. However, I have come to believe that at the time of writing, UK university students, whether or not more vulnerable to mental illness, do face unique disadvantages when they need to access treatment.

By definition, illnesses make people less able to cope with life, and mental illnesses often impair judgment in general and judgement and ability about help seeking in particular. The time of life from puberty to the mid-twenties is the period of highest risk of onset for many major mental disorders, The question of how students at different institutions access treatment, whether in a home setting, a university setting or both, is a further question in itself, which is addressed further in Chapter 18.

What Is the Prevalence of Mental Illness in Students?

As we have discussed, the language used to describe mental disorders is constantly shifting. This conceptual diversity leads to widely discrepant figures for the prevalence of mental disorder in students. A further problem is the practice of asking students themselves to describe their mental health. For those who have not been formally assessed there is a risk that psychological distress of any sort may be described as a mental disorder, particularly if it is likely to provide a route to extra support and consideration, although on the other hand, there are still groups of students who keep a serious psychiatric history secret for fear of it adversely affecting career prospects or stigma.

Even before the COVID pandemic there was already more demand for consideration of mental health amongst students. Higher education institutions have experienced significant increases in demand for student counselling and disability services over the past decade. The number of students 'disclosing' a mental health 'disability' to their higher education institution increased to about 12%, whilst disclosure of physical disability remained stable (Thorley, 2017). I do regret the choice of the words 'disclose' and 'disability', which have to stretch to cover the experience of 12% young people applying university. In fact, studies that examine symptoms in samples of students rather than relying on their own declarations (Macaskill, 2013) suggest that the figures are nearer 20% than 12%. The lowest rates of 'disclosures' are in students of medicine, dentistry engineering, law and business – classically 'macho' disciplines and in some cases still male-dominated.

It is generally the case that when people in the community are screened for illness, it turns out that there are large numbers of people who would test positive but are not receiving treatment. It's not surprising then that some studies have shown high rates of student mental ill health when this was assessed by screening instruments such as the general health questionnaire (GHQ). Monk (2004), also using the GHQ, found that 52% of a cohort of students scored positive. Macaskill (2018) carried out a cross-sectional survey of undergraduates in which students were assessed at entry to university and at the mid-point of years one, two and three of their courses. The presence of mental disorder was assessed using the GHQ-28. The overall prevalence of 'psychiatric caseness' was 17.6%, which is similar to the general population. Rates were higher in women and highest in the second year of study.

Prescribing Medication for Students with Mental Disorders

Psychotropic medication has a disproportionately bad press considering the damage done by untreated disorders. It's important, too, to remember that 'talking therapies' and group treatments also carry risk of serious side effects as well as power to do good. It makes sense that anything powerful enough to effect significant change will have risks. When I work with people with diagnosed mental health conditions, I find that it often takes both medication and psychotherapy to bring about recovery. I often spend some time discussing the pros and cons of medication, and building trust with patients in each other's judgment and willingness to monitor the effects. Usually, my wish for them to try medication is precisely so that they can benefit from the sort of psychological work they were unable to do without some pharmacological support. Patients have often told me too that once they started to feel the benefits of medication they no longer needed a therapist; they could do the psychological work for themselves in the processes of their daily life.

It may be quicker, cheaper and less disruptive to a student's or staff member's life to start medication than to refrain from doing so while they wait on a long waiting list for a therapy they may be too disabled to benefit from. Most GPs are experienced in prescribing the main psychotropic medications, and usually happy to do so whilst a student is attending counselling, rather than insist on waiting for a specialist psychiatric opinion first.

That said, there are reasons to take particular care when prescribing for the mental health needs of students. Some conditions do not so far respond to medications, and others require considerable expertise and time to find the right medication – sometimes one the GP does not have the experience to initiate – and in the right dosage. Medications don't work if the student is unable to take them, perhaps out of forgetfulness, fear or misinformation. It is important to know how long it will take for benefits to emerge, what is the likely pattern of adverse side-effects, and the risks of suddenly stopping treatment or missing doses. In England, people over age 19 must pay for their prescriptions, which may be a problem on a student budget. Those who need more than one prescription a month could find it might be cheaper to get a Pre-Payment Certificate. Some students are also eligible for the NHS low-income scheme, and should ask a GP or university welfare team about the 'NHS HC1 claim form'.

Cost and inconvenience may result in less ideal practice in some cases – for instance, continuing antidepressant treatment beyond the resolution of symptoms can significantly reduce the risk of relapse, but it can be hard to persuade a student who 'feels perfectly fine' to persist with medication. Some medication has abuse potential, and drugs for ADHD are 'controlled' so that there can be stigma and bureaucracy around the prescribing and dispensing.

A final caution is that these days around half of all students are young women of childbearing age. Attending to good contraceptive practices is important, and it is also important to prepare for either accidental pregnancy or planned pregnancy at a later stage. There are certain medications that can protect the health of both mother and unborn child if taken in pregnancy, but others where the risk benefit balance must be calculated mindfully with input from experts. For instance, we are now aware of high risks of damage when a mother is taking valproate drugs in pregnancy. There are usually safer options for treating bipolar disorder and even seizure disorders. The SSRIs have a good safety record in the treatment of depression and anxiety in pregnant women, especially sertraline, but some older or very new drugs are not so favourable. Prescribers who raise these issues with young women can use the opportunity to discuss contraceptive measures, and should be ready to hear about relationship problems and even abuse issues.

Practice Points

At a Societal Level

- It is taking time to reach a climate of respect for mental disorders on a par with physical disorders.
- The blurred concept of 'mental health' suppresses the fact that there are many recognised and very different disorders, not all preventable, and not all responsive to the same approaches.
- The university student age group tends to enjoy good physical health but often poor mental health. This is costly to society and to general practice.

At the Level of University Authorities and Policies

- Mental disorders bring implications for admissions policies, rights and responsibilities, fitness to study and to practice, provision of services and links with NHS and third sector. This is discussed further in Chapter 18.
- Institutional policies and practice on information-sharing agreements should be reviewed to consider permissions about when to contact next of kin.
- Formal documentation should be available to allow those who declare a mental illness on admission or later in their course, so that they can agree in advance to the limits of confidentiality and nominate a 'named person' to contact if there is concern.

NHS and Related Services

- GPs and specialist mental health services should consider designating student mental health a specific subspeciality and area of expertise.
- Networking with university in-house mental health services is essential.
- Arrangements to hold GP and psychiatric clinics on the university premises are to be welcomed.

Families

- Maintaining contact with the student is particularly important when there are signs of social withdrawal, academic failure or low mood.
- Institutional policies and practice on information-sharing agreements should be reviewed to consider permissions about when to contact next of kin. Families may wish to check their university has done this.
- When a student child is involved in counselling or mental health treatment, they should be encouraged them to give permission for parents to be contacted in case of concern, and those parents should prioritise being available to attend meetings with them if invited to do so.

Teachers, Tutors, Directors of Studies, Fellow Students

- It is absolutely not the role of lay people to diagnose, treat or case-manage a student's or colleague's mental illness.
- Some background awareness of the nature of mental illnesses – as with physical illnesses – can inform a compassionate and wise response.

- Chapter 13 examines the role of academic and teaching staff in student mental well-being and the nature of mandatory training.
- Guidelines are needed to ensure students who have to take time out of academic studies – or who need to leave their course – are provided with monitoring and support, as this is a time of high risk.

Individuals Seeking Help and Support

- The key to accessing all NHS treatment is to be signed on with a local GP.
- 'Disclosing' a mental health condition to the university provides rights to support, services and finance (i.e, the disabled students' allowance).
- The option of mental health mentorship, funded by the disabled students' allowance, can be transforming (see Chapters 9 and 18).
- It is important to keep an open mind about both medication and psychological treatments.
- People with all types of illness have rights to both respect and privacy. Disorders don't have to define who you are. There should be no obligation or pressure for a student to become a poster boy or girl for students with mental illness!

References

Cadge, C., Connor, C. & Greenfield, S. (2019). University students' understanding and perceptions of schizophrenia in the UK: A qualitative study. *BMJ Open*, 9, e025813. https://doi.org/10.1136/bmjopen-2018-025813

Carr, E., Davis, K., Bergin-Cartwright, G., et al. (2022). Mental health among UK university staff and postgraduate students in the early stages of the COVID-19 pandemic. *Occupational & Environmental Medicine*, 79(4), 259–67. https://doi.org/10.1136/oemed-2021-107667

Giedd, J. N. (2008). The teen brain: Insights from neuroimaging. *Journal of Adolescent Health*, 42(4), 335–43

Hughes, G. & Spanner, L. (2019). *The university mental health charter*. Leeds: Student Minds

Macaskill, A. (2013). The mental health of university students in the United Kingdom, *British Journal of Guidance & Counselling*, 41 (4), 426–41. https://doi.org/10.1080/03069885.2012.743110

Macaskill, A. (2018). Undergraduate mental health issues: The challenge of the second year of study. *Journal of Mental Health*, 27 (3), 214–21.

Monk, E. M. (2004). Student mental health: The case studies. *Counselling Psychology Quarterly*, 17(4), 395–412.

Morrish, L. (2019). *Pressure vessels: The epidemic of poor mental health among higher education staff*. Oxford: Higher Education Policy Institute. HEPI-Pressure-Vessels-Occasional-Paper-20.pdf

Patton, G. C., Sawyer, S., Santelli, J. S. et al. (2016). Our future: A Lancet commission on adolescent health and wellbeing *The Lancet*, 387(10036), 2423–78.

Power, R. A., Steinberg, S., Bjornsdottir, G., et al. (2015). Polygenic risk scores for schizophrenia and bipolar disorder predict creativity. *Nature Neuroscience*, 18(7), 953–5.

Thorley, C. (2017). *Not by degrees: Improving student mental health in the UK's universities*. London: Institute for Public Policy Research.

World Health Organization (2008). *The global burden of disease: 2004 update*. https://apps.who.int/iris/handle/10665/43942

'Psychotic' Disorders
Schizophrenia and Bipolar

PERSONALITY DISORDERS

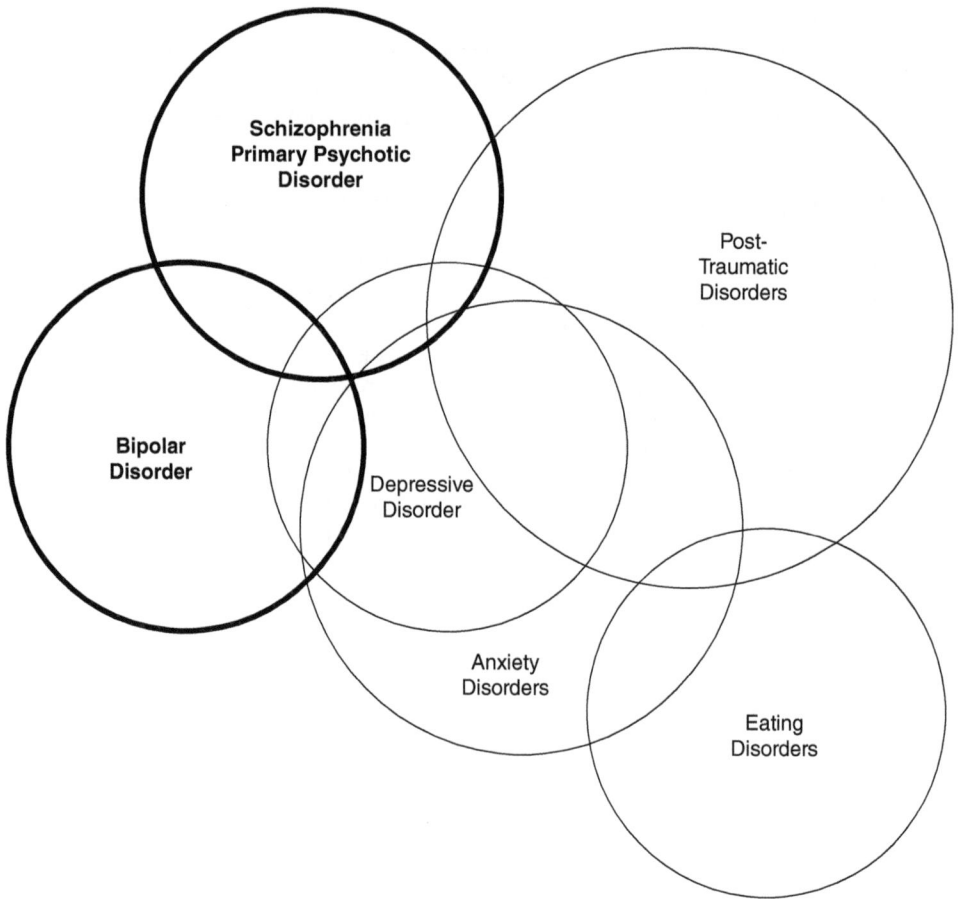

Figure 15.1 Psychotic disorders and their relationships with other mental conditions

AUTISTIC SPECTRUM + NEURO DEVELOPMENTAL

'The Psychoses'

In the technical psychiatric sense of the word a 'psychotic' disorder or experience occurs when the individual loses touch with the reality that is generally perceived by healthy members of the community or communities in which they live. Leaving aside all the philosophical questions, we describe disorders as 'psychotic' when sufferers consistently have beliefs or experiences that prevent them from coping with life and cause distress to themselves or to other people. In theory, many mental illnesses can affect us to such an intense degree that they could be described as 'psychotic' in intensity. For instance, someone with severe depression may seriously come to believe they are cursed, or someone with anorexia nervosa may genuinely believe they have gained weight when they continue to starve, and someone with obsessive–compulsive disorder may believe they have AIDS after a midge bite.

However, those disorders are not specifically characterised by their psychotic intensity, whereas two classes of mental disorder – schizophrenia and bipolar disorder – are classed as 'psychoses'. They are uncommon in the university population but require special accommodations, and they can be too easily overlooked in the current climate of focus on mental health, prevention and non-medical interventions.

These conditions may come to attention when the student is attending university or sometimes on a 'gap year' or abroad as part of their course. When a young person falls severely ill in a country that is foreign to them it is traumatic, whether the student is an international student studying in the UK or a UK student studying abroad. Indeed, both the experience of becoming mentally very ill and the experience of inpatient treatment in an adult psychiatric ward can add a burden of traumatic injury to a mind already convalescing from a serious illness.

Although the highest incidence of onset is in this age group, the prevalence in the student population is generally low. Psychotic disorders – both schizophrenia and bipolar – can be associated with difficulties in intellectual functioning. Problems with thinking and studying usually emerge earlier, before it becomes clear that the young person is ill. They tend to be more severe in schizophrenia than bipolar conditions. In fact, recent epidemiological data suggest that exceptional intellectual ability may be associated with bipolar disorder, placing the student population at higher risk of developing this illness. In one study, individuals with excellent school performance had four times the risk of developing bipolar disorder compared with those with average grades (MacCabe et al., 2010).

The overall prevalence, then, is fairly low, but there are many more students with bipolar disorder at university over the past decade. Approximately 1% of us has the condition, so a moderate sized university of 20 000 students will potentially have 200 individuals with bipolar disorder. If these individuals' disorder becomes destabilised there will be serious personal, social, clinical and administrative challenges for the university community.

Young people with primary psychotic disorders participate in postsecondary education at much lower rates than their healthy peers and those who do matriculate are less likely to achieve high grades. Students with psychosis take more time out of their studies and so take longer to graduate. However, it is possible for most of these students to participate fully in university life if they are provided with appropriate modifications and supports.

James was hall warden on call when two students asked him for urgent help. They were worried about Julian, a quiet but friendly student who had seemed withdrawn and low, recently. James had tried to engage him in conversation the previous evening, but he seemed preoccupied. He wondered whether he was using drugs.

When James arrived, Julian was wandering around the kitchen, unplugging devices and muttering to himself. Julian hushed his greetings and said 'Listen!'. He became tearful and then angry that the others could not hear what he was hearing. He warned them that they were all in danger and tried to usher then out of the building.

James called emergency services and Julian allowed himself to be taken by two gentle but firm police officers to a place of safety at the psychiatric hospital. A nurse later called James to confirm that Julian had agreed to stay on the ward and allowed staff to contact his parents. She took details from James of Julian's director of studies and of the counselling centre where it appeared Julian had already sought help.

James was relieved that the situation was resolved so calmly, but concerned for the two young women who initially summoned him, and found them weeping together. He made hot chocolate while they told him what they had seen and about their worries. He offered to meet them again later and to contact student support or the chaplaincy centre if they would like that. In fact, they opted to stay together and FaceTime their own parents.

Staff Response to Students' Needs When There Is a Psychotic Disorder

When a student experiences a psychotic destabilisation they will need modifications to their academic requirements and advocacy in relation to those in charge of their course. They will not be in a position to manage their own applications for mitigating academic circumstances. Family members might normally be excluded from taking on this sort of advocacy for an adult student, but these days most students will have given formal permission for family to be involved in this sort of situation. It is a good idea to appoint a member of university staff to link up with family as advocates for the student's situation and to guide requests for any confidential reports or medical certificates that are needed.

In an acute episode the disturbed behaviour of a fellow student can be frightening and distressing, and can lead to embarrassment and even avoidance in the relationships later on if not acknowledged and managed. As the case of Julian illustrates, acute psychotic symptoms can sometimes result in behavioural disruption in university teaching or residential settings. Staff and fellow students may need support afterwards, respecting the confidentiality and dignity of the unwell student. Close friends and flatmates of the affected individual may also need allowances to be made for the disruption involved to their own studies and lives. Strong collaborative relationships between counselling, teaching and accommodation staff help manage the crisis sensitively. Symptoms of mental illness – as of physical illness – can be embarrassing and disturbing. It can help to remember that it is the illness rather than the person that causes the embarrassing or threatening situation.

Often the comfort of friends and fellow students or staff is healthier and more effective support than formal counselling, but staff may need to offer an understanding of how a mental illness can affect someone, provide reassurances that effective care and treatment is available, and describe sources of further update and information. Sometimes staff and students are not well-informed about the nature of mental illness and services available, or may have previous traumatic experiences triggered by a crisis. If the person who becomes ill is a member of staff, young students may need help with the unfamiliar reversal of the usual order of things. The recovering staff member may also experience embarrassment at the prospect of their return to work.

Schizophrenia, Primary Psychotic Disorder

Schizophrenia can be a disabling mental disorder. It affects about 7 to 8 individuals per 1000 during their lifetime. (Saha et al., 2005). People with schizophrenia are at increased risk of suicide, with an estimated rate of 5% to10%. Both genetics and family history are involved in causing schizophrenia. It is considered to be 'polygenetic' – there is no clear pattern of inheritance from one generation to the next, but a tendency for the illness to be more prevalent in some families than in others. In fact, it is possible that there may be different types of schizophrenia each with their own profile of genetic abnormalities. Its peak age of onset in males is in the late teens and early twenties. Women are as likely as men to experience the condition but usually with a slightly later onset. Many of those who develop this condition, particularly young men, will do so in the time that they are in the student age group.

> **Summary of ICD-11 Criteria for Schizophrenia/Primary Psychotic Disorder (WHO 2019a).**
> Significant impairments in reality testing and alterations in behaviour, including:
> - **positive symptoms** such as persistent delusions, persistent hallucinations, disorganised thinking (typically manifest as disorganised speech), grossly disorganised behaviour, and experiences of passivity and control – one's thoughts or behaviour are felt to be under the control of an external force
> - **negative symptoms** such as blunted or flat emotional expression affect and loss of motivation and
> - **psychomotor disturbances** such as impaired attention, bizarre behaviour.
>
> **Symptoms must be present for at least one month.**

Schizophrenia is a condition that significantly alters a person's perception, thoughts, mood and behaviour. Its features fall into two groups: 'positive symptoms', such as hallucinations, delusions, thought disorder, and experiences of being controlled, and 'negative symptoms' where there is a reduction in participation in life, such as apathy, social withdrawal, blunting of emotions, lack of motivation, lack of pleasure and impoverished capacity to think.

Positive symptoms can be extremely alarming to both sufferer and onlookers, but usually respond well to medication. Sadly, negative symptoms can be more enduring and resistant, and bring about most of the long-term disability found in this illness.

Symptoms can emerge very gradually and can be hard to notice. There is often a phase in which the student becomes withdrawn and isolated and stops attending meetings, classes and social events. There may be a decline in their personal hygiene and other areas of social competence. The person often experiences poor concentration and lower motivation. They may begin using cannabis and other drugs for the first time as a way to relieve their symptoms, or sometimes the psychotic experience is triggered by substance use. If the student becomes extremely disturbed and behaves bizarrely, the situation may be plausibly attributed at first to being drunk or intoxicated. When this occurs, an opportunity for early treatment can be missed.

Of course, the interactions between substance use and psychotic experiences are complicated. Cannabis use is well-evidenced as a risk factor for schizophrenia especially in adolescent users and when a variant with a high concentration of tetrahydrocanna-binol (THC, the main psychoactive substance in cannabis) is used (Wainberg et al., 2021). There is now widespread use of synthetic cannabinoid receptor antagonists such as 'Spice' and 'K2'. These have a wide range of chemical compositions and street names and are often more potent than cannabis.

Some of us have a genetic vulnerability to becoming psychotic as a result of cannabis, but it is not currently possible to know whether we fall into that group. In people already diagnosed with schizophrenia, cannabis leads to a worse prognosis, with increased rates of relapse and re-hospitalisation (Wainberg et al., 2021).

Based on the appearances of the brain on scans, and on people's observed ability to cope with life, early treatment is really helpful. It could be that the illness itself is actually toxic to the brain in some way – perhaps analogous to the way that inflammation can damage our joints if allowed to continue untreated. This is on top of the undoubted psychosocial disruptions and traumas that result from a period of mental illness. So far, most (though not all) mental illness has a better outcome if treated as early as possible. The most formal evidence for this has been gathered in the field of research into schizophrenia and other 'psychotic' disorders. Researchers have found that longer duration of untreated psychosis predicts more severe outcome, including an extra risk of suicide (Penttilä et al., 2014). Indeed, in terms of reducing risks of student suicide, one logical line of prevention would be the assertively early treatment of the three mental illnesses that have the highest death rates in this age group: schizophrenia and related psychoses, bipolar disorder, and anorexia nervosa.

Outcomes are highly variable in schizophrenia and range from complete recovery to long-term chronic disability. Between these poles, many people experience recurring episodes of illness interspersed with periods of partial recovery.

Management of Schizophrenia (Primary Psychotic Disorder)

In an acute crisis, a rapid response from psychiatric services is of the first importance and the person may need to spend some time in hospital. For a person without a previous diagnosis, the initial management, assessment and need to experiment to find the right stabilising treatment may mean weeks and even months in hospital or intensive home treatment. Further episodes can usually be treated much more swiftly once the person's particular profile is understood.

Medication

Effective drug treatments for schizophrenia and related disorders include the well-known olanzapine and quetiapine. There is a whole range of both older and newer medications affecting the nervous system in slightly different ways. Some are available as injections, administered by a nurse every few weeks. This is helpful for people who struggle to take oral medication and involves regular check-in with a professional, which is often helpful in its own right. Clozapine has strikingly good outcomes, but requires regular blood tests, as some people's white cells might be threatened by the drug. Regular checks of this sort may be burdensome but may also constitute part of the effectiveness of such treatment – clozapine has been associated with lower suicide rates in those who take it. It is also believed to be more effective than other treatments in terms of the 'negative' symptoms of the disorder.

People are understandably reluctant to take high doses of medication long term, and there are some notorious adverse side effects. Older drugs caused involuntary movements, and stiffness, whilst newer medication is more likely to trigger weight gain. Most of the medications are sedative in high doses, so none of this is an attractive proposition for an image-conscious, hardworking student. Prescribers have to offer careful dose adjustment, assertively provide treatment of side effects, and support healthy lifestyle interventions.

Psychological Therapies

After an acute psychotic episode, the young person faces having to tolerate medication, work through the trauma and grief of developing a serious illness, build a new self-image, repair friendships and other relationships, and either return to their studies or develop new goals. Much more than a series of prescriptions is required. The student – or staff member – needs trusting therapeutic relationships with the mental health team and with lay mentors and supporters.

Cognitive behavioural therapy can help people restructure their lives, opportunities to meet with peers going through similar experiences can provide 'normalisation' and hope. There are also family-based treatments to enable people to develop new communication styles that offer clarity and support without increasing the stresses that could trigger paranoia or confusion.

When Julian returned to university to a new student group, he moved into a new set of halls of residence so that he could have a fresh start with new first years. He was granted extra time for submission of course work. He had managed to complete quite a lot before falling ill, this left him a lot of free time to go to the gym, take walks, and sit in the student union. He was excused participation in the sort of intense small group projects that had become so distressing in the context of his paranoid beliefs the year before. Life was far less stressful than the previous year. As the first term came to an end he was provided with of a private room and individual invigilator to sit examinations.

He had been strongly advised to avoid alcohol and recreational drugs, and found himself mostly socialising with a group of international students who disliked the UK partying culture. When he returned home for Christmas, he had a family session at the local hospital where he had been admitted when he fell ill.

The initial optimism in the meeting was modified somewhat when Julian revealed he had recently stopped taking his medication and was able to concentrate and work much better without it. He said that he valued getting a good degree far more than staying recovered from his mental illness.

After recovery from an acute episode, it is often a dilemma as to whether the student should return to their studies. On the one hand, there is some evidence that students developing a schizophrenic episode in the context of a university are more likely to get speedy help than their non-university peers (Hardy et al., 2018). Moreover, for many young people the whole meaning of recovery is a journey toward attainment of meaningful goals and full human potential, not merely absence of symptoms.

On the other hand, university is demanding and stressful and that this may increase the risk of further breakdown. Concentration may be impaired as a result of medication, and this can combine with diminished motivation to make it difficult to meet the academic demands of the course. Moreover, successful return to college is unlikely to be determined purely by the capacity to do the academic work. Rather a whole host of contextual factors influence educational outcomes. These include self-awareness, managing one's mental illness, and the ability to negotiate social relationships.

A student with a history of schizophrenia will often find it difficult to make new friends and re-integrate into university life. This applies even more so if there are still some residual positive symptoms, such as delusional thinking. In cases such as these, university may not be a happy experience for the young person. Someone studying far from home has to cope with all of this without family and old friends around them. The consequence of these factors in combination is a high dropout rate in students with schizophrenia. The research evidence doesn't offer much guidance in predicting which students will do well – current literature on outcomes after a first episode of psychotic illness shows extremely variable patterns of recovery.

> Julian was persuaded to resume medication before returning to university for the spring term, but left on bad terms with his father, who had threatened to withdraw financial support otherwise. By the end of the academic year, he found himself struggling with workload once again, but had not had any relapse of his psychotic symptoms. He spent some of the summer vacation on campus where international student friends had also opted to remain, and passed his resits. His academic advisors discussed several options with him in terms of the year ahead.
>
> He resisted the option of transferring to the university in his home town, despite good links with his treatment team there, and the prestigious nature of that university. He was more open to the options of taking a less demanding course option, within those available in his chosen subject. Alternatively, he might drop to part time studying, whilst still living in halls, where he felt secure and well-supported.

A recent US study found that although 82% students with a first episode psychosis experienced disruptions to their education after their illness, nevertheless, more than half of them went on to return to their studies. Those students whose diagnosis was of a bipolar psychosis were able to go back to university in an average of about 12 months, whereas for those with a diagnosis of 'primary psychotic disorder – the name given to schizophrenia in this study – it took an average of 2 years to recover sufficiently to resume studies. (Shinn et al., 2020).

The authors helpfully emphasise the importance of allowing for generous time spans for convalescence where the illness is a mental rather than physical disorder. We are used to people taking weeks or even months out of their studies for a severe physical illness. The brain and mind take longer to heal than other body tissues, organs and systems. As I have commented elsewhere in this book, periods of at least one year might be expected to allow for meaningful change. Impatience is understandable in young people, but it's important not to give up hope or to expect young people, families and institutions to make premature demands on recovery.

Bipolar Affective Disorder

Joanna worked in a clothes shop during the summer between school and university. One morning her supervisor was called because colleagues noticed her in the stockroom with a paintbrush. She was giggling and literally 'painting the town red' as she said. She was dressed haphazardly in a random range of the shop's clothing, labels still attached. At first people thought she was intoxicated, and called her mother to suggest she was taken home. It was impossible to calm her or soothe her and at one point she sprinted out of the shop and climbed a fire escape onto a nearby roof. At this point emergency services were called. When asked to come down, she offered to 'fly down'. Eventually her mother arrived and climbed up to take her hand, persuading her to descend safely so that they could go to her favourite pizza shop. She was driven to the local hospital, where she was, as promised, provided with pizza and admitted to the young people's ward.

Bipolar disorder is a serious mental illness characterised by extreme mood swings. They can include extremes of either excitement or depressive feelings. Bipolar disorder is more common in people who have a first-degree relative, such as a sibling or parent, with the condition. The vulnerability is lifelong, but assertive treatment can minimise acute episodes of illness. Symptoms can persist for a few weeks or months, or in the case of the depressive symptoms even years without treatment.

In the population as a whole, 1% to 2% of us experience a lifetime prevalence of bipolar disorder. This makes it one of the UK's commonest long-term conditions. Almost as many people live with bipolar as cancer (2.4%) and certainly it is a major concern in the student age group. The World Health Organisation identifies bipolar disorder as one of the top causes of lost years of life and health in 15- to 44-year-olds.

As we have just seen, young people's mental health services often keep diagnostic categories fairly broad, to allow for uncertainties and to capitalise on shared aspects of evidenced treatments. People who have an acute episode of 'mania' such as that described in the case study of 'Joanne', may be given a diagnosis of 'psychosis' without further classification as to whether it may be a manifestation schizophrenia ('primary psychotic disorder') or of bipolar disorder.

However, many people with a diagnosis of bipolar disorder (also called 'bipolar affective disorder', and formerly known as 'manic depressive disorder') will spend more time experiencing depression than elevated mood states. People with 'bipolar II' disorder will not have experienced the severe psychotic symptoms of a full blown manic episode. Their needs are more comparable to people with depressive disorders who do not have a bipolar diagnosis.

International diagnostic classifications subdivide bipolar disorders into bipolar I and bipolar II disorder. The key feature of bipolar I disorder is experiencing at least one past or present episode of mania. The experience of a lesser form of mania, known as 'hypomania', together with depressive episodes, leads to a diagnosis of bipolar II. Sometimes, the diagnosis has to be revised from bipolar I to bipolar II if the episodes of agitation and 'high' mood become so severe as to be psychotic in intensity.

Characteristics of manic and hypomanic episodes:

Euphoria, irritability or expansiveness, and, increased activity or subjective experience of increased energy

plus several of the following symptoms:

- increased talkativeness or pressured speech,
- 'flight of ideas,' distractibility,
- increased self-esteem or grandiosity,
- sleeplessness,
- impulsive reckless behaviour, such as spending, gambling, substance use
- disinhibition, increase in sexual drive & sociability
- increased goal-directed activity, such a planning grand projects.

Hypomanic episodes are usually shorter than manic episodes – manic episodes persist for at least a week or longer. Hypomanic symptoms, though different from the person's usual behaviour, don't impair completely disrupt working or socialising capacity. The person with hypomania doesn't display psychotic features. Hospitalisation is rarely necessary.

In mania, symptoms are pronounced and intense so that work and socialising are significantly impaired. The person's self-esteem may reach delusional proportions, such as claims of having supernatural powers or a special relationship with God or celebrities. There may be severe psychomotor agitation, like pacing, running or climbing, taking off clothes, or constructing or destroying things. People with severe mania need to be cared for in hospital.

Bipolar disorder has its foot in two diagnostic 'camps' as it were. This means that students who have experienced acute episodes of mania or severe psychotic depression may have been treated in specialist 'early psychosis services' for young people. In contrast, adolescents who have presented with depressive symptoms but not yet any significant elevation of mood, will be seen as part of the large group of young people with a depressive disorder.

Bipolar disorder usually begins in adolescence or early adulthood (commonly with an episode of depression), but quite often it takes many years before a definitive diagnosis is reached. Sometimes this is because the young person first experiences an episode of depression. The best clue that this might be bipolar disorder is whether or not there is a family history of bipolar disorder. Research into Edinburgh students referred to a psychiatric clinic with an episode of depression found that 16% had bipolar disorder (Smith et al., 2005).

The depressive phase is defined by exactly the same criteria as any depressive illness (see below), but one striking feature is that the depressive episode that immediately follows a manic or hypomanic phase can be brutally swift in onset and plumb suicidal depths. When individuals are ill, they experience depressive symptoms 75% to 80% of the time and only a minority of their experience is of being 'high' (Kupka et al., 2007).

Each episode of mania or depression increases the likelihood of more frequent episodes, more severe episodes, and poor response to medication treatment. This same phenomenon occurs in other serious menta illnesses – the faster the illness can be treated, the better the outlook for lasting recovery.

The subtlety of milder hypomanic episodes, particularly if these are diagnosed retrospectively, can pose a dilemma as to whether or not it is helpful to make a diagnosis of bipolar II disorder. Often it this has to be a provisional label. Clinicians are reluctant to raise the fears of a significant lifelong vulnerability that are implied by the name 'bipolar'. On the other hand, having a diagnosis flags up the risk of further extreme mood swings and of suicide risk. It also guides clinicians to prescribe cautiously for depressive episodes, given the risk that certain medications can trigger mania in these individuals.

Joanna's 'breakdown' occurred in the summer holiday before taking up her place at a prestigious university many hours journey away from home. She was still 17 and was cared for in a pleasant local young people's ward, and later as a day patient in the intensive treatment service attached to the same building. A schoolfriend was treated for anorexia nervosa in the same service, and both were determined to put the experience behind them and enjoy a 'fresh start' at university. Jo's family tried to persuade her to take a year out. Her grandfather and aunt had both suffered from bipolar disorder, and the grandfather had taken his own life, whilst the aunt had a turbulent life. They chose not to disclose the suicide to Jo, but did speak to staff about it. Child and adolescent mental health services clinicians felt it was too soon to opt for a definitive diagnosis in Jo's case.

In the end, she spent a year at home, attending art courses at the local College. She took medication on a reasonably reliable basis but did sadly have a further episode of illness, this time followed by severe depression. Now 18, she was treated in an adult ward, which she found frightening. However, she had met a fellow art student who told her 'lithium completely turned my life around'. She persuaded her doctors to prescribe lithium, despite their reservations. She had already gained weight on her previous medication and found that lithium was no worse in this respect. It took some time to adjust the doses and establish stable blood levels, and by this time, another year had passed. She eventually took up her university place 2 years later than originally anticipated. She discovered that there was immense diversity and little stigma among her fellow undergraduates, and flourished there.

There is another side to the coin. Many clinicians question whether the diagnosis of bipolar II disorder is an independent disease entity. Many people with this diagnosis have attracted different diagnoses alongside or instead of the bipolar disorder. These include personality disorders of the 'borderline' or 'emotionally unstable' type, posttraumatic stress disorder, attention deficit disorder, anxiety disorders, and substance use disorders. Around 20% people with Bipolar disorder are diagnosed with comorbid Borderline Personality Disorder (Formaros et al., 2016). It would be unhelpful to focus on the bipolar diagnosis at the expense of attending to other treatable co-existing conditions. Mental health services have to support these patients and those around them to tolerate the uncertainties involved.

Students with bipolar I disorder need to receive treatment within a system that has comprehensive rapid response capabilities. The progression of hypomanic and manic symptoms can occur rapidly, and it is critical for students to be seen swiftly after the onset of symptoms. This is best managed by a tightly integrated professional treatment team. Ideally, the student or staff member benefits from an alliance of integrated psychiatric treatment, rapid response, and specific expertise in working with the needs of university students.

Potential access to an inpatient psychiatric unit is essential when treating bipolar disorder. With the bipolar I diagnosis, intermittent inpatient stabilisation may become necessary in response to acute depression or manic episodes. During these times, it will also be important to obtain signed releases, which facilitate communication with parents or other key family members.

Medication for Bipolar I Disorder

Student counselling services do not offer a specialist inpatient ward and would probably not have the expertise on campus to prescribe and monitor special psychotropic medication. This is a particularly sensitive matter for young women who may become pregnant in the future. In the past we may have overestimated the risks of a foetus developing heart defects if the mother was taking lithium. We still acknowledge an increased risk early in pregnancy, though lower than originally believed, particularly when set against advances in paediatric cardiac surgery. We are also more aware of the physical and mental risks to both mother and baby of untreated bipolar disorder. Sadly, many prescribers and patients may have opted for valproate instead, before the higher risks of that drug were discovered. Research now shows that valproate (an anticonvulsant drug that is used as an alternative 'mood stabiliser') does increase a range of risks to the brains and nervous systems of unborn babies.

Lithium is an extraordinary pharmacological agent, with a growing range of applications in modern psychiatry. It has been found to be mood stabilising, anti-manic, antidepressant, effective in reducing suicide risk, even beneficial against dementia. It is very old, and low-cost and easy to source. In the case of bipolar disorder, it is demonstrated to be the 'gold standard'. However, it is not prescribed as often as we might expect.

As we have heard, there is still the fear of damaging an unborn baby, and lithium dosage is critical, so regular blood tests are needed, particularly in the early weeks and months. Lithium has to be kept at sufficiently high levels to be effective and at sufficiently low levels to prevent dangerous toxicity. There is also the potential for interactions with other drugs, whether prescribed or not. Suddenly stopping lithium can trigger acute relapse. For students who tend to run out of supplies – perhaps on their travels – or who are not committed to the treatment, or who take other prescribed or recreational drugs, lithium is not an appropriate choice.

Even when doctors are happy to prescribe, patients can be reluctant as lithium has a reputation for weight gain. Weight gain is unfortunately a side effect of most of the effective medications for bipolar and psychotic disorders. We can hardly overemphasise the dread of weight gain in the student age population (see Chapter 5).

Alternatives to lithium include a range of 'anticonvulsant' drugs – originally developed to treat epilepsy – such as carbamazepine, lamotrigine and valproate. They also include the 'antipsychotic drugs' such as olanzapine and quetiapine. These have antidepressant as well as mood-stabilising properties, but if extra antidepressant medication is needed then the patient can more safely take the traditional antidepressant medication while the mood stabiliser protects against a manic episode.

Contraception

Contraception is all too easy to overlook in mental health practice. Young people negotiating challenging mental conditions are not best placed to address concerns about pregnancy and parenthood. This is true for young men as well as young women, although their range of contraceptive options is narrower. When people are mentally very ill, particularly if they have psychotic symptoms, it is hard to remember pills, condoms or other barrier methods. In the case of bipolar disorder, there may be sexual disinhibition that makes unplanned pregnancy a real risk – as well as unplanned sexually transmitted infections. When a young person has an established diagnosis, choice of appropriate contraception might involve implants, injections or intra-uterine contraceptive devices. For acute, first episode presentations, it is worth offering blood and urine tests and swabs, and remembering not only the 'morning after' pill, but also the effectiveness of an inserted intra-uterine contraceptive device several days afterwards.

Psychological Therapies·

The art of expert prescribing goes far beyond applying an up-to-date knowledge of pharmacology to a prescription pad. Properly conducted prescribing is only one aspect of good practice. Specialist mental health clinicians take time to construct a formulation of the individual's problems and strengths, in collaboration with the patient. This document can then guide a bio-psycho-social management plan. Choice of medication, dosage, arrangements for monitoring, expectations, warnings and alternative options all have to be decided in the context of a trusting therapeutic relationship. In other words, the context of prescribing is a form of supportive psychotherapy in itself.

Whilst the pharmacological aspects of the overall plan are led by the consultant psychiatrist, the therapeutic context can also be provided on campus, by both counsellors and peers. As Federman (2011) remarks, 'The best medication on the market is not going to be effective if the student is unable to acknowledge their vulnerability and find strong treatment alliances with mental health providers.'

A diagnosis of a major mental illness comes as a particular blow to students. It often has to take place when an acute manic episode has given way to deep depression, and in the context of the trauma and embarrassment of treatment, possibly involving compulsion and perhaps some of it acted out in an all too public place in the university. Students who may have boasted excellent performance and participation, have to acknowledge imperfection. Expectations for the future must incorporate the likelihood of ongoing medication treatment and intermittent psychotherapy. Even when treatment approaches work well, people still remind them of the potential for relapse.

The lifestyle management approach was summarised and delivered as interpersonal and social rhythm therapy (ISRT) (Frank et al., 2000). ISRT combines the basic principles of interpersonal psychotherapy with behavioural techniques to help patients regularise their daily routines, address interpersonal problems, and follow a healthy medication regime. Bipolar disorder confers a particular vulnerability to circadian and sleep-wake cycle disruption, so ISRT fine-tunes biological and psychosocial factors to increase stability and support. Most services use aspects of this therapy, which can be delivered individually or in group form.

These people must make lifestyle adjustments that are diametrically opposed to the lifestyle norms of their peer group. Young students are expected to experiment with a wide range of behaviours, some of which can be potentially risky and unhealthy. This is part of the separation/individuation process of late adolescence and young adulthood. For someone recovering from an acute episode of bipolar disorder, the admonitions about lifestyle stability sound like a step back to the same old nagging messages they heard from parents and teachers through their teenage years: work hard, but not too hard, get enough sleep, do not take unnecessary risks, do not use drugs and alcohol, do not get pregnant. It can be heartbreaking to see students' resistance and denial in the face of this advice.

The truth is that often bipolar students are being asked to accept their diagnosis at a point that is premature in terms of their development and maturity. It is simply too much of a stretch for them. Peer groups can come to the rescue. Like Federman (2011), I would argue for the benefits of both individual psychotherapy, and support groups for 'bipolar students'. This might be a joint venture between the national health service (NHS) and the university. In an ideal world, such a group will take place on the university campus and will be co-led by professionals from the university counselling or mental health advisory services, in alliance with local NHS mental health professionals. The psychiatric co-leader has the advantage of seeing how patients are functioning in the group context as well as one to one in clinic, and can guide treatment adjustments accordingly, as well as being available to provide speedy response to any emergencies.

Students with a history of primary psychotic disorder or schizophrenia could be welcomed to the group too, but given that there are likely to be fewer of them, that their progress is typically slower than for bipolar recovery, and that often they are disturbed by intense dynamics within a small group, they might not benefit so much from being part of such a group and prefer a family or individual setting for therapy.

When an established group has success stories from students who have previously experienced periods of instability, then it becomes more worthwhile and even 'cool' to invest in healthy routines. When fellow students advocate the importance of good sleep hygiene, sobriety, medication compliance and contraceptive practice their message is far more effective than what can sound like 'preaching' or 'nagging' from adults.

Practice Points

At a Societal Level

- Despite improved conversations about depression and other aspects of mental health, we still avoid the very mention of schizophrenia and psychotic disorders. Discussions about the nature of the severe psychoses and on appropriate responses could reduce stigma.
- Three groups of severe mental illness have disproportionately high rates of suicide – schizophrenia, bipolar disorder, and anorexia nervosa – but effective treatment can save lives.

At the Level of University Authorities and Policies

- Students who are mentally unwell can place excessive demands on academic staff.
- Staff – both academic and support staff – should be provided with regular updates about emergency contacts and resources so that they can hand over confidently to appropriate professionals.
- Policies on admissions, fitness to study and time taken out of studies for recovery from a severe mental illness need to take account of the long timespans taken to recover in these disorders.
- Close university links with NHS services and family or other lay carers, are essential for the well-being of people with severe mental illness.
- Integrating care around a student or staff member will involve a series of permissions – preferably arranged in advance – for all involved to communicate with maximum confidentiality, privacy and dignity.

NHS and Related Services

- Students who have to take a break from studies usually need care to be transferred to the location of the student's family home. NHS teams may be able to use telemedicine to communicate with a distant university regarding return to studies, and with a different health trust or board, regarding future outpatient follow up and treatment.

Families

- Maintaining contact with the student is particularly important when there are signs of social withdrawal, academic failure or low mood.
- Bipolar disorder can pose a particular risk of overspending and taking financial risks when unwell. Families are probably best placed to help students take charge of their finances, and support them in conversation with banks, finance advisors, Citizen's Advice and advocacy services.

Teachers, Tutors, Directors of Studies and Fellow Students

- It is absolutely not your job to diagnose or treat a serious mental disorder, but some awareness of the nature of mental illnesses helps demystify and reduce fear and stigma.
- There are effective treatments even for the most severe mental illnesses that affect young students. However, it takes far longer to see recovery than with most physical conditions.
- No single individual should attempt to support a seriously mentally ill person unaided. If you have become the person who takes on all the worry, concern and support, seek help from a person senior to you, or – if you are a senior member of the university – from mental health staff.

Individuals Seeking Help and Support

- Do not lose hope: there are effective treatments even for the most severe mental illnesses, particularly when you are young. Be patient: the brain and mind recover more slowly than the body.
- Except in emergencies, the pathway to treatment is through your general practitioner. If you are not already registered, you should do so, or if there is no time to do so, ask to be treated as a visitor or temporary resident. If you are taking prescribed medication, get advice on the most economic and convenient ways to do this. If you have concerns about medication, be sure to discuss these and ask for alternatives or adjustments.
- It is understandable to feel angry and sad about having an illness and being obliged to interrupt your education. It can help to meet up with other people who have successfully managed difficulties similar to your own.
- Some students with mental illness are encouraged to use their experience in publicity and campaigns. Take your time to decide whether this is right for you. There is no obligation to become a poster boy or girl for students with mental illness!

References

Federman, R. (2011). Treatment of Bipolar Disorder in the University Student Population. *Journal of College Student Psychotherapy*, 25(1), 24–38. https://doi.org/10.1080/87568225.2011.532471

Formaros, M., Orsolini, L., Marini, S., et al. (2016). The prevalence and predictors of bipolar and borderline personality disorders comorbidity: Systematic review and meta-analysis *Journal of Affective Disorders*, 195(2016), 105–118. https://doi.org/10.1016/j.jad.2016.01.040

Frank, E., Swartz, H. A. & Kupfer, D. J. (2000). Interpersonal and social rhythm therapy: Managing the chaos of bipolar disorder. *Biological Psychiatry*, 48(6), 593–604. https://doi.org/10.1016/S0006-3223(00)00969-0

Hardy, K. V., Noordsy, D. L., Ballon, J. S., McGovern, M. P., Salomon, C. & Wiltsey Stirman, S. (2018). Impact of age of onset of psychosis and engagement in higher education on duration of untreated psychosis, *Journal of Mental Health*, 27:3, 257–62. https://doi.org/10.1080/09638237.2018.1466047

Kupka, R. W., Altshuler, L. L., Nolen, W. A., et al. (2007). Three times more depression than mania in both bipolar I and bipolar II disorder. *Bipolar Disorders*, 9, 531–5. https://doi.org/10.1111/j.1399-5618.2007.00467.x

MacCabe, J., Lambe, M., Cnattingius, S., et al. (2010). Excellent school performance at age 16 and risk of adult bipolar disorder: National cohort study. *British Journal of Psychiatry*, 196(2), 109–15. https://doi.org/10.1192/bjp.bp.108.060368

Penttilä, M., Jääskeläinen, E., Hirvonen, N., Isohanni, M. & Miettunen, J. (2014). Duration of untreated psychosis as predictor of long-term outcome in schizophrenia: Systematic review and meta-analysis. *The British Journal of Psychiatry*, 205(2), 88–94.

Saha, S., Chant, D., Welham, J. & McGrath, J. (2005). A systematic review of the prevalence of schizophrenia. *PLoS Medicine*, 2(5), e141.

Shinn, A. K., Cawkwell, P. B., Bolton, K., et al. (2020). Return to college after a first episode of psychosis, *Schizophrenia Bulletin Open*, 1(1), sgaa041. https://doi.org/10.1093/schizbullopen/sgaa041

Smith, D. J., Harrison, N., Muir, W. & Blackwood, D. H. (2005). The high prevalence of bipolar spectrum disorders in young adults with recurrent depression: toward an innovative diagnostic framework. *Journal of Affective Disorders*, 84(2–3), 167–78.

Wainberg, M., Jacobs, G. R., di Forti, M. & Tripathy, S. J. (2021). Cannabis, schizophrenia genetic risk, and psychotic experiences: A cross-sectional study of 109,308 participants from the UK Biobank. *Translational Psychiatry*, 11, 211.

Mood Disorders
Depression and Anxiety

PERSONALITY DISORDERS

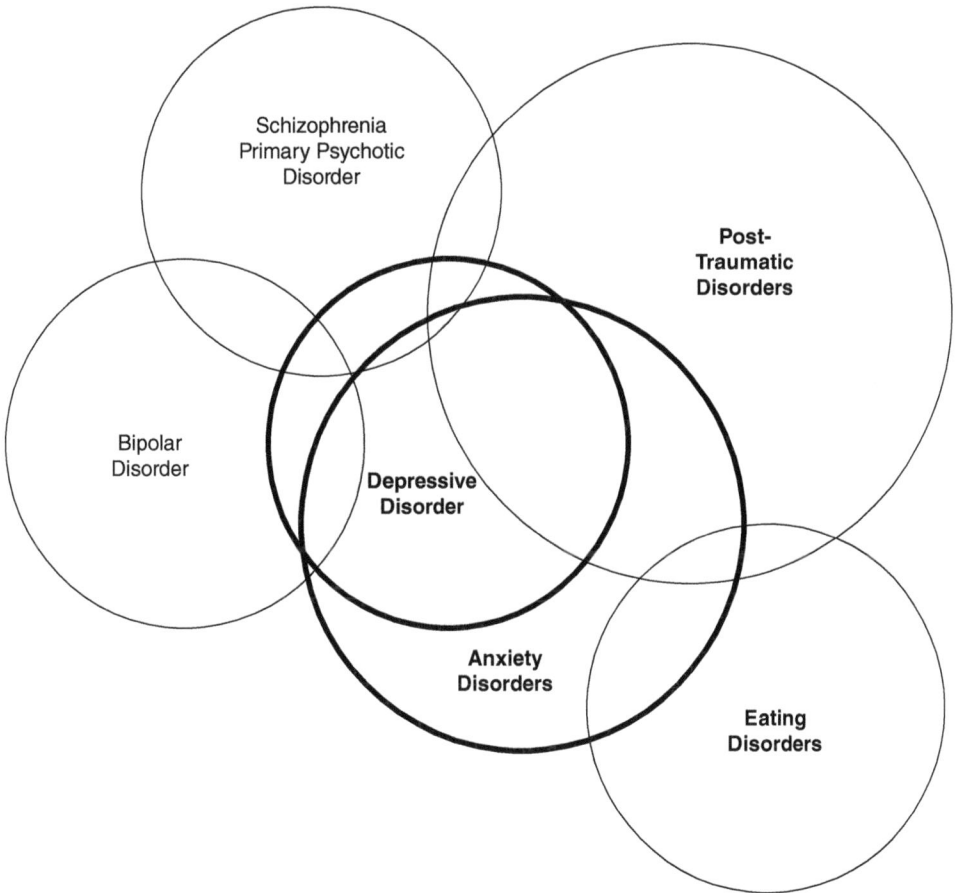

AUTISTIC SPECTRUM + NEURO DEVELOPMENTAL

Figure 16.1 Mood disorders and their relationships with other mental conditions

Mood Disorders and Their Context

For those of us who find it useful to invoke a medical model of mental illness, the words 'depression' and 'anxiety' are misleading. They seem to suggest that feeling low or worried is the same as having an illness and inevitably requires treatment. I sometimes wonder if it would be better to move to different terminology – perhaps resorting to old terms such as 'melancholia' and 'angst'.

The term 'depression' has the further disadvantage in being used almost as a general term to indicate mental disorders and conditions of all sorts. It has become common for instance to call all postnatal mental disorders 'postnatal depression' or to fail to distinguish between the statements 'half of all students are depressed' and 'half of all students have a mental disorder'. This is an important point to remember when we consider the wide range in estimates of what proportion of students experience 'depression'.

Many studies use questionnaires designed to pick up the symptoms of depressive disorder, but they don't usually screen out those for whom the depressive symptoms are a part of another disorder, or perhaps more temporary than the persisting symptoms of a mental disorder. We can better trust those studies that assess the student's experience in a more holistic way, looking for the whole range of mental disorders and then reporting on what proportion of those would be best treated as primarily depressive disorders.

> Jennie was a shy student who had been treated in child and adolescent mental health services as a 12-year-old, when her parents separated. She managed her first year well but found herself struggling in the second year. She ruminated about falling behind in her coursework and couldn't sleep. She hadn't made it into the elite hockey teams, so she left the society. Rock choir clashed with an evening seminar, so she dropped that too. Her friends from hall were now in different flats – her own flatmates were hard-working medics who socialised and revised together. She had drifted apart from her boyfriend that summer and thought no one would ever find her attractive. She was lonely and stressed but was surprised when her general practitioner suggested she had depressive disorder.
>
> As a child she had been warned that young people should not take antidepressants in case they became suicidal, so she was reluctant to accept a prescription. Her general practitioner reassured her that he would see her regularly in the early days, to monitor this. She was also 'fast-tracked' for counselling.

I would absolutely not recommend that lay people attempt to diagnose a student's disorder or to self-diagnose, but I do argue in this book for some improvement in public awareness of the large and subtle range of conditions that can affect the mind. Much of this handbook deals with environmental and routine aspects of well-being. These can minimise the risk of mental breakdown for everyone, and provide the healthiest and most compassionate environment for recovery when people do fall ill.

'Well-being' and 'mental 'health' are overlapping considerations but diagnosable mental illness is a somewhat different matter. Respect for diversity is a crucial in nurturing well-being and mental health: one size certainly does not fit all. Mental illnesses also require treatments tailored to the individuals affected, and different mental illnesses affect people very differently. Well-meaning attempts to offer the same treatments to all people, regardless of disorder, can be disastrous.

In current diagnostic classifications manic, hypomanic and depressive episodes can be all conceptualised as features of different 'mood disorders'. Bipolar disorder –

sometimes called bipolar affective disorder, bipolar depressive disorder or manic-depressive disorder – causes patients to experience both high and low extremes of mood, usually in different episodes. 'Unipolar' depression – major depressive disorder, or just 'depression' – is diagnosed when all the episodes are of low mood, or of a mixture of depressed mood with anxiety symptoms. We discussed bipolar disorder in the previous chapter, with some reflections on the differences and common features with primary psychotic disorders. This chapter is devoted to the extremely common and important condition of 'unipolar' depression in students and university staff.

Features of Depression

There is depressed mood or diminished interest and pleasure in activities most of the day, nearly every day, for at least 2 weeks, accompanied by other symptoms such as:

- reduced ability to concentrate
- indecisiveness
- beliefs of low self-worth or excessive or inappropriate guilt
- hopelessness about the future
- recurrent thoughts (or plans, even actions) of death or suicide
- sleeplessness or excessive sleep
- significant changes in appetite or weight
- physical agitation or slowing down
- fatigue or loss of energy

Depression severity exists along a continuum, reflecting the intensity of the symptoms and their impact on personal and social functioning.

(International Classification of Diseases, 11th Revision)

I have included depressive and anxiety disorders in this same chapter because of the immense overlap of the symptoms. Indeed, despite the separate diagnoses in international classification systems, research suggests that co-occurring anxiety and depression may be more common than either disorder individually (Shevlin et al., 2022). Some researchers argue that we should treat mixed anxiety and depression as the main diagnostic group, with pure anxiety and depression only occurring as special cases.

In 2013, when Ibrahim and colleagues conducted a systematic review of studies of depression prevalence in university students, only one in a hundred of the papers they considered met stringent research criteria (Ibrahim et al., 2013a). Clearly, we need better quality research in the field. Within these well-conducted studies, prevalence rates for depression ranged greatly from 10% to 85% with an average of 30% students having a diagnosable depressive disorder. Half of the samples were entirely composed of medical students. This did not seem to skew the results, and surprisingly the medical students reported slightly lower rates of depression. The studies that examined different rates for male and female students found – as the authors expected – that the rate of depression was slightly higher in women.

Rates of student depression are probably about the same as those of non-students of the same age. A large US study (Blanco et al., 2008) found no significant difference in the prevalence of depression between students and young people of the same age who were not in higher education. Rates were around 8% in both groups using the US diagnostic criteria of the time.

This figure might seem surprisingly low. We should remember that overall the study found that almost half of the young people included met criteria for at least one mental disorder. As I mentioned earlier many people have subjective experience of feeling 'depressed' when they are mentally unwell, although in fact the symptoms might fit better with a different diagnosis. In contrast, a study of UK final-year students (Ibrahim et al., 2013b) found that 58.1% of female and 59.9% of male study participants screened positive for depression. However, rather than interviewing students and assigning a diagnosis, as the US study (Blanco et al., 2008) had done, this study asked participants to complete questionnaires, which picked up depressive symptoms but did not discriminate whether they might be part of a different condition. The Ibrahim et al. (2013b) study did usefully highlight, though, that students from families living in more deprived areas were signifi- cantly more likely to report symptoms. As universities increase access, we need to be aware of the extra vulnerabilities of students from less privileged backgrounds.

For me, there are several important lessons from scrutinising the methodology from different studies. One is, that depressive symptoms are extraordinarily prevalent. The higher figures reported almost certainly reflect high levels of distress in this age group, whether or not they are students. On the other hand, some depressive symptoms may reflect the presence of different disorders. The primary disorder may not respond well to treatment that mainly addresses the depressive symptoms.

Some people who meet the criteria for depressive disorder will already have bipolar disorder, schizophrenia, obsessive–compulsive disorder (OCD), eating disorders or traumatic disorders; may have experienced bereavement; or may be on the autistic spectrum. Depressive disorder may be the most frequently occurring comorbid psychi- atric illness in autism spectrum disorder (ASD) (Ghaziuddin et al., 2002), and often co- occurs with anxiety disorder. People who are high on the autistic spectrum are just one group who need modifications to standard treatments for depression and anxiety. (See Chapter 10 for further discussion of ASD)

The social cost of 'affective disorders' – disorders of mood such as anxiety and depression – is particularly high in young students because they represent the future hope of any community and may be potential leaders. Untreated depression at this stage in life can lead to the accumulation of negative consequences through adulthood, in a range of social and personal domains. Intellectually, depression has been linked to poorer academic achievements (Hysenbegasi et al., 2005) and to poorer work performance (Harvey et al., 2011). This works in vicious spirals. Students often experience academic demands as greater at university than at school. Disappointment with academic performance contrib- utes to the risk of depression and mental health problems (Beiter et al., 2015). Depressive symptoms interfere with successful studying, making academic failure ore likely.

Consistent findings have emphasised the protective role of social support for stu- dents' well-being (Alsubaie et al., 2019). Social support from both family and friends has a substantial impact on the emotional, social and academic performance of university students. About a third of the students in this study reported depressive symptoms on questionnaires. Social support from family, and friends was a significant predictor of whether or not they experienced depressive symptoms, and also of their quality of life.

In this developmental stage of adolescence, friends are increasingly more important as a source of social support compared to family and are more likely to be physically available once a student has moved out of home. Wörfel et al. (2016) found that social support from friends is a significant predictor of depression in university students. Social support from family was not as strong a predictor as support from friends but families do remain an important source of social support (Alsubaie et al., 2019). Parents, and other older relatives can provide maturity and rich experience with life stressors. The maturity of the sources of support is an important factor in the value of the help sought.

It's important to acknowledge that the study of Alsubaie et al. (2019), already mentioned, confirms previous findings about social support. However, like so many studies of student samples, this one was more than 82% female. My experience has been that young women are more likely to volunteer for psychosocial research, to be open about their own mental health history, and to seek and use psychological treatment than their male counterparts. Gender differences have been found in how adolescents experience stress. Adolescent girls report higher stress levels in relationships with parents, peers, and romantic partners. Boys tend to react more to achievement-related events (Camara et al., 2017). We need to be extremely careful about generalising research that is predominantly based on one gender. Obviously the same is true about generalising from data gathered by simply inviting volunteers to participate in research.

Anxiety Disorders

Whilst 'depression' is probably the most commonly discussed mental disorder, in fact the anxiety disorders are probably even more common in the population as a whole. As we have seen, they very commonly overlap with depressive disorders. The presence of anxiety in depressive episodes is associated with higher suicide risks, longer duration of illness and a higher likelihood of non-response to treatment, so it's important to be aware of its presence. As for so many mental disorders, there is evidence that a combination of genetic and environmental factors are involved. Obviously, environmental factors can – and should – be modified to some extent, but people who have inherited an extreme vulnerability usually find that they need to take medication or learn specialist psychological skills to regulate their emotions, and often both of these strategies together are needed.

Features of Generalised Anxiety Disorder

- Marked symptoms of anxiety or apprehensiveness not restricted to any particular circumstance, or excessive worry about negative events in various aspects of life.
- Anxiety with physical symptoms such as: muscle tension, restlessness, gastrointestinal symptoms, palpitations, sweating, trembling, shaking, dry mouth, difficulty concentrating, irritability, sleep disturbances.
- The symptoms are present over several months, for more days than not
- Symptoms are not better explained by another medical or mental condition and are not due to the effects of a substance or medication.
- The symptoms result in significant impairment in personal, family, social, educational, occupational, or other important areas of functioning

(International Classification of Diseases, 11th Revision)

Probably the commonest form of anxiety disorder is generalised anxiety disorder. This is diagnosed in 4% to 8% of general practice patients of all ages. It is almost certainly underdiagnosed (National Institute of Health and Care Excellence, 2022).

Anxiety is exceedingly common in university students. Duffy et al. (2019) showed that amongst US higher education students, almost a quarter had been treated for an anxiety disorder in the previous year. Two thirds had experienced overwhelming feelings of anxiety, even though they had not sought treatment or not been considered to meet diagnostic criteria. This study is impressive in drawing on randomly selected samples of students and examining both symptoms and treatments offered.

Of course, these findings should not be automatically extrapolated to the UK setting, though, or to the changed situation as we emerge from the COVID lockdown and its sequelae.

The authors comment on some of the environmental factors that may contribute to the high levels of student anxiety. They include high use of caffeine, not only in coffee but in cola drinks and other substances students use to remain alert through 'all-nighters' to meet academic deadlines or to stay awake to go partying. Academic anxieties were common and, poignantly, loneliness was cited as an important cause of anxiety. There is a huge amount of overlap here with the predisposing and perpetuating factors of depressive disorders.

As well as recognising generalised anxiety disorder, the International Classification of Diseases 11th Revision (ICD-11) diagnostic system recognises a group of 'anxiety and fear-related disorders' with different categories depending on their 'focus of apprehension'. In other words, certain anxiety disorders involve a particular fear. 'Phobias' for instance involve fear of some individual object – spiders, snakes, heights and so on. Social anxiety disorder is characterised by fear in one or more social situations such as having a conversation, eating or drinking in the presence of others, or giving presentations. The student has an excessive concern that they will be harshly judged by other people. The usual consequence is social avoidance, resulting in failure to develop the necessary skills and 'thick skin' that allow most of us to cope. Despite fearing other people, the student can feel desperately lonely. This is often not a stand-alone condition but part of other anxiety conditions, and often also of a depressive disorder.

Students are also vulnerable to separation anxiety disorder, which is characterised by marked fear of separation from 'attachment figures'. In new students it can take the form of extreme homesickness, beyond what might be considered normal. Separation anxiety in children typically focuses on parents or other family members. In adults, the focus is typically a romantic partner or close friend, and adolescents typically transfer their attachments from family to a friendship group or to individual friends or lovers. Rejection in a romantic relationship can be particularly devastating for a young student. Sometimes the romantic figure represents not only a love object and a hope for a future partnership but also has the status of an emotional carer, and replacement 'attachment figure' at a time of great vulnerability.

Physiology and Psychology of Panic Attacks

A thought or situation – such as worry about giving a presentation – leads to the body generating higher levels of adrenalin and other stress hormones.

Our brains have evolved over the millennia to respond to *physical* threats that might call on us to fight physically or run away or hide. Our stress hormones therefore send as much available blood supply and oxygen to muscles and increase our rate of breathing and sweating. Blood is diverted away from the digestive system.

Unless we harness this physiological change to physical action, we will find ourselves breathless, trembling, sweaty and nauseated. The 'over-breathing' causes changes in blood chemicals that trigger chest pain and even fainting.

The physical symptoms are so alarming that we are now worried about both the presentation AND the fear of serious physical illness. We may even think we are dying! Needless to say, we now try to avoid any situation that might trigger these symptoms again, and we are on constant high alert – which makes us even more likely to panic.

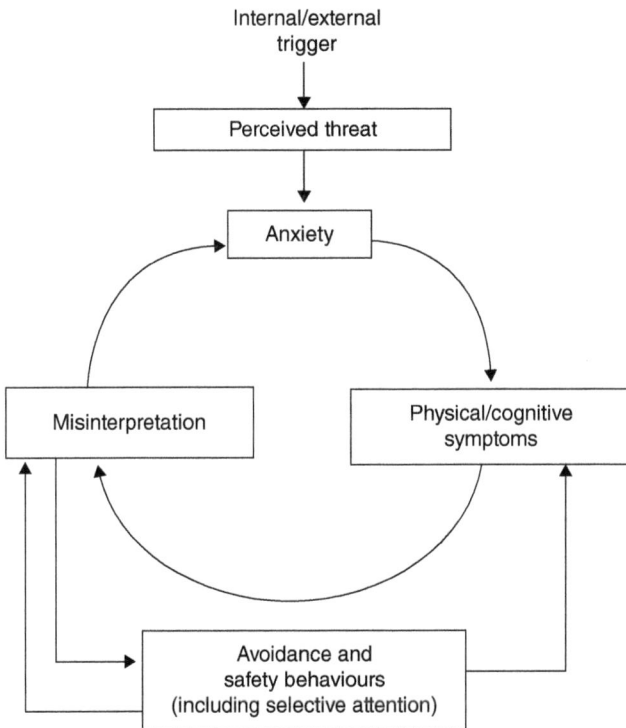

Figure 16.2 The vicious cycle of panic attacks

Anxiety disorders can include the experience of panic attacks, either in association with the feared trigger, or in some cases out of the blue. A panic attack is feeling of intense fear that triggers primitive physical reactions. We then automatically respond to the physical symptoms with catastrophic thoughts such as going crazy, losing control, having a heart attack or an asthma attack, or even dying. Panic experiences can sometimes be triggered by too much caffeine (or other recreational drugs), by hypoglycaemia as a result of not having eaten for a long time, or as a withdrawal effect after having too much alcohol (Figure 16.2).

Panic attacks create fear of future attacks. As a result, the person adopts 'safety, behaviours to avoid them or to ensure they don't have them in an embarrassingly public place. In such cases, a single panic attack gradually transitions into a panic disorder. Whatever the cause, panic is a horrible experience in its own right, and if we don't understand the physiology of panic, it is possible to believe that it represents serious physical illness. Panic can lead to agoraphobia, or it can lead to a form of illness obsession where the patient constantly seeks medical diagnoses for the symptoms.

Diagnostic systems recognise that syndromes such as post-traumatic stress disorder, OCD and the 'eating disorders', are also characterised by anxiety symptoms. In these disorders the 'focus of apprehension' is both specific and wide ranging. People with post-traumatic stress disorder experience fears related to a past trauma. An earthquake survivor, for instance, may avoid travelling to certain parts of the world, and may obsessively practice earthquake safety drills, and check their house's foundations. They may also find that if they are to avoid 'flashbacks' – the horribly realistic involuntary memories of the trauma – they also have to avoid reminders such as wearing a red jacket, if they were wearing a red jacket at the time of the earthquake.

Janine was initially a popular first year student, but she struggled with the messy life of student halls. Her mother was house proud, and she was used to an immaculate home. She ended up completely unable to go into the shared kitchen or to allow anyone else across the threshold of her super-clean bedroom. She was not particularly well-organised or tidy, but admitted that she was terrified of germs, and stayed away from friends who had colds or made any mention of infection. She had never had a romantic partner, and although she identified as heterosexual, she would joke that 'boys are filthy creatures'. She told her counsellor that her fear of infection dated back to being taught about sexually transmitted infections at school, but things had become much worse since COVID. She had felt ambivalent about attending university at all, even though she was vaccinated, and lockdown was now officially lifted.

A student or staff member with OCD who is obsessively afraid of infection, may find it difficult to share accommodation, may have to keep to their own crockery and cutlery, may avoid crowded places or have to wear masks and gloves, and boil wash their clothes when they come home each night. Eventually they may become housebound. During COVID, some patients with OCD initially appeared to be model citizens, but later became so handicapped by their fear of either catching the virus or of passing it on, that they couldn't leave home even to get a vaccination, and struggled more as lockdown was eased than during the worst restrictions.

The so-called eating disorders have much in common with OCD, with the over-whelming fear of gaining weight or body fat, and the exaggerated sense of responsibility for controlling body weight and shape to an unrealistic extent. The eating disorders are discussed further in Chapter 5.

It can be agonising to live alongside people with severe obsessive disorders. They can appear to be 'controlling'. In fact, we all try our utmost to control and avoid extreme danger. The difference is that when we share a healthy perception of what is dangerous, we do not feel controlled. People with extreme anxiety disorders are unable to balance the risks of being exposed to what they fear against the risks of avoidance behaviour. The social and interpersonal difficulties can be crippling.

The prevalence of anxiety disorders is high in people who are on the autistic spectrum (see Chapter 10 for further discussion of this). They are particularly vulnerable to social phobias, separation anxiety, generalised anxiety disorder, OCD and eating disorders. Anxiety around other people is a particular challenge for people with ASD unless they have had support to learn more sophisticated social skills. Their perception of other people's negative responses to them may contain a grain of truth. Students who have not learned 'neurotypical' social signals, can be stigmatised. Happily, the higher proportion of people with ASD in a university environment can make for a more comfortably diverse culture. Society still has to work out how far avoidance and obsessionality should be accepted as part of that diversity, and how far individuals should be encouraged to overcome anxious avoidance to build up mental resilience, emotion management skills and interpersonal effectiveness.

Personality Disorders

Features That Commonly Attract a Diagnosis of Borderline or Emotionally Unstable Personality Disorder
- Deliberate self-harm
- Substance misuse – alcohol, drugs
- Unhealthy attachments to people, either over-idealising or denigrating them
- Eating disorder symptoms such as binging and purging
- Sexually chaotic behaviour
- History of trauma, particularly sexual abuse
- Risk taking.

The term 'personality disorder' is problematic for several reasons. I am still dissatisfied with the term, after many years of training in psychiatry and psychotherapy, and working with scores of people who have attracted this diagnosis. For one thing, it implies that the features incorporated in the diagnosis are lifelong and relatively unchangeable, in contrast with the symptoms of the other disorders discussed in this and previous chapters.

The most commonly diagnosed personality disorder has been known as 'borderline' or 'emotionally unstable' personality disorder. This is most often diagnosed in young women. Research consistently shows that the symptoms that characterise this diagnosis are in fact amenable to change, both as the individual gets older, and in response to treatment. Psychological therapies that teach the skills of emotion regulation, distress tolerance and interpersonal relationship skills can reduce levels of deliberate self-harm and improve relationships with services.

'Maladaptive coping disorder' might be a more accurate way to describe the condition, although I acknowledge that it is not an adequately sympathetic description. We do need a name for the condition to allow it to be validated, researched and treated as effectively as possible – it could be helpful to invite participation of people with this diagnosis to help design a new name. We need to rescue it from being a diagnosis of exclusion, in all senses of that word. There continues to be a risk that when people – particularly young women – fail to respond to standard treatments for depressive or anxiety disorders, or when they present with self-destructive behaviours, they are automatically given this diagnosis.

I'm very uncomfortable with the levels of stigma and rejection shown to people who attract this diagnosis. I'm not the only one. Some colleagues have dropped the 'personality disorder' label in favour of less derogatory terms. Unfortunately, this practice seems to involve diagnosing a condition that looks similar but not quite the same as the condition described as 'personality disorder. 'Chronic trauma' may attract a more compassionate attitude towards the patient, but suggests that treatment should focus on an identifiable trauma. Not everyone with the constellation of symptoms can identify such a trauma or can benefit from addressing it. 'Multi-impulsive bulimia' and 'multi-impulsive eating disorders' have been used by clinicians within eating disorders services to describe a similar syndrome but through the lens of the eating disorder. At least these consciously inaccurate diagnoses allow the patient access to services, but perhaps not to services that address their core difficulties or that have expertise in managing the dynamics of the interpersonal problems involved.

The traditional excuse that there were no effective treatments for 'borderline personality disorder' and that attempts at treatment would inevitably make things worse is no longer the case. Dialectical behaviour therapy (Robins et al., 2004) is only one of the therapies that have been shown to help steer patients towards recovery.

Treatments for Disorders of Depression and Anxiety

Diagnostic systems and formal guidelines still tend to treat anxiety and depressive disorders as separate entities. In practice, there is an overlap in the evidence-based treatments involved. As a result, students or staff with co-morbid depressive and anxiety disorders can often address the whole spectrum of their symptoms within the treatment offered for their primary diagnosis. Therapists can design psychosocial interventions to meet the individual's particular needs. Fortunately, the so-called antidepressant medications are effective in both conditions. Prescribing is slightly different for people who have symptoms of anxiety, trauma or obsessionality, though. They are likely to require higher doses of medication, or they may find that medications that are effective against depressive symptoms are not helpful for the anxiety symptoms.

Some people have a marked preference for either medication or non-pharmacological treatments, and are likely to flourish best with a treatment in which they have faith and commitment. A trusting relationship with the prescriber or therapist is a strong predictor of good outcome. Often the art of prescribing must include a 'therapeutic' stance, and sometimes referral to a psychological therapist to learn psycho-social skills. Meanwhile, the work of psychological interventions may include encouragement to accept medication. Sometime the patient is unable to benefit from the psychotherapy because of disabling symptoms. Both psychological and pharmacological modalities of treatment can involve side effects such as feeling more agitated before feeling better, and the risk of 'withdrawal' effects if treatment is stopped suddenly.

There has recently been a great deal of media denigration of psychotropic medication and particularly of 'antidepressants', so it can be helpful to address this up front. Staff and students outside the psychiatric profession may be alarmed by oversimplistic headlines. 'Talking therapies' are not automatically better or safer than medication. They are often more expensive in terms of the training and provision of therapists, but also in terms of the student's or scholar's own time and effort. Most therapies provide a 1-hour session each week with the therapist, and expect that the patient will devote time between sessions to practice the skills learned. Effective therapy demands effort and courage from the patient. Medication is usually more time-efficient although it too may demand courage and trust. And whilst in an ideal world long waiting lists for therapy would not be a consideration, in practice it may be safer to offer immediate treatment than wait for many weeks or months.

The practice of offering an assessment session and then an 'internal' waiting list is regrettable, and it is often the case that student counselling is restricted to a small number of sessions. For a student with a major depressive disorder, a longer course of treatment, with the continuity of a single trusted therapy is not merely desirable but an essential part of the active ingredient of the treatment.

There is limited research on the specific outcomes of treatments for students living within the UK, with access to the national health service (NHS). We cannot entirely extrapolate results of trials of treatment in places such as the United States – where outcomes may be influenced by participants' gratitude for free treatment in normally fee-paying health services. Conversely, students, having been selected for their cognitive ability, might do better than other members of the community in intellectually-demanding treatments such as cognitive behavioural therapy (CBT) (Cuijpers et al., 2016). The youth of students may also give them a better prognosis than older patients. However, the evidence, such as it is, fails to show any difference in results of therapy between students and the general public.

One of the most rigorous and well-analysed studies of treatment of depression in the young is the Treatment for Adolescents With Depression Study, which examined the benefits of anti-depressant medication and CBT separately and in combination at different stages of treatment (March et al., 2007). This was a multicentre study based in the United States that included 12- to 18-year-olds with moderate to severe depression. They were obviously younger than the undergraduate population and living at home rather than away at university. They did, however, represent a demographic similar to our students in terms of social background, ethnicity, gender and co-morbidity – many of them also had anxiety and related symptoms. For me the importance of the study is in demonstrating the subtle differences and benefits of each treatment in young brains and minds.

The antidepressant medication used in the trial was fluoxetine. This is the only antidepressant medication approved for young people under age 18, because of observations that many others increase the risk of 'suicidal behaviour' in the young. Whilst university students are usually over this age, it is worth remembering that brains do not suddenly mature overnight, so we should be particularly cautious about prescribing the two drugs that had caused particular concern: paroxetine and venlafaxine.

Researchers in the Treatment for Adolescents With Depression Study found that after 12 weeks of treatment, fluoxetine treatment gave the best rates of improvement whether alone or in combination with CBT (March et al., 2007). After 18 weeks, the combination of CBT and medication was doing better than either treatment alone, although after 36 weeks from the start of the project, more than 80% of the participants had responded well to treatment, whatever group they were in – with combination treatment still a little ahead of the other two groups, and fluoxetine still a little ahead of CBT. Suicidal ideation decreased with treatment, but less so with fluoxetine therapy than with combination therapy or CBT. The authors wisely conclude that fluoxetine provides a faster recovery from depression but that adding CBT to medication enhances the safety of medication (March et al., 2007).

Psychosocial Treatments

Cognitive behavioural therapy is one of the leading 'talking therapies' for anxiety, depression and related disorders. The 'behavioural' aspect of the treatment is crucial in both depression and anxiety. For the depressed individual, 'behavioural activation' involves restructuring the day and week, actively participating in activities that used to bring pleasure, even if they no longer do so, and taking physical exercise. For the anxious individual, replacing avoidant behaviour with 'approach' behaviour means gently building up exposure to feared situation – particularly social situations.

Another therapy with a strong evidence base in depressive and anxiety disorders is interpersonal psychotherapy (Weissman et al., 2017). Interpersonal psychotherapy has been specially adapted for the adolescent age group, so younger students may benefit from the adaptations (Mufson & Sills, 2006). A course of interpersonal psychotherapy is often reported as a particularly fulfilling experience for both therapist and patient, perhaps because the interpersonal aspect is so congenial to the student age group, and because there is the option for the treatment to address the highly relevant 'transitions' focus.

There are many apps, books and websites offering CBT and other structured therapies in 'self-help' form, but once a student has a diagnosis of significant disorder it can be impossible to mobilise sheer willpower to follow the course. Face-to-face therapy – including group therapy – can provide the encouragement and accountability to bring about change. Groups can be either stand alone or add-ons to individual therapy, providing a protected 'practical class' to practice psychosocial skills and to acquire an understanding peer group. Superficially they may seem like a more economical way to deliver therapy, but in practice many patients need individual sessions to prepare them for the group experience and sometimes to support them alongside attendance at the group. Others may be too severely affected to tolerate the group experience or may have symptoms that could influence the group in a harmful rather than helpful way.

Medication for Depression and Anxiety

The discovery of the selective serotonin reuptake inhibitors such as fluoxetine, late in the twentieth century made it possible to treat depressive and anxiety disorders without the inevitable sedation that came with their predecessors. Later, the development of serotonin and norepinephrine reuptake inhibitors, such as venlafaxine and duloxetine, also brought activation rather than sedation. For most students and academics this was a crucial benefit, but the older medications are still available. Research in the under-18 age group, though, resulted in cautions against prescribing the shorter-acting medications (in particular, paroxetine and venlafaxine) to younger people. It makes sense to bear this in mind with young students.

Another aspect to consider, particularly when prescribing for young women, is the possibility of pregnancy (and breastfeeding). This is not only in case of short-term unplanned pregnancy. When people need to take medication longer term, or are at risk of future episodes, it is helpful to have established that they respond well to one of the medications that is safe in the perinatal period. A growing body of research suggests that benefits to both mother and unborn child of effective treatments for mental illness outweigh the risks of most medications. At present sertraline has probably the best track record, whilst fluoxetine and citalopram are also recognised as good choices.

Fluoxetine has a long half-life. It takes days and weeks for a single dose to gradually leave the body. This means that withdrawal symptoms are rare. When students divide their time between different locations they may run out of medication. A forgetful student can omit a few days' supply without going into withdrawal – there is a smooth reduction of drug concentration.

Young people are especially likely to stop taking medication when symptoms are relieved, so that monitoring and reminders are needed. It is usually recommended to continue medication for a year after the resolution of symptoms, to reduce risk of relapse. For some students, it is advisable to remain on medication for the rest of their university course, or at least to make the trial of discontinuation during a long vacation, to avoid further disruption to studies.

Fortunately, the selective serotonin reuptake inhibitors, which are effective in both depressive and anxiety disorders, tend to have little street value or abuse potential. The same is true of mirtazapine. This is a chemically different antidepressant. It tends to be sedative rather than activating, so provides a good alternative for students who struggle to sleep. These drugs are fairly safe in overdose – indeed much safer than paracetamol, though the latter is available over the counter. However, it is always worth considering risks of overdose and interactions with other drugs and substances, both for the student who is the patient and in terms of potential access by flatmates and fellow students.

Family Experiences of Treatment for Depression and Anxiety

When other members of the family have a depressive or anxiety disorder, the student may have both genetic and environmental predispositions to experience a similar disorder. Treatments that have helped one family member may be more effective for other family members.

It is always useful to hear about the mental health and treatment experiences of family members, even when the student does not want their parents or siblings to be directly involved in treatment. Students may look on relatives as role models in managing a mental condition – or may prefer to focus on the hope of newer treatments to forge their own recovery.

Jean was a university student with severe anxiety. She taken a year out before returning to take final examinations. Her symptoms reappeared almost as soon as she arrived back on campus, and she felt desperate. Her psychiatrist knew that her mother had also had lifelong depression and that her father was highly perfectionist, but Jean had not wanted her family to be involved in her treatment. However, she now agreed to hold a review with her mother, though not her father, present in the clinic.

It emerged that her father was almost certainly very high on the autistic spectrum, though he had resisted his wife's suggestion to have formal assessment. Jean's mother was able to describe some features of Jean's childhood that would suggest that she too might have ASD. She described her own experience of depression, which had responded best to venlafaxine, a drug which Jean had not so far taken.

All participants felt that the meeting had been constructive and hopeful. This in itself went some way to relieve Jean's anxiety. She was able to embark on her new term with some plans and positive expectations.

Practice Points

- Students have depressive disorders at around the same rate as the rest of society but have unique difficulties accessing treatment.
- 'Depression' and its symptoms may be the observable features of several different mental conditions, which require different treatments. It is particularly important to identify whether there may be a bipolar vulnerability.
- Use of alcohol and other recreational drugs can cause or worsen depression and anxiety (See Chapters 6 and 7).

- The eating disorders can be manifestations of depression or anxiety, but can also bring about these conditions, so that treatment of the whole vicious cycle is needed (See Chapter 5).
- There are a wide range of anxiety disorders, and anxiety is very often present alongside depression too. When this is the case, higher doses of the so-called antidepressant drugs are required.
- People who are high on the autistic spectrum or otherwise not 'neurotypical' may be particularly vulnerable to these disorders.
- A student may have both genetic and environment predispositions to mental disorders. Treatments that have helped a family member may be more effective for them.
- Including medication in the treatment plan has much to recommend it. Young people can recover faster, can benefit from the ready availability and convenience of medication and can access psychotherapies alongside medication to enhance benefits.
- Prescribing needs to take account of the youth of the student, and for female students, consideration of treatments that would be safe during any future pregnancy.
- Students with a significant level of depression or one of the more severe anxiety disorders are likely to require longer courses of therapy than Counselling services routinely offer.
- Discussions with local NHS clinics are needed to share care appropriately and provide therapeutic continuity. Arrangements for treatment during vacations are essential, whether the student is taking medication, accessing psychosocial treatments of a combination of these.

References

Alsubaie, M. M., Stain, H. J., Webster, L. A. D. & Wadman, R. (2019). The role of sources of social support on depression and quality of life for university students, *International Journal of Adolescence & Youth*, 24(4), 484–96, https://doi.org/10.1080/02673843 .2019.1568887

Beiter, R., Nash, R., McCrady, M., et al. (2015). The prevalence and correlates of depression, anxiety, and stress in a sample of college students. *Journal of Affective Disorders*, 173, 90–6.

Blanco, C., Okuda, M., Wright, C., et al. (2008). Mental health of college students and their non-college-attending peers: results from the National Epidemiologic Study on Alcohol and Related Conditions. *Archives of General Psychiatry*, 65(12), 1429–37. https://doi.org/10.1001/archpsyc .65.12.1429

Camara, M., Bacigalupe, G. & Padilla, P. (2017). The role of social support in adolescents: Are you *helping me* or *stressing me out? International Journal of Adolescence and Youth*, 22(2), 123–36, https://doi.org/10.1080/02673843.2013 .875480

Cuijpers, P., Cristea, I.A., Ebert, D.D., et al. (2016). Psychological treatment of depression in college students: A metaanalysis. *Depression & Anxiety*, 33(5), 400–414.

Duffy, M. E., Twenge, J. M. & Joiner, T. E. (2019). Trends in mood and anxiety symptoms and suicide-related outcomes among U.S. undergraduates, 2007–2018: Evidence from two national surveys, *Journal of Adolescent Health*, 65,(5), 590–8. https://doi.org/10.1016/j.jadohealth.2019 .04.033.

Ghaziuddin, M., Ghaziuddin, N. & Greden, J. (2002). Depression in persons with autism: Implications for research and clinical care. *Journal of Autism & Developmental Disorders*, 32,

299–306. https://doi.org/10.1023/A:1016330802348

Harvey, S. B., Glozier, N., Henderson, M., et al. (2011). Depression and work performance: An ecological study using web-based screening, *Occupational Medicine*, 61(3), 209–11. https://doi.org/10.1093/occmed/kqr020

Hysenbegasi, A., Hass, S. L. & Rowland, C. R. (2005). The Impact of Depression on the Academic Productivity of University Students *The Journal of Mental Health Policy and Economics*, 8, 145–51

Ibrahim, A. K., Kelly, S. J., Adams, C. E. & Glazebrook, C. (2013a). A systematic review of studies of depression prevalence in university students, *Journal of Psychiatric Research*, 47(3), 391–400,

Ibrahim, A. K., Kelly, S. J. & Glazebrook, C. (2013b). Socioeconomic status and the risk of depression among UK higher education students. *Social Psychiatry & Psychiatric Epidemiology*, 48, 1491–501. https://doi.org/10.1007/s00127-013-0663-5

March, J. S., Silva, S., Petrycki, S., et al. (2007). The Treatment for Adolescents with Depression Study (TADS): Long-term effectiveness and safety outcomes. *Archives of General Psychiatry*, 64(10), 1132–44.

Mufson, L. & Sills, R. (2006). Interpersonal psychotherapy for depressed adolescents (IPT-A): An overview. *Nordic Journal of Psychiatry*, 60(6), 431–7.

National Institute of Health and Care Excellence (2022). *Depression in adults: Treatment and management*. www.nice.org.uk/Guidance/NG222.

Robins, C. J., Schmidt III, H. & Linehan, M. M. (2004). Dialectical behavior therapy: Synthesizing radical acceptance with skillful means. In Hayes, S. C., Follette, V. M. & Linehan, M. M. (eds.) *Mindfulness and acceptance: Expanding the cognitive-behavioral tradition* (pp. 30–44). The Guilford Press.

Shevlin, M., Hyland, P., Nolan, E., Owczarek, M., Ben-Ezra, M. & Karatzias, T. (2022). ICD-11 'mixed depressive and anxiety disorder' is clinical rather than sub-clinical and more common than anxiety and depression in the general population. *British Journal of Clinical Psychology*, 61(1), 18–36. https://doi.org/10.1111/bjc.12321

Weissman, M. M., Markowitz, J. C. & Klerman, G. L. (2017). *The guide to interpersonal psychotherapy: Updated and expanded edition*. Oxford University Press.

Wörfel, F., Gusy, B., Lohmann, K., Töpritz, K. & Kleiber, D. (2016). Mental health problems among university students and the impact of structural conditions. *Journal of Public Health*, 24(2), 125–33.

Chapter 17

Suicide at University

This chapter offers a perspective on the nature of suicide and self-harm in the context of mental disorders in the broader community and within UK universities in particular. There are no simple answers. Even addressing the topic raises powerful anxieties. I would like to promote a climate of subtler understanding and compassion towards everyone involved in trying to prevent and survive suicide: students, families, social groups, staff, clinicians and authorities.

There have been welcome attempts to investigate suicides and other adverse outcomes in a spirit of learning rather than blaming and shaming. It is important to appreciate good care, as well as to clarify gaps and failures of responsibility. We're now learning how important it is to go beyond this and ensure reparative and supportive action for survivors too. This process has been called 'postvention' and is a welcome but sadly not yet universal approach. Readers may wish to access postvention resources by both Papyrus UK (www.papyrus-uk.org/) and Samaritans (www.samaritans.org/). UK readers who have time for longer accounts than this chapter are also directed to Mallon and Smith's (2022) recent book, Preventing and Responding to Student Suicide.

After Ian's death by suicide, his brother felt despair and knew that life would never be the same again. He had lost the person closest to him in the world and blamed himself for not picking up on things. He felt close to suicide himself at times but would not do anything to cause his parents further grief.

The junior doctor, Dr Shaw, who had decided not to admit Ian to hospital on the day of his death felt shame and despair and that her life would never be the same again. She faced fatal accident inquiries, trust investigations, the pity and avoidance of peers, and a fear that the General Medical Council would strike her off the register of medical practitioners. Her identity as a doctor – in a medical family – was so threatened that she felt close to suicide. She had recurrent nightmares of the encounter with Ian.

The vice principal at Ian's university felt seriously worried. He feared damage to the university's reputation and to his own reputation for being a caring leader, a 'safe pair of hands'. He was afraid student recruitment would suffer.

National health service (NHS) managers meanwhile were terrified that Ian's family would pursue complaints against the trust that operated health services responsible for Ian. This would be expensive in a difficult financial climate, and the effects on staff morale might make staff recruitment and retention even harder than before. They were reluctant to have any contact with Ian's family without the advice of lawyers. It did not occur to them that Dr Shaw might herself be at real risk of suicide.

What Is 'Suicide': What Does It Mean to Us?

Any 'illness' or 'disorder' poses a risk to the quality of life and may threaten life itself. Acknowledging this and balancing risks of the illness with those of any interventions is the very stuff of medicine and the other healing arts. We are most likely to think of 'risk' in the context of emergencies and acute situations. This is particularly the case in Mental Health situations, where threats of harm to the patient's own self or others are enormously feared.

Finding Words

Ironically, in the very context where we need to talk, available lay terms, old terms are often pejorative and unhelpful, and we are tempted to avoid engaging out of a 'fear of saying the wrong thing'. This list is not prescriptive but a suggested expansion of our vocabulary so that we aren't obliged to be inarticulate.

- *'Committed suicide'* implies that to do so is still a crime.
- *'Completed suicide'* was a popular expression for a while but its portrayal of 'completion' misses out on the shocking sense of a life interrupted and cut short.
- *'Died by their own hand'* is a slightly ceremonious expression, often seen in obituaries. The dead person is credited with agency for the manner of their death, which is only sometimes accurate.
- *'Killed him/herself'* may be used by someone close to the dead person, with its nuance of the aggression detected in the act. Those of us with less claim to know the person who died may feel it's too brutal a description to use in the first instance.
- *'Died by suicide'* is a graceful neutral expression commonly used by people whose loved ones have died in this way. It allows for a separation of the late person from the mode of their death somewhat like the expression 'died of a heart attack'.

Suicide, though it has not been a crime since 1961, still generates a sense that someone is to be blamed. The expression 'committing suicide' is still in currency. It seems that at some level we still hang onto the idea that someone has killed our fellow citizen/child/family member/friend/student. That person – even if they are the same person – is somehow a murderer, at the same time as being a victim, and we have trouble integrating our two views of the person.

I have seen a similar struggle in my perinatal patients who have experienced a miscarriage, stillbirth or loss of a young baby. The mother is so closely identified with the baby, and the loss such a physical matter, that she is undoubtedly a victim, yet so many women in this situation search for something they did wrong to 'kill' the baby. Families who have lost a loved one to anorexia nervosa find themselves in this dichotomy too, where they feel fury with dead person for starving themself to death as well as pity with the individual for being starved to death by anorexia.

Seeing the dead person as the agent of the death also plays into some religious and moral views that underpinned old laws, whereby a person who dies by their own hand has 'sinned'. In the past they would not have been granted a ceremonial funeral or burial in consecrated ground, and their soul would not reach heaven. The tragic and shameful feelings generated by these beliefs do not depend on our rationally still holding them as true, but continue to lurk unspoken.

Side by side with old religious feelings, there were institutional and feudal considerations. A servant or soldier did not own their own life as it was in thrall to their lord.

Modern society and especially modern universities cannot avoid commercial concerns, which are closely linked to reputational considerations. Universities may feel that suicide is a sort of perverse 'league table' indicating the health or disorder of the whole institution.

The way we think and speak about suicide is important. It reflects our assumptions, communicates them to others and can shape the way the discourse is held. One of the most important myths to dispel is the one that suggests that asking whether someone is feeling suicidal can 'put ideas into people's heads'. It may have the opposite effect in allowing them to think things through and accept support.

Some of us find it helpful to 'externalise' the cause of suicide away from the person. Just as we might see how external abuse or bullying might drive someone to despair, so we understand that mental illnesses can 'bully' a person from within their own psyche. We might say 'she died as result of bipolar disorder' or 'from a depressive illness'. For some people though, this sort of thinking goes a step too far in taking away the person's own agency.

Dr Rachel Gibbons, a medical psychotherapist who has worked on suicide for many years, believes that 'suicide is a human condition not a mental health condition' (personal communication). She says, 'suicide results from an incapacity to mourn'. She sees it as 'an acting out event' and explains that, 'You act out when you cannot put your emotional experience into words.' When forms of non-destructive communication are available people can translate their experience into words, images, actions or music, and a whole range of alternatives can help less verbal individuals. Staff and students have to be academically literate and articulate to get into university in the first place, but they are not always able to use emotional language. Non-verbal therapies and opportunities could include art, music, dance, animal therapies, gardening and sports.

Suicide and deliberate self-harm are among a whole range of 'acting out behaviours' – including risk-taking behaviour and harm to property or to other people – that particularly characterise immaturity. The process of acquiring maturity involves finding non-destructive and preferably positively constructive ways to metabolise pain, frustration and loss. A university education may be seen as part of the process of young people's development into greater maturity. In that sense it could even be considered as a mass suicide prevention intervention. However, moving into maturity involves successfully mastering challenges that are just about within one's capacity, or where there are services to teach and support coping strategies.

How Common Is Student Suicide?

Youth suicide rates, particularly those for young men, rose rapidly in Western countries in the second half of the twentieth century but then fell, at least in England and Wales. The 2005 rate of 8.5 per 100 000 for 15- to 24-year-olds was the lowest for nearly 30 years (Biddle et al., 2008). More recently, suicide rates have climbed again, and we still await clarity about the effects of COVID, particularly in terms of the effects on students, who were uniquely affected by lockdown.

The suicide rate among men is over three-times higher than for women, but the rate in female students has increased faster than for male students and it is now the leading cause of death for both genders in this age group. It may be a surprise to discover that the rate of suicide amongst young people attending UK universities is considerably lower than the rate amongst their non-university peers. In England and Wales the rate of suicide in students of age 18 to 20 is 2.8 per 100 000, compared with 9.7 per 100 000 in the age-matched population (Gunnell et al., 2020). Scotland, though, has higher suicide rates.

External social factors may partly explain the rise in the figures. There have been increases in student numbers, so that more of those who would not in the past have had the privilege of higher education are now doing so. We also need to observe that recent figures reflect the 2010 shift in the legal standard of proof used to determine a death as suicide in England and Wales. It used to be necessary to prove 'beyond all reasonable doubt' that suicide was the cause of death, but the standard is now 'on the balance of probability'.

Generally, where harm is significantly reduced in one particular environment, we find ourselves looking to identify protective factors and evidence of good practice, to apply these to other environments, too. However, young people who attend university are not really comparable to those who don't. They are already more likely to already experience factors (social, financial, educational and health privileges) that are make them more likely to get to university and also protect them against mental illness, distress and suicide. We would therefore expect a cohort of university students to have lower rates of suicide.

A further complication arises when we consider that figures quoted for 'UK suicide rates' often turn out to be for England and Wales and do not include Scotland and Northern Ireland, which are known to have higher rates of suicide. Moreover, universities are often more ethnically diverse than the communities around them, and with different patterns of diversity. For instance, the proportion of wealthy young Asian people studying at the University of Cambridge is markedly higher than in the local Cambridge community.

We have seen that interpretation of the numbers may not be straightforward, so why do they matter so much? We need to collect accurate data so that we can track the effects of efforts to improve things. For both students and their peers, suicide is now the leading cause of death for young people in the age group (Office for National Statistics, 2018b). Each individual case represents a unique nexus of suffering. Moreover, each individual suicide in a closely connected environment (connected by electronic media as well as face to face interactions) can influence a whole constellation of damage. This goes beyond 'copycat' suicides and self-harm, through the post traumatic responses of family, friends, classmates and staff, to the longer-term attitudes and responses in the community. These may be avoidant and defensive or creative and reparative.

Institutions also understand that the media use suicide rates as a sort of proxy for the mental health of a university, so there are important reputational considerations. It is a nightmare scenario for a university to experience a cluster of suicides in a short space of time, as happened in Bristol in the 2017–18 academic year, and more recently in Cambridge. This can generate extreme anxiety and anger, demands from some quarters to tackle the problem, and dread and demoralisation in university staff with responsibilities for pastoral care. A logical response is the search for common factors in these tragic deaths, such as risk factors in the particular institution concerned, although this can lead to a blame-and-shame culture, and underlying reasons can be missed if the investigation is not handled thoughtfully.

We are still some way off empowering most university personnel to discuss and manage issues around suicide. The very word 'suicide' carries almost superstitious power, so that it is often felt safest to avoid saying it altogether. The fear of 'putting ideas into their heads' persists. Dazzi et al. (2014) conducted a review of studies examining whether asking about thoughts of suicide induces suicidal ideation in adults and adolescents, and in both general and at-risk populations. None of the research showed a statistically significant increase in suicidal ideation when people were asked about their suicidal thoughts. In fact, it appeared that acknowledging and talking about suicide can reduce, rather than increase suicidal ideation.

Can Suicide Be Prevented?

The growing 'zero-suicide movement' seeks to proactively identify and care for all who may be at risk of suicide rather than only react when someone reaches crisis point. A zero-suicide ambition for mental health acute services was added to England's national suicide prevention strategy in 2018 (Department of Health and Social Care, 2019). I applaud the initiatives and resources of the movement, but I do regret the term for its implication that suicide is always unacceptable, intolerable and preventable. It imposes an impossible 'target' that potentially sets up blame and defensiveness in an area where those characteristics are already destructive. There is a risk that everyone involved treats suicide as an outrage rather than as a complex tragedy. Compassion may be lost.

We're still wrestling with a very limited evidence base to guide prevention efforts. When it comes to focussed psychological interventions, most studies use 'suicidal behaviour' or 'suicidality' as the outcome measure, rather than deaths by suicide. This is understandable given that suicide is too rare an occurrence to provide a ready sensitive indication of the effectiveness of interventions. Unhappily we have no proof that reducing the prevalence of reported desire to die, or reducing observed episodes of deliberate self-harm, will actually result in a reduced suicide rate, reasonable as that may seem.

We can't always be sure to what extent interventions are saving lives and to what extent they are causing unwanted and even harmful side effects. It would be mistaken to imagine that a psycho-educational group intervention could not possibly be harmful on the basis that it is not a drug treatment. We already know that irresponsible media reporting can trigger suicides, so this is an area where an unthinking approach of 'raising awareness' is not a safe stance.

In 2016, Zalsman et al. (2016) reviewed 1797 studies of suicide prevention, but only 40 of these were the 'gold standard' randomised controlled trials. Some awareness-based programmes in educational establishments were shown to reduce 'suicide attempts' and 'suicidal ideation', though not necessarily deaths. They found insufficient evidence to assess the possible benefits or harms of suicide screening in primary care, in general public education and media guidelines.

For people already in treatment for a mental illness, the authors emphasised the preventative benefits of prescribing effective pharmacological and psychological treatments. They found that two medications – clozapine and lithium – appear to have particular 'anti-suicidal' benefits. These are medications that tend to be reluctantly accepted by patients when other treatments have failed, as both require intensive monitoring with regular blood tests. The intensive nature of monitoring and care may of course be part of the protective power of these treatments.

Known risk factors for suicide	
In the general population	In higher education students
Being male	*As for general population plus:*
Middle-aged, especially 40–55 age group	2nd year at university or later
Use of alcohol/other substances	Undergraduate rather than graduate
Interpersonal loss – bereavement, relationship	student
break-up	Socially isolated
Previous deliberate self-harm, especially if with	Leaving university before the course is
suicidal intent	finished
Recent or current mental illness	Perceived academic failure
Chronic or severe physical illness	Financial hardship/difficulties
LBGTQ+	
Neurodiversity – ADH or ASD	

Suicide and the Environment

In with the uncertain evidence for psychosocial interventions, the Zalsman et al. (2016) review found that evidence for restricting access to lethal means in prevention of suicide has strengthened since 2005, especially with regard to controlling the sale of paracetamol and other analgesics (overall decrease of 43% since 2005) and fencing off hot spots for suicide by jumping (reduction of 86% since 2005). Our physical environment can keep us safe in many ways from legislation on seat belts and motorcycle helmets to toddler-proof lids on cleaning chemicals. Mental hospitals are spending large sums to remove potential 'ligature points' from their buildings. It's well known that veterinarians, anaesthetists and farmers are at higher risk of suicide because of access to lethal chemicals, and in addition farmers have access to hidden 'outbuildings' to make it less likely they will be found in time. One classic change that reduced suicide rates was the replacement of household 'coal gas', which contained deadly carbon monoxide, with 'natural gas'. Many authorities have also equipped bridges and other high places with barriers to discourage jumping.

Students use the same means of suicide as other age groups. In the UK, hanging accounts for roughly half of deaths, followed by self-poisoning, drowning and jumping. It seems likely that university buildings and halls are already aware of risks, because Gunnell et al.'s (2020) analysis found that students did not acquire the means of suicide from university premises. In fact, half of the deaths occurred away from the university city, including in the home town of the student.

Researchers seem surprised that suicide rates are lower during the first year at university, despite the stresses and vulnerabilities of that time. It would be worth investigating whether living in halls of residence, a common feature of first year, is associated with protection from suicide.

Qualitative Research on Student Suicide

Numerically based reviews of the literature on suicide are essential in measuring outcomes and effectiveness, but detailed descriptive studies of student suicides can guide our under-standing too. Stanley et al. (2009) reviewed 20 UK student deaths by suicide. All were young men, mostly in their early twenties. The researchers were not allowed by university authorities to include the deaths of international students in the study because of concerns about contacting the families and differences in cultural understandings of suicide.

Most had died of violent methods such as hanging or jumping from heights, which have a high likelihood of fatal outcome. Most students were living in private rented accommodation at the time of death and only one student who jumped from a high place on campus. Three died while staying at their parents' homes.

Seven students had previously attempted suicide, although not all had received hospital treatment or were assessed as making a serious attempt at the time. Eight had discussed suicide with their parents or girlfriends but again, the seriousness of their intent had not always been evident. Two were known to have self-harmed in the period leading up to their deaths. Six had no history of a mental health problem. Four were deemed to have been influenced by 'suicide transmission', where knowledge of another person's suicide is a motivator (Stanley et al., 2009).

This chapter will repeatedly turn to findings from the Stanley et al. (2009) study to shed light on different aspects of student experience that may be closely associated with death by suicide.

How Is Deliberate Self-Harm Linked to Suicide?

The three case studies that follow show what diverse intentions and difficulties lie behind deliberate self-harm (DSH). DSH used to be called a 'failed suicide attempt' or 'parasuicide' but is more likely today to be seen as 'maladaptive problem-solving behaviour' – the 'acting out behaviour' referred to by Rachel Gibbons (personal communication). Suicide prevention programmes are often addressed at people presenting with DSH. They explicitly teach alternative and more mature skills for managing distress. DSH does increase the risk of future death by suicide, but many people who die by suicide have never engaged in DSH. There is a certain amount of overlap but considerable difference between the two groups of people involved. For instance, male students are more than twice as likely to take their own lives than females. However, more women than men have been found to self-harm.

Mental health services often assign a 'personality' diagnosis to people who frequently engage in DSH. It is often part of a range of immature self-destructive behaviours that are undertaken in a self-defeating attempt to regulate intolerable emotions. Our understanding of the so-called personality disorders is still evolving and was discussed at greater length in Chapter 16. Some of the interventions offered to people attracting these diagnoses are proven to be effective in improving emotional regulation and distress tolerance. There is often a reduction in DSH and in emergency presentations at hospital, but it is not proven that there is any reduction in deaths by suicide. We may focus on the needs of people who present with DSH in their own right, but such interventions fail to address the needs of the majority of those who die without any history of DSH.

Juliette, an 18-year-old first-year student, enjoyed both the academic and social aspects of university life but towards the end of each night of clubbing she would quickly lose her confident demeanour and wail to her friends that she was fat and stupid, and that no one would ever love her. Her caring flatmates would take her home, but she would then secretly scratch her arms and legs until she drew blood.

Her friend Mo found her in the bathroom one night with a razor and blood on her arms and took her to hospital. Her cuts were stitched by a tired and resentful junior doctor. On her return home she ripped off the bandages and opened the cuts again 'to punish herself'. She said she felt like two people, 'the strict, angry judge and the stupid klutz'. Other times, looking at her body, she felt like a customer who had been sold an inferior product and demanded that this one be ripped apart and replaced by a pristine new one.

Counselling helped her to treat herself and her body with more kindness and tolerance, and she gave up alcohol for a while. It was not easy to do this in her social circle, but Mo gave up drinking herself as she had been badly scared by Juliette's self-harm. In time, though, Mo came to resent the time and attention she devoted to 'keeping Jules safe'.

John was a second-year student previously suspended for inappropriate sexual behaviour, and readmitted on condition that he undertake mentoring. He did not at that stage have a formal autism spectrum disorder (ASD) diagnosis, but this was being assessed.

His mentor was called to his halls where he stood roaring and brandishing a badly bloodied fist. He had identified Louise, a fellow student, as a potential girlfriend, approached her in her room and suggested that they have sex. She refused, horrified, whereupon he burst into the communal sitting room and began to punch walls and furniture. The mentor checked first on Louise's well-being, summoned help from a concierge then took John to a separate room away from the scene to understand what had happened.

John's actions represented distress and frustration but also a demonstration of his power and fury. At home he had been used to having family members do whatever he wanted by engaging in such behaviour and hadn't learned other ways of meeting his needs.

Meanwhile the young woman was supported by the mentor's colleagues to take her concerns to university authorities. She was offered transfer to another hall of residence, but John's mentor protested that this gave the wrong message and that the young man should be moved because it was his behaviour that had disturbed the security of the residence. The move would also allow him a fresh start to learn new social skills.

The (fictionalised) case of Juliette is an example of how therapies focussed on teaching emotion-regulation skills can reduce the likelihood of DSH, whereas the case of John indicates the importance of assessment of autistic spectrum conditions and an individual assessment of the meaning of DSH in that context.

The third case study, that of Janet, represents a situation that may easily have been lethal, yet she is the individual who had not come to the attention of mental health services before the potentially lethal event.

Janet took a year out of her business studies course to care for her mother, a single parent who was dying of cancer. When she returned to university for her final year, her year group had moved on, and she found herself sharing a flat with strangers who enjoyed partying more than she now did. She had got out of the habit of regular studying and found it hard to concentrate. She put in extra hours at her paid job in a local shop, and often felt too exhausted to study. She was surprised to find herself so low, as she had no mental health history. She felt guilty that it was not the loss of her mother than preoccupied her, but rather the stress of examinations and assignments.

One night in the week before examinations began, Janet wrote an apology on a Post-it note, bought a packet of paracetamol from the local shop and added that to what she found in the bathroom at the flat. She washed it down with vodka and later woke up in hospital on an intravenous line. Her flatmates had called an ambulance after finding her unconscious. She told the nurses that she just needed 'a break from it all' and really wouldn't care if she died.

The Role of Mental Health Services in Student Suicide Prevention

Only 33% of people in the general population who die by suicide were known to the mental health services at the time of their death, and for students who die by suicide only 17% had contact with such services (Gunnell et al., 2020). It may be the case that students fear stigma and 'fitness to study' questions, and so avoid mental health services. It is probable too that not all suicides arise from a formally treatable mental illness. Nevertheless, we do know that mental illness and mental distress are risk factors for suicide. It is hard to know how far the students concerned are deliberately avoiding mental health services, and how far there are gaps in the provision of such services, or obstacles to accessing them. As the world emerges from COVID it seems likely that there are gaps and blocks to students in extremis receiving the help they need.

Since the COVID pandemic and lockdown, both general practitioners (GPs) and their patients have raised alarms about shortages in primary care. For students, who may not even have registered with a GP, accessing formal psychiatry is difficult. Waiting lists can mean it takes a crisis for a student to be seen – if at all. Students with pre-existing mental illnesses, face immense disruption in the transitions to universities – these are discussed further in Chapters 2 and 3. Information sharing between agencies has been problematic too, although in theory electronic records should have improved this situation. Communication between the NHS and student well-being services is not routine, and in fact GPs and NHS specialist clinics do not share the same record systems.

There have long been concerns that even students who do register with a new GP most likely split their year between different addresses. Students who have to take breaks from studies are most vulnerable of all to these disruptions and discontinuities to support and treatment.

Zalsman's (2016) review of suicide prevention found that for people already in treatment for a mental illness, effective pharmacological and psychological treatments reduce suicide risk. Bipolar affective disorder, a mental condition described in more detail in Chapter 15 is particularly prevalent amongst high-achieving academics and carries a uniquely high lifetime suicide risk. Students and staff who are known to have this disorder may benefit from extra monitoring and intensive treatment to keep them safe and to protect their quality of life.

The eating disorders are the other group of mental illnesses that have a high mortality rate, both from the physical consequences of starvation, other weight losing behaviours, and from suicide. These disorders are particularly prevalent in the student age group. Demand for eating disorders services has increased markedly as we emerge from lockdown.

Suicide Risk for People with ASD or ADHD

There have been anecdotal reports that people with autism are more likely to die by suicide. These are now validated by a large study based on Danish data. Koves et al.

(2021) used a nationwide database to analyse data of more than 6 million people from 1995 to 2016. More than 35 000 people had a diagnosis of ASD. The key finding was that people with ASD had more than three-times the rate of both 'suicide attempts' and of death by suicide than people not diagnosed with ASD. 90% of the people with ASD who attempted suicide or died by suicide had also been diagnosed with a mental health condition. The researchers also found that 'high-functioning' autistic people (previously described as having Asperger's syndrome) were at even higher risk of suicide. The authors speculated that this may be because they were less likely to be closely monitored and supported.

Balazs and Kereszteny (2017) conducted a systematic review of evidence, and confirmed previous suspicions that attention deficit hyperactivity disorder (ADHD) confers an increased risk of 'suicidality' in both sexes and in all age groups. As in the case of ASD, the risk is mediated by the increased occurrence of comorbid mental disorders in people with ADHD. It was interesting that in both forms of neurodiversity, females had an increased risk of dying by suicide compared with the predominantly male deaths in the 'neurotypical' population.

How Useful Are Formal Individual Risk Assessments?

A university – like a school or place of work – can protect people by highlighting instances where a member of the community is not engaging in expected structures. Alert systems can detect patterns of difficulty, such as not attending classes, failing to hand in work, showing a sudden drop in grades, not paying rent, fees or fines, and disciplinary issues. Such loss of function is not specific to being suicidal but can provide a useful constellation of reasons to be concerned about an individual's well-being. These concerns may be protective in themselves.

Even when an individual is identified as at risk, the search for reliable 'risk assessments' and responses continues to frustrate. Institutions often insist on the use of unvalidated measures; staff carry these out and document them largely out of professional self-defence. They may well be useful prompts to consider the risks that a person's psychosocial state currently poses to themselves or to others. Unhappily, we have no proof that individual scores on any measure can accurately predict the risk of suicide (or indeed homicide).

For instance, the Columbia suicide severity rating scale is 'a validated and reliable instrument that measures current and past suicidal ideation, suicide attempts, preparatory behaviours as well as non-suicidal self-injury' and was 'found to predict future suicide attempts among adolescent and young adult psychiatric emergency department patients'. However, as we have seen, reducing 'suicidal behaviour' and 'suicidal attempts' is not the same as reducing deaths. There are cases where a death by suicide was preceded by a risk assessment that concluded the risk was not high. In any case, many people who die by suicide do not present beforehand to any place where a risk assessment might be conducted.

At present the risk factors we know about are too general to provide useful 'red flags'. Student and staff suicides often happen 'out of the blue'. Rachel Gibbons (personal communication) uses the useful analogy of an amateur footballer suffering a sudden cardiac arrest on the football field. The young man may have an invisible weakness that has never been evident until sudden extra stress triggers a life-threatening event. Routine medicals may have failed to identify the vulnerability, and everyone is deeply shocked by the occurrence. People clamour for better risk assessments and screenings, but these are imperfect, and are often undertaken to defend organisations against responsibility rather than with conviction that they work.

I am saddened by Stanley et al.'s (2009) detailed portrait of 20 student deaths by suicide. But I also find myself wondering what findings might be if the authors were to randomly select 20 living male students of the same age and conducted 'risk assessments' on both groups. The romantic disappointments, use of alcohol and other drugs, and levels of perfectionism might not be significantly lower in the living students than in the students who had died. It may emerge that those with ASD and ADHD, or mental disorders, whether or not diagnosed, were generally at higher risk, but not to the extent that individual risk assessments would predict which young men would die.

Suicide and the Use of Alcohol and Other Substances

Chapters 6 and 7 of this book acknowledge that heavy use of alcohol and recreational drugs is culturally embedded for young men in particular and may be normalised within student populations. After depression, alcohol use is the commonest modifiable factor in prevention of suicide.

In the Stanley et al. (2009) study of 20 students, five of them who had a diagnosis of depression were also described by parents or friends as having alcohol 'problems'. Heavy cannabis use in three cases was associated with both alcohol problems and depression. Other researchers (Smalley et al., 2005) explored the interaction of substance misuse and affective disorders in relation to young male suicide. Substance misuse makes the symptoms of mental illness worse, and tackling this could result in a decrease in levels of violence to self and others.

After a death by suicide, it is hard to reconstruct and understand the dead person's final experiences. A recent study from England (Bailey et al., 2021) used toxicological analysis to examine patterns of alcohol and cocaine use prior to suicide in a large sample of people – not specifically students. This confirmed the finding from international data (Norström & Rossow, 2016) that alcohol and cocaine use disorder are independent predictors of suicide. The study also found that that people with very high levels of blood alcohol at the time of the suicide were nearly six-times more likely to have used cocaine than those not using alcohol.

The authors of both of those papers call for increased public education and interventions to address alcohol and cocaine use in suicidal acts. For example, *Talk to Frank*, the public health advice website about substances, does not mention that alcohol or cocaine use is associated with suicide. The otherwise helpful training programmes produced by the Zero Suicide Alliance fail to address substance use and intoxication, and don't acknowledge that conversations with people at high risk of suicide may be hampered by the difficulty in communicating usefully with a person who is drunk or high.

Suicide and Academic Competition and Stress

Student suicide in Japan is closely linked to the shame of academic failure (Uchida & Uchida, 2017). The culture of suicide and shame is known to be more extreme in that country, but there is much to suggest that academic difficulties are an important factor in the UK too, particularly as student culture becomes increasingly international in character. We acknowledge academic 'stress' involves long periods of challenging study, difficulty finding enough time in the day to master a demanding syllabus, and for some students juggling studies with paid work, and other obligations.

Universities address the more mundane experience of 'stressful' studying, especially around examination times, bringing in extra counselling, drop-in sessions, pet therapy and advice packages. In contrast, UK universities are less likely to acknowledge the concept of individual academic 'shame'. This is the result of real or expected failure to achieve high marks, failure to progress to the next stage of the course, failure to qualify as a professional course, or to achieve a degree, being shown up as inferior to one's peers and 'letting down' or 'disappointing' one's family, school and supporters. We are not so good at relieving the reputational injuries, shame and isolation of students after poor examination results.

When a shame experience occurs, it is likely to be after the end of university term, or after the student has left or dropped out. Once they are off campus, they are off the radar of protective university structures and services. It may be that part of the reason for lower suicide rates in first year students, is that they have so far accumulated only a modest backlog of overdue assignments and resits to be taken, and there can be little evidence of academic failure on their record or their self-image.

Turning back to the Stanley et al. (2009) study, we find that 11 of the 20 young men were described by their relatives and friends as perfectionists or as having an extreme fear of failure. The authors describe 'an increasingly intolerable state of existence where the prospect of failure loomed large.' They point out that most of the deaths occurred either at the beginning or at the end of the academic year. The end of the academic year is when the structure and support offered by the academic timetable are removed, friendship groups dissipate, and support services become less accessible in vacation periods. The start of the academic year presents fresh challenges and obstacles, which students have been able to put behind them during the vacation.

Recent figures from the Office for National Statistics (2018a) have also suggested a clustering of suicide deaths when students leave before completing the course. It is likely that figures for student suicide may be an underestimate because the definition of the word 'student' excludes those who have now left the university.

The availability, visibility and assertiveness of student support services at these times needs to be reviewed. Some student counselling services operate in vacation periods, but students may be unaware of this. Students already known to be at risk, either because of a previous history or because of academic failure, could be helped by proactive approaches to engaging them with supportive services at these times. There is also work to be done in collaboration with careers advisory services in association with counselling, mental health and academic staff to identify alternative 'escape routes' for students who are particularly distressed by the experience or possibility of academic failure.

Relationships

Interpersonal relationships with peers are amongst the most salient and turbulent aspects of adolescent life, with the university years often a time when lifelong friendships and sexual partnerships are established. For most, though not all, students, the family of origin represents a haven to return to when peer relationships rupture or disappoint, but living away from home, elements of pride and shame, or the pessimistic overlay of a depressed frame of mind, can reduce that safety net. Chapter 12 of this book considers the challenges of the sexual dimension of life at a modern university. Close sexual relationships can represent an important source of support and self-esteem, but that support can prove precarious.

In the Stanley et al. (2009) case series, 12 of the 20 students who died by suicide were reported to have relationship problems. Six had experienced the break-up of a relationship shortly before their death, three were experiencing difficulties in a relationship and a further three were described as suffering from 'unrequited love'. Friends and parents spoke of 'turbulent' and 'emotionally charged' relationships and the authors describe 'young people with limited experiences of intimate relationships struggling to manage the emotional vulnerability and losses they experienced'. It is obviously impossible to make retrospective diagnoses, but these descriptions should make us particularly careful to support people with ASD around relationship problems.

Media, Social Media and Suicide

Emotionally powerful networks are nothing new amongst young intellectuals. The term 'Werther effect' comes from reports of an epidemic of 'copycat' suicides after the publication of Goethe's 'The Sorrows of Young Werther' in 1774. The novel provides detailed descriptions of Werther's mental state and concludes with his death by suicide. More recently, a systematic review (Sisask & Värnik, 2012) supported the idea that media reporting and suicidality are associated. The phenomenon of 'cluster suicides' has been addressed by media guidelines. Typically, they urge reporters not to glamorise or glorify suicide, not to reveal or discuss specific suicide methods, and to limit the amount of reporting about the same suicide. But specific information on individual deaths by suicide continues to be published, particularly if a celebrity figure is involved – the suicide of the actor Robin Williams is one example of some reporting not fully following guidelines.

A positive phenomenon has been identified, known as the 'Papageno effect'. This occurs when media focus on helpful resources to promote healthy coping with crisis and trauma, provide information on the role of treatable mental illness, where and how to seek help for suicidal thoughts, and a message of hope that suicide is preventable. Evidence that this may be associated with a reduction in suicides was empirically confirmed by an Austrian group (Niederkrotenthaler et al., 2020).

The mushrooming of social media this century has blurred the distinction between the media authors (to whom guidelines are aimed) and media consumers (who may be influenced and harmed by the material). The same person will be both an author of posts and a consumer of the material. Online communications are much more speedily interactive and harder to monitor. The nature of search engine algorithms is to assertively offer further details of topics a person is searching for. Unless this is moderated, searches can automatically generate information on suicide methods and interest groups for those who appear to be interested. Chapter 8 of this book provides a broader consideration of social media in university life.

When schoolgirl Molly Russell took her life in 2017, her Instagram account was found to contain graphic posts about suicide and self-harm. Her family mobilised public demand for regulation of the internet and a formal duty of care by tech companies. The Online Harms Bill is currently going through Parliament. Molly was only 14 years old, but students do not suddenly become streetwise as they turn 18. We need to campaign for nuanced and effective regulation, which offers realistic protection to all vulnerable people.

Side-by-side with the dangerous potential for triggering further suicides, social media can be comforting in the aftermath of bereavements, including those by suicide. It can be helpful to share memories of the person who has died and to send messages of support to others. However, using social media comes with the risk of online rumours and unkind messages about the person who has died or their friends and family. It can be helpful if designated members of the university 'postvention team' offer some sort of moderation and support around online messages that cause distress. University press offices can also be helpful in both protecting the reputation of the Institution and advising bereaved family and friends about dealing with the press. Some families like to prepare a statement to have more control about what is said or written. Samaritans have a communication team who can offer support and help make complaints if it is felt that press enquiries were intrusive or that the coverage may affect other people's safety.

Supporting Students Who May Be Considering Suicide

As a psychiatrist I routinely discuss my patients' worst fears and feelings and ask about their thoughts of suicide now and in the past. I can ask, secure in the knowledge that I can always call on someone to help, to stay with the patient, to observe and soothe them, perhaps even in a hospital ward. I can prescribe medication to treat symptoms, and share responsibility with a team of professionals, as well as calling on the friends and family of the patient. I would feel very different in a real-life situation on campus, without my 'doctor' status, considering how to ask similarly intrusive questions to a person who might walk off at any time, might be intoxicated or dismissive of me, or might need resources I do not have as a private individual.

If people in a university community are to effectively support someone at risk of suicide, there has to be support that we can all confidently invoke. Fortunately, we have all heard of Samaritans, and could call their number at any hour, for help and advice. Some excellent university webpages will appear in response to typing 'how can I help a suicidal student?' into a search engine. You can often get specific advice by adding in the name of your own university. Even if you find yourself unexpectedly needing to support someone who may feel suicidal, there is support and advice online.

There is a huge difference in confidence, however, that comes from being prepared in advance, not only by gathering information and materials, but preferably talking with others about their approaches and experiences. Pastoral and academic staff should have regular training that includes consideration of suicide, but all of us need to speak about the issue from time to time so that we are ready to hold difficult conversations effectively and compassionately, rather than avoiding them.

Information to Keep on Hand When Supporting Someone Who May Be Considering Suicide

- Contact details of the nearest accident and emergency department
- NHS mental health crisis team
- Student counselling/out of hours contact

- Your own line manager
- Local taxi

These helplines are free, confidential and open 24 hours a day, 365 days a year:

Samaritans telephone 116 123
National Suicide Prevention Helpline UK telephone 0800 689 5652.
Text SHOUT on 85258.

We may dread hearing that someone has already taken an overdose, hurt themself or is about to do so. In fact, this is a relatively straightforward scenario. In this case they need to be taken to hospital for treatment. Someone should go with them to ensure they do not leave before being seen, to provide useful information to staff and find out what follow up arrangements are needed. If at all possible, the burden of all this should not fall upon a single individual, specially not on a fellow student.

More often, the person is not at immediate physical risk but is strongly considering suicide. There is more time to arrange support, reduce stress and set up monitoring to keep the person as safe as possible meanwhile. It is important to hold the conversation with respect for privacy and dignity, but you should not put yourself in a position of being isolated as the sole holder of responsibility. It is reasonable to ask for agreement to contact a person's doctor or counsellor, and their next of kin. If they cannot agree, then if you believe life may be at risk, you have a duty to breach confidentiality – doing so in as boundaried and private manner as possible. If your relationship to the student or colleague is not a professional one, then you are not bound by confidentiality in any case, but by human respect and concern. In practice, people usually appreciate compassionate 'breaches' of confidentiality, particularly if the other person is honest about what they are doing and why. The student may feel 'overruled' but not betrayed. There are various protective factors that can be considered to help people whilst the crisis is addressed (see Box).

It is most difficult when someone insists that they are not at risk of suicide, and you are left wondering whether your gut feeling was mistaken, whether perhaps something else is going on, or whether the person is at even greater risk than you thought, but unable to accept help. It worth checking whether they are afraid of someone else. You will be left with feelings of anxiety and embarrassment, but rather than 'backing off' completely, it's a good idea to leave the conversation as an open one that can be resumed. You are still there to help if things do get difficult, and you will check in again later.

Whatever the scenario, and your role in it, you will need to look after yourself through all of this, recognising that it is extremely difficult to support another person who is at risk of suicide. Your concerns and behaviour need to be shared with someone senior, thoughtfully and in a boundaried way. It can be helpful to confidentially write down a short account of what happened, both to help make sense of the encounter and for later reference.

Possible Protective Factors for a Person at Risk of Suicide

Staff, friends and next of kin are aware of the vulnerability
The person is registered with a GP and referred for any necessary treatment OR seen as emergency by accident and emergency or crisis team

Refrains from alcohol/recreational drugs, but takes prescribed medication
Takes a break from social media
Has support to organise and manage any financial concerns/debts
Examinations/deadlines have been modified to allow realistic study time, or if necessary academic deadlines suspended completely
Follows a structured timetable, with most time spent in company of other people, regular mealtimes, physical activity, sleep
Instillation of hope – plans for future counselling/careers advice/leisure activities with family and friends.

Coping after a Death by Suicide: The Practice of 'Postvention'

In the aftermath of death, even sudden or violent deaths, there are bureaucratic and routine tasks to be undertaken. If these are bungled, further trauma is added to the burden of survivors. When well-rehearsed preparations are in place, the bereaved community can benefit from the structures and obligations involved. There can even be some comfort in knowing that society recognises that we sometimes find ourselves in these 'unimaginable' situations and has developed ways to go on with life.

Readers of this chapter are referred to Mallon and Smith's (2022) book Preventing and responding to student suicide, and in particular to Responding to Student Suicide, the chapter in which Nic Streatfield (2022) provides a blow-by-blow account of a fictionalised case response. Streatfield (2022) emphasises the benefits of pre-planning and providing checklists. In the couple of days after the death, regular meetings are called at a high level, sometimes several times a day, to ensure a co-ordinated response. Timing is crucial.

Streatfield's (2022) account shows how confident management of practicalities and formalities allows space for humanity and containment to be offered. In contrast, a later chapter of the same book describes the bleak isolation of a bereaved family, who were provided only with written information. Staff who had been involved with the dead student were too nervous, overwhelmed and uncertain of their rights and responsibilities to make themselves available.

Each institution should have a plan for sudden death response and postvention, including a notification protocol showing who should be informed and by whom. The plan needs to cater for eventualities such as night times and weekends, or for key people being on leave or unavailable. It should include operationalised checklists accessible to those who will need them. It is vital to plan this in advance rather than relying on decision-making in a crisis. The university should identify and train a 'suicide postvention team'. This might include the Chief Executive Officer, the head of student support, head of student services, dean of the student's academic school, director of communications, president of the student union and head of chaplaincy – or their deputies.

The Chief Executive Officer will call a major incident team meeting at an early stage. The team may draw up a draft communication to let students and staff know about the tragedy and detail support available. Meanwhile, other staff have the important task of ensuring university life continues as normally as possible for other students.

Police and other emergency services have to be on the scene of the death as soon as possible and will take the role of first informing the next of kin. University staff should appoint a lead to liaise with the lead police officer. If the death occurs at the university, any students and other witnesses at the scene of the death should be offered support, for instance from student support and chaplaincy, in the time they are needed by police to give statements. Practicalities such as hot drinks, snacks and blankets are comforting.

Those who are now aware of the death should be advised of the importance of social media silence. Police need to inform next of kin first – it is traumatic to discover the news on social media. At a later stage the press may also need some guidance on responsible reporting practices (Samaritans, 2013; Walker et al., 2014). Once police have informed the next of kin, a senior and psychologically skilled member of the university support services should contact the family and provide continuity of support for them for some time ahead.

In England and Wales, sudden and unexplained deaths are reported to the coroner, an independent judicial officer (usually a lawyer or a doctor). The coroner may decide to hold an inquest to investigate, in which case the death cannot be registered until this is completed. It is not a trial, and its purpose is to discover the facts of the death, not to apportion blame. If the person died while under the care of mental health services, there will be an investigation ('serious incident investigation') in parallel with the coroner's inquiry. The aim will be to find out if the death could have been prevented and to learn for the future. Some universities may wish to hold their own meetings, or series of meetings, to allow serious reflection with different groups of people involved.

Staff and students who were close to the dead person may need to take time out of teaching or support work in the aftermath of a suicide. It is also important to remember the needs of those who may not have known the student personally but have been involved in the aftermath of the death. Secretaries typing up distressing details for reports have been known to become vicariously traumatised and need help.

It is usually appreciated if permission is sought from the family to send formal representation of the university at the student's funeral. The period after the funeral can be particularly painful for survivors, as the structures and interpersonal supports of the ritual are now over. Further ahead, the one-year anniversary of the death is a time when survivors struggle, and some acknowledgement and offers of help are timely.

Grieving after a Suicide

The responses experienced immediately after a trauma, though they may range from florid distress to numbness, do not in themselves constitute a mental illness. The compassionate closeness of the community, and the ceremonial and memorial rituals can be healing in the presence of grief. There are excellent online resources for both staff and students, but the live presence of fellow humans is more powerful. Universities should take particular care that their lists of resources are up to date, as in-person groups often have short lives, and websites can be unavailable. It is particularly distressing at a time of trauma to be offered a resource that doesn't exist.

The process of mourning a significant death is a matter of months and years, but when the death was by suicide it is estimated to take up to three-times as long. It may be more likely to become 'stuck'. Dr Rachel Gibbons (personal communication) says that after a suicide many survivors construct a 'delusional narrative' whereby they could and should have predicted and prevented the death. Sometimes the idea that we failed is more tolerable than the terrifying threat of unpredictable uncontrollable destructive forces.

People bereaved by suicide often receive little support even though they are at increased risk of suicide themselves. Some survivors find themselves jumping to conclusions about the meaning of the suicide. One student said, 'I don't want to go on living in a world that was so awful Ben took his life.' Another wrote on social media, 'I couldn't give him the love he needed, I am such a bad girlfriend.' Bereaved people often experience an obsession with attributing or shifting blame. This stands in the way of healthy adjustment and promotes mental illness and psychosomatic disorders.

In contrast, bereaved survivors who have received focussed support, particularly in the form of group therapies, speak of posttraumatic growth, where the process of reflecting on life and death enhance their own wisdom and maturity.

David Mosse, whose 23-year-old son killed himself, says 'someone who dies by suicide becomes unknowable because of the way they died'. Suicide, homicide, war, and other major disasters can all lead to the person being remembered more for the manner of their death than the unique nature of their life. We owe it to those people to work towards a better perspective on their humanity that includes but is not dominated by the manner of their death.

> After Martin's death by suicide, his family wanted to create a memorial that would be tangible and bring comfort. They contacted the university chaplaincy to discuss possible projects but ended up offering to contribute to refurbishing and refurnishing the rather shabby chaplaincy premises. Their memorial projects raised an impressive sum of money so that the environment could be attractively transformed, and the remaining money bought information leaflets, electronic screens and other resources for the building.

Parents who have formed groups to mourn their child's death by suicide often transform the energy of their grief into altruistic campaigning and helping others. James Murray, father of Ben, quoted in the Papyrus UK guidance says, 'Our grief is accompanied by the conviction that had we known his predicament at university, we could have done something and by the determination that we learn from Ben's death to help prevent others.'

Practice Points

At a Societal Level

- Suicide is one of the leading causes of death in the student age group, especially in young men, and is probably increasing in prevalence.
- We can monitor the built environment to guard against 'suicide hotspots' such as towers, bridges and car parks. Ensure access to chemicals and drugs is secure. Limit access to analgesics in campus shops.
- Use of alcohol and other substances is not only a predisposing factor to an individual's risk of suicide, but alcohol and substance use overwhelmingly occur around the time of death itself.
- Social media and other aspects of the internet interact in complex ways to increase the likelihood of suicide. Effective regulation and research are needed.

Families

- Maintaining contact with the student is particularly important when there are signs of social withdrawal, academic failure or low mood.

- If your student child is involved in counselling or mental health treatment, encourage them to give permission for you to be contacted in case of concern, and make yourself available to attend meetings with them if invited to do so.

At the Level of University Authorities and Policies

- The university campus and halls can be screened for 'suicide hotspots', access to chemicals, drugs and weapons, access to analgesics in campus shops.
- Excessive consumption of alcohol and other leisure drugs in universities needs review and debate.
- Websites should be kept updated and linked with helpful resources, including very simple instructions for people in a crisis.
- An institution's policies and practice on information-sharing agreements should be reviewed to consider permissions about when to contact next of kin.
- Support pathways for distressed students should be developed, implemented, and regularly reviewed, both in terms of support within the university and in terms of collaborative local care pathways into statutory mental health services and NHS crisis intervention teams.
- A suicide 'postvention' plan and team should be always prepared and regularly updated.

Teachers, Tutors, Directors of Studies and Fellow Students

- Asking about suicidal thoughts does not increase the likelihood of a person acting on them, and in fact is more likely to be protective.
- Staff should be prepared with regular updates about emergency contacts and resources. A range of online and real life training courses is available. The best training involves conversations with colleagues or peers about how to cope when you suspect that a student or member of staff may be suicidal.
- Guidelines are needed to ensure students who have to take time out of academic studies – or who need to leave their course – are provided with monitoring and support, as this is a time of high risk.

Recommended Resources

- The Zero Suicide Alliance (zerosuicidealliance.com) has good materials including a free suicide awareness training, in versions for adults, university students, and other situations.
- Papyrus UK (www.papyrus-uk.org) offers support and advice to young people who may be at risk of suicide and to those concerned about a vulnerable young person.

    Helpline: 0800 068 4141
      Monday to Friday, 10 a.m. – 10 p.m.
      Weekends and bank holidays, 2 p.m. – 5 p.m.
    SMS: 07786 209697
    Email: pat@papyrus-uk.or

- Help is at Hand (www.gov.uk) is an excellent online booklet for those bereaved by suicide, and covers what to do and how to access support from the early days through to years ahead in the grieving process. (The legal advice is specific to England and Wales.)

References

Balazs, J. & Kereszteny, A. (2017). Attention-deficit/hyperactivity disorder and suicide: A systematic review. *World Journal of Psychiatry*, 7(1), 44–59. https://doi.org/10.5498/wjp.v7.i1.44

Bailey, J., Kalk, N. J., Andrews, R., et al. (2021). Alcohol and cocaine use prior to suspected suicide: Insights from toxicology. *Drug & Alcohol Review*, 40(7), 1195–201. https://doi.org/10.1111/dar.13260

Biddle, L., Brock, A., Brookes, S. T. & Gunnell, D. (2008). Suicide rates in young men in England and Wales in the 21st century: Time trend study. *BMJ*, 336(7643), 539–42. https://doi.org/10.1136/bmj.39475.603935.25

Dazzi, T., Gribble, R., Wessely, S. & Fear, N. (2014). Does asking about suicide and related behaviours induce suicidal ideation? What is the evidence? *Psychological Medicine*, 44(16), 3361–63. https://doi.org/10.1017/S0033291714001299

Department of Health and Social Care (2019). *Cross-government suicide prevention workplan*. HM Government. www.gov.uk/government/publications/suicide-prevention-cross-government-plan

Gunnell, D., Caul, S., Appleby, L., John, A. & Hawton, K. (2020). The incidence of suicide in university students in England and Wales 2000/2001–2016/17: Record linkage study. *Journal of Affective Disorders*, 261, 113–20.

Mallon S. & Smith J. (eds.) (2022). *Preventing and Responding to Student Suicide*. London: Jessica Kingsley Publishers.

Niederkrotenthaler, T., Braun, M., Pirkis, J., et al. (2020). Association between suicide reporting in the media and suicide: systematic review and meta-analysis. *BMJ*, 18(368), m575. https://doi.org/10.1136/bmj.m575

Norström, T. & Rossow, I. (2016). Alcohol consumption as a risk factor for suicidal behavior: A systematic review of associations at the individual and at the population level. *Archives of Suicide Research*, 20, 489–506.

Office for National Statistics (2018a). *Estimating suicide amongst higher education, England and Wales: experimental statistics*.

Office for National Statistics (2018b). *Leading causes of death, UK: 2001 to 2018 Registered leading causes of death by age, sex and country*.

Samaritans (2013). *Samaritans' media guidelines for reporting suicide*. www.samaritans.org/about-samaritans/media-guidelines/media-guidelines-reporting-suicide/

Sisask, M. & Värnik, A. (2012). Media roles in suicide prevention: A systematic review. *International Journal of Environmental Research and Public Health*, 9(1), 123–38.

Smalley, N., Scourfield, J. & Greenland, K. (2005). Young people, gender and suicide: A review of research on the social context. *Journal of Social Work*, 5(2), 133–154.

Stanley, N., Mallon, S., Bell, J. & Manthorpe, J. (2009). Trapped in Transition: Findings from a UK study of student suicide. *British Journal of Guidance & Counselling*, 37(4), 419–33.

Streatfield, N. (2022). Responding to student suicide: A student services perspective. In: Mallon S. & Smith J. (eds.) *Preventing and responding to student suicide* (pp. 289–306). London: Jessica Kingsley Publishers.

Uchida, C. & Uchida, M. (2017). Characteristics and risk factors for suicide and deaths among college students: A 23-year serial prevalence study of data from 8.2 million Japanese college students. *The Journal of Clinical Psychiatry*, 78(4), e404–e412.

Walker, C., Davidson, F. & Duncan, S. (2014). *Responsible reporting on mental health, mental illness and death by suicide*. National Union of Journalists. www.nuj.org.uk/resource/nuj-guidelines-for-reporting-mental-health-and-death-by-suicide.html

Zalsman, G., Hawton, K., Wasserman, D, et al. (2016). Suicide prevention strategies revisited: 10-year systematic review. *The Lancet Psychiatry*, 3(7), 646–59.

Mental Health Services on Campus and in the NHS

This chapter examines what can be expected in a modern university in terms of prevention, early intervention and treatment of mental ill health. Some of the names and assigned role descriptions may vary between institutions. Not all help is formal. Students often informally assign carer roles onto people not necessarily officially appointed to fill them, including peers, teachers and family members. It can sometimes be hard to pinpoint whether a student is simply interacting in a healthy way and making normal use of interpersonal support, or whether they are receiving explicit support for their mental health, albeit from unofficial sources.

Jasmine, a second-year student, had moved out of halls into a flat with two friends. They noticed she had become increasingly withdrawn and asked what was wrong. She admitted to feeling constantly anxious and often unhappy without any particular trigger. After a couple more weeks of this her friends took her along to the counselling service.

She was given a prioritised assessment where it was found she had a restrictive eating disorder as well as social anxiety and low mood. With her agreement, the counselling service contacted her general practitioner (GP) and arranged referral to the national health service (NHS) eating disorders clinic. Unfortunately, things became worse before she could be seen there. She returned home and received treatment in her former home town.

Before she returned to university the following year, she was encouraged to declare a 'disability' and apply for Disabled Students' Allowance (DSA). This paid for weekly appointments with a specialist mental health mentor who encouraged her to keep appointments with the eating disorders clinic and to follow their advice. The mentor helped her with strategies for when she 'slipped up', and ways to socialise better and make sure the disorder didn't interfere with her studies.

One of the most important skills for helpers is knowing when to introduce the person to more formal support. This matters for the well-being of both helper and helped student. In fact, much of the effective work of helping with mental health difficulties involves steering paths through the myriad different options available.

For those who require more formal help, it is essential to have an idea of what is available both within the university, and beyond its walls, and for all helpers to be able to coordinate care effectively. This chapter outlines formal service provision and its recent developments, as well as progress in its integration and networking capacity. Finally, it examines some examples of projects and pilots of interventions in different UK universities that show promise.

A Time of Change and Growth: 'Step Change', 'The University Mental Health Charter' and the Work of the World Health Organization

At the time of writing this chapter, support for student mental health is in a phase of striking expansion. In the past, the main sources of pastoral support for students were academic personal tutors, hall wardens, and chaplaincy services. Student health services, counselling services and disability services supplemented this support These have been close to being overwhelmed as student numbers have risen overall and with proportionate increases in rates of those who need support with their mental health. This was the case even before the COVID pandemic and lockdown further exacerbated the situation.

There was already a 50% increase in the demand from students for mental health and well-being services between 2010–11 and 2014–15. Several reasons for that increase were hypothesised: reduced stigma around disclosure, widening participation, reductions in NHS support and increased financial stressors, such as student loans. During this period, the number of undergraduate students recorded as declaring a mental health condition trebled from 0.4% to 1.3%, but there was still a high level of non-disclosure and low levels of help-seeking relative to known levels of need (Macaskill, 2013).

Counselling was the most consistently offered effective intervention, and positive results were also demonstrated in services offering psychodynamic therapy, structured brief therapy and integrative therapy. However, the capacity of one-to-one counselling services to offer support to large numbers of students was too limited to be appropriate as a first-line intervention for all who seek help. Waiting lists lengthened, and alternative approaches, were suggested, particularly cognitive behavioural therapy and mindfulness. These were often in online and self-help formats, although some studies reported poor uptake and high dropout rates for these (Brown, 2018).

The expansion in student mental health services has occurred in the context of growing dissatisfaction with NHS services. There has been some unease about whether student mental health services are being called upon to make up for shortfalls in the NHS. In contrast, NHS specialist services point out that the mental health needs of students are often closely entwined with the academic and social environment built up by university institutions. Universities make considerable profit out of bringing a large extra temporary population into an NHS Trust area during termtime. It may be reasonable to expect that some of the students' fees be invested in supporting their mental health.

COVID and its aftermath have created a climate of further pressure, both on GPS as service gatekeepers and referrers, and on NHS mental health provision. There are risks that without considerable extra resource, student mental health referrals may not be prioritised unless they reach emergency point. NHS waiting lists are often unrealistic in terms of the length of the course and semester dates that students work to. Vulnerable students should not be expected to be their own care co-ordinators in such a climate.

It is understandable that authorities such as governments and university governors might see the answer to student mental ill health as mobilising resource to employ more 'student counsellors'. This was indeed the response of the Scottish Government in 2018 when their Programme for Government invested £20m to provide more than 80 additional counsellors in further and higher education institutions over the subsequent four years. Such increase in counselling staff is welcome, but far from being the whole answer. Counsellors cannot reach out to the whole community to provide preventative interventions, nor can they prescribe or manage severe episodes of mental disorder.

This book, like The University Mental Health Charter (Hughes & Spanner, 2019), concludes that a 'whole university approach' is needed to address the dynamic and complex situation. Such an approach depends on high-quality research and integrating whole networks of response to the diverse needs of the student population – both undergraduate and graduate – and also the needs of the staff groups. Chapter 13 considers further how staff, both academic and non-academic, at all levels of seniority, can benefit from mental health support and treatment in their own right and in in their important roles as culture carriers, role models and pastoral carers within the university.

One approach to improving services is to increase the capacity of existing services. Another is to add in completely new services, either to replace current structures, or more commonly on top of current provisions. This latter approach has the benefit of plugging gaps whilst preserving – or adapting – the resource that is already in place. There is, though, a real risk of increasing confusion and difficulties in communication. Clarifying, publicising and facilitating pathways between services can be a worthwhile action in itself. It can be a risky venture to dismantle longstanding services, even if they are inadequate, but remodelling and improving them has to be done with regard to the morale and wisdom of staff involved.

Jeannette worked for more than 20 years in a university counselling service, where she was recognised as expert in the support of people with traumatic backgrounds. She provided long-term support, sometimes extending beyond the time when a student graduated or dropped out of academia, and was admired and loved by her colleagues, to whom she provided both formal and informal supervision.

After a critical review, the university decided to increase student access to counselling by limiting treatment to a norm of two sessions, with a maximum course of six sessions. Training was provided, in which the training team from a prestigious university presented compelling evidence for the benefits of the new way of working.

Jeanette had not been personally consulted in the changes, and decided to leave the service rather than adapt to a way of working that would not recognise her particular skills. She felt demoralised and deskilled by the implication that research had shown her style of counselling was not effective, but she was headhunted to work in a military trauma service. Meanwhile, many of her colleagues became uneasy without her support and supervision in the service. So many left that there was effectively a complete changeover in staff, and a period where the service was not working at full capacity and not attracting staff. No one knew whether outcomes for the new way of working were any better than before, as the measures used to assess this were not comparable with previous data.

In September 2017, a working group published new guidance for leadership in the report 'Stepchange: Mentally Healthy Universities' (Universities UK, 2020). This offers a wide perspective beyond the usual focus on counselling. The document points out the publicised increase in student suicide and highlights the duty of care of higher education institutions to their students. It urges universities to see themselves as health-promoting environments, adopting mental health as a strategic priority with a 'whole-university approach', embedding good mental health across all university activities, including greater investment in university mental health services, digital interventions and suicide prevention. Stepchange (Universities UK, 2020) recommends that universities collaborate with parents, schools and employers to prepare students for transitions and that they work closely with the NHS to explore how mental health services should be commissioned, co-ordinated and delivered to students.

The report's principles have provided the basis for a charter award scheme to measure, validate and appreciate excellence in this area of student well-being. As mentioned earlier in this book, The University Mental Health Charter (Hughes & Spanner, 2019) allows university applicants and their families and other funders to take this crucial aspect of university life into account when deciding on choice of university (Chapters 2 and 3). Regular reviews are required to keep services appropriate to the changing student population and the dynamics of society itself.

Social change means that treatments that were effective for one cohort of students may not continue to be so over time. For instance, the guided self-help we offered in the 1990s to students with bulimia nervosa was strikingly effective, using paperback books and minimal input from trainee psychologists. Today, such books and manuals are less effective. They fail to address social media and online influences on eating disorders. Books and print formats are less acceptable and appropriate to modern students, who expect online modules and interactive apps. Such texts appear dated in their implicit assumption that all patients are young white heterosexual women. It is primarily psychological therapies that become dated in this way, but it's also crucial to prescribe drug treatments in accordance with updated knowledge of options, interactions and adverse side effects.

Teaching and Academic Staff on the Front Line of Supporting University Mental Health

The role of academics in managing their own and their colleagues' and students' well-being, mental health, and mental disorders, is discussed further in Chapter 13. Students' mental health difficulties often arise in the academic context; the students concerned may prefer to access support from a familiar and sympathetic teacher than seek formal help. They also tend to return to trusted teachers and academics while they are on the waiting lists for services and or when they feel that services don't meet their needs. In this situation students are receiving support from unqualified academic staff, weakening appropriate boundaries and placing both academic and student at potential risk.

Chapter 13 provides further recommendations for the sort of training that could support staff's own well-being, foster more effective help for students, and build close constructive relationships between teaching staff and mental health staff to share responsibilities appropriately.

Awareness and Information on Campus and on the Internet

Any visitor to a university campus will be struck by the number of leaflets in piles, posters on toilet doors, stalls offering home baking, and awareness-raising information about mental health initiatives and help contacts. Browsing university and student websites and social media pages, also brings up a bewildering range of help options ranging from phonelines and charity websites to peer support groups. It is like being in a huge supermarket, wondering which foods are in fact substantial and nutritious and which are more a matter of attractive packaging. Universities can provide a great service to their members by subjecting some of these initiatives to rigorous scrutiny and investing in properly evaluated interventions whenever possible.

Mental Health Services Typically Found on University Campuses

Student Mental Health Support Services and What They Offer

- Student health service – physical AND mental health advice and input – contraception, sexual health, vaccination, travel advice, 'signposting' nurses, perhaps doctors
- Student counselling service – mental health – trained counsellors, no prescribing
- Mental health mentors – mentorship (rather than therapy) for students with a self-declared mental disorder. Funded by ringfenced government money (DSA)
- Student funding or financial services – advice, loans, emergency funding, debt management, advice on DSA (See Chapter 9)
- Disability services (including neurodiversity – attention deficit hyperactivity disorder, autism spectrum disorder, dyslexia and dyspraxia – diagnosis and adjustments to study) (See Chapter 18)
- Multifaith chaplaincy
- Student inclusion service – international students, those from different ethnic or non-traditional backgrounds, 'first gen', LBTGQ+ minority groups (See Chapters 11 & 12)
- Hall wardens, senior hall residents, security staff and administrators often find that a significant part of their work involves pastoral care.

Names and structures differ, but most UK universities offer free access to general 'disability services', specialist learning support, counselling services, mental health mentors, financial services, accommodation services and chaplaincy. They may be grouped loosely with international student support and careers service, sometimes sharing buildings, and often linking with the student union.

According to The University Mental Health Charter (Hughes & Spanner, 2019) virtually all universities report having well-documented and robust frameworks and procedures for responding to an incident or crisis affecting staff or students. Students experiencing a mental health crisis are generally referred directly to NHS services. Several institutions highlighted the effectiveness of security staff in dealing with crises. This is analogous to the role usually played by police.

In an acute mental health crisis in the wider community my experience has been that police officers show evidence of good training and display remarkable compassion and kindness to our patients. University security staff also need mental health to be part of their training and supervision.

Outside acute crises, most staff and students told Hughes and Spanner (2019) that they preferred help that was bespoke to academic pressures. NHS mental health services – particularly psychological and counselling services – involved longer waits than on campus services.

Counselling Services

In the clamour for more counselling to be made available to students it can be all too easy, to overlook the important issue of how effective the counselling actually is when accessed. This is yet more important as the length of contact is increasingly cut down to a maximum of six sessions or even fewer. We need to specify what is meant by 'counselling', what the 'dose' of treatment needs to be, and what outcomes have in fact been measured.

There have been laudable attempts to assess effectiveness of student counselling. These include an analysis by Murray et al. (2016), who used the respected Clinical Outcomes in Routine Evaluation (CORE) questionnaire scores to assess outcomes in 305 individuals attending a large UK university counselling service. At the end of the course of counselling, 63% of individuals showed a reliable improvement. However, these were students who completed the course. It is important to include evaluation of everyone who was referred, if the overall effectiveness of the service is to be properly evaluated.

> The history of providing counselling in higher education institutions goes back more than 70 years.
>
> In 1948, Mary Swainson began to offer personal counselling in the Postgraduate Department of Education at University College Leicester. By 1955 the College had recognised this 'psychological advisory service', though undergraduates were only offered the service if referred by their head of department.
>
> In 1964, Audrey Newsome set up the first fully developed student counselling service at the new University of Keele.

This has been achieved in a well-designed recent study by Broglia et al. (2021) who evaluated progress of over 5000 students referred to counselling at four universities. On average, the students waited 14 days to be seen, then spent around 13 weeks in contact with services, during which they attended between four and five counselling sessions, excluding the initial assessment.

The students concerned were mostly undergraduate, female, UK white, and had not declared a 'disability'. The students received one-to-one, face-to-face in-house counselling sessions from professionally accredited therapists. Staff were trained in humanistic, psychotherapy, cognitive behavioural therapy, psychodynamic, and integrative approaches. The measures used were versions of the CORE or Counseling Center Assessment of Psychological Symptoms (CCAPS) assessment tools (Locke et al., 2011). These questionnaires are both respected validated measures.

In this study, outcome measures were completed at every visit, so it was possible to demonstrate that students who ended therapy prematurely had poorer outcomes. Even allowing for the inclusion of these students in the overall results, the change in depression scores was substantial. The combined rate for severe and moderately severe distress fell from 60% before counselling to 27% after counselling. 66% students who completed the planned number of sessions showed 'reliable improvement' – a comparable figure to previous studies' findings.

The study is important in being a first step towards developing a national dataset of student counselling outcomes, which could ensure we provide students with the most effective known treatments and speedily evaluate new ones. Examining the features of the clients carefully can also allow us to consider what works for whom. Only by using similar measures across national samples will we get big enough numbers to evaluate what works for minority groups too.

Meanwhile it is heartening to observe that students who presented to counselling with low levels of well-being and functioning, and high levels of depression, anxiety, academic distress and trauma could be treated so effectively in so few sessions, and may leave us understanding why governments are ready to invest in more of these impressive services on campus.

Adaptations to University Counselling during COVID

At the time of writing, research is only starting to emerge on adaptations to student counselling services in lockdown, and their effectiveness. Psychological support, like academic teaching and meeting, transferred to online platforms. There were delays and obstacles while platforms worked to ensure confidentiality and access for both counsellors and their clients.

Some early studies from Italian universities describe experience that can be generalised to the post-COVID climate. One study (Savarese et al., 2020) emphasises how the use of the online mode significantly changed the professional work of the therapists. They held daily team meetings to address unfamiliar issues, including the modification of the setting and the professional reflections that this activated. However, they succeeded in providing not only individual counselling but also small groups for anxiety management and study skills.

Ierardi et al. (2022) in Milan exploited the situation to measure the effectiveness of online versus in-person counselling for university students. They identified two groups of students with comparable mental health difficulties and demographics. The first group was treated face to face just before the pandemic, the second group was treated online during lockdown. The good news is that online counselling reduced symptoms of depression, anxiety, obsessiveness–compulsiveness, and interpersonal sensitivity to a similar extent as in-person counselling. However, the online intervention was less effective in reducing 'total psychopathological distress'.

The authors observed that both therapists and students were by now well used to using technologies in their daily lives and had little problem creating a good therapeutic alliance based on empathy and listening. There did appear to be extra benefits to in-person counselling. This was associated with reduction in discomfort, anger, and somatisation (bodily symptoms of mental distress) and increase in life satisfaction. They admitted, though, that the pandemic situation itself and the resulting lockdown, might be responsible for how resistant to change these symptoms were in the second group. It would be helpful to repeat the comparison of face-to-face versus online treatment with two groups of students after lockdown. Now that people are better equipped to use technology for therapy, this could allow treatment when students are on vacation or away on placements.

Chaplaincy

All universities host chaplaincy services offering quiet spaces for reflection and prayer, and compassionate support. Students and staff have told me that they appreciate the warmth – sometimes literally on a cold winter day on campus – and informal opportunities for non-pressured, non-judgmental conversations. Others have felt wary that if they engage in this there will be an ulterior motive of 'converting them' to a religious faith. However, most chaplaincies welcome staff and students of all faiths or none, calling themselves 'non-denominational' and 'multi-faith'. Chaplaincies continue, as they have done for centuries, to provide listening, religious services, meditation opportunities, tea and coffee, even lunch, and low-key social events to counter loneliness. A straightforward view of the campus chaplain is as a representative of a particular faith tradition who works in a secular environment – similar to the work of chaplains in hospitals, prisons and the armed forces.

> The word 'chaplain' is thought to originate in the legend of St Martin of Tours. While serving Rome as a soldier deployed in Gaul, in the third century AD, he cut his military coat in half to share it with a ragged beggar. That night Martin dreamed of Christ wearing the half-cloak he had given the beggar. The half he kept became a holy relic to which people would pray. The relic's guardian was called a 'chapelain'.
>
> One of the earliest known instances of a chaplain in a university dates back to the year 1256, when the University of Cambridge was granted funding for two full-time chaplains to serve its students.

In contrast with the increasingly regulated and measured structures in university counselling services, the practice of chaplaincy services has always been less defined, and open to the creative responses of individual chaplains to the circumstances they find. Chaplains engage with academic departments to varying degrees depending largely on individual relationships and common points of intellectual interest, but this is often uneven and unstructured. Increasingly, they are integrating themselves with more formal university structures, providing websites and regular programmes, as well as providing services to academic and pastoral staff. Some offer meeting places, hosting for meetings on sensitive topics such as suicide reviews, supporting bereaved students, and collaborations with student services. Some student support services use chaplaincy premises to hold some of their clinics and meetings.

A profession characterised by goodwill and very flexible job descriptions may find itself called to fill gaps in other provision. This may be positive and creative but also risky and controversial. In some institutions for instance, chaplains have been approached to lead on legal responsibilities around counter terrorism. Chaplains may be assumed, rather than explicitly qualified, to have the necessary expertise in religious politics and pastoral diplomacy.

Chaplaincy can be treated as a sort of overflow service for oversubscribed professional support departments. Nolan (2021) claims that 'What began as a Christian ministry is visibly morphing into a secularised form of therapeutic service'. This is a precarious arrangement, based on an assumption of good communication and trust between all parties. Most chaplains are part time, many are volunteers, some are paid by their church or religious organisation, some by the university and others by some combination of funding. They are unlikely to have the same line-management or training opportunities as counsellors. Their job descriptions tend to specify membership of a religious organisation rather than a professional body, so they are not usually within the systems of accountability, safeguarding and quality control that university managers demand of mental health staff in student services.

This recontextualising of the campus chaplaincy – both as non-denominational spirituality and as a form of mental health care – is felt by some chaplains to pose problems of balance even as it has helped to renew attention to the office. They are happy for students who aren't in any world religion to they come in, have tea and meditate. But some still wish to prioritise the needs of students who identify as having specific spiritual and religious needs.

In the context of this book, it is not appropriate to debate the balance between religious and mental health input that should be expected of our university chaplains, though we need to be aware of that potential conflict. Almost by accident, chaplains may be being expected to undertake advanced mental health practice without the appropriate training, supervision and indemnities. I have been unable to find a legal view of this situation.

It is not clear what mental health training should be provided to chaplains both before and after appointment. Both recruitment criteria and provision of continuing professional development are needed, particularly where the role overlaps considerably with social work and counselling. Gloria Woodland, who directs the Associated Canadian Theological Schools Seminaries, defines the role of the chaplain as 'spiritual health practitioner'. She says it takes more than the usual clergy training – 'It's going to take interpersonal skills, as well as skills in the field of psychology, mental health, and a theological perspective.'

There are costs associated with expecting previous training or providing it for appointees. Currently, the salary for university chaplains (when they are not volunteers) is around £25 000, in comparison with £40 000+ for university counsellors. It is unlikely that religious organisations could fund chaplaincy at that level but might instead expect universities to consider taking over costs and governance arrangements. Chaplains remain accountable to their religious organisation, but those undertaking mental health work might benefit from additional membership of a professional body such as the University Mental Health Advisors Network.

Chaplaincy is particularly suited to well-being interventions rather than specific treatment for people with mental disorders. One university chaplain hosts an annual guided walk through the city's sacred places – churches, temples, synagogues and mosques. The walk follows a lunch of bread and soup and is attended by students of all faiths and none. International students are particularly welcomed.

One year, as they visited a temple, one new Hindu student was moved to tears to have found her own place of religious worship. Many of the students from the walk became 'regulars' at the Wednesday lunches hosted by the chaplaincy centre. These were continued through the Christmas vacation to support students unable to return home to their families.

University Mental Health Advisors

The role of mental health advisors (MHAs) is to assess the impact of mental health needs on academic ability and provide information about mental health issues and the services available to support them. They work alongside disability advisers, mental health mentors, well-being advisers and counsellors. MHAs normally either have a postgraduate qualification in mental health or a professional qualification, and many have extensive experience of working in the public sector. The professions represented include occupational therapy, mental health nursing, social work, psychology, counselling, psychotherapy and people with a portfolio of extensive experience of supporting people with long-term mental health conditions.

The role involves co-ordination and case management rather than direct counselling or therapy. The job title and remit of their role may differ across each university, but typically, a MHA acts as a point of contact for the student throughout their course. Confusingly – but also conveniently – many MHAs also work as specialist autism mentors, or provide specialist one-to-one study skills and strategy support. Since 2003, there has been an overall professional association for MHAs, the University Mental Health Advisors Network. This association also functions as a campaigning body to improve services and increase the appropriate uptake of DSAs for students with mental health conditions.

Meeting the Extra Costs of a Mental Disorder at University: DSA

The DSA is a government-funded allowance designed to ensure that students who have a longer-term health condition or 'disability' are not disadvantaged in accessing their university studies. When a student discloses their mental health disorder to the university, this generally sets off the process of inviting them to apply for DSA, but a student who later decides to request help or develops their disorder later on, may of course apply.

It is an important part of the role of university mental health professionals to help steer students through the complicated pathways to help. Further details about applications and the financial context of mental health are described in Chapter 9.

For many students with mental health problems, the greatest benefit to receiving DSA is being able to access one-to-one support from a specialist mental health mentor. Counselling and some other university services often have limited, fairly short duration of contact, whilst psychotherapy and psychology services in the NHS usually have very long waiting lists. Specialist mental health mentoring, on the other hand, provides regular, flexible long-term input from a qualified mental health professional, and usually from the same individual for the length of the university course.

Mental Health Mentors

Mental health mentors (here referred to as 'mentors' but not to be confused with peer-mentors), like MHAs, work with students for the duration of their studies to help them achieve their full potential at university while also mitigating the impact their mental health condition might have on them. Unlike MHAs, mentors do deliver regular substantial face-to-face appointments typically weekly, over at least 30 weeks of the academic year. These are not strictly therapy for the disorder, but therapeutic in terms of ensuring that the consequences of the disorder are managed in the context of the student's university life.

Students who have disclosed a mental health condition or autism spectrum disorder can apply to Student Finance England, who then allocate DSA to pay for a certain number of hours of mentorship. Most mentors are paid for by the students' DSA but international students and others not eligible for DSA can often be supported by university or charitable funds – such referrals are increasing.

Mentors are qualified mental health professionals (this is one of the requirements of DSA funding) who can work with students with a range of mental health conditions, help them come to terms with their diagnosis, and help them improve their self-management competences. They can help explore the underlying causes that prevent effective study, such as perfectionism, fear of failure and anxiety. They can provide support with timetabling, goal setting, workload prioritisation, and managing expectations about appropriate levels of study. They will work with the student on short- and long-term targets, providing them with the tools and the mindset to achieve personal academic goals.

Jagesh had been diagnosed with bipolar I disorder after an alarming 'breakdown' in his second year at university, when he believed he had 'superpowers' and had invented a machine that would bring fortune to his family. At the time he was engaged to be married, but this was called off, and he was on bad terms with his family in India.

He was provided with a specialist mental health mentor through university funding, and was allowed to repeat second year. He had been a high-achieving student up to that point. He now had depression and was concerned that the medication he was prescribed was slowing his brain and causing weight gain.

He took a whole term to warm to his mentor, partly because she was a woman of the same age as his strict and disapproving mother, but eventually developed a trusting and appreciative attachment to her.

One simple intervention that transformed his academic recovery was for her to phone him each morning for a week to help him get up, take his medication and attend lectures. The following week he called her to confirm he was up and about, and after that he would text.

Another useful habit was the 'practice interviews' they conducted together before his appointments with the psychiatrist. Initially, Jagesh felt he should simply agree with everything his doctor said, even though he would not necessarily be able to follow the advice afterwards. With his mentor's help, he learned to courteously but firmly express his own point of view.

Eventually, they discussed rebuilding the relationship with his family. His improved grades gave him a greater confidence in taking up the communication again.

The University Mentoring Organisation (UMO) has conducted a large and detailed online survey of all students on their books between 2011 and 2019, focussing general life functioning, academic performance, and the experience of mentorship (Matthews, 2020). 90% responded very positively and endorsed the service they received as having a profound influence on all these areas of university life.

A smaller qualitative study explored the experience of mentors as well as the students they mentored (Lucas & James, 2018). Again, mentees' satisfaction levels were high. Mentors reported that in the 1-year mentorship they had developed their personal skills, had a strong relationship with their mentee and were positive about the mentoring role within the university. As with counselling, mentorship moved to online platforms during COVID lockdown and is now coping with the challenges of post-COVID mental health problems.

Students Who Flourish without Formal Support

Despite concerns about deteriorating student mental health, and even in the aftermath of COVID, remarkable numbers of young people thrive with only minimal therapeutic input, often without formal referral at all. Research described in Chapters 2 and 3 of this book examines some of the features that characterise those flourishing students, including strong peer relationships and engagement in physical activity.

> Jakob was an Australian geography student whose whole life seemed sunny. He made friends very quickly at his UK university, and whilst he was not an ambitious sportsman, he joined several 'social' sports societies and engaged in a great deal of volunteering work. He had the knack of remaining friendly with ex-girlfriends, and found a more lasting relationship with a fellow Australian in his third year.
>
> He had a tendency to leave his academic work until the last minute, and his teachers sometimes felt he was underachieving, even 'cruising'. He surprised everyone by getting a good 2.1 degree before the couple returned to their home country to take on postgraduate studies.

Even students previously diagnosed with a formal mental health condition may flourish without formal mental health support, particularly if their needs are anticipated. Young people usually prefer to talk to friends and family and people they know rather than professionals. There are risks though that students may come to rely inappropriately on psychological support from academics and teachers at the expense of both parties. This is explored further in Chapter 13.

> Jacinda was diagnosed with obsessive–compulsive disorder (OCD) and severe anxiety at age 9, so her school and family expected she might have some struggles at university. She had been discharged from child and adolescent mental health services (CAMHS) at age 15 on medication, which she continued to take, and decided to disclose her mental condition on her application. To everyone's surprise she required no formal counselling or hospital appointments. She says,
>
> > My mental health OCD and anxiety was dealt with very well whilst at university. It did not affect my studies directly. I have heard of stories on the news of students who committed suicide after not receiving support over their mental health, which has raised questions around mental health support at some universities. I had times where I had issues surrounding OCD and anxiety. However, this was dealt with very well at the university health centre and at my local GP clinic. My medication was reviewed and I took it regularly. and whilst there were likely peaks and troughs, I cannot recall any particular cases where it deteriorated significantly.

Preventative and Early Intervention Input

Researchers have learned from the characteristics of flourishing students and designed interventions to reinforce strong peer relationships. The Oxford University peer support programme trains undergraduate and graduate peer supporters using qualified peer support trainers. They teach the skills of being a good listener, helping others feel more comfortable with social and academic relationships, helping others to manage and communicate sensitive issues, learning one's own limits in a listening situation and knowing when to refer the person being supported (Crouch et al., 2006).

Byrom (2018) examined a six-part peer-led course for mild depression, based on behavioural activation. This showed promising evidence of effectiveness in those who attended most of the sessions but attrition was relatively high with only 28% completing the six session course.

Recent Developments at the University of Bristol

2016 launch of new Vision and Strategy to review student pastoral support. £1milliion per annum to fund new student well-being service embedded in academic schools to proactively support well-being and to identify and ensure access to specialist services when needed. Review of pastoral support in residences

2016–17 Cluster of student suicides prompted new suicide prevention and response plan (University of Bristol, 2018c)

2018–19 Pilot of *The Science of Happiness* – a first year formative rather than summative course on mental well-being, examining the science of well-being from multidisciplinary viewpoints with and supervised small groups to put principles into practice. Student who took the course in their first term, reported higher levels of well-being than those waiting to take the course in their second term

'Single session one at a time' approach (Dryden, 2019) Students are offered a single session of counselling only, albeit with the option of booking a further session after reflection. This has reduced waiting times, an aspect of care particularly appreciated by students.

Single point of access designed so that the university, not the student, manages the complexities of assessing, allocating and co-ordinating support (Ames, 2022). Students to apply for mental health support using a single online form.

E-Mental Health and Apps

Bristol, like other universities, has experimented with embedding mental health improvements into all students' curriculum using youth-friendly methods such as 'apps'. The Fika app (www.fika.community/) is specifically focused on mental 'fitness' – not mental health. The app designers have embarked on research in which participating universities map and embed their 5-minute 'emotional workout' app across the curriculum. Though they refer to it as an 'emotional' workout, in practice, there is more focus on cognitive rather than affective aspects of health. It is too early to endorse particular apps without further studies, but conducting such studies is essential and overdue.

There is a concerning abundance of apps that are readily accessible by the public without the means to quality assess or determine their appropriateness. A review of mental and physical health apps found that only 14% had been designed with input from a healthcare professional (Sedrati et al., 2016). The majority of apps for physical health had been designed for medical professionals rather than patients, but the majority of apps for mental health had been designed for direct use by clients or patients.

So far, I have not heard of any lawsuits brought against apps providing inappropriate advice, but I have seen harms. Young people with anorexia eating disorders for instance have followed advice to increase exercise and avoid 'unhealthy' food as ways to improve their mood. Potential users could benefit from having professional guidance on the appropriate use of apps. Mental health authorities might consider using a hallmark of some sort to endorse appropriate apps. It is usually relatively easy for professionals to spot harmful apps, but in order to recommend effective positive apps we need more research.

Parents, Families and Lay Carers as Mental Health Support

There is no doubt that today's students are able and willing to stay in closer contact with their parents than were previous generations, thanks to digital technology. More than ever, this makes those parents informal partners in the mental health care of students.

A 'cluster' of students suicides at Bristol University triggered discussions about changing contracts about sharing information with parents. Bereaved parents took a lead in campaigning for the change. The university created a new student emergency contract procedure (Ames, 2019) that allowed students at the time of registration with the university to nominate an emergency contact in the event of serious concerns about their well-being. More than 90% students provided this consent, suggesting that students do expect people close to them to be involved in caring for them when they need help. There is now more of an onus on universities to justify any decision to not use the emergency contact, rather than a fear of 'breaching confidentiality' if they do make contact. The views and roles of students' families are considered further in Chapter 4.

How Services within the University Connect with the NHS

Mental Health Services That Students and Staff May Need to Access Off Campus

NHS Services That Are Particularly Relevant to Students
- General practice (also called 'primary care')
- General adult outpatient services
- Adult eating disorders services
- Psychotherapy services
- Psychological therapies
- Early psychosis teams

Gaps in NHS Provision for Students
- Sheer amount of resources – to allow shorter waits, more regular appointments, longer courses of treatment and better integration of services when the student has several different disorders or where the disorder manifests in different ways.
- Developmentally appropriate services. This is not only a matter of respecting 'transition age youth' but also of acknowledging that the needs of intellectually and academically active students are different from those of non-academic middle-aged adults with more chronic disorders, particularly in the case of inpatient wards.
- Services for misuse of alcohol and other substances that may not (yet) reach criteria for addiction or severe chronic disorder.
- Services for 'Borderline' or 'Emotionally unstable' personality disorder, including chronic trauma services.
- Services for people with sexual difficulties, both for those who have been victims of sexual aggression and for young disturbed or confused perpetrators.

The role of in-house university mental health and counselling services is to support the short-term mental health needs of students and staff, with special acknowledgment of academic demands in a university. In contrast, NHS services are designed to support citizens' severe and often longer-term mental health needs and support their clients towards recovery.

For most of us in the UK, access to specialist services, including NHS mental health services, is through our GP. Strictly speaking, GPs are not NHS employees but are financed by the NHS to provide primary care, and then to be 'gatekeepers' or 'conduits' where their patients require more specialist input. There has been growing concern about inadequate GP numbers for the population need, and we have already seen in Chapters 2 and 3 about the transition to university life that students do not always manage to sign up with a GP in their university city.

GPs and Student Mental Health

Universities UK (2020) asks universities to develop regular high-level links with NHS commissioners and services, and with local authorities and the third sector, with a particular focus on the dangerous transition periods. Universities UK (2020) report that, in 2018 before COVID, about 45% of institutions had a student GP based on site and in 33% of institutions, students can access NHS mental health practitioners on site. Universities might consider hosting more primary care, secondary care and third-sector mental health provisions on campus. As GPs are the gatekeepers to most NHS services, signing up with an on-campus GP could be readily facilitated at Student Registration.

Specialist student GPs quickly become expert in the student culture of the moment. They often provide longer than usual appointment times and hold joint meetings and reviews with other services. Student medical practices develop expertise in dealing with situations common in university life, such as eating disorders, drink, drugs, relationships, procedures for coursework extensions and contacts with the best people to speak to about other matters of concern. At the moment, though, GPs are not properly appreciated or resourced for expertise in student mental health.

Funding is allocated to GPs via a formula based on the general medical services contract, weighted by deprivation and age then distributed according to number of registered patients. Additional funding is mostly based on long-term physical rather than mental conditions. Students are within an age group that is physically very healthy and unlikely to make large demands on the GP practice in terms of their physical health. However, mental conditions are becoming increasingly dominant parts of a GP caseload, especially after COVID. Practices with a high number of registered students are faced with substantial gaps in funding for their workload. This could be changed to recognise mental as well as physical disability on general practice.

IAPT and Its Relevance for Universities

Improving access to psychological therapies (IAPT) is an initiative introduced in 2008 by NHS England to improve outcomes for 'low-level' mental health difficulties. It was developed and introduced by the Labour government of the time, based on economic evaluations by Professor Lord Richard Layard, therapy guidelines from the National Institute for Health and Care Excellence (NICE) and input from the eminent clinical psychologist David M. Clark. There are over 200 IAPT services across England, making it the largest publicly funded implementation of evidence-based psychological care in the world. Patients are initially offered brief, low-cost, and low-intensity guided self-help based on principles of cognitive behavioural therapy, delivered over the telephone, via computerised cognitive behavioural therapy, in large groups or in a one-to-one format.

There is much to commend IAPT. The initiative included regular collection of standardised data. This allows critical evaluation and adjustment of the project. Saunders et al. (2020) found that outcomes were improving up to and beyond the government's 50% recovery rate target. This was linked to patients receiving more treatment sessions, delivered in a more condensed period of time, and reduced non-attendance.

In contrast, the project has been criticised for failing to appoint enough qualified therapists, resulting in high caseloads, long waiting lists (6–18 weeks after referral) and short treatment times. It has also been noted that the goals of getting people back into the workplace and reducing the need for antidepressant prescribing have not been achieved. In fact, both antidepressant prescribing and psychiatric disability claims have continued to rise. Most university students would be able to access specialist student counselling more conveniently and effectively than using IAPT. Timimi (2015) found that recovery rates, as a percentage of patients referred, was lower for IAPT services than for university counselling services.

Diversity of Service Provision

Universities do not all offer the same mental health services – and nor should they. Until we have better evidence about the benefits and risks of different interventions, it is healthier for different institutions to creatively set up and research services that respond to the observed needs and collaboratively incorporated demands of students and other members of each unique university. It's healthy too, that some institutions 'borrow' examples of good practice that work in other university communities, and discover whether such models work in their own environment.

The size of the institution is an important factor. Initiatives developed in Manchester may work well in other large cities where there are multiple higher education establishments and very large student populations, but may not in smaller or more rural settings. Conversely, there may be extra problems for the London universities, where the student population is spread over several different health boroughs.

Universities, like schools, have different profiles, different special areas of excellence, and attract different ranges of diverse applicants What works for one setting may not work for another, and the existence of different ambience and pace allows individuals choice – provided that they are aware of the diversity. There is an important caveat to this, however. New and un-researched services and interventions should be carefully researched in terms of outcomes and economic costs. Ineffective treatments are potentially harmful in their own right and also by dint of taking up resource that could be used effectively elsewhere.

Integrating NHS and Student Services in Greater Manchester

Greater Manchester has one of the largest student populations in the country, with around 100 000 people attending the city's five higher education institutions. Just before the COVID pandemic, it became the first place in the country to establish a dedicated centre to help support higher education students with mental health needs when higher education forged new links with the health and social care partnership.

The centre – jointly funded by all the partners – takes referrals directly from the different counselling centres, so that the student has only seek help once. Whether the student presents to the NHS mental health system, third sector or university they receive the same standard assessment, and are then directed to appropriate intensity of care. Their treatment plans take into account important demand factors such as examination periods, and the specialist experience of the centre is an extra benefit.

A university setting is ideal in providing expertise and eagerness to practise research and evaluation skills, so it is disappointing when proper evaluation is not in place from the start of any new plan. Feedback from a self-selected group of participants is not a substitute for the use of painstaking application of objective and subjective outcomes.

Creating a New Mental Health Speciality?

This book has repeatedly emphasised how university students are disadvantaged in NHS mental health services, largely as a result of the multiple transitions they face on leaving home and CAMHS services, and continue to experience as they travel between home and university, or spend time on placements elsewhere or abroad. However, it would not be ethical for students to expect privileged queue jumping within the NHS at the expense of other patients. Moreover, it can be of concern that students present with different needs from the majority of NHS psychiatric patients, who tend to be considerably older, and in many cases more disabled by their conditions.

It has been argued elsewhere that the expertise of CAMHS clinicians may still be relevant to this group of 'transition aged youth'. Some CAMHS services in the NHS are experimenting with extending their age group up to age 25, but this doesn't necessarily solve the problem of geographical moves, and is pragmatically difficult to manage. There are legal and social differences involved in treating people under age 18 with those who are legally adults. Finally, the staff shortages in CAMHS services are already worrying. Expecting CAMHS to take on the large numbers of mentally ill individuals from age 18 to 25 is frankly unrealistic.

There are other communities whose particular mental health needs are catered for in ways which respect their needs without disadvantaging society – the armed forces have their own clinicians, with ring-fenced budgets. Older adult mental health services are a separate specialism within NHS Psychiatry, and of course there is CAMHS itself. Other specialist mental health services include eating disorders services, substance misuse services, and psychotherapy departments. Their models would have much to teach us about networking on a regional and national basis to cater for special needs groups.

Women in the perinatal period have been another group of young people for whom existing 'general adult' services have been problematic. Again, time constraints involved in pregnancy mean that many months on a waiting list fails to keep up with the need. In the same climate that has seen growing pressures on NHS staffing, the new speciality of perinatal psychiatry is flourishing.

One feature of all these relatively small specialities is the crucial role of communicating with other services around the patient. They regard managing transitions as a powerful part of the work, rather than as a mere inconvenience to the treatment. We have to protect access to confidential records, but the current scattered nature of electronic records doesn't so much protect confidentiality as fragment communication. GPs do not automatically have access to their patients' hospital records or vice versa, clinicians in different health trusts and boards cannot access previous records, and too much responsibility is placed on individuals to remember and repeat their medical and social history, even at times of mental illness.

In principle, management of transitions involves handing over care from one service to another, but in practice, students experience fluctuating transitions. They do not completely leave their home and spend all their time at university. If they become seriously mentally ill, their condition may sometimes require inpatient hospital care, more often outpatient care, and sometimes only the support of the university mental health services. Multiple handovers and handing back can interrupt the course of recovery. It can work much better if everyone involved in the individual's care remains informed and potentially available to hold planning reviews.

Integration, communication and cohesion of different mental health services with each other and with other specialities and disciplines is crucial. In the outside world, adults are usually expected to provide their own integration of care between work, doctors, hospitals, social care and so on. This is always difficult when a person is vulnerable as a result of illness. All the more so if the illness concerned is a mental illness and the patient is still very young. However, it can be a challenge for outside agencies to manage the networking and integration for them when confidential record keeping is not shared across different services and different geographical locations.

I would strongly suggest that each university hosts forums where NHS mental health services can share with universities their experiences, methods and campaigns. Taking this further, I would strongly urge the construction of national and UK-wide specialist groups devoted to expertise in university mental health. The College of Psychiatrists of Ireland does have a Faculty of Youth and Student Psychiatry. I would urge the Royal Colleges of Psychiatrists and of GPs to create faculties of university mental health. This would recognise the specific challenges and expertise and workforce required to meet them. This expertise could then be explicitly taught as part of the medical curriculum and tested in examinations.

Practice Points

- Students and staff are provided with a large range of mental health support, many of them boasting excellent outcomes, but the multiplicity makes for confusion rather than clarity
- Counsellors, mental health advisors and mental health mentors are available without fee to most university students. These are well researched and evidenced in the treatment of mild to moderate mental illnesses and in the support of people with longer-term disorders.
- Students with a significant level of depression or one of the more severe anxiety disorders are likely to require longer courses of therapy than counselling services routinely offer.
- Chaplaincy takes many forms and is also a widely available but so far less well evidenced
- There is still much work to do in terms of dovetailing and integrating different services around a vulnerable student. The challenge is greatest when NHS as well as in-house university services are needed.
- Discussions with local NHS clinics are needed to share care appropriately and provide therapeutic continuity. Arrangements for treatment during vacations are essential.
- Integrative models such as that piloted in Greater Manchester show promise, but different universities and geographical locations may need different solutions.
- More than half of universities do not have a GP on campus. Workforce shortages make it ever more difficult for GPs to co-ordinate the care of their student patients.
- GP funding needs to be reviewed to acknowledge the extra burden of mental health care.
- The Royal College of Psychiatrists and related organisations could focus expertise in the field of university mental health by creating a new faculty of university mental health.

References

Ames, M. (2022). Supporting student mental health and wellbeing in higher education. In: Mallon S. & Smith J. (eds.) *Preventing and responding to student suicide* (pp. 208–223). London: Jessica Kingsley Publishers.

Broglia, E., Ryan, G., Williams, C., et al. (2021). Profiling student mental health and counselling effectiveness: Lessons from four UK services using complete data and different outcome measures. *British Journal of Guidance & Counselling*, 1–19.

Brown, J. S. L. (2018). Student mental health: Some answers and more questions, *Journal of Mental Health*, 27(3), 193–6. https://doi.org/10.1080/09638237.2018.1470319

Byrom, N. (2018). An evaluation of a peer support intervention for student mental health. *Journal of Mental Health*, 27(3), 240–6.

Crouch, R., Scarffe, P. & Davies, S. (2006). *Guidelines for mental health promotion in higher education*. Universities UK/GuildHE Committee for the Promotion of Mental Well-being in Higher Education. www.umhan.com/resources/15-guidelines-for-mental-health-promotion-in-higher-education

Dryden, W. (2019). *Single-session 'one-at-a-time' therapy: A rational emotive behaviour therapy approach*. Routledge.

Hughes, G. & Spanner, L. (2019). *The university mental health charter*. Student Minds. www.studentminds.org.uk/uploads/3/7/8/4/3784584/191208_umhc_artwork.pdf

Ierardi, E., Bottini, M. & Riva Crugnola, C. (2022). Effectiveness of an online versus face-to-face psychodynamic counselling intervention for university students before and during the COVID-19 period. *BMC Psychology*, 10(1), 1–10.

Locke, B. D., Buzolitz, J. S., Lei, P.-W., et al. (2011). Development of the counseling center assessment of psychological symptoms-62 (CCAPS-62). *Journal of Counseling Psychology*, 58, 97–109.

Lucas, R. & James, A. I. (2018). An evaluation of specialist mentoring for university students with autism spectrum disorders and mental health conditions. *Journal of Autism and Developmental Disorders*, 48(3), 694–707.

Macaskill, A. (2013). The mental health of university students in the United Kingdom, *British Journal of Guidance & Counselling*, 41(4), 426–41. https://doi.org/10.1080/03069885.2012.743110

Matthews, A. (2020). *The role and impact of specialist mental health mentoring on students in UK higher education institutes*. University Mentoring Organisation (UMO). www.umhan.com/resources/100-the-role-impact-of-specialist-mental-health-mentoring-on-students-in-uk-heis

Murray, A. L., McKenzie, K., Murray, K. R. & Richelieu, M. (2016). An analysis of the effectiveness of university counselling services. *British Journal of Guidance & Counselling*, 44(1), 130–9.

Nolan, S. (2021). Religious, Spiritual, Pastoral. . . and Secular? Where Next for Chaplaincy?. *Health and Social Care Chaplaincy*, 9(1), 1–10.

Saunders, R., Cape, J., Leibowitz, J., et al. (2020). Improvement in IAPT outcomes over time: Are they driven by changes in clinical practice? *The Cognitive Behaviour Therapist*, 13, e16. https://doi.org/10.1017/S1754470X20000173

Savarese, G., Curcio, L., D'Elia, D., Fasano, O. & Pecoraro, N. (2020). Online University counselling services and psychological problems among Italian students in lockdown due to Covid-19. *Healthcare*, 8 (4), 440. https://doi.org/10.3390/healthcare8040440

Sedrati, H., Nejjari, C., Chaqsare, S. & Ghazal, H. (2016). Mental and physical mobile health apps. *Procedia Computer Science*, 100, 900–906.

Timimi, S. (2015). Children and young people's improving access to psychological therapies: Inspiring innovation or more of the same? *BJPsych Bulletin*, 39(2), 57–60.

Universities UK (2020). *Stepchange: Mentally healthy universities*. www.universitiesuk.ac .uk/what-we-do/policy-and-research/ publications/stepchange-mentally-healthy- universities

University of Bristol (2023a). *Student's emergency contact*. www.bristol.ac.uk/ students/support/wellbeing/policies/ emergency-contact/

University of Bristol (2023b). *Suicide prevention and approach*. www.bristol.ac .uk/students/support/wellbeing/policies/ suicide-prevention-and-approach/

19

Students of the Professions and 'Fitness to Practise' Issues

> During one of my many marathon study sessions in my third year, my bleary eyes took in the diagnostic criteria for depression. It was almost an exact description of how I felt and behaved . . . I thought that I was weak and wouldn't be allowed to be a doctor if I mentioned this to anybody. I read that as a young man the thing most likely to kill me was myself. I wrote this down on flash cards and carried on studying.
>
> After graduation, these pathological thoughts and attitudes continued. I felt that being a doctor was all that validated my existence. . . . I was completely unaware of the need to care for myself and of the support services that are available both as a medical student and after graduating. . . . If this was something more openly discussed and that you were signposted to support for, it would have reassured me that professionals had experienced this before, that I wasn't an anomaly, and that help was there for me and I wasn't weak by asking for it . . . this is an area in which my medical school failed me, and I doubt that I'm alone in this. . . . Having our seniors and people we respect teach us about this as a hazard of the job rather than an abstract headline would remove some of the stigma. To hear another doctor – somebody I could relate to – talk openly and frankly about what they went through, how they overcame it, and the lessons they learnt would have helped me so much.
>
> Crofts (2020)

As Crofts' (2020) story illustrates, the 'stigma' of mental illness continues to exist amongst university students, despite the greater openness of intelligent young people. Above all it exists amongst medical and other professional students, who fear that if they were known to have a mental disorder, they would lose their vocation. The work needed to qualify for entry to such courses is immense, exceeded only by the intensity of studying and practical work demanded by the long and arduous training involved. Individual identity often becomes subsumed in the professional role. Family and friends can invest heavily in the student's aspirations too, so it's hardly surprising that students and trainees desperately defend their career against perceived threats.

This chapter considers the fear that disclosure of a mental illness is damaging to the pursuit of a cherished career, and whether there are ways we could make disclosure more helpful, with outcomes that creatively harness the contributions of professionals with mental disorders and disabilities. It is essential to distinguish between bad practice on the one hand, and the unintended reductions in work skills resulting from an illness on the other. It is not a crime to have a mental illness, but students describe feeling that it is a guilty secret. The public is not well served and protected when the perceived response to professional behaviour concerns is to shame and reject highly skilled people.

Previous chapters of this handbook have addressed concerns of mental health and mental illness amongst students and university staff. In this chapter, our concern extends to the mental health of qualified members of those professions for which the students are training. This is because the culture in the professions themselves may influence student attitudes and behaviour more than the culture of the university itself.

Are Our Professions Fit to Practise in and to Train in?

Students of medicine and other high-prestige disciplines may have extra mental health needs. Characteristics that lead people to train for – and be successful in – such professions may make them unusually vulnerable to certain mental illnesses. These professions have ingrained subcultures, which disparage disclosure of vulnerability and tacitly encourage dysfunctional coping strategies such as heavy drinking, use of illegal drugs, partying, unwise sexual activity, gambling and risk-taking. These are difficult behaviours to assess, not always meeting criteria for a formal treatable mental illness, though sometimes symptomatic of an underlying disorder.

The evidence we have suggests that medical students have a high prevalence of mental disorders compared with matched peers. There are several reasons why this might be the case. One plausible theory is that the high grades required to enter medical schools – and even more so schools of veterinary medicine – select for people who have a genetically programmed predisposition to high achievement. It is known that families where there are many high achieving individuals also display vulnerabilities to autistic spectrum, obsessional, or bipolar disorders. These families then also provide an environment with a strong work ethic. Growing up like this prepares people well to achieve the high grades required by many professions. It can also predispose some people to disabling depression, shame and anxiety.

Jolyon studied Law, like his parents before him, whilst his sisters were training to be a doctor and a vet. Their mother had noticed that whilst most of her in-laws had achieved prominence in demanding careers, they were also prone to periods of breakdown and depressive symptoms. She consciously protected them from ambitious family expectations and bought them up to enjoy low-key pleasures and follow family routines. She found that nevertheless they showed great competitive drive, even amongst themselves.

Jolyon enjoyed high energy levels and excelled at sport as well as academic studies. When he left home for university he found he could study through the night for days on end alongside playing for the university soccer team and partying too. Without the restraining structures of home life, he became slightly manic, over-spent his student loan and lost a lot of weight in a few weeks. His flatmate spoke to Jolyon's parents (this caused an irritable fallout between the flatmates), but when his parents arrived, they recognised the signs of a pattern they had seen before. They took Jolyon home where his mood immediately crashed, and he spent days in bed. He was referred urgently to an NHS clinic. He was relieved that doctors advised 'watchful waiting' and lifestyle advice rather than pushing him to start medication.

Even if we hypothesise that this group of students is unusually sensitive to certain mental disorders, environment factors are powerful in deciding whether frank disorders are triggered or not. In particular, the culture of 'stoicism and bravado' in medical and other professional trainings may precipitate or exacerbate mental illness (Carr, 2008). Not only students but also qualified members of the professions describe a fiercely competitive and hierarchical culture, with interpersonal tensions, bullying, high levels of sexism, racism, shaming and blaming. This adds to the trauma that those in such professions are exposed to. Regularly facing life threatening suffering and death is known to predispose one to post-traumatic stress disorder. The way such trauma is managed within the culture profoundly affects the rate of disorder manifestation. Individual 'resilience' is limited. Indeed, many junior doctors find the term objectionable. They see it as a way to turn responsibility on the sufferer, instead of striving to improve working culture and working conditions.

Unhappily, our professional cultures make mental illness more likely and perpetuate the fear that seeking support will result in punitive fitness to practise (FTP) procedures. There is scope for improving the culture for our students and trainees. This takes on even greater importance if we believe that mental disorder in doctors and other professionals affects the quality of care that they provide to us all as their potential patients, pupils and clients.

A study of depression rates in more than 120 000 medical students across a spread of continents (Rotenstein et al., 2016) found that more than a quarter of them experienced depression. This is between two- and five-times the rate of peers who are not medical students. Less than 16% of the depressed students actually received treatment for their depression. The study did not include UK students and examined only depressive disorder, but it seems reasonable to suspect that this finding would apply to the UK and to other mental disorders. In line with these rates, a 2015 survey of more than a thousand medical students in *Student BMJ* had found that 30% of respondents had received treatment for a mental disorder. 80% of these described the treatment as poor or barely adequate. There was a widespread attitude that it was detrimental to career prospects to officially disclose a mental disorder.

In 2019, the British Medical Association conducted a qualitative analysis of interviews with individuals and groups of medical students and junior doctors (Sykes et al. 2020). Findings included:

> issues related to hierarchy and bullying, the stigma around mental health, erosion of peer support networks and a perceived natural tendency of doctors to be type-A personalities (i.e., perfectionism, fear of weakness or being seen to fail).
>
> Compared with qualified doctors, the medical students in this study generally felt well supported by their medical school/university in terms of preventative measures and initiatives . . . Peer-to-peer networks were often set-up during the student induction process and most students had been offered well-being services.

This may indicate improvements in recent years, but the group of students was very small indeed, so hard to consider as representative.

There has been clear evidence internationally and for many years now, that medical students and qualified but 'junior' doctors have high rates of suicidal thinking and more than usual access to lethal methods of self-harm – as of course do students and practitioners in nursing, dentistry, veterinary medicine, farming and pharmacy.

Students in related disciplines also report high rates of perceived mental illness. Psychology students in Florida described mood disorders, eating disorders, anxiety disorders, substance misuse, burnout, personality disorders and interpersonal problems in their peers (Oliver et al., 2004). These students experienced resentment towards their impaired peers, and anger that their seniors allowed such trainees to continue into the profession. In other studies students felt they could identify 'problematic' student peers better than staff. They told researchers that the main problems they saw involved interpersonal skills and emotional regulation (Rosenberg et al., 2005).

There are several psychological therapies that can effectively improve interpersonal and emotional regulation skills. Doing so would be a more constructive approach to protecting the public than pejorative labelling of people who lack such skills. The teaching of such skills could make the difference between wasting the potential and investment in trainees who have become impaired, and providing the necessary supports and treatments to allow them to continue. Some students may be unable to learn academically, emotionally or interpersonally, until a mental illness has been addressed. Repairing skills deficits and treating illness could shift blame and shame and peer frustrations like those described in the studies of Oliver et al. (2004) and Rosenberg et al. (2005).

Misuse of Alcohol and Other Substances

Amongst qualified doctors, the identification of a chronic problem like addiction, is often precipitated by a crisis – drink-driving, error at work, stealing drugs from the workplace. This was the case in the study of the specialist drug and alcohol treatment service for healthcare professionals at the Maudsley Hospital in London, where referral was often observed to follow an incident involving persistent absenteeism or intoxication at work (Gossop et al., 2001). Certainly, substance misuse figures very prominently in FTP concerns about students and qualified professionals.

It is controversial as to whether, or at least when, the misuse of alcohol and other substances constitutes a mental disorder in itself. In some cases, it is a cause of mental damage, and in some it is a consequence of a mental disorder, whether as 'self-medication' or because of reduced inhibition and control. Doctors and nurses, like members of the armed forces, turn to alcohol as the preferred resource for 'destressing' after traumatic experiences. The fact that it has become enshrined in social rituals brings the power of interpersonal soothing and comfort to the (short-term) chemical effects of relaxation and mental escape. What is not controversial is the observation that there is a massive culture of alcohol in medicine. One student remarked 'Medsoc is not about medicine at all but about drinking!'

At an age when the drinking culture is being established, medical students share many common but increasingly diverse cultural backgrounds. Researchers in Glasgow (Dr Fatemeh Nokhbatolfoghahai, personal communication) collected qualitative data from 30 students, who confirmed that alcohol is the central focus of many social programmes in medical school. Although the drinking culture is embraced by many, others such as younger/older students, those recovering from alcoholism and religious students feel excluded and obliged to create their own niche groups. They call for education about the socially excluding consequences of the drinking culture as well as negative physical health consequences of excessive drinking.

Medical students are certainly not the only group with a heavy drinking culture. There is some evidence suggesting Law students may be even more likely to drink to excess. There is more consideration of the issues of drug and alcohol misuse in universities in Chapters 6 and 7. Health professionals need to be able to recognise drug and alcohol problems in themselves, their clients, and their colleagues. Concepts relating to the misuse of alcohol and other drugs are already an integral part of student education, medical training, continuing medical education, and professional development. But like Crofts (2020), in the opening vignette to this chapter, individuals don't always achieve the same insight about their own problems as they do about the problems of their patients.

Treatment of Mental Health Conditions and Professional Function

Professionals and those aspiring to such vocations have the advantage of extremely powerful motivation to work hard on their recovery. This is vitally important for mental disorders, as recovery involves more than being a passive recipient of care. Psychiatric patients have to muster courage to comply with medication despite side effects, to prioritise appointments and to undertake the 'homework' demanded in between psychological therapy appointments. The evidence is positive. Doctors who have had appropriate care for any mental illness are less likely to take extended sick leave or to retire prematurely (Department of Health, 2008)

Another study of doctors and medical students (Miller, 2009) found that after a period of mental ill-health, most doctors are able to return to full-time or part-time work. They considered that with improved support even more doctors could recover and return to work. A Canadian study examined outcomes for medical practitioners after treatment for substance misuse problems (Brewster et al., 2008). Long term recovery rates were substantially higher than for the general population, often exceeding 85% in this clearly highly motivated group.

Hays et al. (2011) analysed profiles and prognosis of UK and international medical students who were struggling with their course. The study observed different key problems – poor learning skills, immaturity, poor organisational skills, major personal crisis, poor mental health, and poor insight. All groups except for the last had a positive prognosis with appropriate support, though they sometimes needed some time out from their studies. The group who showed poor insight – believing that they had no problems, or that their poor performance was not their problem but the fault of others – were 'difficult to remediate'. For students with mental health conditions, then, particularly for those who receive treatment, we can afford to be positive about their achieving FTP.

In Hays et al.'s (2011) research, poor insight was not limited to the students with diagnosable mental illnesses. Some mental illnesses, though, do notoriously involve at least temporary loss of insight. This is not necessarily something that improves with maturity and experience; rather, it may be a direct casualty of the way in which the disorder – or a substance of misuse – affects the brain. People experiencing severe depression, anxiety or obsessive–compulsive disorder can lose insight into their own competence and goodness, whilst those suffering from a manic episode can experience inflated ideas of what is possible.

Fortunately, there are ways to plan in advance to deal even with loss of insight. Just as people can make legal provisions to entrust decisions to a trusted proxy if they lose capacity, psychiatric patients are increasingly encouraged to write a formal 'advance statement' while they are well. This describes how their 'healthy self' would wish to be cared for during an acute relapse. At St Thomas's Hospital in London, medical staff who have bipolar affective disorder can write a formal plan whereby one of their trusted colleagues is empowered to report immediately to the named clinician if they think the doctor or student is behaving differently. Immediate assessment, sick leave and treatment can then be provided.

Legal Protections for People with Mental Disorders and Disabilities

All UK citizens have legal protections applying when they are ill either physically or mentally. These are harder to invoke in the case of mental disorder, though. Mental illness is diagnosed clinically by doctors, often those qualified as psychiatrists. In the UK, diagnosis does not have to conform to precise national or international classifications. This is different from those countries where insurance companies demand precise classification. A diagnostic 'label' can be helpful in validating the illness and providing guidance to likely effective treatment. Most experts would agree, though, that the science of psychiatric classification is still evolving and far from perfect.

Students with a mental health diagnosis will have rights during their education and training and as employees, particularly if the condition constitutes a disability. Working as a psychiatrist has constantly challenged my vocabulary in terms of the conflicting meanings, implications and expectations of using particular words. The law moves at a different pace, and often uses different definitions from those current in my specialty or in common speech. Legal definitions of 'disability' are amongst such terms. Students can be embarrassed or incredulous to claim 'disability' if they are not wheelchair bound (and some even then). The word suggests chronic, long-term loss of function.

The website www.lpmde.ac.uk/professional-development/fit-for-work-guidance/further-information breaks down aspects of medical work and matches it with specific demands on physical and mental health. There is also a video available on Vimeo: https://vimeo.com/user4672630/review/97931030/2ae27c2de4

The legal term 'disability' is defined more precisely. Someone has a disability if they have a physical or mental impairment with a substantial and long-term adverse effect on their ability to carry out normal day-to-day activities. (For instance, people with anxiety disorders may find rush hour travel on public transport unbearable. People with bipolar disorder may not be able to take on night shifts because major sleep disturbance can trigger an episode of illness.) It is valuable for the student to have an up to date note from their doctor and/or another professional to explain:

- The diagnosis and nature of the mental health problem
- how the problems and their treatment affect the student's life,
- what treatments are needed and the demands on the student to attend appointments and
- what adjustments might help them undertake their work.

The Disability Discrimination Act 1995 (amended 2005) was designed to protect UK employees against discrimination. Under the Act, employers have clear duties to make reasonable adjustments to the workplace before they can assert that the applicant's or employee's mental health prevents them from doing the work. All public sector employers, including the NHS, are required to promote equality for people with mental health problems and disabilities within their workforce and in their services. The have a duty to publish and implement a disability equality scheme to proactively ensure equality in the recruitment and retention of staff with mental ill health.

For those senior people with responsibility for predicting and managing behavioural risks associated with mental illness, there are some useful guidelines available. Good background information then needs to be supplemented with information about the individual's situation, provided by the student and by others who know them well. It would be helpful for all professional students to be aware of this legal context, both to support their own patients and clients, and to support for their own health and that of their colleagues. Two real-life cases vividly exemplify the need for all of us to know what rights people have and how easily they may be overlooked or over-ridden in the workplace.

Case 1:   Health Professions Council (HPC 2007)
An applicant to a speech and language therapy course said in her application that she had bipolar disorder. The admissions staff received an occupational health assessment and more information from the applicant. They were confident that they could accept the student, who met their admissions conditions. However, from informal discussions with colleagues who worked in clinical practice, they felt that there was little likelihood of a speech and language therapist with bipolar disorder being employed within the NHS. They felt that employers could be worried about her contact with children or vulnerable adults. So, they did not offer her a place on their course. This would be likely to be unlawful, because such a judgement may be discriminatory and could be based on assumptions or stereotypes about disabled people.

Case 2:   The Farnsworth Case (London Borough of Hammersmith and Fulham v. Farnsworth)
Ms Farnsworth was rejected by the London Borough of Hammersmith and Fulham Council for a post working with children with special needs, because of an earlier history of clinical depression. The Employment Appeal Tribunal held that the employers had discriminated against her. They could have made reasonable adjustments such as placing her on a probationary period, supervising her closely during this period and monitoring her work and her absence record.

Barriers to Professional Students Seeking Treatment and Care

Despite high levels of mental distress and illness in students of medical and other public service professions, and evidence that treatment is particularly effective for such highly motivated individuals, there are obstacles to their obtaining the necessary treatment. There is fear that disclosure of a mental disorder will not be kept confidential, but will cause stigma and loss of career. Students and senior professionals alike perceive referral to FTP procedures as catastrophic in themselves. They fear that harsh action will be inevitable. Such risks appear to outweigh any perceived benefits.

In 2012 the General Medical Council (GMC) commissioned research on how to best support medical students with mental illness. Findings revealed beliefs – often without empirical evidence – that medical schools excluded applicants on grounds of mental illness, and that it was an FTP issue. Winter et al (2017) explored these beliefs and found that UK medical students commonly felt that medical school 'support' systems were in fact punitive and that mental illness was unacceptable within medicine. They had invested so heavily in the idea of qualifying as a practising doctor, that this was the only acceptable future for them. They feared FTP proceedings as likely to lead to expulsion, failure and parental disappointment, and distrusted medical school offers of assistance.

Winter et al. (2017) identified strong beliefs that were powerful in reducing disclosure and help-seeking. These included 'Mental illness is weakness that won't be tolerated', 'FTP covers every aspect of your life and is a system designed to exclude the weak, including those with mental health issues' and mental illness 'will be on my record forever'. Taking time off for treatment would break the code of 'presenteeism', which expects medical students, like doctors, to attend even when unwell and only book in self-care in their own time.

Many application forms for university, and especially for caring professions courses, use different and distinct sections to request information about mental illness as opposed to physical illness. This implies – perhaps correctly – that the information will be used differently. There is an implication that mental illness is more likely to cause impairment of function than 'physical' illness, without there being clear evidence that the two can be so neatly separated or that mental illness does in fact cause more impairment.

Students are rarely well-informed about exactly who will have access to the information they are asked to provide and under what circumstances. It is ironic that professionals seeking to help and support students with mental disorders often complain about barriers in accessing information and communication, whilst students themselves fear that all information gathered about them will be collected in a single great 'record' that is then passed on to everyone in authority over them for the rest of their lives. Whilst such views may appear slightly immature and a little 'paranoid', it is the nature of mental illnesses such as depression and anxiety to negatively colour all our evaluations and increase our sense of helplessness. Just when we are greatest need of help and support, we are most likely to fear stigmatisation.

It is likely that students are in fact informed, but in small print on websites and during the hectic induction sessions of freshers' weeks, about the differences between academic and health records and their respective levels of privacy. It would be more helpful to provide written and spoken reminders each academic year, and always in the information supplied when students are signposted to services. Concrete examples are most helpful.

Poignantly, the students in this study appealed to the concept of the 'investment' that they and their families and teachers – even society – had made in their training as doctors. Wasting this would be a shameful failure. Many of their teachers and trainers are aware of the same pressures and beliefs, and therefore hesitate to act in any way that might trigger the shame of a potential colleague or 'waste' the investment in their education.

Records and Boundaries of Confidentiality

Time pressures add further obstacles to treatment, on top of fears of stigma. Students training in these disciplines have extraordinarily intense timetables with lectures, practical classes and placements all the working day, and hours of private study required to pass the relentless assessments and examinations imposed. (This workload contrasts starkly with the paucity of face-to-face teaching that students find so disappointing in other disciplines.) Often there are requirements to spend time away from the campus or city where the university is based to go on clinical attachments, teaching practice or professional placements. This contributes to strong bonding between students on the course, but perhaps isolates them from the wider university community. It also makes it extraordinarily difficult, as well as embarrassingly obvious, to access help in working hours – 'the whole world wants the Wednesday afternoon appointments' said one student. Clinics offering evening or weekend slots are hugely appreciated. Virtual appointments can facilitate contact too, despite some disadvantages.

Some students are embarrassed to access on-campus clinics. Medical and nursing students may even prefer to be referred out of area, to avoid being treated by clinicians they are likely be on placement with and later work with. It is embarrassing for them to think they may later need to ask for references from the very doctors who treated them when they are mentally ill. They may also encounter fellow students who are on the ward or in clinic for their teaching placements.

> Joe, a nursing student, had been treated for depression at school and recovered with treatment. End of year university exams were coming up and he was feeling stressed, dreading that the depression might be coming back. His friend was concerned and offered to go along with him to the general practitioner (GP).
>
> Dr Kendall explained that she would record his symptoms and treatment in his medical records, but that these could only be seen by other GPs. She did think he had symptoms of depression and would like to refer him to the hospital psychologist for a top up course of cognitive behavioural therapy, as this had worked well in the past. That would mean there would be further confidential records at the hospital. She would put in a request for these records to be kept in a special store for records of colleagues.
>
> GPs and the hospital psychologist could share information with each other about his progress, but this would not be available to the university. He could request a letter from Dr Kendall explaining extenuating circumstances around his exams, but the university would still not be given access to his NHS medical records.

One UK study examined potential models of personal (as opposed to academic) support, drawing on evidence from the websites of the 32 UK medical schools (Grant et al., 2015). They observed that medical schools functioned very much as a separate institution within the university, signposting students to services within the medical school rather than to generic university services.

The GMC has consistently advised that academic and personal support roles should be separated out, but not all medical schools manage to do this. The ideal arrangement would be mental health services that are conveniently located for busy medical student but at the same time assured of confidentiality and guaranteed separation from the clinicians with whom they study and work.

Reciprocal out-of-area arrangements with neighbouring services are time-consuming to put in place. They involve travel and disruption to studies. However, the COVID situation has normalised use of telecommunication in mental health delivery. This could revolutionise access for busy students. For students who attend university away from home, there could be benefits from their having treatment from their own home services. There has been controversy as to whether the medical records of healthcare students should be held with an extra level of confidentiality. Shame is a powerful obstacle to help seeking, but at the same time there are disadvantages to having one's records unavailable to admitting doctors in an emergency. At present the decision is generally taken out of the student-patient's hands. Perhaps they could be consulted individually about the risks of each option.

Evening clinics would be tremendously helpful both at GP surgeries and in mental health facilities – perhaps special outreach evening clinics on campus in convenient, non-stigmatising environments – student unions, careers departments, chaplaincies and libraries. Clinicians who provide mental health care to students of the health professions need particular support and supervision. They may over-identify with the professional culture and automatic assumptions. A tight circle of confidentiality has to be maintained in order to protect professionalism and assure trust. At the same time, healthcare students should not be expected or allowed to manage their own illness.

One possible solution is the provision of a mental health clinic specifically for health care students, sited conveniently within the medical school, offering extended opening hours, guaranteed standards of confidentiality and privacy, and perhaps staffed by visiting clinicians from another board or trust who are not involved in the home training setting. Such models are already being trialled in some of the large London institutions.

The Concept of Fitness to Practise

Most universities declare expectations that all students, like their seniors, should behave considerately in real life, in public and online, respecting the safety, security and well-being of others. Institutions have slightly different frameworks and procedures for considering breaches of these expectations, in respect of either academic or general conduct. For most students these will invoke the notion of 'fitness to study'. This includes consideration of other people's rights and needs, basic honesty, academic integrity and behaviour compatible with the university's reputation.

For students of healthcare, legal, educational and related professions meeting expectations of 'fitness to study', may not be enough to meet standards of conduct required by the profession. There is the additional expectation that their conduct complies with the expectations of the professional, statutory or regulatory body with which they will be eligible to register upon successful completion of their qualification. These regulatory bodies seek to safeguard the public interest and maintain confidence in the profession concerned. The regulatory body is not generally the regulator of student conduct, but it is linked closely in terms of advice to universities so that decisions about a student's progress are informed by both professional standards and the educational and developmental expertise of the higher education institution. The concept of FTP is invoked.

Professional Regulatory Bodies

Medicine: General Medical Council (GMC): www.gmc-uk.org
Nursing: Nursing and Midwifery Council (NMC): nmc.org.uk
Teaching: General Teaching Council (GTC) for England: www.gtce.org.uk
Social Work: Social Work England: www.socialworkengland.org.uk
The Law: The Law Society: www.lawsociety.org.uk

Formal Regulation of Fitness to Practise in the UK

'Fitness to practise' is a formal term used in professional settings, drawing on several overlapping concepts and invoking related notions and assumptions. 'Professionalism' is a narrower term than 'FTP' because it assumes freedom from 'impairment'. Professionalism, then is a concept of ideal practice, whilst FTP concerns itself with minimum acceptable standards. Parker (2006) offered a definition of FTP as having three parts:

1 *Freedom from physical and mental impairment, so that duties can be performed*
2 *'Professional conduct and behaviour', complying with codes of conduct and ethical behaviour*
3 *Clinical/practitioner competence, in terms of skills and knowledge.*

The notion of 'freedom from physical and mental impairment' is an unrealistic concept, and could be usefully rephrased as 'sufficient physical and mental ability to perform duties'. With this modification, the three-part structure could provide a useful framework for considering what professionals require to be 'fit for practice'. It can inform appraisals and revalidation exercises, for instance. However, there is little sense that FTP panels are for assessment and remediation. Rather they appear as disciplinary procedures for people who are unfit to practice because of habitual calculated self-serving behaviour at the expense of others. For professionals who depend on their reputation for their livelihood and personal self-respect, the risk of association with such procedures is anathema. Often, they would suffer in silence rather than risk this.

There may be a case for re-naming existing FTP bodies to better reflect their focus on misconduct, whilst separating out facilities that support greater FTP, particularly in terms of health. This might help build a reality where health conditions can be spoken about more freely, setting aside any conduct issues that can result, rather than such conditions being dealt with in a context that stifles discussion due to the fear and risk.

If we distinguish concerns about illness from concerns about academic failure and from concerns about misconduct, we are better able to discuss and solve some genuine problems relating to the employment of people with health problems, mental and physical. For instance, frequent sickness absence is expensive for employers. Employing a workforce with high anticipated levels of sickness absence involves planning and budgeting for higher staffing levels. Otherwise, workforce pressures contribute to a culture of 'presenteeism' in which staff – and trainees and students – experience compulsion to work to their own detriment and at the expense of reduced standards.

This may be why colleagues report that on the whole there are higher levels of acceptance of an illness or disability in large 'centres of excellence' in contrast with small, poorly funded services where management feel they cannot afford investment in talented people with high sickness rates. Even where finance is not the main concern, smaller populations often have difficulty recruiting staff and high levels of vacancies. We need to advise students about this as they plan to go into the workplace. We also need to develop solutions for employers, so that professionals with health problems are not excluded from making a valuable contribution on the basis that they cannot guarantee 100% attendance. If we are unable to do so, healthier staff are repeatedly asked to cover for their sick colleagues. This might generate resentment expressed as prejudice against those colleagues.

Risks to the Public: Patients, Clients and Pupils

Unsurprisingly, the public at large takes a harsher view of professional misconduct than do members of the professions. In research that sent different case scenarios of medical behaviour to three groups of people, medical students were the most lenient in their judgment of the protagonists' behaviour, whereas qualified doctors took a stricter view of what was permissible, and members of the general public were most draconian in finding conduct unacceptable (Brockbank et al., 2011). The public might reasonably expect that professionals in positions of great trust should have appropriate treatment for any physical or mental disorder, so that their illnesses do not compromise patient safety.

Professionals in the age of social media expose their private lives to public scrutiny more than ever before. Society is still learning to put appropriate checks in place, so this generation of students may be uniquely exposed online (see Chapter 8 for more discussion). For this reason, most medical schools provide explicit advice and discussion about online behaviour. Meanwhile, evaluators struggle to assess the status of inappropriate personal or public material posted by students and professionals.

The equation of mental disorder and risk to the public is hard to address. No-one can claim to be entirely 'non-dangerous' and being asked to prove a low level of danger is impossible. It may seem convenient to use evidence of past behaviour from criminal records or medical records as a straightforward way to screen out 'undesirables' from our professions. We should not succumb to the temptation to assume that either is an accurate and lasting assessment of fitness to practise within a profession. It would discriminate against people who can practices safely whilst failing to flag up individuals who pose high risks. Addressing the implications of a criminal record is not within the scope of this book. Medical history of a mental illness certainly should not disqualify a potential professional from training, but rather prompt assessment of what treatments and support the person may need in order to meet professional standards and remain as well as possible.

Disappointingly, risk assessment in psychiatry is still a very fraught and imperfect art, despite clamour for it to be undertaken. Whatever formal risk assessment tools are used, past behaviour still tends to be the best – though imperfect – predictor of future behaviour, and even this can be balanced by protective factors, treatments and the growing maturity of young individuals. Risk of harm can arise from many sources; it is both lazy and prejudiced to imagine that either a diagnosis or a tick-box risk assessment will reliably identify 'dangerous individuals' and offer protection to the vulnerable.

Risk is not the fixed characteristic of an individual or of an illness, but a dynamic entity that varies over time in terms of the person's maturity and insight, presence or absence of treatments and supports, the characteristics and protective factors associated with any potential victims, the opportunities available for inflicting harm or neglect, including self-harm and self-neglect, and the nature of the environment and culture in which all parties live and work.

Risks to Others from Professionals, Trainees and Students with Mental Illness

Terms like 'risk' and 'harm' are often too general to be useful. In the case of physical risks, we are more likely to identify and consider the specific dangers to the person themselves and to others – the risk of falling as a result of an arthritic condition, the risk of mistakes in surgery if a surgeon's eyesight fails, or the risk of life-threatening diabetic coma in someone with inadequately controlled diabetes. Too often, we fail to clarify exactly which elements of the mental disorder concerned, or the treatment prescribed for it, might impair occupational functioning in the particular role that is under consideration.

The consequences of mental illness may be more nebulous and abstract than those of physical illness but that should not prevent us from trying to envisage and plan around them. Someone with bipolar disorder may become disinhibited without realising this, resulting in embarrassing or even offensive comments or behaviour, or may be more cavalier in recommending treatments. A professional with severe untreated obsessive–compulsive symptoms may be unduly risk averse, or classically may engage in time-consuming, skin-damaging hand-washing rituals. However, some professionals and students demonstrate no such behaviours in their professional practice despite suffering from these conditions, often because they respond well to treatments or supports.

Many studies have focused on the cognitive effects of depression, such as reduced concentration and attention, and fatigue, which is known to have a particularly deleterious effect on occupational performance (Lam et al., 2013). Changes to motivation and sleep pattern may also be important. These problems can be compounded by the effects of medication.

All too few guidelines and treatment studies examine occupational outcomes. The Cochrane Collaboration did conduct a systematic review of available randomised controlled trials of work-directed interventions for depression (Nieuwenhuijsen et al., 2020). This found that a combination of a work-directed intervention and a clinical intervention probably reduces the number of sickness absence days in the shorter term, but with no improvement in the longer-term rates of return to work for depressed individuals. Unfortunately, as we have just discussed, amount of sickness absence taken is only a poor proxy measure of actual occupational performance when at work. This study did not focus on the professions addressed in this chapter, however.

Work can be an aid to, as well as proxy indicator of, recovery from mental ill health. There is evidence for the benefits of work to mental health, and well-being (National Institute for Health and Care Excellence, 2022), leading to increased self-esteem, reduced symptoms of ill health, lowered dependency and risk of relapse. This is likely to be true for work-based training as well as for paid employment, and is particularly relevant in the support of students with a highly valued vocational drive. In my own practice I have seen young people able to tolerate the distress of weight gain in order to recover, fired by their passion for the profession they yearned to pursue.

Background to Student Fitness to Practise Concerns

This chapter is dominated by experience and evidence regarding students of medicine. In 1995 the GMC and UK Medical Schools Council established a Student FTP Working Group, which was in the forefront of FTP in students and trainees, and has influenced many disciplines across the world. The issues discussed do also pertain to students in other disciplines where high standards of behaviour and judgment are required to serve and not harm vulnerable individuals. Departments of nursing, clinical psychology, dentistry, pharmacy, other health care disciplines, social care, teaching, veterinary science and the law, observe similar FTP procedures.

Universities are expected to adjudicate fitness to enter these disciplines, and to provide training towards achieving such standards. This demands developmental and pedagogical wisdom, ethical judgment and sophisticated risk-assessment skills. The ultimate aim cannot be to identify and exclude some theoretical minority of 'flawed' individuals, but rather to examine whether students are healthily aware of their own levels of psychosocial vulnerability and to draw on appropriate supports and treatments to manage these maturely. When this is the case, students will be able to carry compassion and awareness into their profession, understand the importance of contributing to a mentally healthy workplace and well-functioning team, and acknowledge mental as well as physical disorders in a supportive constructive manner in themselves, their colleagues, clients, patients and pupils.

Many mental illnesses occur in acute episodes, even though there may be a lasting vulnerability to such disorders. Between episodes there are periods of healthy function. Only rarely does an illness become a chronic impediment to good functioning. Strangely, many acknowledged lifelong disabilities such as amputations, insulin dependent diabetes, or dyslexia, are regarded as compatible with high functioning given good supports and adjustments. Severe and enduring psychotic disorders certainly exist but it is a myth that all mental disorders are relentless lifelong impediments. In practice, most are episodic and subject to both treatment and suitable environmental adjustments. Even when a person is impaired by an illness so that they are unable to work at one time, it does not follow that this is a lasting state of affairs.

Within medicine, specialities such as psychiatry and general practice will require highly tuned skills in psychological thinking and interpersonal relations. The same is true of mental health nursing, teaching and some legal specialties, so that students who are able to function effectively in other disciplines may not be well-fitted to these. Paradoxically, it is often those individuals who have themselves experienced mental illness who are most effective as practitioners, but this may not apply during periods of acute illness.

The conflation that a person suffering from a mental illness automatically poses danger to the public is both outdated and prejudiced but seems to linger despite guidelines that suggest more sophisticated attitudes. Being 'unfit to practice' may not involve mental disorder. Indeed, it is an oversimplification to place responsibility for ethical practice entirely onto single individuals. In the real world, professional practice depends on whole systems working together, continuing to train together, looking out for each other to correct each other's biases, and working in environments that provide adequate rest and nurturing. We cannot demand individual 'resilience' in chronically challenging conditions.

Modern practice does acknowledge that a culture of individual blame is unrealistic in many settings, and a more systemic approach to critical incident reviews is appearing in professional contexts. However, it is still sometimes the case that an individual should not be allowed to proceed immediately in a professional context if they are clearly at risk of contributing to harm to themselves or others. Many clinicians remember seeing colleagues struggling dangerously but feeling unable to help or intervene for fear of the punitive blame culture.

What is fitness to practise? – The Nursing and Midwifery Council

Being fit to practise requires a nurse, midwife or nursing associate to have the skills, knowledge, health and character to do their job safely and effectively.

The Code sets out the professional standards that nurses, midwives and nursing associates must uphold in order to be registered to practise in the UK.

We will investigate whether someone on our register is fit to practice if an allegation is made that they don't meet our standards for skills, education and behaviour.

If necessary, we will act by removing them from the register for a set period of time or in some cases, permanently. This is called being 'struck off' our register.

The Nursing and Midwifery Council (www.nmc.org.uk/concerns-nurses-midwives/dealing-concerns/what-is-fitness-to-practise/)

Implications of the Word 'Fitness'

We use the word 'fit' in diverse contexts, with favourable implications – 'fit for purpose', 'survival of the fittest', 'keeping fit' or even to describe an sexually attractive person as 'fit'. When we use it negatively there are subtle or not so subtle morally pejorative implications – 'not fit for purpose', 'unfit for practice' and simply 'unfit'. I have not heard physically sick colleagues or students described as 'unfit' or 'not fit' to work or study, nor have I heard of concerns for professionals who are experiencing visual loss being taken to FTP tribunals, Physical health concerns seem on the whole to be handled separately.

We might argue that all health issues should be managed in a separate forum from disciplinary procedures that investigate repeatedly concerning conduct, and that mental health disorders should not be in themselves regarded as red flags. Rather, psychiatric diagnoses should be considered as part of mitigating or potentially treatable factors when misconduct is examined. The legal professions, at the time of writing (in 2021), base such enquiries on conduct, but some lawyers have criticised the system for failing to address the contribution of mental illness and disability to apparent misconduct, and have proposed the setting up of separate bodies to examine 'fitness'.

Whatever the nomenclature, there appears to be an acknowledged problem with the conflation of blameworthy misconduct and mental illness or disability. We need apparatus in both professional and university bodies to separate disciplinary tribunals dealing with misconduct – where mental illness might well be raised as a potential factor – from supportive reviews – where students with any disorder or disability could discuss progress, obstacles to progress and facilitation of studies.

M and N are classmates at medical school. Both have diagnoses of depressive and anxiety disorders. They compared notes and found that both were obliged to report to the Occupational Health Department every 3 months.

M: 'I feel that they're monitoring me as a potential public enemy rather than offering supports to my study and work.'

N: 'They tell me I shouldn't take on optional projects or even give presentations in case it's too 'stressful'.

M: 'But you've published papers and talked about them on TV! It's the same for me – they don't want me to opt for a high prestige speciality, like surgery maybe. They see me as weak and less intelligent because I have a mental history. I don't know if they really could stop me from getting a Surgical job, but I do wonder if maybe I should have kept quiet about my breakdown at school. This is no good for my self-esteem.

N: 'I thought disclosing my depression would get me more help and support but I've spent most of the last 3 years on waiting lists'.

Maturity Issues: Fitness for Professional Training and Study versus Fitness for Independent Practice

A further complexity is inherent in the concept of 'student' status. Healthcare students in particular have privileged clinical contact with patients, and access to confidential documentation, but are not yet independently responsible clinicians. In the UK, initial qualification brings only 'provisional' registration with the GMC for the first year. Thereafter, 'trainee' and 'junior doctor' status persists for many years, under the mentorship and supervision of a responsible consultant. and informal supervision is provided by colleagues in their teams and peer groups. Other professions operate similar structures. University structures apply to the assessment, support and discipline of students, but once they become qualified professionals, they are subject to the disciplinary oversight of the GMC or relevant professional body. Common ethical and practical principles apply to all groups.

'Immaturity' is readily understood in younger students, fresh from school. Professional 'immaturity' can occur at any age when an untrained person first acclimatises to the expectations of a responsible profession. Further developmental considerations arise when people are subjected to extreme stress, and temporarily regress to immature behaviour, dark humour and silliness as a form of stress relief. There is no need to label stress-relieving or merely immature behaviour as 'unprofessional' provided it is undertaken in private, protected situations. The armed forces tolerate a degree of immature behaviour as part of the cost of exposing professionals to extreme stress. Each profession has to set its own boundaries pragmatically and exercise wisdom in expectations as professionals progress, rather than setting arbitrary standards that are too harsh to reliably and fairly enact.

Academic Achievement versus Professionalism

Universities can focus so much on academic evaluation that they become confused by the idea that a student can still fail a course without failing academically. It can seem alien to enact gatekeeping processes without grades and marks to justify this. Staff members are not always aware of options for addressing FTP concerns. They may believe that the only options are for the student to drop out of training or else invoking heavy-handed disciplinary measures.

Students and those who work with them should be aware of the philosophy and practicalities around the concept of FTP, so that when concerns arise the situation is not aggravated by confusion and panic. The idea of a disciplinary tribunal arising catastrophically out of the blue could be replaced by the idea that there is a range of structures supporting good practice.

Training programmes do currently include teaching on ethical and moral aspects of practice, though one student described their teaching on this as 'the lecture on how to stay out of trouble'. More open debates could ensure that both students and staff are kept informed about professional guidelines and about each other's interpretation and attitudes. The discussion of up-to-date FTP documents from the professional body concerned would be a good starting point for such discussion. For instance, medical students, debating the document *Achieving good medical practice: Guidance for medical students* (General Medical Council, 2020), raised the difficulties they perceive in being expected to report conduct concerns about their seniors.

Involving students themselves in collaborative discussions allows them to provide feedback to those who update policy, both at the level of the university and the professional body. Ultimately, though, attendance and participation in workshops and even the submission of reflective essays, might demonstrate intellectual and theoretical skills rather than professional propriety.

Jac was a prize-winning medical student, but as third year progressed, he became anguished about clinical placements and sought help through his GP. His grades were still good, but he ruminated about his responsibility for life and death, and lost sleep worrying how he would cope with the responsibilities of a qualified doctor. Peers offered kindly but ineffectual reassurances and did not visibly feel the same way. He was seen at the psychiatric out-patient department, having been reassured of the measures taken to prevent him meeting people he knew during his attendance. He was diagnosed with anxiety and obsessive–compulsive disorder.

At first, neither therapy nor medication helped, but when he finally agreed to take a year out, he found that outside the hospital environment his symptoms almost vanished and he enjoyed taking on voluntary work. At the end of the year, he took advice from university careers advisors and pursued an 'intercalated' honours year in business studies, to keep his options open. After this he decided to graduate to work in management in a large international medical charity.

It is always worth bearing in mind that a university is entitled to bestow – and a student to receive – the accolade of a degree or other award, without accrediting that student as professionally competent or fit to practice. For example, an individual might achieve an honours degree in Medical or Nursing Sciences and pursue an outstanding career in research, particularly if they don't have the appropriate stamina or interpersonal skills to safely or happily work in clinical practice. We can support students who would not work well in their chosen profession by facilitating them to exercise their intellectual talents in other directions. Closing the door on a chosen career will be painful but it should not be enacted as a punitive gesture, or be accompanied by needless waste of talent and learning.

Paradoxically, the climate of over-arousal around FTP and the sense that FTP procedures are punitive and adversarial leads to less effective protection of both public and practitioners. There is little point having powers and procedures that are too confusing or too distasteful to be invoked. Structures need to be both firm and benign. For instance, one major barrier often cited to terminating a student's enrolment for non-academic reasons is fear of litigation. Teachers find it very hard to make a case for failure of a course or placement, and may be conflicted between their roles as mentor and facilitator versus being gatekeeper or evaluator.

Proactive Approaches to Fitness to Practise: Changes for the Better

FTP processes risk seeming reactive, adversarial and punitive. Whatever we decide to call them, it's important that there are clear criteria set for FTP and supporting policies, and that students themselves are involved in the collaborative development and regular review of such documents. The 'professional' students to whom they apply could be asked to sign agreement to the policy on enrolment to the source, and review their agreement at least each year of training. Whilst FTP panels will never be invoked lightly, they can be normalised by clarity and proper consultation and representation.

Students should have the right to be accompanied at the panel hearing by a lawyer or support person and to have a representative of the student union is in attendance. Students need to be kept fully informed about their rights and options and the available adjudications, and provided with thoughtful feedback. Those cases where the student lacks insight or denies responsibility for demonstrated difficulties will almost inevitably attract appeals and complaints. An institution is better able to defend and assert its decision-making when the system has been set up as democratically and openly as possible.

Transparency and collaboration can do much to improve both student mental health and FTP issues, but it is essential that 'collaboration' involves more than having a token student union representative at tribunals or involved in policy writing. Each individual student has to be assertively involved in discussions, opportunities for self-assessment and encouragement to seek appropriate levels of support. This is not just a matter for those with mental illness and those who have to adjudicate FTP.

It may be challenging to integrate students into both the university culture and into a professional community that values safe practice and a healthy workforce. In the field of physiotherapy, Lo et al. (2018) piloted a proactive initiative in which students are invited at the start of training to confidentially self-declare any issues that they feel could impair their FTP. If they do so they are offered a meeting with a member of staff, using principles of Motivational Enhancement to promote healthy behaviour change. Students were actively involved in setting up the pathway for self-declaration and support, so that the whole initiative fostered reflective practice, and promoted help seeking behaviour. Feedback from both students and clinical educators was positive, with one remarking they learned '... that it isn't "wrong" to have an FTP issue – everyone has them at some stage in their professional/personal lives'.

The primary focus of this chapter is not to examine the effectiveness or otherwise of how to protect the public from malpractice, but rather to discuss better ways to enact such protections. It acknowledges that we may currently be contributing to mental harms rather than mental health in the population of students of the professions. Improvement of FTP policies and processes can only be one aspect of supporting the special mental health needs and fears of this group of students. The other aspect of supporting mental health in professional students involves promoting a healthier, less 'macho' culture.

An important first step is simply to refrain from laughing about alcohol and drug excesses, and to refuse to take part in scorning weakness in colleagues and students. A second step is for students in the Health Professions, Education and Law to be provided with training in approaches such as mental health first aid (Kitchener &

Jorm, 2004). This training was originally developed in Australia, but has since been used in Scotland, Ireland, Hong Kong and the USA. It was especially well received in public sectors, and successful in increasing knowledge and understanding of mental health issues, including participant's own mental health, and in enabling people to talk more comfortably about mental health (Stevenson & Elvy, 2007). I am always wary, though, of adding yet more to an already heavy student curriculum, and would put in a plea for another piece of teaching to be dropped to make way for this – a plea that will surely be controversial.

Meanwhile, rather than waiting for FTP concerns to be raised, each individual member of staff and the student body should find out who is the appropriate person to turn to when they have concerns about either behaviour or illness or both, and to check out what are the likely options open to that person in following up concerns. A book like this cannot save trouble by supplying the 'right' answer, since different institutions have different pathways. University counselling services may not themselves assess such concerns, but they will usually be able to identify those who can.

Alliances of current students and recently qualified professionals with senior faculty members can be powerful in building and repairing trust and refreshing guidelines. Young trainee doctors have a powerful role as ambassadors for a culture of openness and constructive support. Students benefit from talks from trainees and senior students who can describe strategies to cope with vulnerability, relapse, or a period of illness. There may be a risk of 'tokenism' when eminent senior professionals retrospectively disclose their struggles with mental illness, however well-meaning this is. Students point out that such individuals are no longer vulnerable in the same way, or question the severity of the disorders they describe. Nevertheless, such disclosures model courageous, open behaviour and bring hope, as well as demonstrating that mental illness is absolutely not synonymous with inability to contribute to one's chosen career.

I'm a consultant psychiatrist. I have a job I love, in the specialty I love, and it probably all looks like I've been living the dream. But it isn't as straightforward as it might look. My career in psychiatry actually started on the other side, as a psychiatric inpatient going through multiple admissions, medications and courses of electroconvulsive therapy. . .

I felt driven to do well and to show people I could be a good psychiatrist, as well as a patient, and I worked very hard, probably too hard. But despite my anxieties, I experienced little stigma or discrimination, and ultimately gained the consultant job that I wanted most, in my home city – in the very hospital where I had been a patient. . . I have been ill again, over the years, but am lucky enough to usually be well in between. I have also had huge support from colleagues, all of whom know about my illness. . .

The risk of becoming unwell again casts a cloud and can make me hesitate to take on new projects. I was last treated with electroconvulsive therapy 2 years ago, and continue to take lithium and antidepressants. But the truth is that I love my work, and with the support I have, I usually feel able to take those chances. . .

I want other trainees to know what happened to me, so that they can see what is possible. So every few months I give a short talk about my illness, how I got through, what helped me. After the first time I did it, I thought I could never do it again, it felt so exposing. But the feedback was good, and I haven't looked back.

One in four people experience a mental health problem of some kind each year. To demand that psychiatrists come from among the mentally unblemished is not only unrealistic, it would mean a potential waste of talent and empathy that we can scarcely afford. If my story helps anyone unsure of their capacity to take on the job, or worried about the "dark secret" of their own psychological troubles, then I think it's worth telling.

Dr Rebecca Lawrence, The Guardian (Lawrence, 2020)

We have emphasised throughout this handbook, that a majority of the population will have met criteria for at least one diagnosable mental illness by midlife, with half of these disorders manifest by age 18. Having a mental illness is in fact 'normal'. An individual's FTP in a demanding profession may not depend so much on whether they are coping with a disorder as to what coping strategies they are using. Some hallmarks of good professionalism are having insight to recognise one's disorder, humility to admit the need for help and accept treatment, and courage to declare the situation to authorities. Most professional guidelines do acknowledge this, but in practice, institutions and human beings struggle to enact the spirit of what is written down.

Practice Points

Society, Professionals and Students

- We expect professional institutions to provide training, support and scrutiny for their membership so that we can trust them with confidential and precious matters.
- Mental illness is not synonymous with occupational impairment, and someone can certainly be unfit to practise without being mentally ill. However, most FTP regulations conflate by implication the ideas of mental illness and irresponsible behaviour.
- Most of us experience mental illnesses in our lives, so it's impractical as well as unethical to exclude students from the caring professions on such grounds.
- The phenomenon of 'intersectionality' means students who are already disadvantaged as result of culture, race, class, poverty or gender, are likely to be disproportionately affected by FTP stigma. These groups need extra information and supports to alleviate catastrophic assumptions and highlight benefits of mental health supports.

Parents, Families and Schools

- Parents and other family members, as well as schools, should be wary of investing too heavily in children's ambitions to become doctors, nurses, lawyers, teachers or members of other prestigious professions.
- If the chosen career turns out to be unsuitable for the student's well-being, they will survive their disappointment better if it is not amplified by a sense that they have let down the whole family.

Professional Bodies and Disciplines

- Individuals drawn to these careers may be constitutionally vulnerable to mental illness.

- The close-knit student cultures within the specialities may encourage unhealthy coping strategies. The cultures may also raise obstacles to accessing the mental health supports we need to build optimal FTP.
- The current culture of medicine and related professions increases rather than protects against mental illness. We need to shape professional cultures to be more fit to train and practise in.

University Governance, Fitness to Practise Tribunals and Panels

- Universities need clear, well-publicised policies and pathways for disciplinary FTP concerns. These should be clearly demarcated and explicitly separated from mental health services.
- FTP regulations may be perceived as so threatening that students judge it safer to suffer mental illness in silence.
- Fears are embedded in student mythology rather than necessarily reflecting university practice. However, since stigma and mistrust have passed into the culture, there is a real risk of untreated mental illness leading to avoidable suffering and impairment, with paradoxical consequences for quality of service to the public.
- FTP is everyone's business! Policies should be regularly reviewed and redeveloped in collaboration with students and recently graduated trainees as well as faculty policy makers.
- Students have much to learn and to offer in collaborating in FTP panels and reviews, in creating and revising protocols and publicising resources.

Well-Being and Awareness for Students of the Professions

- The most intractable issue in FTP concerns is where a student or practitioner lacks insight into the consequences of their own behaviour. Insight can often be improved with a combination of maturity and regular discussion. Episodic loss of insight during a mental illness can be managed with forward planning.
- Students in the professions should be encouraged to learn mental health first aid and self-help cognitive behavioural therapy techniques. This can help the students themselves and benefit to peers and clients.
- Interviews for entry to medical schools and later job interviews should invite candidates to discuss what benefits might come from experiencing illness personally or in those close to them, and to provide examples of good practice in supporting sick colleagues.
- Students speak highly of the benefits of hearing from practising professionals with psychiatric diagnoses about their own experiences and advice.

References

Brewster, J. M., Kaufmann, I. M., Hutchison, S. & MacWilliam C. (2008). Characteristics and outcomes of doctors in a substance dependence monitoring programme in Canada: Prospective descriptive study. *BMJ*, 337, a2098.

Brockbank, S., David, T. J. & Patel, L. (2011). Unprofessional behaviour in medical students: A questionnaire-based pilot study comparing perceptions of the public with medical students and doctors. *Medical Teacher*, 33(9), e501–e508.

Carr, D. (2008). Character education as the cultivation of virtue. *Handbook of Moral & Character Education*, 99–116.

Crofts, P. (2020). Studying medicine affected my mental health – here's what I learnt.

BMJ, 370, m3664. https://doi.org/10.1136/bmj.m3664

Department of Health (2008). *Mental health and ill health in doctors.*

Gossop, M., Stephens, S., Stewart, D., Marshall, J., Bearn, J. & Strang, J. (2001). Health care professionals referred for treatment of alcohol and drug problems. *Alcohol & Alcoholism*, 36(2), 160–4.

Grant, A., Rix, A., Winter, P., Mattick, K. & Jones, D. (2015). Support for medical students with mental health problems: A conceptual model *Academic Psychiatry*, 39, 16–21.

Hays, R. B., Lawson, M. & Gray, C. (2011). Problems presented by medical students seeking support: A possible intervention framework. *Medical Teacher*, 33(2), 161–4.

Kitchener, B. A. & Jorm, A. F. (2004). Mental health first aid training in a workplace setting: A randomized controlled trial [ISRCTN13249129]. *BMC Psychiatry*, 4(1), 1–8.

Lam, R. W., Malhi, G. S., McIntyre, R. S., et al. (2013). Fatigue and occupational functioning in major depressive disorder. *Australian & New Zealand Journal of Psychiatry*, 47(11), 989–91.

Lawrence, R. (2020, 16 September). *I thought mental illness meant I'd never be a doctor. Now I'm a consultant psychiatrist.* The Guardian.

Lo, K., Francis-Cracknell, A., Hopmans, R. & Maloney, S. (2018). Online fitness to practise specific module alters physiotherapy students' health knowledge, perceptions and intentions. *New Zealand Journal of Physiotherapy*, 46(2), 79–87. https://doi.org/10.15619/NZJP/46.2.05

Miller, L. (2009). Doctors, their mental health and capacity for work. *Occupational Medicine*, 59(1):53–5. https://doi.org/10.1093/occmed/kqn111

National Institute for Health and Care Excellence (2022). *Mental wellbeing at work.* www.nice.org.uk/guidance/NG212

Nieuwenhuijsen, K., Verbeek, J. H., Neumeyer-Gromen, A., Verhoeven, A. C., Bültmann, U. & Faber, B. (2020). Interventions to improve return to work in depressed people. *Cochrane Database of Systematic Reviews*, (10), CD006237.

Oliver, M. N., Bernstein, J. H., Anderson, K. G., Blashfield, R. K. & Roberts, M. C. (2004). An exploratory examination of student attitudes toward 'impaired' peers in clinical psychology training programs. *Professional Psychology: Research and Practice*, 35(2), 141.

Parker, M. (2006). Assessing professionalism: theory and practice, *Medical Teacher*, 28(5), 399–403.

Rosenberg, J. I., Getzelman, M. A., Arcinue, F. & Oren, C. Z. (2005). An exploratory look at students' experiences of problematic peers in academic psychology programs. *Professional Psychology: Research and Practice*, 36, 665–73.

Rotenstein, L. S., Ramos, M. A., Torre, M., et al. (2016). Prevalence of depression, depressive symptoms, and suicidal ideation among medical students: A systematic review and meta-analysis. *JAMA*, 316(21), 2214–36. https://doi.org/10.1001/jama.2016.17324

Stevenson, R. & Elvy, N. (2007). *Evaluation of Scotland's mental health first aid.* Edinburgh: NHS Health Scotland. www.healthscotland.com/uploads/documents/5015-RE037FinalReport0506.pdf

Sykes, C., Borthwick, C. & Baker, E. (2020). *Mental health and wellbeing in the medical profession.* British Medical Association. www.bma.org.uk/media/1361/bma-mental-health-and-wellbeing-medical-profession-research-summary-oct-2019.pdf

Winter, P., Rix, A. & Grant, A. (2017). Medical student beliefs about disclosure of mental health issues: A qualitative study. *Journal of Veterinary Medical Education*, 44(1), 147–56.

Summing It All Up
Seven Key Challenges for UK University Mental Health

This final chapter summarises themes that have recurred repeatedly when we considered mental health in UK universities. It emphasises the ways in which their interactions amplify and complicate the effects of each single issue. It calls for thoughtful action, rather than suggesting 'quick fixes', and appreciates the potential for mental well-being and human development in university communities.

As a child psychiatrist in the early years of this century I read the book *Toxic Childhood* (Palmer, 2006). Sue Palmer, a schoolteacher and writer, described the loss of traditional childhood freedoms, and of traditional routines and rhythms of eating and sleeping. She flagged the dangers of what she called the 'electronic village' where children roamed unprotected by their elders. I recognised many of the features she described in my patients and in their peers, regardless of whether or not they were suffering from a diagnosable disorder. I was both curious and anxious to see how that generation of children would fare as they grew into young adulthood. In writing this book I have had the opportunity to examine how life has turned out for those children.

Many of the problems Palmer described have intensified rather than been resolved over the past 16 years. Late adolescence is also the time of life when most of the severe mental illnesses occur. The problems we see in psychiatric clinics today are not only the direct results of mental 'disorders', but also the interactions of illness and vulnerability with environmental and developmental factors.

The process of researching and writing this book has left me deeply concerned by the environment – in every sense of that word – in which young people grow and develop. I hope the book may inform and encourage discussion, and suggest different options for action on UK university mental health. Some key issues have emerged repeatedly in my experience, in my study of the literature, and in conversations with the many academics, students, staff, parents, patients and politicians who have contributed their experiences and views.

Key Challenges to UK University Mental Health

Seven Key Challenges for UK University Mental Health

1. **Transitions** – into university, through university life, out of university (Chapters 2 & 3)
2. **The need to belong** – family as secure base, new peer groups, embracing diversities (Chapters 2, 4, 8, 10, 11 & 12)
3. **Finance** – equity for all backgrounds, commercialisation of university life, individual financial savvy (Chapter 9)

4. **Mental illness** – prevention, diagnosis, management, need for a joined up approach (Chapters 13–18)
5. **Routine and structure** – sleep, nutrition, exercise, organisational skills (Chapter 5)
6. **Social media** – and online gaming (Chapter 8)
7. **Intoxication** – alcohol, drugs (Chapters 6 & 7)

The evidence from a range of topics accumulated during the writing of this handbook to focus on seven key issues that struck me as most salient in determining the overall mental health of university communities in the UK. The broad headings for these challenges are: transitions, the need to belong, finance, routine and structure, social media, mental illness and intoxication (box). The rest of this chapter considers their importance and their interactions. Researchers, regulators and university students and staff have paid attention to some of the challenges, even over the time it has taken to write and edit the book. For instance, the importance of transitions, with the associated recognition of developmental issues, has attracted interest from mental health and educational specialists, and is guiding the realignment of services. This is also a result of the campaigning by parents who have lost a student child to suicide.

Transitions and Attachments

Universities getting better at recognising parental emotional as well as financial participation in the lives of their student children. They are finding ways to ensure that where parents are supportive, they can be consulted about students who are at risk, whilst respecting principles of privacy and confidentiality. Some universities have also understood the plight of 'estranged students' and those who are themselves carers. These young people suffer a range of financial, academic and social obstacles to a fulfilling university experience.

As we acknowledge the power of a secure family base – and the secure base provided by schools – there has been more focus on providing secure and consistent new attachments at university. 'University families' and other forms of mentorship are fostered, not least the excellent mental health mentorship scheme, which provides consistent specialist mental health mentorship for students disclosing a mental health condition. We are getting better at encouraging students to declare their health needs and to register with a general practitioner (GP), and universities offer the remarkable benefit of in-house counselling and support services, free of charge. These are not yet optimally linked up with the NHS, although ambitious projects such as that in Manchester are pioneering schemes to address this.

There is UK-wide debate about reconfiguring NHS mental health services to better manage the transition from child and adolescent mental health services to adult services. For most students, the move from school, and often away from home, to university brings about a natural transition that has to be managed in any case. It would be helpful if the move of services could be allowed to happen more flexibly at the point of moving to university rather than rigidly on the 18th birthday.

Moreover, there is another inevitable transition when the student completes their course or leaves in an unplanned way. This transition is so far relatively neglected, despite being an equally dangerous time in the young person's life. Again, I suggest matching the service transition to the life event rather than to some arbitrary age. As I have proposed in Chapter 18, professionals in mental health could benefit from a faculty and speciality of university mental health, which as its hallmark would teach and deliver expertise in the management of transitions, and support the development towards maturity that characterises this stage of life. There would also be special attention to treatment that allows optimal academic performance.

It would be wise to reassess the workloads of GPs who treat more mental than physical ill health, so that those who have a younger caseload are not disadvantaged. Since the COVID lockdown experience, we're also in a better position to provide realistic appointments for the mobile university population, using telemedicine or even simply telephone appointments.

The Current State of UK Universities: The Business Model

The very institutions addressed in this book – UK universities – have been a moving target. They have changed even over the past few months and years, and are very different institutions from those that existed in previous decades. As a result, older research may be outdated unless it addresses very general and fundamental issues. Often the changes are welcome – the fresh diversity of university membership can be a social and academic strength, and broadening access to poorer students and staff is a worthy aim. The scale and speed of change has disturbed me, though.

It has been fascinating to turn the spotlight on our universities from my current perspective in later life. When my mother went to university after the second world war, she was supported by a generous grant, seen legally as a child because she was under 21, and guided by staff who were 'in loco parentis' When my siblings and I attended university in the 1970s, there were still free tuition, government grants and institutional canteens and facilities, but we were deemed adults, demanded political powers, and felt privileged. Many of today's universities were then accounted 'training colleges' or 'technical colleges' and did not award degrees.

By the time my children and their cousins went to university this millennium, virtually all their classmates who had stayed on after age 16 expected to attend university. Half the UK population now attends university, and most of the institutions concerned are dominated by the teaching of young students. Scholarship for its own sake is an exception, and research may be valued more because of its business potential than as the core task. The shift to charging tuition fees and the replacement of grants by loans has been another factor in universities' following commercial pressures.

It is clear (Chapter 9) that there are well-evidenced interactions between finance and mental health at different levels of university life, with implications for staff, students, families, scholars, the government and the wider community. Young students face pressures to be 'consumers' of education, accommodation and other aspects of a student lifestyle. They receive only patchy training and support to manage their finances confidently. Students from affluent and supportive families are greatly privileged in contrast with those without, and this is not sufficiently recognised by university finance bodies.

We can theorise alternative ways to finance higher education on this scale. They would require significant changes to student experience, or alternatively increases in our taxes. For instance, young people might be expected to attend their home university, to avoid accommodation expenses. Tertiary education might be funded as a further level of schooling, paid for by the taxpayer. Such a model might be followed by the reconfiguration of some institutions as graduate schools, as in the United States, to accommodate more advanced specialist scholarship and research. At the undergraduate level, teaching might be shared between resident higher education tutors with special interest and training in pedagogy, by visiting lecturers from graduate institutions, or some combination of these.

Now that universities have moved into the business model, though, it is likely that 'consumer' demand rather than assertive redesign will determine their evolution. My hope is that however they change in the coming decades, the well-being and mental health of the whole population should be a priority in redesign.

Meanwhile, individual students arrive at university with differing levels of financial concern and confidence. Many go on to graduate (or leave prematurely)with increased financial stresses. Evidence suggests that financial stress in itself contributes to the onset of mental illness, while established mental disorders in turn feed into vicious spirals of decline. In these cases, treatment should involve financial counselling and well as psychological and medical treatments.

The combination of financial stress with maladaptive coping strategies such as gambling, sex working and drug dealing can lead students into association with a criminal culture, which is destructive to individual and community well-being. Debt and financial concern are associated with poorer mental health and academic underperformance at university and after graduation (See Chapter 9). As the whole world emerges from COVID and is stricken by war and climate emergency, it is not realistic to merely call for more money for all students. It is essential to promote greater financial equity and to teach and support students as individuals to develop confidence in managing finance and necessary debt.

Changes in How We Think of Mental Health and Mental Illness

The twin focus of the book, the climate of mental health and mental disorders, has been in flux too. Only this year (2022) the UK has moved from old diagnostic systems to the new World Health Organization's eleventh revision of the International Classification of Diseases. This dry fact reflects enormous amounts of debate and research, advancing attitudes to the very nature of mental illness and its management. Universities have hosted much of the research, in partnership with health services or by recruiting students themselves as study samples.

Policy has shifted towards supporting the whole university, rather than solely those students experiencing mental health difficulties while recognising this group still requires specialist support (Thorley, 2017). Research often focuses on factors linked to poorer mental health in individuals, rather than institutional level understanding though.

Mental health is not synonymous with a state of constant happiness, though it includes experiences of happiness in its range, but closer to the term 'maturity'. Indeed, recognising a person's level of maturity and providing support and challenges appropriate to that level, is key to maintaining well-being. The opponents of 'therapeutic education' point out that we can inhibit more mature behaviour by failing to expect it of young people. This is true only up to a point. The terms 'transition aged youth', 'thresholders' and 'emerging adults' remind us that 18-to-25-year-olds are not yet on a plateau of 'adulthood'. It is already a demanding task to get used to the internal changes in the brain and mind at this age. Imposing more external change and transition can lead to regression or breakdown in some individuals, even though it can stimulate personal growth and positive transformation in others.

Young people and their own representative bodies (including but not limited to student unions) are pioneers in their openness about mental ill health and their emphasis on its importance. In contrast there has been opposition to too much provision of 'therapeutic education'. This need not be a binary debate, although the phenomenon of 'cancel culture' associated with social media can shut down healthy discussion.

There is increasing understanding of the sheer range and difference of mental conditions and mental disorders, showing that more people than ever before can identify a treatable or manageable mental condition. There are two strands for consideration. On the one hand there is 'well-being' and on the other 'mental illness', with considerable overlap when it comes to experiences of anxiety, depression and trauma. We'll never abolish mental illness completely but can minimise environmental contributions to falling ill and also improve services to treat mental illness as well as make an environment where it's easier to recover.

In writing this book, I noticed a third dimension, as well as the polarities of well-being and mental disorders. People experience individual difference that are not defects or disorders but bring suffering if diversity is not nurtured. People in minority groups in terms of ethnicity, neurodiversity, sexual preference and gender identity, may all find themselves in such contexts. People feel insulted if their belonging to a minority group is treated as if it were a disorder, but we should formally recognise and mitigate the disadvantages of living with difference in a powerful mainstream culture.

Examining the consequences of significant mental illness for students and university staff has emphasised for me the helpful role of diagnosis. We might want to 'spare' our patients the distress or stigma of diagnosis, but in doing so we underplay their suffering, deprive them of evidenced treatments, support and benefits. In the past, a mental health diagnosis was often in itself a poor prognosis. Today it is a signpost to potential recovery, the more so for young intelligent adults.

The Current State of UK University Mental Health

The mental health of young university students is not very different from that of their peers who don't attend university, once due allowance is made for social advantage or deprivation and levels of education. The differences relate to a number of potentially modifiable factors, but currently those factors are not always taken into account. Unhealthy binge cultures around alcohol and drugs are condoned, at the same time as encouraging greater openness about mental health. Larger numbers of counsellors and other mental health support staff and being provided. Such services are shown by research to be effective in addressing common conditions such as depressive and anxiety disorders. However, they are still insufficiently linked up to our overstretched NHS mental health services.

The mental health and well-being of university staff, whether academic or support staff, is certainly a cause for concern. Staff are far less likely than students to 'disclose' a diagnosable mental condition to their university and to be provided with adjustments to their role. When staff suffer in their own right, there are further adverse effects on the university culture and on their capacity to provide pastoral care. Ironically, the increased burden of pastoral care is a big factor in their distress.

University policies should ensure academic and teaching staff don't have disproportionate responsibility for student well-being and clarify that staff well-being is an integral part of duty of care. Institutions should acknowledge the inevitable pressures of balancing pastoral support with the other expectations of academic roles. Formal university recognition for academics who provide pastoral support – financially and in terms of status – would be an excellent start in destigmatising and valuing mental health.

Why Mental Health Matters in UK Universities

I have spent my working life in the service of human mental health and healing, but can't take it for granted that everyone shares my assumption that this is a supreme priority. Universities do not exist to improve our mental health, but rather to employ it in the service of other goals. Increasingly these goals are financial as well as academic or service-related goals. Students, academics and their families are likely to choose an institution for reasons that may scarcely involve their mental well-being record, and be more swayed by indices of scholarly achievement, or for their record of graduate employment. Student satisfaction scores, indices of student retention on courses, the financial success of the university and rankings in various 'league tables' all affect profitability, both for the university itself and for those investing in the education offered.

Now that universities are businesses, resourcing mental health is more likely to be seen as a desirable investment if it increases the achievements, rankings and prestige of the institution. Happily, current research on student well-being suggests an indissociable and bi-directional relationship between mental and academic performance. As we might expect, positive well-being is associated with enhanced cognitive and psychological functioning. Successful treatment of mental illness has been repeatedly shown to improve academic performance, too.

Some of our highest achieving young people are predisposed to certain mental illnesses or to conditions of neurodiversity. Since more than 50% of all mental illnesses starts in the teens and early twenties, supporting the mental health of staff and students is a massive investment in the achievement and success of the university. Choice of a university that will reliably provide such support is also a good investment in the student's or staff member's own mental health and academic and career success. I would hope the university UK Mental Health Charter scheme can guide all involved in providing students with a psychological environment in which education can be most effective.

Early Assertive Diagnosis and Treatment of Mental Disorders in Students and Staff, Recognition of Longer Recovery Times

It is taking time to reach a climate of respect for mental disorders on a par with physical disorders.

The university student age group tends to enjoy good physical health but often poor mental health. This is costly to society and to general practice. Three groups of severe mental illness have disproportionately high rates of suicide – Schizophrenia, bipolar disorder, and anorexia nervosa – but effective treatment can save lives.

There are effective treatments even for the most severe mental illnesses that affect young students. However, it takes far longer to see recovery than with most physical conditions. The mind and brain take a long time to recover and heal – months and years rather than days and weeks. Policies on admissions, fitness to study and time taken out of studies for recovery from a severe mental illness need to take account of the long timespans taken to recover from these disorders. Students who have to take time out of academic studies – or who need to leave their course – need extra monitoring and support, as this is a time of high risk.

The key to accessing all NHS treatment is to be signed on with a local GP, which may prove challenging in the current climate of GP workforce shortages. However, for students, there is a parallel source of free mental health support – though not psychiatric treatment as such. Students and staff are provided with a large range of mental health supports, many of them boasting excellent outcomes, but there is still work to do to dovetail different services around a vulnerable student. The challenge is greatest when NHS as well as in-house university services are needed. Integrative models such as that piloted in Greater Manchester show promise, but different universities and geographical locations may need different solutions.

'Disclosing' a mental health condition to the university provides rights to support, services and finance – the disabled students allowance (DSA). The option of mental health mentorship, funded by DSA, can be transforming. Students with a significant level of depression or one of the more severe disorders are likely to require longer courses of therapy than counselling services routinely offer. They may also require prescribing of medication from a GP or psychiatrist.

For students with a diagnosed mental illness, including medication in a treatment plan has much to recommend it. Young people can recover faster, can benefit from the ready availability and convenience of medication and can access psychotherapies alongside medication to enhance benefits. Prescribing needs to take into account the youth of the student, and for female students, treatments that would be safe during any future pregnancy.

Individuals drawn to professions such as medicine, nursing and the law may be constitutionally vulnerable to mental illness. The close-knit student cultures within the specialities may encourage unhealthy coping strategies and increase rather than protect against mental illness. Fitness-to-practise regulations may be perceived as so threatening that such students judge it safer to suffer mental illness in silence.

Suicide Prevention and 'Postvention'

Suicide is one of the leading causes of death in the student age group, especially in young men, and is probably increasing in prevalence. Use of alcohol and other substances is a predisposing factor to an individual's risk of suicide, and alcohol and substance use overwhelmingly occur around the time of death itself. Social media and other aspects of the internet interact in complex ways to increase the likelihood of suicide. Effective regulation and research are needed.

Asking about suicidal thoughts does not increase the likelihood of a person acting on them, although it may be difficult to converse usefully with an intoxicated person. All members of the university, particularly staff, need regular updates about emergency contacts and resources. A range of online and real-life training courses is available, but links with counselling staff and clinicians to discuss concerns provide greatest confidence in helping when a student or member of staff may be suicidal.

Websites should be kept updated and linked with helpful resources, including very simple instructions for people in a crisis. Institution's policies and practice on information- sharing agreements should be reviewed to consider permissions about when to contact next of kin.

The distress of a death by suicide does not end with the life taken. If we are to learn from tragedies, and in order to support survivors, institutions need 'postvention' plans with a dedicated team to address the tragedy (See Chapter 17).

Social Media

The role of social media in suicide provocation and prevention is being intensely debated. Our online virtual life can dominate every aspect of our existence, but is often a secret and intimate experience, unshared with carers and mentors. When we are concerned about someone's mental health or well-being, it is helpful to include questions such as 'what's going on for you online?' We are only just waking up to the relentless commercial interests – rather than our best interests – driving online interactions. Legal and institutional regulation are still inadequate to protect young people from exploitation and harm, particularly when they are deemed 'adults'.

There is progress in evidence-based online interventions to protect school pupils in the digital world. These might be adopted and adapted by university staff and unions. Meanwhile student use of social media is not only a potential threat to the reputation of the individual and the university but is insidiously damaging student well-being and academic performance.

Body Image and Its Disorders

Society's preoccupation with body image is amplified in the media, including social media, and can threaten well-being in a community even when it stops short of a mental disorder. Universities inevitably host many young people with diagnosable eating disorders, given the demographic involved. Specialist eating disorders services have reported a further increase in referrals since the pandemic.

Every university should build links with the local specialist eating disorders service – usually the adult eating disorders service. An adolescent with an existing eating disorder is likely to become much more vulnerable to relapse after the transition to university unless this is carefully managed. However, eating disorders can develop at any age. Staff as well as students may experience these conditions. Eating disorders do not all take the same form, and require tailor-made treatments. It is worth recognising that anorexia nervosa is the most lethal of all psychiatric disorders. This is only partly due to deaths relating to the physical consequences. There is also a high rate of death by suicide.

Loss of Rhythms and Routines

Even young resilient bodies and brains suffer when our inherent 'biorhythms' are not respected. Modern society provides all too many opportunities for dysregulation – jet lag, shift work, 24-hour lighting, availability of fast food, international online gaming at all hours, smartphones in bedrooms – and the looser timetables of university life compared with school permit further loss of rhythm.

There are demonstrated benefits in having routines around regular social mealtimes, adequate sleep and physical activity. These contribute to good grades and better relationships, which in turn improve self-respect and well-being and protect against mental illness. Older academics have suggested the restoration of subsidised university canteens, dining halls, and tearooms, where staff and students meet and socialise together. These could go some way to providing an alternative way to socialise to the current dominant binge-drinking culture.

Universities could make modest contributions to re-establishing an environment more friendly to healthy biorhythms. These might include high-quality institutional staff and student dining rooms and a restructuring of student timetables so that lectures start after 10 a.m. This would accommodate the sleep patterns of the young brain. Good enough nutrition is important, though obsessive attention to calories is not. Physical activity, including outdoor activity, is important for physical and mental health – it shouldn't be just a competitive activity for the elite.

New Recognition of Diversity

Better nurturing of ethnic diversity in university communities can be associated with improved academic achievement as well as improved well-being. However, it goes beyond these considerations in being ethically and humanely right. Those of us enjoying white privilege face the challenge of recognising our defensiveness and discomfort, as 'white fragility' blocks progress and justice. The stance of respectful curiosity is a more helpful approach.

Universities have experimented with a number of interventions to improve awareness of prejudice and to reduce racism. All too often they merely pay lip service to an anti-racist stance. Newer approaches could include –

- actively seeking to appoint more Black, Asian and minority ethnic (BAME) staff
- providing assertive welcome and support to staff from minority groups of all sorts and ensuring they are not left out of pathways to promotion, recognition and grant applications
- signing the university up to Advance HE's race equality charter
- providing 'reverse buddying' to pair up senior staff with juniors and students from diverse backgrounds, to expand their understanding of the issues faced
- recruiting more BAME counsellors and health practitioners, not necessarily to match them with clients of the same background, but to improve the ethnic diversity of the clinical group.
- Providing extra support for a return to studies after a mental illness for all students from minority backgrounds, as they are at increased risk of dropping out

Students who identify as belonging to minorities in terms of sexual orientation or gender identity can experience increased vulnerability to mental health difficulties and diagnosable conditions. Like other minorities they can find too much focus on the differences between their experiences and those of the 'mainstream' and too little focus on human commonalities. Virtually all students who leave home discover liberation to experiment with sexual behaviour and identity. For some students, this poses problems for trust and communication with the family of origin. The sexual dimension of life is so particularly important to the student age group that this should be part of any assessment and treatment plan.

School pupils and students alike have commented on the emphasis of educational input on the mechanics and physical risks of sexual behaviour and too little discussion of ethical and relational concerns. They report that such classes show inadequate awareness of the context to their sexual concerns. In contrast, some school sex education is shown to protect students from gender-based violence throughout their university career and beyond (see Chapter 12).

Students with neurodiversity may need extra support to negotiate the role of sexuality in their development, and this significant minority group is particularly vulnerable to developing mental health disorders and to have an increased prevalence of suicide. There is almost certainly an underdiagnosis of both ASD and ADHD in girls and probably in ethnic and other minority groups.

Culturally-Endorsed Intoxication: An Elephant in the Room

The most striking experience in writing this book was the frequency with which student use of alcohol and other recreational drugs cropped up in the research evidence. This is more marked in the UK than in the United States, and perhaps even more than elsewhere in Europe. The long-term risks are of concern to public health specialists. For the purposes of this book, I have focussed on the culture of deliberately setting out to become as acutely intoxicated as possible and its acute consequences.

The book provides separate chapters on the use of alcohol and of other drugs of recreational and voluntary use. This was based on the different legal status, regulation, and research evidence relating to them. There are aspects that do not overlap, but the outstanding message for me was that the UK university culture fosters the activity of regular acute intoxication.

I feel obliged to strongly recommend serious consideration of the use of alcohol in our universities. We are not necessarily talking about reduction in the overall amounts of alcohol consumed. I am convinced that significant reduction in binge drinking could result in improvements in many areas of well-being and in academic performance. It is an extremely uncomfortable topic to raise with people within or outside the walls of our universities. The message is not about demanding a new temperance movement, but a focus on the acute risks of the growing and entrenched binge culture.

My impression is that the activity I observe to be dangerous – acute communal intoxication – is one that is engaged in very deliberately and valued for its own sake despite, or even partly because of, the risks involved. It can feel almost as if I were to question practices such as mountaineering, cycling or water sports, on the basis of their dangers and associated deaths.

Alcohol use at UK universities is associated with

- increased risks of unwanted and unprotected sexual behaviours
- misuse of other drugs and substances, and with gambling and gaming to excess.
- social exclusion of non-drinkers – often women and ethnic minority groups
- poorer academic performance
- disinhibition
- fitness-to-practise concerns in students of the professions
- worsening of existing mental illness and potential interaction with prescribed medication
- increased frequency and severity of deliberate self-harm
- death by suicide.

At present there is widespread anxiety about mental disorders, suicides, sexual trauma and offensive behaviour, alongside apparent acceptance of an intoxication culture that increases their prevalence. We need to acknowledge the connexions so that we can balance our values and approaches.

How Can We Ensure Mental Health Is a Priority in UK Universities?

The UK population as a whole has become more interested in the mental health of students. This very interest will help prioritise the issue, but will require some form of measurement to hold institutions to account in terms of achievement. Currently such measures of success include indices of academic achievement, research league tables, figures on employment rates and salaries after graduation, student satisfaction scores, figures on student retention on courses, and awards to individuals or institutions as a whole. Some universities now subscribe to charter marks such as the Athena Swann gender fairness programme, and more recently we have The Mental Health Charter. This is one way for universities to enhance their reputation and prestige in the service of mental health on campus.

It may be even more powerful as motivation for institutions to know that mentally healthy students (as measured by a variety of criteria) are more likely to thrive academically, to complete their courses and achieve good grades. We may appeal to financial incentives. Analyses repeatedly show that the costs to society of providing medical and mental health treatment are significantly lower than the costs of neglecting to do so. The financial cost to society, though, is not directly borne by universities. Government intervention may be needed to co-ordinate re-direction of resource.

Universities are ideally placed to conduct research into the whole range of mental health and to provide critical commentary on results. There are already organisations linking such research across the UK, such as the 'SMaRTeN' projects (www.smarten.org.uk/about.html) Both research agendas and audits of university mental health policies could usefully bear in mind the seven key challenges I have outlined.

This book, and in particular this chapter, has attempted to integrate the current concerns about UK university mental health and extract some key features. It has not done so through systematic research methodology, but there are scientific ways to extract themes for research, which could be usefully applied. There is value in identifying headline issues, to inform both further research and current practice. For instance, I use a list of prompts to try to capture the most relevant challenges to troubled students and university staff.

Using the Seven Key Challenges to Better Understand the Experience of Staff or Students

This is not a script for an interrogation, but a prompt to include key well-being issues in conversations with troubled students. Carers, counsellors, clinicians and staff might want to prepare possible responses and local resources so that they can respond most helpfully.

What's going on for you just now? Have there been any big changes in life lately, or anything coming up? What are you afraid might happen?

What's going well? What are your potential resources and strengths? Who can you rely on?

How are you getting on with other people, is there a group of people you feel you belong to? Have there been any fallings out? Are you worried about someone else?

Have you got any money worries?

Is there anything troubling on social media or online?

How are you sleeping? Eating? Are you physically active? Are you managing to study/research/teach and get things delivered on time?

How much do you drink? Any other recreational substances? Medications?

Have you had any mental health conditions in the past? What helped you cope with those?

Has it been so bad you felt life wasn't worth living?

It has been a moving experience as I have written this book to find myself contemplating the ways in which diverse students and their academic and support staff negotiate their development together. Young adults pass through a sort of initiation from being relatively passive recipients of adult care, to being agents of their own well-being, subject to the support of their chosen groups and to the rulings of university authorities. They can benefit from the influences of past and present wisdom and experience, from philosophical and environmental structures, and as they emerge from adolescence into adult life, they are empowered to bring their own contributions to the structures that serve them.

The Royal College of Psychiatrists, to which I belong, says 'There is no health without mental health'. The mental health of today's students and their peers determines the social, emotional, academic, economic, physical and spiritual health of our future, as a human race and as a planet. There could scarcely be any more worthwhile investment.

> University life brings huge pressures. They act like a pressure cooker and reveal the cracks in anyone's psyche. But this is true of any rite of passage, and though I see a lot of distress, most of all I SEE THE GROWTH.
>
> Elrika, University Counsellor

References

Palmer, S. (2006). *Toxic childhood: How contemporary culture is damaging the next generation and what we can do about it.* Orion.

Thorley, C. (2017). *Not by degrees: Improving student mental health in the UK's universities.* London: Institute for Public Policy Research.

Index

YOG

In
Synergy With
Medical Science

Acharya Balkrishna

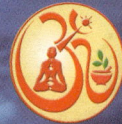

DIVYA PRAKASHAN

Divya Yog Mandir (Trust)
Patanjali Yogpeeth, Hardwar

|| OM ||

Publisher	:	**Divya Prakashan** Patanjali Yogpeeth Maharishi Dayanand Gram, Delhi-Hardwar Road, Bahadarabad Hardwar 249 408, Uttarakhand
E-mail	:	divyayoga@rediffmail.com
Website	:	www.divyayoga.com
Telephone	:	(01334) - 244107, 240008, 246737
Fax	:	(01334) - 244805

First Edition	:	25,000 Copies (June 2007)
Printer	:	Sai Security Printers Pvt. Ltd. Faridabad, Haryana E-mail : sspdel@saiprinters.com, saipressindia@yahoo.com
Distributor	:	Indian Postal Department This book is available at all main Postal offices in India. It can also be obtained at home, at no additional cost through your Postman. Diamond Pocket Books New Delhi E-mail : sales@diamondpocket.com

191 (06-07)

CONTENTS

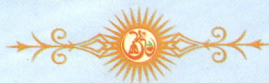

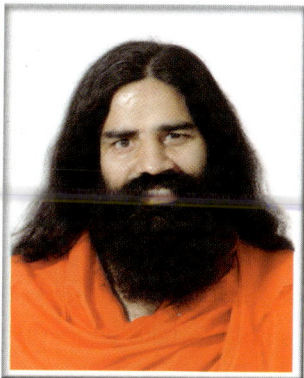

FOREWORD

The veracity of modern medical science is based on controlled clinical trials. Seeking and establishing the same in a scientifically unknown area is indeed a challenging responsibility. The benefits of Yog or Pranayam is a truth established from personal experience and regular practice. To demonstrate this, we have experimented with Pranayam directly and indirectly first on thousands then on millions of people. These experiments have revealed some amazing facts. The participants in these individual and collective experiments were normally healthy people as well as patients. This individual and extensive practice of Yog was attended by both healthy people and the patients of cancer, heart, diabetes, hypertension, obesity, asthma, thyroid and other serious diseases who were searching for a healthy and disease-free life. It is an undisputed fact based on the results of these experiments that people got cured of diseases that are normally considered terminal. The evidence comes from the clinical examination of the patients of cancer, hepatitis and other serious diseases performed before and after the practice of Pranayam. The results of medical examinations and direct health benefits derived by millions of people reveal facts about Yog that cannot be denied. This work would definitely point out a new direction to the research and practice in medical science. People tired of and frustrated with life will find in Yog a basis for hope, faith and vigour in life.

Adopting a new system in life is very difficult. Indians had adopted Yog as a life-style since the beginning of civilization. The practice of Yog became less popular during middle ages but the present Yog revolution is like reviving the past, as millions of people are again practicing and getting its benefits. We want that Yog should become a philosophy of life for everyone and people with any disease should take to Yog for regaining health. The practitioners of Yog should be able to experience ultimate happiness and blissful state of samadhi; those feeling lost should find some direction. Those feeling dejected, insecure and, therefore suicidal, may get on the path of self-awareness. A self-aware person can not take his/her own or somebody else's life. A Yogi is above crime, corruption and violence, and contributes to building a creative, positive, qualitative and productive society. A yogi is beyond terrorism, casteism, regionalism, communal passions and follows the path of nation building. Today, through Yog, the strong humanistic, nationalistic, spiritualistic forces and those standing for truth and righteousness in the world are coming together, paving the way for world peace and welfare. Yog is a blessing for those who because of financial constraints are unable to afford allopathic treatment not only in India but also abroad. Yog is a solution for incurable diseases and this truth shall be unraveled as you go through the pages of this book.

If we look at the figures included in the United Nations (UN) report for the year 2005-2006, we find that India spends around Rs.4,79,520 crore rupees on various medical services annualy and the World Bank report (Page No.11) represents a bitter truth about the same. The truth is that only 35 percent of Indians are able to afford medical treatment and 65 percent (71 crore population) are not able to afford the cost of medicines and treatment. If we assume that every Indian is able to take allopathic medicines then the total expenditure would be to the tune of Rs. 13,70,057 crore. Assuming that Indians stop using the traditional medical systems like Yog and Ayurved and follow the allopathic system like the USA, then every Indian would have to spend $5,277 per year for medical facilities. If we attempt to provide medical facilities at a similar level in India then the total expenditure would be a whopping Rs. 7,52,67,514 crore, which would not be met even after using up the entire GDP (Gross Domestic Product) of the country.

Every Indian has to bear 93 percent of the medical expenses and the government's contribution is a negligible seven percent. In this context, every person in the country and even the world requires such a medical system, which can provide good healthcare with no or very minimal cost and it cannot be anything except Yog. We are very confident that as we proceed at Patanjali University on the path of genetic research and controlled clinical trials for Ayurved and Yog with full determination, wisdom and scientific approach, we shall be able to demonstrate through scientifically results that these two provide the needed medical system.

This book 'Yog In Synergy With Medical Science' is our first attempt. The process of scientific documentation and research would continue with the support of millions of fellow citizens. We will be able to establish Yog as a health building solution and philosophy of life through scientific research. We are also confident that we would be able to give a new definition, meaning and a new knowledge to the world in the realm of Yog and Ayurved. It will also start a new debate and discussion internationally and truth shall prevail at last. The dream of sage Charak **Sadaaiv Yuktam Bheshjayam Yadarogyaya Kalpate** ǀ will become a reality. The whole idea is to give priority to physical health involving minimum expenses and thus to take the society in the right direction. It will be able to provide simple, easy, effective and scientific treatment with the help of Yog to around 500 crore people who are unable to get medical facilities due to poor economic conditions. Revered Acharya Balkrishna has written this book with considerable devotion, hard work and dedication. This will prove to be a milestone in the history of Yog and guide the future generations. I am confident that this work will be able to remove the misconceptions and doubts present in the minds of people due to ignorance and resistance to change, and shall unveil the truth. This will begin a fresh revolution in the society and we will be able to bring Yog and Ayurved along with other Indian medical systems into the mainstream systems currently in use in the world. Whenever people think of this health revolution, they will certainly appreciate the noble efforts of revered Acharya Balkrishna.

I extend my heartfelt wishes to revered Acharya Balkrishna Ji, all the medical practitioners and dedicated individuals who have contributed in the preparation of this book.

Swami Ramdev

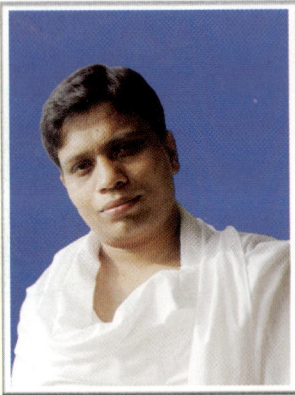

Today, Yog has acquired global recognition and an exalted status as an ancient health-building system. While many medical practitioners and intellectuals are keen to test it using scientific evaluation methods, there are several others who are resisting this trend and inclusion of Yog in medical science. The welfare of patients is being overlooked for the sake of personal, commercial and business interests. Unfortunately, today medical science is taken mainly as allopathy, world's health concern is more of an allopathic concern and World Health Organization (WHO) could be taken as an organization supporting and working for allopathy. We are not trying to question the ethos behind existing medical/health system but we aim to start a healthy debate about health concerns internationally and secure right to health for the common man. We are aware that we have a mighty challenge to deal with. With this objective in mind, revered Yog Rishi Swami Ramdevji Maharaj has committed himself to the objective that, "no person should die of disease and nobody should die on account of being poor." We have decided to proceed in this direction so as to put a check on the large scale exploitation going on in the country in the name of providing health services. In this age of science, we are committed to firmly establish Yog as a science using scientific tests. It is true that Yog is powerful and contains the solutions for all the global problems. From time immemorial, millions of people have immersed themselves in this pious ever flowing Ganga of Yog. But never ever neither the power holders nor any voluntary organization or a resourceful individual has come forward to work on Yog from a scientific perspective. Although some holy saints, a few dedicated institutions, and small groups have made attempts in this direction, their work has not received international recognition. We ascetics decided to drive away the misconception that Yog is simply exercise for physical fitness, created by people out of ignorance, selfishness and resistance. In fact, these people have their own agenda for not letting Yog, a glorious and time-tested tradition, to get its due recognition and rightful place on the world health map. Despite the lack of proper resources, we are committed to deal with such impediments on the path of Yog getting its due recognition. We have been able to take up this Herculean task for the sake of welfare of mankind with the unflinching support and trust of millions of people in this world.

Today, we have reached a stage where every intellectual of the world has greater appreciation for Yog as a complete medical science and philosophy of life and accepts its scientific reasoning and basis. Yog is not just a physical exercise but a holistic medical science; it is a philosophy of life, a spiritual knowledge. it is a profound philosophical thought process, but it is also about having a simple, easy and balanced life-style. It is the path to gain eternal wisdom, ultimate truth and to unite the inner soul with the supreme soul through self-realization. It is a tradition in which sages have attained immeasurable bliss, indescribable happiness and inexplicable peace by entering the supreme conciousness which is present beyond mind. It is the science that inhibits the agitations of the mind and takes it to its highest level. Yog is the spiritual journey from ignorance to knowledge, mortality to immortality obvious to hidden, peace to ultimate tranquility. It is the inner journey from thoughtfulness to emptiness, subjective to objective concentration, from determinate to indeterminate samadhi and extrovertedness to introvertedness and being firm in judgement (gifted with unshakable mental equilibrium). It is a holistic and scientific process to transform body, mind and life. It is an experience of complete silence and calm based on self-realization, Tadēva arthamāatra nirbhasaṃ Ṣwarōopa śōoṇyamiva Samāadhiḥ It is devotion that transcends desire and a state of nothingness attained by self-realization, which is very different from emptiness caused by intoxication. It is an understanding of truth of life and rationality. There is a need to appreciate Yog, Ayurved and all Vedic traditions in totality. Life becomes a celebration once it imbibes Yog that leads to making of an equity-based, simple, developed, healthy and happy society. Yog brings forth the indisputable truth that the solution to any problem lies within and can't be found outside. Yog activates the healing strengths within our bodies. Āavāata vāabi bhēṣajaṃ, vivāata vāahi yaḍ rōopaḥ, Ṭwaṃ hi viṣthava bhēṣayo dēvāanāaṃ dōota iyasē || (Rigveda). The Vedic verse of yathāa Piṇḍē tathāa brahmāaṇḍē I leads to the same conclusion that solutions lie within not without. All the chemicals, salts, hormones, which we take in the form of medicines can actually be harmful instead of being beneficial until we surrender ourselves to Yog. When we start practising Yog, one does not need external stimulations as the body itself secretes required hormones and balances the internal chemical processes. The anabolism, catabolism and metabolism processes in the body, i.e. vata, pitta and kapha are maintained in equilibrium. Mind becomes calm, bringing happiness and helps in overcoming depression One feels a sense of fulfillment in life and this is the glorious truth and essence of Yog.

We are committed to get Yog accepted internationally as a medical science. We are determined to achieve this goal through the Patanjali Yogpeeth and Patanjali University. At the same time we are committed to build a healthy and disease-free world in accordance with Indian ethos of Vasudhev Kutumbkam and Sarvē bhavaṇtu sukhinaḥ I and thus contributing to the cause of promoting and conserving rich Indian cultural and spritual traditions. This book is an humble attempt in this direction. We are determined to obtain more scientific evidence and build a science perspective not only for

Yog and Ayurved but for the entire vedic knowledge and wisdom. We shall lead the world in finding solutions for complex problems besetting humanity through the fusion of science and spiritualism.

Writing this book has been a very challenging, difficult and responsible work for me. The task of scientific documentation, analysis of benefits of Yog, representation of Yog as per scientific standards, compiling the experiences of people and psychosomatic study of effects of Yog on about 12.5 million people was very complex and labour intensive. Today, Yog has reached more than billion people and 200 nations with the help of media and is being practised extensively the world over. The self-centred, ill-minded and egoist people with power have been questioning the benefits of Yog in the absence of scientific evidence. This is our first attempt to present Yog backed by currently available scientific evidence obtained with our limited resources. The goal is far more ambitious and the task of scientific documentation and research is an ongoing process. We will continue with the research and shall present new facts as they become available. We are also determined to carry on this mission till Yog reaches each and every individual of the world and gets complete scientific recognition. We aim to conduct research and analyse the benefits of Yog at personal, social, economic and international levels at the Patanjali University. This book is the outcome of meticulous work put in by us in order to present various scientific standards used to test and validate this ancient system of Yog, demographic study and personal experiences of several hundred people along with sufficient supporting proofs and documents. When the task is so huge, possibility of errors cannot be ruled out. Therefore, we humbly request the learned readers, intellectuals, and scientific and medical fraternity to come forward with their suggestions and point out the mistakes so that they can be rectified in the next edition. I invite you all whole-heartedly to participate in this noble mission for the welfare of all human beings.

Ramnavmi

Monday, 26 March 2007

Acharya Balkrishna

REMEMBRANCE

I remember the Almighty who has made an ordinary person like me the medium to accomplish this huge task of representing ancient knowledge and wisdom of sages in the present form with scientific evidence and documents, though He himself is the cause behind this grand task. I dedicate this book to the sages like Patanjali, Jaimini and several others who underwent a lot of hardships, practised austerity and prayed for all to be free of disease (sarve santu niramayah)'. They spent their lives striving for and attaining the supreme bliss and preached Yog in order to make them healthy both physically and mentally. It gives me great pleasure in bringing out this book. I hope, my commitment for establishing ancient cultural and spiritual knowledge through scientific parameters and perspective will be realized through this book to some extent.

Had sage Dayanand not been born in this age, we would have forgotten the Vedic science and traditions. I bow to such a sage and express my gratitude to my mentors who with great love and constant efforts helped this young mind to embrace vedic knowledge and traditions. I think of revered Acharya Baldevji, revered Swami Raghunathanandji Avadhut and all other mentors with sincere gratitude.

I am indebted to those great devotees, sages, saints and holy souls who came into my life as my gurus, friends and brothers. What can I offer them when I am just a small link in the whole process? It is impossible to express in words the enormous significance of efforts made by these people to place Yog and Ayurved on international platform; and to acknowledge their efforts for the upliftment of Indian culture. This book is just an effort to appraise and evaluate the extensive work carried out by these learned people internationally. I remember Yog Rishi Swami Ramdevji and seek his blessings. He has taken me as a younger brother and I always have his guidance and affection. Whatever I am today, I owe everything to having his companionship and patronage.

I remember my venerable mother, Shrimati Sumitra Devi who nurtured me in her womb for nine months. She inculcated pure and noble virtues in my mind and gave me the the burning desire to make something of life. Though illiterate, hardwork, fearlessness, will power and sincerity are her main characterstics, I am sure I have imbibed some of these characterstics. I pay my obeisance to my very loving and respectable mother. I also remember my father revered Shri Jay Vallabhji who despite facing all kinds of hardships led the life of a saint and wanted to remain celibate. He remained so for 30 years at a time when child marriage was prevalent in the society. People used to consider him wild because he sported a long beard, big moustache and had long hair. Later he entered the life of a householder as family members pleaded with him to do so. I am indeed blessed to be born as his first child. It is the result of his noble deeds and self-control that I am devoid of stress, weariness and fatigue, and enjoying a disease-free and healthy body despite having hectic daily schedule and mounting work pressure. My father took all the hardships with courage and never let it affect our upbringing. I bow down at the feet of such admirable parents and remember them from the core of my heart.

I remember all those pious people who have given me inspiration, cooperation, good wishes and blessings all through my life; and when I think of those people it feels like recalling memories from past many lives. I feel proud of my fate when I recall memories from the past. I am fortunate to have the company and affection of many holy people. I also offer my respects to Shrimati Gulab Devi and Shri Ramnivasji, who gave birth to a saint in the form of Swami Ramdevji. I also remember revered sages Swami Shankardev, Mahant Rajendra Das, Swami Narayan, Anand Chaitanyaji, Acharya Pradyumanji, Swami Satyamitranandji, Swami Chidanand Muniji, Swami Hansdasji, Jivraj Bhai Patel, Mata Jyotika, Suresh Chilllar and others with deep respect.

I would also like to remember my colleague Swami Muktanandji who has always loved me like a brother and supported me in the mission of Yog. I also offer sincere thanks to Rambharat, Dr Yashdev Shastri for their dedicated work in the Ashram. I also remember Dr B. D. Sharma, Dr Bishvjeet Mukherjee and his wife Shrimati Mahua Mukherjee who let him take time off from household responsibilities to offer his services to the Ashram.

When I think of the initial challenges involved in documenting research work on Yog, I remember the helping hands of so many others without whom this work could not have been completed. I believe this work could become possible on account of deep committment held by Shri O. P. Shrivastava. Bahen Renu Prakash who along with discharging her family responsibility, remained at the forefront to make this work possible. She made her son Rajat Prakash to be available at the service of Swamiji. I offer my heartfelt thanks to her, Shri Alakh, Dr H. P. Kumar, Dr R.K. Gupta, Dr R. K. Mishra and the team of doctors of SGPGI, Lucknow, and Saharashri Subroto Roy for making services of his Sahara Medical team available for this work. The concept of compiling the records and presenting it in this form was ours but it would not have been completed without the efforts of Dr Rajendra Vidyalankar and his wife Dr Suman Rajan. I offer my gratitude to the devoted couple. I would also like to express my thanks to Dr S. K. Tijariwala, Prof. Umrao S. Bist, Sumegha Agarwal, Dr Srikant Bhave, Dr Dharamvir Rai and Dr Kulveer Chikara for the work of writing and compilation, Priyata and Raghavan family and Shashi Bhushan for finishing the entire printing work within a very short time. I sincerely appreciate the services of Late Mata Kantaji and Ajay Aryaji who retired from government services and dedicated their time and energy to the services of Yogpeeth and the Ashram.

I also thank all the Ayurvedic doctors, volunteers and colleagues who have contributed their time and energy for this assignment including Gagan, Lalit, Arvind, Jaishankar

Mishra, Col. Dheer, Sharmaji, sisters Ashu and Parul, Vaidya Rajendra, Vaidya Avnish and Subhash. It is the result of their dedicated efforts that today more than 1,000 volunteers are offering their services to the Yogpeeth. They are keeping the flag of Yog flying high internationally with committment and unwavering dedication.

The task of construction of a huge pharmacy in a short time would not have been possible without the support by Shri S.K. Garg, Chairman of ELDECO Group. He is following in the footsteps of his Late mother Hemlata Garg in the service of people. I would like to thank Manoj Singhal and sister Jyoti and the whole team for their contribution.

I would also like to remember several lakhs of patients who regained good health and thus a new life; who became the main source of inspiration for the conceptualization and accomplishment of this work. It was the cry from their hearts, their blessings, their strong desire, which made it possible to rise above the self and do something good for the mankind.

I thank every person who has contributed to bring out this book in some form or the other. I also thank them for having committed themselves to the service of the nation, public welfare, culture, spiritualism, Yog and Ayurved. Several retired people contributed 50 percent of their pension for fulfilling this dream, several mothers contributed their daily wages obtained from tailoring or from doing other petty work. It brings tears of joy to my eyes when I think about all these people and about their sincere and unselfish efforts. I also want to thank all the negative forces that were trying to sabotage the mission of making this country and the world disease-free. Whenever these forces tried to unleash hurdles on our path, we surged forward with greater vigour and strength.

I would like to remember all those people who have worked diligently to extend this mission to each and every person, those who got a new ray of hope, those who are concerned about national and cultural heritage, and those who are ready to be a part of this movement to generate public awareness. I pray to the Almighty to give strength to all such people so that they can relieve the pain of sick and suffering people. They should become lamps and enlighten the life of others to bring back happiness. I would also like to express sincere thanks to the Yog teachers whose only mission is to extend Swami Ramdevji's Yog to each and every household and individual.

I dedicate this book to the divine energies and once again express gratitude to all those who have contributed in whatever way possible with limited resources to mould this creation in the present form.

Ramnavmi

Monday, 26 March 2007

Acharya Balkrishna

Chapter 1

HISTORICAL BACKGROUND OF YOG

Yog is the greatest Indian concept annunciated to the world. For a civilized society and for a successful individual, Yog is perhaps the finest and most clearly laid out uplifting system available so far. The human tendency to find their sense of accomplishment within their family, caste, community, region, nation, language and religion will only lead to anarchy for others. In their particular reference framework, this whole quest is about finding one's identity, not eternal peace. The ongoing popular discourse in the world is guided by populist slogans for religion, country and community. It's selfish, misleading and is about one-upmanship. Most often, support is sought for the so called fight for identity in the name of religion and justice.

Do we have any other methodology to achieve social equality and equity? Is there any one methodology which can be followed by the entire humankind? A methodology that does not destory the unity and integrity of a nation and its people. A metodology which every individual can adopt and practise to attain ultimate happiness, tranquility and bliss in life. Yes, we do have one that can be followed by all the people all over the world fearlessly and independently, to meet all the above needs.

It is none other than Saint Patanjali's Ashtang Yog.

It is only Ashtang Yog that can stop the bloody wars going on in this world. It deals with every stage and phase of life from mundane to the most exalted. It guides one not only in day-to-day activities but also in reaching the highest stages of meditation and Samadhi. Anyone in the search for self identity and the ultimate truth should practice Ashtang Yog.[1]

Yog is indeed an easy, simple and most effective method of meeting one's material as well as spiritual objectives. It arouses the dormant inner vision within us. A person without inner vision takes on the charming path, full of thorns, of pleasure seeking which only leads to destruction, instead of taking the higher path of righteous living leading to eternal peace. Such a person improves neither this life nor the next. Yog can make mind free of prejudices, ego, inflexibility, and misconceptions which are the biggest hurdles in the path of individual's development and thus of the community and the nation. Yog fills mind with divinity, makes it more steady than a mountain and deeper than the ocean. The practice of Yog provides tranquility in times of depression. It removes all doubts and suspicions and assures the attainment of supreme bliss. The history of world is replete with the stories of such people who were able to achieve self-realization with the practice of Yog. Such great personalities have rid themselves of the negative feelings of jealousy, hatred, unhappiness prevailing in the society and brought peace on earth.

The gigantic advances made in the field of literature, philosophy, science, religion and spiritualism have been possible only because of meditation, concentration and hard work of some very determined individuals. We need high degree of concentration and dedication in order to understand the spiritual truths and hidden secrets. At the same time the concentration of scientists who enlighten the world with inventions and unravel the secrets of nature cannot be underestimated. If those who sought answers to existential questions as they contemplated on mantras are sages, then scientists who make new discoveries and discover the laws of nature are also sages. The person who accomplishes various tasks with full concentration and awakened consciousness acts like a sage. Such people have constant awareness and are always striving to reach new heights; they are called pioneers.

India's precious texts like Brahmsutra, Aranyaks, Upanishads and classics on medicine, astrology are the result of supreme wisdom. The treatises on the nature of dualities like wisdom-ignorance, heaven-hell, active-inactive, virtue-vice, etc. are very precise because they are the products of conscientious minds. The feeling of collectiveness in place of separateness, 'We' instead of 'I' is the biggest gift of this wisdom. When the person understands these facts, the individual's mental and internal quest comes to fruition. Undoubtedly the blessing of Yog is supreme among the gifts of Vedic sages. It is a knowledge, which is free of disputes and controversies, it is an art which is multidimensional, and it is a science, which assures abundant happiness even when there is a paucity of resources.

Yagyavalkya has made a humble appeal in 'Yagyavalkya Smriti' and said, Ayaṃ tu paramōdharmō yadyōgēnāatmāadarśanaṃ ।[2] It means self-realization with the help of Yog is the supreme duty. It gives us insight into how vedic society was so much taken up to Yog. It can be said that Yog came about propelled by the human desire to understand and unveil the secrets of life and nature. We cannot deny the fact that before saint Patanjali, this glorious tradition of Yog was not organised in a scientific and systematic manner in great detail. A question may arise as to why sages needed to compose more texts when Vedas were already available. Sage Yaska opined that owing to intellectual lethargy people became disinterested in studying metaphysics considering it too complex to deal with. Sages presented

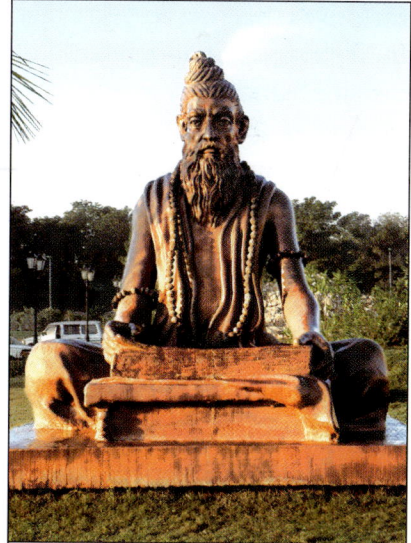

A statue of Saint Patanjali situated at Yogpeeth Hardwar

such seemingly complex knowledge in a very interesting manner in various texts. In any case, today we are not in a position to know or declare the exact period when Yog shastra acquired an independent entity. However, there are many references available in parts of Vedas and Puranas. Many Vedic Samhitas discuss directly or refer to various aspects of Yog. Although in these places the discussions on mind control, prana (vital energy), and sadhana (regular practice) are not detailed and systematic, they do catch our attention. Rigveda mantras (1.18.7, 1.34.9, 10.13.1) mention Yog. Some mantras included in Yajurveda describe the concentration of mind and the results obtained thereby. Mantras 1-5 contained in chapter 11ᵗʰ of Yajurveda talk about Yog in detail and probably no other Samhitas could present it so wonderfully.

Yuṇjatē mana utayuṇgatē dhiyō viprāa viprasya vasatō vipaśchitaḥ।

Revered sage Dayanand says that ujjate means 'to make steady'. Yujayate Mana purports to stabilizing the mind. Yujayate Dhia refers to making the intellect steady. Here the word vipashchita stands for wise persons with discriminating intellect.

Let us look into the following mantra included in Yajurveda:

Yuṇjāanaḥ prathamam manastv vāaya savitāa dhiyāaḥ।

In his Rigvedadi-bhashya-bhumika Swami Dayanand interprets the word 'yujjanah' in the above mantra as "yogam kurvanah san (manushyah)" which means "(men) performing Yog". All the five mantras of Yajurveda mentioned above are discussed in greater detail in Shwetashwatar Upanishad and appear there exactly as in the Veda. In vedic texts, we find extensive references to Yog's highest aspect of Pran vidya or the science of vital life energy. In Yajurved, we find reference of five prans- Prana-controlling respiration; Apan-excretary system; Saman-digestive system; Vyan-circulatory system; Udan-reactions and finally ejection of Pran. Although Pran as vital energy includes all these five that have been given different names related to the position, function, and purpose in the body. In Yajurveda we find reference to these at different places individually or collectively. However, Yajurveda describes mainly the first four mentioning Saman only briefly. In Atharvaveda, vital life energy and upward movement and circulation and expiration have been discussed to a great extent. It is also necessary to understand that Atharvaveda contains the most detailed description of also the first four are discussed even in greater detail in chapter 11. Here, the different basis and actions of Pran from isolation to collectiveness have been discussed in detail. The first mantra of this chapter stresses the all-inclusiveness of Pran and says, 'We all bow down to Pran, which controls everything. It is the God to all living beings and contains the entire universe'.[5]

One of the verses of Yajurveda addresses Pran as Rishi or 'sage'.[6] The vital life energy present in the body develops and nourishes the mana (mind) and brain. Here 'sage' or 'Rishi' means one who understands the hidden secrets and foresees the future. The ability to comprehend and interpret the facts and their deeper meaning is termed as Rishi Drishti. The ultimate state of analytical and intellectual faculties is called Rishitava. Without this faculty of the mind and intellect, it is almost impossible to clearly understand the knowledge buried in the scriptures. It is clear therefore that only a highly conscious mind developed through Yog can fully comprehend the contents of Vedic texts and treatises.

Ahirbudhnya Samhita mentions Hinranyagarbha as the originator of Yog. It classifies Yog into two types-external and internal or physical and disciplinary, which includes the Yama-Niyam. In Yagyavalkya Smriti and Mahabharat also Hiranyagarbha is stated as the originator: "Hiranyagarbhah yogasya vakta nanyah puratanah", i.e. Hiranyagarbha was first to speak of Yog. In another context in Mahabharata, Hiranyagarbha has been described as omnipresent and powerful.[9] The 121st verse of 10th chapter of Rigveda is known as Hiranyagarbha verse. The Hiranyagarbha as mentioned in Mahabharata is none other than the Almighty Brahma of Hiranyagarbha sukta. Ramayana declares Him as the soul of the entire universe. This whole description makes it clear that Vedic tradition accepts Yog as the one propounded by God himself.[10] Some scholars have expressed different opinions with respect to Hiranyagarbha. Some learned men believe that the propounder of Sankhya Shastra, Kapila is Hiranyagarbha. While some others say that a sage called Hiranyagarbha propounded Yog. Saint Patanjali presented the philosophy of Yog on his own basis. Upanishads contain advanced form of Yog as propounded by Hiranyagarbha but it has not been compiled properly. As mentioned earlier we find all the descriptions with reference to Yog in Upanishads. When the highest aspiration of self-realization has been the inspiration behind various Vedic texts, how can they remain indifferent towards the grand conception of Yog? The main objective of Yog is the restraint of mental modifications. In fact, this is the stage of Samadhi of self-realization which is also the main objective of Upanishads. The ardent appeal by Yagyavalkya to Maitreyi is the highest level of aspiration for self-realization.[11] Ishopanishad asks for removing the golden veil for meeting the truth. In Yog Shastra, this golden veil is none other than five afflcitions as expounded in Yog and all other afflictions included under the five types of misconceptions and the root cause for all these lies in ignorance. In Ayurved too, afflictions of the intellect are taken as the root cause of all diseases. Brahmavidya as expounded in important Upnishads like Kena, Chandhogya, Brihadaranyak, Maitreyani, Koushitaki and Shwetashwatar is no different from Yogvidya. Many Upanishads begin the subject with Ḃrahmavāadinō vadaṇ̣tiı

Upanishads clearly mention about posture, Pranayam or breath control, belief system, Dhayan and Samadhi of Yog. We also find ample references to cleanliness, contentment, devotion, self-study, non-violence, truth and celibacy in Upnishads.

The Indian philosophical texts have given a lot of emphasis to Yogsadhna. Yog is described with prominence in various texts and treatises of Indian streams of Darshan (philosophy).

In terms of subject commonlaties, 'Yog Darshan' is an associate of Sankhya Darshan. The latter is considered to be more ancient than Yog Darshan. However, the two are considered to be complimentary to each other for having many commonalities. Gita proclaims that any person who considers these two Darshans separate from each other must be having intellect that of a child.[12] In Sankhya Darshan, Asana, belief system, Dhayana and other aspects of Yog have been codified as separate sutras and often these are similar word-by-word with sutras as stated in Yogdarshan. In Yogdarshan, descriptions about asanas, inclinations of mind and impact of resisting them or blocking them, five types of afflictions, measures and practices for subjugating unfavourable tendencies of mind, detachment, Kriya Yog, Dhayana and Samadhi are simialr to what has been stated in Sankhya sutras.[13] According to Sankhya Darshan, a person by nature with pure living in close proximity with nature becomes bonded with it. Imprudence causes the state of being attached to nature, till imprudence prevails person will remain bonded and thus shall remain troubled by sorrows and confusions and remain in the cycle of life and death. The only cure available for this imprudence is Samadhi or state of deep meditation. When the soul is able to differentiate between the conscious and unconscious, there can be no scope left for imprudence. With imprudence gone, proximity or bondage with nature goes too and then comes Moksha or final deliverance.

This exemplifies the deep similarity with Tara Drishtu Swarupeavasthanam. The Nayaya Shastra has stressed the need for restrained conduct and strict observances in order to achieve the objective of Samadhi or deep meditation. The Vedanta Darshan prescribes many Yogic practices including Dhayana to stabilize the mind. Besides, ancient texts contain extensive description of Yogic practisces. Various episodes of Mahabharata especially in Shanti Parva, Asvamedh Parva and Anushasan Parva contain various important references to Yog. Gita is a living account of various radical definitions and declarations about Yog. The way Gita has used the word 'Yog ' in various contexts, gives a ground breaking broad base to Yog. The definition of Yog and discipline of Yog, its elements like Tapa (devotion), Karma (action), Sawadhaya (self-study) , Dhayana (meditation), concentration, practice, non-attachment, diet, conduct and daily routine have been described in a very interesting and informative manner in Gita and it is almost impossible to find in any other text. Multidimesional aspects of Yog as GyanaYog, KarmYog, BhaktiYog, RajYog have been expounded in great detail in Gita. Puranas are the most controversial among Indian classic texts. Many learned men, scholars, reformers and analysts have alleged that Puranas led Indian Dharma and Darshan on the path of degradation. They also contain several references to Yog like Vayu, Shiva, Brahma, Garuda, Vishnu, Agni and Lingam. The 14th Chapter of 'Garuda Purana' mentioning about Dhayana Yog, KarmaYoga (Yog of action) as mentioned in Agni Purana, resistance towards passion, observances of Ashtang Yog as mentioned in Vishnu Purana easily draw the attention of seekers. The 10th Chapter of Vayu Purana introduces us to the merits and demerits of different parts of Yog. However it needs to be mentioned that many a times these references have been exaggerated and are inappropriate.

References and Comments

1. *Yog Sadhna Va Yog Chikitsa Rahasya, Swami Ramdevji, pp. 1-11*

2. *Ayam tu paramo dharmo yadyagenatmadarshnam. Yagyavalkya Smriti 1.8*

3. *Yajurveda - 18.2, 6.2, 22.33. 1.2, 7.27, 13.19*

4. *Pranpano chakshu Shrotrakshitischa ya*
   Vyanodano Vangamanaste va Akutimavahan. Atharvaveda 11.1.4

5. *Pranpano chakshu Shrotrakshitischa ya*
   Vyanodano Vangamanaste sharirena ta iyante. Vahi 11.8.26.
   Pranya Namo yasya Sarvidam Vashe
   Yo Bhoota sarvasyeshvaro yasmintsarvam pratishtitam. Atharvaveda 11.4.1

6. *Saptarishaya Pratihita shashire sapta rakshanti sadampramadam. Yajurveda 34.55*
   Almost all the authors have explained the word saptarishaya as seven Prans or vital life energies.

7. *Yagyavalka Smriti 125*

8. *Mahabharata 12.349.65*

9. *Mahabharata 12.342.96*

10. *Hiranyagarbho Jagadantaratma. Adhbut Ramayana 5.6*

11. *Atma Vayare Drashtavya Shrotavyo Mantavyo Nididhyasitavya*

12. *Sankhya Yogo prithak bala pravadanti na manishina. Gita 5.4*

13. *(A) Sthir Sukhmasanam. Yogsutra 2.46 and Sankhya Sutra 3.34*
    (B) Vrittaya panchataya klishtaaklishta. Yogsutra 1.5 and Sankhyasutra 2.33

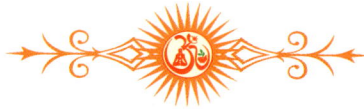

Chapter 2

DIFFERENT DIMENSIONS OF YOG

It is true that Yog and human body are complimentary to each other. The tired, weary body becomes energetic, the person becomes active and gets a new direction with regular practice of Yog. It helps in reaching the stage of deep meditation. Great poet Kalidas targeting physical body comments in his work 'Kumar Sambhav': Śareeramāadyaṃ khalu dharmasāadhanaṃ । that is taming the body is the very first goalpost on the path of Dharma (religion). In Indian context, every good and positive deed is about fulfilling one's Dharma. If the body is not healthy, whether one is on the path of spiritual or material fulfillment, nothing can be accomplished. The state of physical well-being shapes and influences other aspects of personality.

In a not tamed and disturbed body, higher aspirations for life do not exist and will never be aroused. The Atharvaveda describes the body in a very respectful manner and qualifies it as Ayodhya[1], Hirnyayi Puram,[2] Aparajitam[3] and Amritenavrutam Puram[4] (that which is covered with nectar). The body is the medium through which we engage with this world or attain salvation. Everyone recognizes the centrality of body for enjoying pleasures of life and release from the cycle of life and death is taken as the end of bodily existence. When a seeker fails repeatedly in the path of devotion, he/she gets very frustrated for not being able to have control over sense organs. The seeker punishes the sensory organs, keeps them deprived of nourishment and eventually destroys them. A Vedic mantra cautions us towards this attitude stating that treating the body in this manner is not the solution, but it is moving towards from darkness or ignorance to greater darkness or ignorance. Destroying in any form or cutting off the sensory organs from the body does not bring an end to sorrows but denotes to having a basal state of mind. It is a fact not an illusion that we cannot run away from our body or senses. They are not our enemies but friends. They can only be guided with love and understanding not with disrespect.

The sages in Upanishads were deeply hurt to see the immature behaviour of their disciples towards the sensory organs and hence they declared the sensory organs to be full of divine elements and advised the disciples to protect and preserve them. They talked about the constitution of the body and explained that fire entered the mouth in the form of voice; Sun entered the eyes in the form of vision; the various directions became sound and entered the ears; food, medicine, vegetation entered the skin through pores, the Moon entered the heart in the form of mind, death became Apana (life force) and entered the navel and water entered the sexual organ in the form of semen.[5]

The main objective of describing the constitution of the body with the entry of various Gods into sensory organs was to stop the immature behaviour of disciples who ignored their importance. Every action, which makes the sensory organs weak prematurely, is an act of violence. Yog is just opposite to violence. One who practises Yog, incredibly, is not intolerant towards sensory organs or senses but still can remain attached with the society. A yogic mind is enlightened with the dutifulness, which makes all retrogressive engergies directed towards creativity. Sense of dutifulness is the starting point of self-realization.

Physical Aspects of Yog

Constitution of Body: Anatomical Perspective and Yog Sadhna Perspective

The constitution of our body is purely scientific. Anatomy and science of Yog classify it in different ways. The former studies the macro aspects, whereas the latter studies the origin of micro aspects and their functioning. It is necessary to understand the constitution of body before understanding the effect of Yog on it.

At the time of birth the soul resides into three types of body. Yog Sadhna terms it coarse, subtle and causal. The coarse body is visible, whereas subtle and causal body are invisible. Coarse body is the abode of the other two bodies. All the three bodies are closely related to each other. Enjoying luxury, practising Yog and attaining salvation is possible by activating all the three bodies. In order to understand the functioning of the body from the perspective of luxuries and practice of Yog, we can refer to Taiteriya Upanishads where the sages have divided it into five sheaths (koshas). They are namely Aannamay Kosh (consisting of the physical limbs), Pranmay Kosh (of vital energy), Manomay Kosh (of mind), Vigyanamaya (of intellect) Kosh and Anandmay (of bliss) Kosh. In these five sections, different stages and various active body parts are described in a very systematic and organised manner. The coarse body and its functioning is described in Annamay Kosh, the activities and characteristics of subtle body are described in Pranmay, Manomay and Vigyanmay Kosh and finally causal body and its characteristics are enumerated in Anandmay Kosh.

The two main elements of our coarse body, i.e. five sensory organs and five organs of action are included in the Annamay Kosh. The outer skin, bones, fat, skeleton, flesh, bone marrow and all elements get nourishment from food and constitute Annamay Kosh. Before taking birth this body develops from the food as eaten by the mother. Every part of the body for its development is indebted to nourishment obtained from the mother. Our arteries, nerves, lungs, heart, teeth, tongue, brain and its composition - all are included in this section. The size of Annamay Kosh is proportionate to the size of the body. The ant's body has very small Annamay Kosh, whereas an elephant has a bigger Annamay Kosh. All those parts of the body that can be weighed are included in Annamay Kosh.

*Read Yog Rishi Swami Ramdevji's Yog Sadhana Evam Yog Chikitsa Rahasya for more information on this topic.

Very important constitutents of Annamay Kosh are five organs of action, five sensory organs, heart, lungs and brain. Our five sensory organs namely eyes, ears, nose, skin and taste are all situated on the face except skin. We need to remember that the sensory organs do not belong to somebody else. Sensory organs are invisible tools, which give the experience of different emotions within us when they are used. No one can see his/her own eyes, ears, nose (in totality) and even tongue directly. The eyes and ears can see and hear the things situated at a distance respectively, nose can smell within a limited range while taste and touch need proximity or closeness. There are miniscule parts on the tongue which actually get the taste of a particular thing like bitter, sour, salty etc. It is interesting to note that the things, which can evaporate emit smell and the things, which can be dissolved in water give taste. This is the reason that our tongue is always wet and contains sufficient amount of water. The food that we eat first dissolves in this water and then we get the taste of that particular thing. The five different feelings obtained through sensory organs are called rudimental elements namely taste, voice, smell, form and touch. The five elements giving rise to these rudimental elements are fire, ether, earth, water and air. Like sensory organs the organs of actions are also five in number they are hands, legs, feet, face, rectum and reproductive organs.

Heart is an important organ of physical body (Annmay Kosh). It is a machine, which provides pure blood to the whole body. The blood enters from one side and comes out from the other. The heart beat indicates the circulation of blood in the body. The automatic organ made from involuntary muscles is secured between both the lungs in the chest area. The shape and dimensions of the heart in each individual is equal to the size of his or her fist. The heart lies in between two sticky sacks like things made of two layers, which are known as covering. The heart is hollow from inside; it contains a veil of flesh, which divides the heart into two sections. Each section has two smaller sections. The upper section is called auricle and the lower is called ventricle. In this way, the heart has four sections, one auricle and one ventricle on both right and left side. The auricle receives the blood and ventricle throws it out. When the blood is pumped in not much pressure is exerted on the muscles but while throwing it out a lot of pressure is exerted. Surprisingly we find that the walls of left auricle are three times thicker than the right ventricle. Therefore, the left ventricle circulates pure blood in the whole body. The pumping and throwing of blood is performed by the expansion and contraction of heart. According to an estimate a healthy person's heart beats 72 times in a minute, whereas it beats 140 times in case of a child. Emotional conditions like sex, anger, fear, happiness and physical exercise increase, the rate, whereas fasting, weakness and unhappiness slow down the rate. Annamay Kosh also contains skull, the spine constituting 26 vertebrae making the vertebral column extending from neck to the rectum and lungs, these will be later explained in the context of Pranayam.

Three guiding Principles for good health

It is essential to control and conserve the coarse or physical body in order to achieve success on the path of Bhog to Yog. The regular practice of Yog makes this large body energetic and regulated. Good health is the biggest gift in this world. Many great people have defined health in different ways but the famous Ayurvedic text Sushrut is more appealing. According to this book, the body - which has all the three doshas i.e. vata, pitta and kapha in equilibrium; the digestive fire is neither more nor less; the seven Dhatus (gross tissue elements of the body) are in correct ratio - Rasa or essence, Rakta (blood), Mansa (flesh), Medas (fat), Asthi (bones), Majja (bone-marrow) and Sukra (semen); the faeces matter is excreted properly; mind, soul and all the 10 sensory organs are happy - is said to be a healthy body.[6] Sushrut's definition of health measures the body on three different levels. A person cannot be called healthy unless the body is in equlibrium at all the levels – physical, mental and spritual. If the body is healthy and yet the person suffers from lust, anger and other negative emotions and becomes the victim of bad thoughts and deeds; then the body begins to deteriorate and spiritual progress also slows down. It is clear that the last two stages of health, i.e. mental and spritual are affected through Yog, whereas Yog clearly contributes to overall physical fitness. Ayurvedic text Charak explains three main basis of health; they are diet, sleep and celibacy.[7] In Mahabharata, when Arjuna becomes fearful and despondent having to fight with near and dear ones in the battle, he seeks Lord Krishna's counsel. Lord Krishna tells him that the devotion is said to be successful when the main factors that determine success, namely diet, actions, thoughts, behaviour, good intentions, sleep and awakening is meaningful.[8]

Diet

Among three guiding principles for good health, diet is the base which cannot be neglected at all. Until or unless a proper diet regime is adopted, one cannot think of achieving good health. In fact diet itself is Bheshjaya (medicine). We can keep the diseases at bay by understanding the science of diet and its effects. The Indian sages and seers have classified food very minutely. Almost all the dieticians in the world prescribe a diet keeping in mind the coarse body's nutritional needs and preservation requirements. Whereas Chandyogya Upanishad cautions us that diet controls our mind as well as the body.[9] The effects on mind become a part of our mental and thinking process, and ultimately we perform according to what we decide at the mental level. Surprisingly diet is a determining factor behind our actions and world view. It is clear that diet nourishes our sensory organs, strengthens the vital energy and it also nourishes the attitude of our mind.[10] Indian sages have proclaimed in the context of diet and its affects – the good and bad intentions with which we consume food, the happy or sad environment in which we eat our food and other minor factors play a very significant role in the personal development. Although in biochemistry, it has not been possible so far to document such effects and influences of diet on human body, diet does have a decisive effect on our thoughts and mind.

Once when the propounder of Ayurved, Sage Charak probed his disciples about health-related issues, one of the disciples Vagabhatt made this remarkable comment: Hithbhuk, Mitbhuk, Ritabhuk, i.e. a person should cosume healthy, balanced and seasonal food in tune with individual nature. Charak recommends that a learned person having restraint over senses should always eat healthy food in sufficient quantity in all seasons. Eating against these principles can generate various serious diseases.[11] We eat food to satisfy three physical needs – first is formation and development of physical organs, second to compensate the physical degeneration caused by day-to-day work and third to develop immunity, energy and vitality and make it capable for work. However, these guidelines are very conveniently forgotten when we sit down to have food. When we partake food making taste as the deciding factor for selection, it may not prove beneficial for health. In the context of above said guidelines about food and its cosumption we can develop three guiding principles that are; what to eat, how to eat and when to eat.

The food that we eat in the form of fat, protein, sugar, water, and salts helps the body in preparing around two thousand different useful compounds. These compounds reach different body organs and parts through blood and give nourishment. We need to select the nutritious items in tune with our nature and bodily needs in order to get best out of this process. We also need to remember that all these nutritious items should be obtained from natural sources and not from meat. Along with the selection of food we also need to pay attention to how and where we eat. While simple food consumed with a peaceful, happy, tension and stress-free state of mind gives excellent results for physical and mental development; most nutritious food consumed in a fearful, stressful and troubled state of mind can lead to several dangerous diseases. The food quickly fixed and eaten in a hurry is not beneficial for body and mind. We need to remember that the teeth are in the mouth not in the intestine. Those who make intestine, in a way work as teeth cannot expect to have good health for a long time. Hence every morsel should be properly chewed and then swallowed after it is mixed with saliva and other juices. Such a person lives longer and remains healthy. Another important point is that eating when one is not hungry or is suffering from indigestion is like taking poison.

Sleep

Sleep is the second most important factor for having good health. It is one of the best gifts of God. Not allowing a person to sleep and keeping him awake is the biggest and most severe punishment in the world. Just imagine the consequences if God takes back sleep from mankind, the whole world will turn into a big asylum in a few days. The weary and tired body needs sleep to get back the energy and strength to work. All the living things on this earth go to sleep after day long work. Therefore, our mental and physical health is dependent on sleep. Every living being in both animal and plant kingdom surrenders to sleep as devised by nature. In fact, our physical and mental health is very much dependent on having a good night's sleep. Early to rise and early to bed has remained the corner stone of Indian life-style. However, widespread industrialization and urbanization have severely impacted upon the daily routine. An individual and a system needs to give due consideration to the fact that sleeping for six to seven hours during any time of the day is not sufficient but we need to sleep at the right time for six to eight hours.

Celibacy

Celibacy is the third pillar for good health. The amount of description made in ancient literature about celibacy, its scope, its basis and importance has not been done in any other subject. The person who follows celibacy with complete austerity develops incredible physical, mental and spiritual abilities. Celibacy constitutes worshipping God, attaining knowledge and protecting and conserving semen. Sage Charak has appealed for promoting celibacy as a kind of favour to society; he declares celibacy to be the biggest virtue that protects the body against diseases, increases vitality, gives happiness to body and mind and makes an humble appeal to propagate in the world.[12] The author of Shatpath also says that a celibate is never unhappy.[13] As a matter of fact, celibacy controls the continuous reduction in mental and physical strengths. It is the strong foundation for having a good life. This applies equally both for men and women. Let us forget yogis for a while, even those enjoying pleasures of life should undertsand that in the absence of a sound body and happy mind, the person cannot even enjoy the luxuries of life. When a person is suffering with fever even delicious sweets taste bitter. Similarly in times of depression the auspicious blessings also sound like curse. Those who wish for well-being should practise celibacy and supporting factors. The first two pillars of good health, diet and sleep play an important role in supporting celibacy. A monogamous man and a monogamous woman (except for days of menstrual cycle), is considered to be a celibate. Sex eduction is not the solution for the problem of HIV/AIDS epidemic, world is grappling with. Indian value system of practising monogamy can certainly help.

In conclusion one can say that the Almighty has gifted us with this physical body (Annamay Kosh), which is a work of art, science and organization. However, we in a way are always eager to destroy and distort this amazing faultless creation on account of personal misconduct, social pressures and mental exertion. Our scale of measuring accomplishment or success in life is flawed. We generally tend to become illogical while dealing with this beautiful body that works like a machine. We continuously ignore the directions to be followed to protect it. As a result, life becomes hellish and then only we realize the pain. Without getting into theoretical discussion, we should try to understand and accept the fact that dietary imbalance, irregular life-style and thinking which is needless are in the root of diseases. Any process and system of the body is directly related with other processes and systems. If we try to meddle with a particular process or system, it's sure to have impact on other processes and systems. From holistic point of view, it is better to treat the body as one unit instead of being constituted of different parts. Dietary imbalance, irregular daily routine, disequilibria of vata, pitta and kapha, imbalance of humours of the body and excess or deficiency of digestive fire has deep impact on the health of the body. It also affects the functioning of various glands. Various diseases are the result of this irregularity.[14] According to Acharya Vagbhatt, the accumulation of faecal matter in the body is also the reason for diseases.[15] The faeces and other waste accumulate in the body due to digestive disorders which are mainly caused by decrease in digestive fire. Because of decrease in digestive fire, food is not properly digested and starts accumalating as faecal matter.

Transformation of Physical Body with Yog

From the very outset, Yog transforms the physical body. Self-discipline, celibacy, cleanliness and austere devotion, posture, and Pranayam play an important role in transformation of the body. Practising Yog helps in keeping the coarse and subtle organs active in its natural state. Needless to say that natural functioning of body organs is the basis of good health. The health maintained through artificial things cannot be ever lasting. Consuming medicines especially allopathic not only reduces the sensitivity of physical organs but also eliminates the chances of reinstating the natural processes. It so happens that in the process of curing one disease, a particular medicine can cause another. These physical diseases slowly lead to mental diseases.

Different yogic processes – posture, breath control or Pranayam, austere devotion, Mudrabandh and Shatkaram – purify different glands, blood, vital energy or Pran and other organs. All the faecal matters, the root cause behind all distortions and diseases get removed from the body. The body, which is maintained with proper diet, sleep and celibacy, does not fall sick. The first two stages of Ashtang Yog, Yama-Niyama (resistance towards passions and observances) actually forms the basis for a healthy human being and a healthy society. Yama (resistance towards passions) in other words non-violence, truth, not to steal, not collecting unwanted things give a momentum to the development of a disciplined society. Niyama (observances) – cleanliness, contentment, austere devotion, self-study and deep devotion towards the Almighty determine individual accomplishment. It should never be thought that non-violence has no role to play in individual progress. Eventually, individual's acceptance will be akin to acceptance by the entire society. Except celibacy, non-violence and other restraints are useful for society whereas cleanliness applies to the individual. In this context, Saint Patanjali calls Yama having universal significance and thus universal application. That is, a nation inclined towards Yog, should not slacken in following non-violence and other restraints using the excuse of time and circumstances. Although cleanliness, devotion, self study and other observances could be in concurrence with the time, circumstances and needs of the nation. The word 'devotion' has attained a larger perspective in the Indian literature.

Saint Patanjali's brief regime of Kriya Yog gives great emphasis to self-study, deep devotion towards the Almighty and also to austerity or Tapa. It is evident that Tapa or devotion is about continuous enhancement of physical and mental energies and is not about maltreating physical body. According to Patanjali, devotion is about dealing with the mental conflicts; and having more physical energy and analytical faculties imparts an individual with tremendous capacity to deal with such conflicts. The Indian sages have recognized hunger, quest, cold and hot conditions, happiness-unhappiness, loss-gain, fame-disrespect and victory- defeat as the confusions going on at the physical and mental level. The ability to deal with conflicts eventually depends on the amount of patience one has. Patience is the ultimate virtue considered to be the core quality of family, social, political, religious and spiritual life. Gita gives a much broader perspective to devotion. It classifies Yama-Niyam (integral elements of Tapa or devotion) as of physical, verbal and mental in nature. The luxurious life style full of pretence depreciates the natural strengths rapidly. The human being who has become used to a comfortable life-style cannot imagine to live without the luxuries. He feels like a handicapped person in the absence of these comforts despite having all the organs. Due to such thinking, the body becomes a bundle of diseases. Devotion is an invitation to sacrifice luxurious life lived in contradiction with the nature.

Asana (posture) is an important part of Yog to maintain the proper physical balance. Saint Patanjali defines it in a very simple manner and says that sitting comfortably and straight is Asana. Different writers have different opinions about posture. Out of these the most interesting is from 'Dhyanbindupanishdkar'. According to it the types of Asana are as many as there are number of living species.[16] We need to nourish the nerves and muscles in order to keep the body healthy for a long time. Asana and exercise give strength. Exercise plays a very important role in providing nutritional elements to different organs and parts in the form of food that we eat. In the absence of physical exercise the body does not develop in a balanced manner. Asana and light exercise also strengthen the respiratory system. Many Yog experts are being successful in curing different types of diseases through Yog Sadhna. Asanas are very effective in curing the diseases related to spine, neck, stomach and knees in a very simple and effective manner.

Pran (Vital life force) and its Role

Vital life force (Pran) and mind (Mana) inspire our physical body. Vital life force has the major responsibility to keep the physical body active round the clock. Development-deterioration and protection- nutrition of the body from birth to death are all dependent on it. The sage in Vrihadranyak Upanishad declares the Pran being most important over voice, eyes, ears, intelligence and semen. The sage says that when all these organs failed in front of demons, vital life force rescued the gods and goddesses, and it began working for the glory of the Gods. When the demons saw this they charged ahead to destroy Pran. The demons collided with the selfless Pran and broke apart into pieces. All the gods and goddesses won as they capitulated to the power of Pran. The person who recognizes the value of Pran and makes it the very base, certainly wins over enemies.[17] The sage of Chandyogya Upanishad echoes the same view. Practically speaking the person can live without all other sensory organs but life is unimaginable in the absence of Pran. The mind and sensory organs become strong with Pran and weak in its absence. The strength of Pran gives rise to self-confidence. The vital energy is the basis of disease-fighting capacity and life. Pran makes the whole body energetic and healthy besides the glands, heart, lungs, brain and spine. Controlling (Sadhna) of vital life force is at the base of all successes and accomplishments in life; it plays an important role in ensuring physical well-being, mental strength and concentration of mind. Controlling the vital life force automatically controls the mind and sensory organs. The process of controlling the Pran or vital life force is known as Pranayam in Yog. While the physical or coarse body is constituted with food, Pran has been separately recognized as a separate section (Pranmay Kosh) constituted with vital energy or essence of life. As a matter of fact, vital life force and mind (mana) work in synchronicity and are combined with the coarse body. It is only the Ananmay Kosh or coarse body which develops and grows in size, while the extension of Pranmay and Manomay Kosh occurs owing to its after effects.

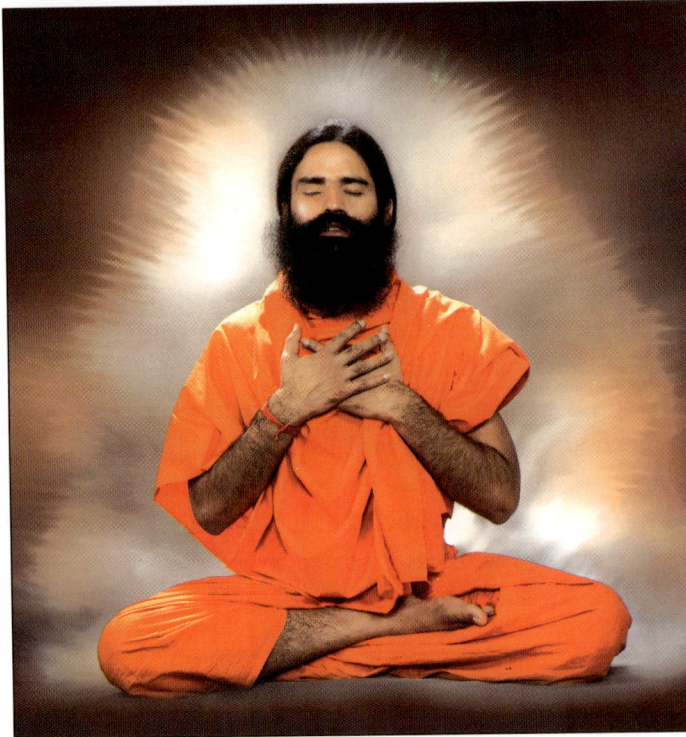

Swami Ramdevji practicing Pranayam

We need to understand that there is only one Pran, which inspires the coarse body but based on the different physical processes and actions Pran has been given different names. On this very basis Pran has been classified into 10 types. Basically it has five main divisions and five sub-divisions. The main divisions are Pran (vital energy), Apana (expiration), Samana (uniformity), Vyana (circulation) and Udana (upward movement). In the sub divisions we have Naga, Kurma, Krukal, Dhananjay and Devdutt. It needs to be specially mentioned that the Vedic literature contains of many references to the five main classifications of vital energy but Kurma and other secondary vital energies did not get much importance. Pran remains in the upper part of the body. It gives momentum to our sensory organs and also activates the lungs, heart, food pipe and respiratory system. The continuous process of inhaling and exhaling is actually Pran. The Apana or air that moves upwards resides in the rectum area. It plays the role of a cleaner. The evacuation of faeces and polluted air is possible with the help of this air.

Various processes carried on from heart to navel are performed through vital energy called Samana or uniformity. It resides in the navel region and controls all the functions related to liver, intestines, spleen, pancreas and other digestive organs. It supplies the juices made from food to different parts of the body. Vyana (circulation) is spread all through the body including the sensory organs. It sends the emotions from all the systems to mind and from there the messages are transmitted to the sensory organs and organs of action. It is circulated all over the body and gives energy and activates the muscles, glands, nerves etc. Udana or air that moves upward remains active from throat to head. It gives energy and inspiration to organs present in the upper body and directs and gives energy to the upward movement of brain. At the time of death the soul separates from body and proceeds into the other world or into a womb. Small processes like sneezing, feeling sleepy, thirst, hunger, feeling satisfied, belching, hiccups and swelling are controlled by sub-Pran like Naga, Kurmadi etc.[18] Till these natural processes continue in the body it gets energy and remains energetic mentally. However, with the bad conduct, bad food habits and bad thoughts the Pran becomes polluted or disturbed and normal functions of the body like digestion of food, formation of blood, evacuation of faeces and other functions are obstructed. The process of purification of polluted air is called Pranayam. Pranayam removes all the physical and mental diseases and makes life easy, simple and joyful. Pranayam is like a magic wand, which rejuvenates, activates and energizes the inactive body. Pranayam is about igniting the will to live; it is the greatest medicine of all medicines. The main objective of Pranayam is production, protection, usage and management of vital energy to the optimum. The better management of Pran both at physical and mental levels shall lead to having better success at achieving one's goals.

Pran controls and inspires different processes of body because Pran or vital energy is spread in it and therefore it is necessary to understand its constitution in order to understand the effect of Pranayam for the purpose of nourishing the Pran. Even if we do not understand the entire constitution, we should at least know the constitution of that organ with which the Pran or vital energy is directly related to namely lungs. Our body has two lungs, one on each side of the chest. The left is slightly wider and heavier than the right lung. The air reaches the throat through the nostrils and from its lower part it reaches the left and right lungs. The throat circulating air to lungs consists of small pores; they are so sensitive that the dust and foreign particles are removed through cough and sneezing. This natural process protects the lungs from dust and food particles. The constitution of lungs plays an important role in the process of blood circulation. The lungs consist of innumerable minute pouches of air and blood cells. The walls of both the lungs are so thin that only gas can pass through it. The blood flowing within these walls takes oxygen from these pouches and gives carbon dioxide to outside air after exhaling. In this way the blood gets purified with continuous flow of oxygen . When oxygen enters in the blood it becomes dark red in colour and is known as pure blood, whereas it turns blue when it mixes with carbon dioxide.

Lungs carry on the respiration in the body. When we inhale the chest muscles expand along with air pouches and this fills them with pure air. When the air is exhaled these pouches and lungs contract along with the muscles. In this process, while exhaling entire air present in the lungs is not removed and sufficient amount of air remains. As we live a fast-paced life, process of respiration becomes fast and shallow as a result the air left over in the lungs keeps on increasing. This remaining air remains inactive, i.e. doesnot become part of respiratory cycle giving rise to many diseases. Pranayam, most importantly purifies this left over air only. While practicing Pranayam we take a long and deep breath and more amount of air reaches the lungs. When we breathe out with the same depth the polluted air present in the lungs is thrown out.

Why We Need Pranayam ?

According to an estimate our lungs contain air in the density of 180 - 200 cube inches. When we inhale we take in 30 cube inches air and exhale the same amount. In this way we can see that out of the total air inhaled around 150 cube inches remains in the lungs all the time. If we take a deep long breath then we can manage up to 100 cube inches of air. With the help of Pranayam we can influence major part of this air present in the lungs. If the air becomes pure the food is digested properly, the body organs become strong, the body as a whole is purified and rejuvenated. Whatever food we eat comes into the contact of oxygen that is inhaled in the process of respiration. The process prepares several important elements required for the body. The carbon present in the food becomes carbon dioxide. It mixes with nitrogen, another gas that is present in the food and is thrown out when we exhale. Phosphorous present in the food comes in contact with oxygen and becomes phosphate, which builds bones in our body.

Here it needs to be mentioned that short, incomplete and shallow respiration is generally fast and the person taking short breaths does not live long. Longer (deeper) and slower the breath, longer the life. This is the secret behind the long life of tortoise, which lives up to 200 years or even more. It takes three to five breaths in a minute. Pigeon, pigs and other animals take 34-37 breaths per minute and live for 10-12 years. Human beings take 15 breaths in a minute and by practising Pranayam they can increase the life span. Controlling the breath gives the ability to control the sensory organs, leads to intellectual and spiritual attainment. History is full of references about glorious stories of many practioners of Pranayam. Pranayam for individual practice should be selected in accordance with the objective one could be striving for. Saint Patanjali has specified Pranayam that is useful for devotion. The other texts and classics describe Pranayam techniques with can strengthen the body and cure it of diseases.

Mental Aspects of Yog

The mind is like a mirror, which reflects the image of an individual. It is the mind that creates peace in war and war in peace, harmony in disharmony and vice-versa. Mind is the biggest problem and eventually solution to all problems lies in the mind only. Psychology has been developed to study mind only. But do we still know what is mind? The conclusion is yet to be arrived at. The Indian sages categorized sensory and vital energy as Ananmay Kosh and Pranmay Kosh respectively and then recognized the activities of mind as Manomay Kosh. Mind (mana) is the contact point between individual's internal and external worlds. It is also the mediator and is in the middle of the physical and etheric body, mental body and causal body. It cannot be measured in dimensions of length, breadth and thickness. We can call it as the window open to the knowledge in that particular point in time.

The mind analyzes all the external information sent by the sensory organs and synthesizes it and the same mind analyzes various experiences of soul and brain and sends it out. It controls the physical and etheric bodies. It is the soul of the etheric body.[19] It comes from nature. It makes one of the four factors along with intellect, reason and ego (Buddhi, Chitta, Ahankar) of the innerself. When we go into the depth we realize that actually the other three are different forms of mind only and are known with different names due to different functions they perform.

The functions of innerself have been classified very minutely. On the inner self, along with Manomay Kosh, also dependent is Vigyanmay Kosh. The main basis for its conceptualization is element of intelligence; and can be termed as the enlightened area of mind. When dealing with confusion about whether to do something or not to do it, it is the intelligence which becomes active. The mind brings forth some logic and counter logic in this confused state of mind creating a situation, which helps us in taking a decision. The mental processes (mana) take us towards forming various relations, at the same time intellectual processes help us in coming out of those situations. The intelligence makes a right or wrong decision solely depending on the level of mental development and ego. Ego full of passion does not let the highest level of consciousness express itself. The low level of consciousness and ego obstructs the decision-making capacity of mind. This process of understanding the struggle between resolutions and alternatives is very difficult to understand but technically it is very simple and natural. Budhi, Chitta and Ahankar are various dimesions of mind. Saint Patanjali uses the word Chitta for Mana as well. Swami Atmanand Saraswati has classified the constitution, composition, functioning of different elements of mind very minutely in his book, Shivasankalp and Vedic Psychology. According to Swamiji the mind works at five levels namely divine, Yaksha or demigod, wisdom, consciousness and equanimity. The equanimity has been further classified as pertaining to soul, universe and subjugating the mind. The divine mind compiles all the information with the help of divine sensory organs and sends it across different parts of body. The mind in the form of demigod supervises the organs of actions. This mind keeps the movement of the organs of action and decides whether the internal orders have to be followed or not. The wisdom makes a logical analysis of the information received through wisdom and takes a decision. The supervisor of organs of actions introduces the mind in the form of demi god to take decisions to be followed. The mind element active at this moment is element of intelligence. The conscious mind keeps an account of the influence of actions and experiences values. The fifth mind, i.e. equanimity works on three different levels and is the centre of knowledge free of confusion, for developing a worldview and of committment for divine personal conduct.

What is mind? It is difficult to control it in complete form but what does mind do and how? In this context we can understand the analysis of sages in a better manner. Sage Gautam gives an interesting information with respect to mind; he says mind does not generate two types of knowledge or experiences at the same time.[20] In other words mind does not grasp the smell or its essence at the same time when it is grasping the form of an object. But it all takes place in a fraction of second and we do not realize the whole process.

The complete engagement of mind with the welfare and development of individual depends on its health. Diseased mind is the biggest hindrance in the path of development, peace and happiness. Saint Patanjali made an in-depth analysis of different illnesses arising in mind in the form of depression, disappointment, worry, illusion, fear etc. at different points in time. The study done to understand the foreground of mind, its conditions, feelings, five types of anguish are indeed pioneering.

According to Yog our mind can be in five different states or conditions. They are inaction, destruction, confusion, distraction, concentration and deep meditation. When we are worried, angry and sad our mind is lost somewhere or totally insensitive. In this state the passion is predominant and the mind is hence wandering in external world. It is engrossed in meaningless activities. When our body is weak and unconscious due to some disease then the mind is said to be in a state of confusion. In this stage the mind is generally dominated with negative feelings like jealousy, hatred etc. and is the result of Tama or anger arising in the mind. In this stage the person forgets his responsibilities and gets angry at every small thing and the mind is always inclined towards negative actions. The man who controls the feelings like loss-gain, fame-defame, victory-defeat, happiness-unhappiness, life-birth and other worldly factors partially is said to be associated with distraction. When the person is able to concentrate on one particular subject totally, it is called concentration. Ahead of this stage is deep concentration when the mind is free from all kinds of conditions in the mind. Out of these the first five are not useful for the practice of Yog. Although, after reaching the third stage, i.e. distraction the person starts experiencing the possibility of concentrating the mind on one subject. In this stage the person tries to concentrate his mind on one goal or aim. When the mind wanders in this state for some time it automatically gets into the stage of deep meditation. This is the highest point of mind; it is the ultimate stage of purity and positive thinking. The person then reaches the stage of deep meditation and experiences happiness or Ananda. When he remains in this stage for some time he experiences different levels of deep meditation or Samadhi and ultimately attains salvation.

Saint Patanjali has explained different conditions of mind while being in these stages. He has categorized them in five types – evidence, transformation, alternative, sleep and memory. According to Saint Patanjali they give both happiness and unhappiness. If we look at the mental and worldly actions then we will be surprized to know that there is no mental or worldly action, which does not fit into these five conditions. The different conditions prevailing in the mind from time to time create disturbances and confusions. These conditions get involved in subjects and transform into lusts. These change the virtues into sins. But if we try to control the conditions with calm mind then we will get positive results. When the conditions of mind are suitable to the environment, which is the beginning of concentration, then the different changes taking place in the environment lead to disappointment or lean it towards worries and does not allow it to prepare for defense. On this matter Dr Radhakrishnan has said: 'We cannot change the sequences of incidents happening in the world and the disturbances taking place in our mind according to our desire but we should have strong will power that none of these can influence us and we do not deviate from it in any way'.

Our behaviour in the world is accomplished through these mental conditions and it is necessary to be controlled in factual and positive manner. The factual and positive state of conditions is a good indication for upliftment of an individual. It is also necessary to understand that factual state guarantees positive state. Saint Patanjali gives it a lot of significance. The objective is of placing evidence, transformation and alternative in the first three places. These three stages stress on the factual and positive bent of mind.

Ultimately evidence is fact. The factual knowledge is based on three factors. They are: perception, inference and testimony (word). Gautam's 'Nyaya Darshan' carries on detailed study on Indian philosophy. Normally, the knowledge obtained from sensory organs is known as perception, the knowledge obtained on the basis of some direct evidence (hetu) is called inference and the knowledge after hearing the Vedas or reliable persons is called testimony. We also need to understand that evaluating a thing on the basis of its form or error is juxtaposed to its practicality. According to Saint Patanjali this notion is an error. Therefore, it is extremely important that a thing should be used without thinking about evidence. If knowledge is judged on the basis of evidence or inaccuracy then it will be error. When something becomes superior due to its evidence or proofs and contains errors then we think of alternative. Hearing or learning something about a thing and its constitution gives rise to the condition of alternative in the mind. All the three conditions namely evidence, mistakes and alternative are related to the conscious mind of the person, whereas all the mental conditions arising when the person is dreaming has been termed as condition of sleep by Saint Patanjali. The mind is extremely calm and peaceful during sleep and many desires and aspirations arise in the mind when it is in the state of dreams. This state is either beneficial or harmful for us. The state of dream is full of many unsolved queries arising in the mind. The dreams are nothing but the combined representation of desires and aspirations present in our mind since ages, which were suppressed when the mind was awake.

Saint Patanjali has recognized the incidents, experiences that took place in our life and the attitude of remembering the past happenings as another condition of mind called memory. This condition of mind is a live document of our past. Thousands of pieces of information present in the mind comes out during conscious or unconscious state and either proves to be beneficial or harmful for the person. This condition is both inspirational and provocative. It can also be the basis of violent nature and also self-defence. The memories, which are based on some resolutions, become inspirational and some negative ones give rise to turmoil in life. Saint Patanjali calls them as giving rise to happiness and unhappiness. Careful supervision of these conditions decides whether it is difficult or simple. The propounders of Yog made a humble appeal to the people who desire to lead a happy and satisfied life to control the flow of such conditions disturbing mind. They have also cautioned people to stop the inflow of negative elements that hinder the process of removing the conditions from mind. There are nine such negative elements; they are disease, confusion, carelessness, suspicion, laziness and desire for peace, illusions, jealousy and uncertainty. Besides, there are also four types of secondary elements namely unhappiness, wickedness, egotism and respiration.

Saint Patanjali has also described about five negative conditions that influence the functioning of mind. They are ignorance, pride, enmity, hatred and attachment that created different types of conditions in the mind and make it diseased. These five negative conditions that remain attached to the mind are very big hindrances. These conditions always make us feel inferior and ruin the life. In this context there is an important reference made in Yog classics that ignorance is the root cause of all the other four types of anguish. This is known as the field of area of other anguish. Pride, enmity, hatred and attachment arise from ignorance and can also be called as the branches of ignorance or half knowledge. It is the root cause of all unhappiness, tensions, anger, ill intentions, bad behaviour and meanness. Indian philosophers believe that ignorance is the hindrance in the way of all attachments. Ignorance is the root cause for inaccuracy. Pride is a passion which gives rise to egotism of lower level. The high aspiration for fame, anger and vengeance when it is not fulfilled is carried on in the shadow of pride. Enmity arises due to the strong desire for a thing with a feeling of comfort. Desire and aspirations are also one of its form. Enmity gives rise to involvement in worldly affairs. Non-attachment is one of the ways to recognize the superiority of ascetics who sacrifice involvement in worldly affairs. Hatred is the fourth anguish and is actually the form of enmity. Enmity gives birth to hatred. Enmity itself means attachment with some things and hating some other things. Enmity cannot arise without it. Attachment is the fifth and last anguish that gives birth to desires and fears. The social reformers of the world have dreamt of fearless people and fearless society. Crime and atrocities can be carried on in the society only under the veil of fear. A Vedic prayer desires for revealing fear that we should not only be fearless of the natural incidents occurring in the universe and earth but also from friends, enemies, known, unknown, direct, indirect, night, day etc. All the desires should be our friends. Western philosophy has conducted a lot of research on phobia. It says that if a person is afraid of a particular thing it attacks the person's mind with the same intensity in other words the person develops extreme fear in his mind towards that thing for example towards exams, height etc. The person becomes over protective and tries to feel secure. He wakes up in the night and checks whether the doors and windows are properly locked or not, whether the night watchman is patrolling or not. He wakes up hearing slightest sound and feels as if somebody is attacking him. Saint Patanjali sees this as the ultimate condition of fear of death. Actually the root cause of all fears is the fear of death.

Sage Vyas advises to burn all the anguishes in the fire of wisdom. A seed burnt in fire is not suitable for sowing, in the same way anguishes burnt in the fire of wisdom will not give rise to unhappiness and other negative thoughts. Anguishes should be nipped in the bud before they attack the mind. When anguish is not controlled in the first stage it becomes a habit and a part of our life. It becomes extremely difficult to remove the conditions at this stage. Yog Darshan includes the description of these anguishes arising in mind at different levels due to ignorance. Mental ailment, depression, phobia, disappointment etc. arise in the mind in the form of conditions. Irregular daily routine and life-style give birth to negative conditions on a conscious mind. The tough competition and high work pressures are making it even more complicated.

The conditions keep on transforming due to social, economic, political, cultural and religious happenings but there is practically no change in the basic nature of the person. Reflection of conditions in mind is the only solution. The reflection of conditions in mind begins with the transformation. The outward flow of conditions from inner self is actual transformation. If the person cannot stop thinking about the subject then destruction begins. At first we think of subjects then we get attracted, which leads to lust, anger, attachment, illusions, loss of intelligence and finally destruction. This chain which has no control over the conditions leads to sorry tale of destruction of the person. Hence it is extremely necessary to transform these conditions with the help of reflection. An individual or society lacking peace of mind does not deserve happiness or satisfaction. The sage of Kathopanishad declares that a person who is involved in sins, lacks self control and is unable to control the sensory organs such a person cannot attain internal peace despite understanding the verbal meaning. We understand that controlling the conditions of mind is an important factor in practice of Yog. This is one point, which helps the person in entering the inner self from external world. Although it is not easy, leave aside an ordinary man, even Arjuna had expressed his inefficiency in practising it by saying that it is equal to collecting air in a bundle when Lord Krishna had advised him to practise self control. The difficulty for Arjuna was the strength and strong determination of mind more than its playfulness. Had the playful mind been mild, weak and soft then it would not have been dangerous but the strong determination, dedication and concentration prove to be challenges for the playful mind in the process of self control.

Mental conditions establish physical and mental needs in the form of lust. When the person satisfies his hunger the desire for fame arises in his mind. It sometimes arises in the most dangerous forms and becomes the cause of serious acts. The mental dissatisfaction is expressed in its worst forms and gives rise to inhuman acts. When the desires arise in the golden veil of ambitions then they make the person egocentric. The tasks, which are done with the feeling of ego or pride, become destructive. The society dominated with egocentric people reacts in a negative way. The person or society full of negative reactions cannot be calm and cultured. It loses compassion, auspicious thoughts, productivity, and creativity. The person acts like a machine, the society is nothing but a crowd, the voice appears to be chaos, discussions become debates, groups becomes criminal troupes. This process goes on developing. We understand the seriousness of the situation when the religion becomes violent. The religion become a subject of mockery and places of worship develop as centres of destruction. We need to bring all this to a stop at some point. Yog is the invitation to people to control this condition of mind, which is working on the basis of people and society's thinking. This is not easy but does that mean that we accept defeat looking into the difficulty and complexity? Kalidas encourages us and says that one totally committed towards achieving their goal cannot be stopped just like the flow of water moving towards the slope cannot be stopped. All that is needed - strong determination and committment to achieve anything.

Yog classics have described controlling, removing and getting free from different conditions arising in mind as a scientific process. When the person adopts the external sources of Yog, the mind is encouraged towards deeper involvement in Yog. He develops the social understanding with the help of Yama-Niyama which includes cleanliness, resistance towards passion and practising non-violence. The auspicious feelings in the form of resistance towards passions weaken the ill-intentions present in mind. Yog plays an important role in controlling the mind and making it strong. Saint Patanjali advises for attaining concentration of mind with regular practice and sense of non-attachment. Continuous efforts to keep the mind free of conditions and negative thoughts is called Abhayasa or practice and non-attachment is about deep disinterest in material goods and having a mind free of desires.

Lord Krishna had inspired Arjuna, who expressed that self-control is impossible, to do Abhayasa and practise non-attachment. Practice will give good results only when it is done for a long time with will power and determination. If we violate this rule then practice weakens. We need to practise a lot in order to become proficient in various things for the sake of existence in the world. Therefore, we can understand the seriousness and carefulness required to practice self control and make the mind free of conditions. We cannot pretend to be free of attachment. It is an internal feeling. When the mind is totally free of desires both visible and heard only then we can achieve ultimate state of non-attachment. When the person experiences the contradiction between the mind and his/her true nature then he/she develops the feeling of non-attachment. The person engrossed in the world considers the mental condition to be his condition and mental aspirations to be his aspiration due to ignorance and but then the light of knowledge removes this illusion and enlightens him with wisdom.

We have already discussed about the hindrances coming in the way of removing the conditions from the mind. Sage Patanjali has not prescribed norms for social behaviour in order to walk on the path of Yog. Yog classics talk of four kinds of social behaviour viz. friendship, empathy, ignoring and happiness, which support pursuit of Yog. In day-to-day life, pursuit of different kind of behaviour in accordance with the person dealt with, is an important factor in freeing our mind from conditions. These factors make life easy which otherwise is full of favourable and unfavourable conditions. Friendship with happy people, being empathetic and kind towards the sick, feeling happy with pious people and ignoring the ill-minded and sinners helps us to stay stable on the path of Yog.

Practice of Yog destroys all the anguishes and strengthens the mind. Yog practice improves resoluteness in a surprising manner and as a result, life becomes balanced and and joyful naturally. The directions, prescribed by modern science for having a balanced life are too superficial when compared to Yog Sadhna. The resoluteness generated from practise of Yog embellishes a person with extraordinary qualities. The biggest challenge before an ordinary person is to maintain balance and harmony in this age of complexities and adversities. Yog presents a scientific method by giving analysis for all the mental confusions and for making the mind free of these confusions.

Stress is spreading like an epidemic in the metropolises owing to increasing desire for material comforts, problems at home and work place, unfulfilled ambitions leading to frustration and sad memories. Restlessness, anger, anxiety, depression, stress, lack of concentration, non-productivity, loss of memory, irritability and insomnia are the results of stress. Stress leads to high blood pressure and other diseases.

Kalhan had mentioned in the classic titled, 'Rajtarangini' that clouds in the sky give an illusion and appear in the form of lion, tiger, elephant, demon, snake and other different shapes. In the same way different conditions arising in the mind at different moments give rise to tensions. Stress has its own body language. We can easily recognise stress as indicated through changes in behaviour, body movements etc.

Specialists all over the world recommend meditation in order to get rid of stress. The Western psychiatrists are using Yog to a great extent. The patient under stress is asked to practise Shavasana and control his/her actions and mental conditions with the help of Pran and mind in the form of guided relaxation. This is another form of meditation, but it is very beneficial. Yog has provided a fixed method to make the mind bright, intelligent and energetic through meditation and concentration. Gaining knowledge is concentrating the mind on to internal or external with the help of devotion, celibacy and Pranayam. The places in the body where mind is focused is called concentration of mind in that particular place. Therefore, we can say that concentration and meditation are complimentary to each other. Meditation is a very broad term. Although saint Patanjali uses it for a definite purpose, he says meditation is a process of self-realization. However, he does not have any issues in considering a person who does his/her work with extreme care as being in meditative state of mind.

Yog mentions different methods of meditation and gives the freedom to select any one. The person selects the method of meditation according to his or her interest. Meditation and interest are closely related to each other. A person, who selects what he is interected in, can attain concentration very easily. With the regular practice of meditation the person develops the quality of diverting the mind from one condition to another. He quickly changes his mind during stress. The thoughts, which obstruct the state of rest or sleep, are immediately controlled with the help of meditation. He controls the feelings of victory, defeat, loss, gain, respect, disrespect etc. A person develops patience with the help of meditation.

Spiritual Aspects of Yog

According to saint Patanjali Yog has three main objectives:

■ To remove all types of anguish present in the body

■ Attain the stage of deep meditation by removing the conditions of mind

■ Attaining salvation of mind by self-realization.

The person is able to remove the physical anguish with the help of yoking Annamaya and Pranmaya kosh and conditions of mind with the help of Pranmaya, Manomaya and Vigyanmay kosh. As has been mentioned earlier, the process of mind making decisions in called Buddhi (intellect). The actions are performed taking inspiration from the intellect. The sharpness of brain or dullness is due to the performance of this part of the body.

Successes achieved in the world are the primary determinants of Buddhi, the secondary determinant is the removal of conditions of mind, and the highest concept of Buddhi is attaining knowledge and higher most is attaining the stage of deep meditation. Lord Krishna had described this condition of the mind as the stage of wisdom to Arjuna. This stage of intellect is described as having attained superknowledge or supernatural wisdom in Upanishads. The pure mind obtained with the help of this practice helps in removing the anguishes such as ignorance present in the mind easily. When the ignorance and other anguishes are removed from mind and the conditions become calm, the devotee moves towards the path leading to the stage of deep meditation. He is able to enter the stage of deep meditation and attain spiritual fulfilment. The mind does not face hindrances after reaching this stage. After reaching the stage of deep mediation the mind gets very refined and is revolutionary which has been termed as having Ritambhara Pragya.

 After reaching this stage the seeker remembers only his goal, the seeker and what is sought get merged. In this stage of Samadhi, source of Ananda, the Almighty God becomes the ultimate aim to attain. The seeker does not remember anything during this stage, neither about self nor the fact that he is in the stage of deep meditation. He only thinks about supreme soul. He has already attained the stage of happiness. The sages of Upanishad also recognize this as the last stage of happiness. The stage of happiness also changes along with the stages of deep meditation. The seeker gets firm in this stage and moves towards the form of God.

Saint Patanjali classifies Samadhi in two main categories as Sampragyat (determinate) and Asampragyat (indeterminate) and in further sub-categories. All these classifications and subdivisions represent different levels of deep meditation. One should remember that wisdom arises from the stage of deep meditation. Once in a state of determinate Samadhi, the devotee need not to make efforts to gain wisdom from other sources. In indeterminate Samadhi even the Ritambhara Pragya or the virtues attained from it also lose their value.

In determinate Samadhi conditions of mind are in control but not totally destroyed while in indeterminate Samadhi all afflictions of mind are completely destroyed. The soul is in direct intercourse with the Almighty and it reconises its true nature. This is the stage of salvation, state of meeting the supreme soul, this is nirvana or emancipation. This is the end of all problems. This is the end of accomplishment of life. This is the permanent fate. This is the last achievement of spiritual life. This is the biggest gift of devotion of Yog.

References and Comments

1. *Aṣṭachakrāa navaḍwrāa dēvāanāaṃ purōyōḍhyāa,*
    Taṣyāaṃ hiraṇyaḥ kośaḥ ṣwaṛgō jyotiṣāavritaḥ।   *Atharvaveda* 1o.2.31

2. *Prabhrāajāanāaṃ hariṇēeṃ yaśasāa Sampaṛēevṛatāaṃ ।*
    puraṃ hiraṇyamayēeṃ brahmāa vivēśāaparāajitāaṃ ।   *Atharvaveda* 1o.2.33

3. *Ibid*

4. *Yō vai taaṃ brahmanō Vēdāaṃritēnāavṛitāaṃ puraṃ ।*
    Taṣmāa brahma ca brāahmāaścha chakṣuḥ prāaṇaṃ prajāaṃ daduḥ ॥   *Atharvaveda* 1o.2.29

5. *Agniṛvāagbhōoṭwāa mukhaṃ prāaviśaḍ, vāayuḥ prāaṇō bhōoṭwāa nāasikē prāaviśaḍ,*
    Āadityaśchakṣuṛbhōoṭwāaaskśinēe prāaviśaḍ,
    diśaḥ śṛōṭraṃ bhōoṭwāa kaṛṇau prāaviśaḍ,
    Aṇṇō-śdhivanaṣpata yō tōmāani bhōoṭwa ṭwachaṃ prāaviśaṇśchandramāa manō bhōoṭwāa nṛidyaṃ
    prāaviśaṭ mṛityuṛapāanō bhōoṭwāa nāabhiṃ prāaviśaṭ, āapōrāto bhōoṭwāa śiṣnaṃ prāaviśaṇ ।
         (Ait. upa. 1.2.4)

6. *Samadōṣaḥ samagniśca samadhāatu malakṛiyaḥ ।*
    prasannāatmēndriyamanāaḥ ṣwastha ityabhidhēeyatē ॥   *Sushrut -Sanhita sutra*

7. *Trayōpaṣṭambhāa āahāaranidrāa brahmacaṛyamati ॥*   *Charak*

8. *Yuktāahāaravihāarasya yuktacē ṣṭasya karmasu ।*
    Yuktaṣwa prāavabōdhasya yōgō bhavati dukhahāa ॥   *Gita 6.17*

9. *Amamaśitaṃ trēdhāa vidhēeyaṇtē taṣya yaḥ ṣthaviṣṭhō dhāatuḥ tatpurēeṣaṃ bhavati yō*
    madhyaṣtanmāansaṃ yō 5nitaḥ tanmanaḥ ।

10. *Āahāara śudhāu satwaśudhiḥ ṣatwaśudhāu ḍhruvāa ṣmṛitiḥ ।*
    Ṣmṛitiṛlabdhē saṛva granthināaṃ vipramōkṣaḥ ॥   *Chandyogyopanishad*

11. *Hitāaśēe ṣyāaṃmitāaśēe ṣyāat kāalabhōjēe jitendriyaḥ,*
    paṣyaṇ rogāaṇbahōoṇ kaṣṭāaṇbudhimāan viṣamāaśanaat ।   *Charak*

12. *Charak. ch-1, Rasāayanapāade-4*

13. *Brahmachāarēe na kāaṇchanāaṛittimāaṛcchhati ॥*   *Shatpath .5.4.3*

14. *Vāataḥ pittaṃ kaphaścēti trayō dōṣāaḥ samāasataḥ ।*
    Vikrataavikritāaḥ dēhaṃ ghnaṇti saṃvaṛdhayaṇti ca ॥
    kupitāanāaṃ hi dōṣāaṇāaṃ śarēerē paridhāavatāaṃ ।
    Yatra sagaṃ khatu vāiguṇyāad vyāadhiḥ tatrōpajāayatē ।   *Sushrut*

15. *Rogāaḥ saṛva5pi maṇdē5ghō sutarāamudarāaṇica ।*
    Ajēeṛṇāanyatināuśchāaṇtaiḥ jāayaṇtē malasaṇchayāat ॥   *Vagbhatt*

16. *Āasanāani ça tāavaṇti yāavaṇtyō jēevajāatayaḥ ।* Dhyanindupanishad Verse 42

17. *Brihadāaraṇyakōpaniśaḍa 1.3.7*

18. *Niḥśwāasōççhhwāa sakāasāaśca prāaṇakarmēti kēerṭitāaḥ ।*
Apāanavāa yō karmatat viśmōoṭrāadi visarjanaṃ ॥
Hāanōpāadāanachēṣṭāadi vyāana karmēti çhēśyatē ।
udāana karma taṭ prōktaṃ dēhasyōṇnayanāadi yaṭ
Pōśaṇāadi samāanaṣya nāagakōormēti çhōçhyatē
Nimēetanāadi karṇaṣya kṣutaṃ vaī krikaraṣya çha।
Dēvadaṭāaṣya viprēṇḍrataṇḍēe kōormēti kēertitaṃ
Dhaṇanjayaṣya śōphāadi sarvakarma prakēertitaṃ । Yogi Yagyavalkya 4.66–69

19. *Taṣmāaḍvāa aītaṣmāaḍ prāaṇamayāadatyō5ṇtara āaṭmāa manōmayaḥ ।*
Tanāiṣa pōorṇaḥ । (Tāittēerēeya upa. Valli II)

20. *Yugpaṭ jgyāanāananutpaṭṭirmanasō liṅgaṃ ।* Nyaydarshanv.1.16

21. *Avidyāa kṣēṭramuṭṭarēṣāaṃ prasuptatanu viçchhainōḍāarāaṇāaṃ ।* Yogdarshan 2.4

22. *Abhayaṃ na karaṭyantarikṣamabhayaṃ ṭyāawāapritshavēeubhē imē ।*
Abhayaṃ paśçhāadabhayaṃ puraṣṭāaduṭṭarāadadharaadabhayaṃ nō aṣtu ।
Abhyaṃ mitrāadabhayamitraadabhayaṃ jgyāatāadabhayaṃ purō yeḥ ।
Abhyaṃ naktamabhayaṃ divāa naḥ sarvāa āaśāa mama mitraṃ bhavaṇtu । Atharvaveda 9.15.5–6

23. *Dhyāayatō viṣayāaṇpunṣaḥ saṅgaṣṭeṣōopajāayatē ।*
Saṅgāaṭsaṅgāayatē kāamaḥ kāamāaṭkrōdhō 5bhijāayatē ।
krōdhāaṭbhavati sammōhaḥ sammōhāaṭsmriti vibhramaḥ ।
Ṣmritibhraṇśāaḍ budhināaśō buddhināa śāaṭpraṇaśyati ॥ Gita 2.62–63

24. *Aśāaṇtaṣya kutaḥ sukhaṃ ।* Gita 2.66

25. *Nāavirātē duścharitaaḥnāaśāaṇtō nāasamāahitaḥ ।*
Nāaśāaṇtamanasō vāapi praggyāanēnāinamāapnugaaṭ ॥ Kathopanishad 1.2.24

26. *Chaṇchalaṃ hi manaḥ kṛiṣṇa pramāathi balavaḍḍriddhaṃ ।*
Taṣyāashaṃ nigrahaṃ manyē vāayōriva suduśkaraṃ । Gita 6.34

27. *Kaḥ jpsitāarṭha sthiraniśçhayaṃ manaḥ*
Payaśça nimnāabhimukhaṃ praṭēepayēṭ ॥ Kumarasambhav Fifth Ch.

28. *Tadēvāarṭhamāaṭra nirbhāasaṃ śwarōopaśōoṇyamiva samāadhiḥ ।* Yogsutra 3.3

29. *Chhāandōyōpaniṣaḍ।*

30. *Taṣyāapi nirōdhē sarvanirōdhāa ṇnirbēegaḥ Samāadhiḥ ।* Yogsutra 1.51

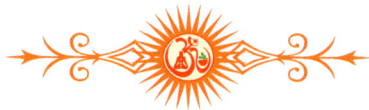

Chapter 3

ROLE OF PRANAYAM IN YOG PRACTICE AND ITS EFFECTIVENESS

Both the words 'Yog' and 'Pran' have broad meanings. Pran or vital life energy can have several meanings such as inhalation, breathing, life, vibrancy, consciousness, air, energy or strength. The word 'Soul' also to some extent represents the same meaning. Generally vital life force/energy carrying oxygen, necessary for life, is referred in several ways. 'Ayam' or dimension means length, extent and resistance. In this way, Pranayam means controlling the breath. This control is achieved when all the functions of breathing are completed. For example inhaling (Poorak) is filling air in lungs, Exhaling (Rechak) is evacuating/removing the air from lungs and holding the breath is known as Kumbhak. In Kumbhak stage there is no inhaling and exhaling. In 'Hath Yog' the word Kumbhak has a wider meaning. Here all the three actions of respiration namely inhaling, exhaling and stopping the breath are assimilated in Kumbhak.

Kumbhak means a pot, tub or container. A pot can be totally emptied and filled with water or all the water can be removed and can be filled with air. In the same way Kumbhak has two conditions. First, after inhaling the process of respiration halts for some time, the lungs are full of vital life energy. In the second condition, the respiration stops for some time after exhaling and the lungs become free of air. In the above processes when the air enters the lungs the respiration stops but air does not go out and is known as 'Antar Kumbhak'. In the second stage when the air is exhaled completely then breathing process stops for some time but air is not taken in and is known as 'Bahya Kumbhak'. 'Antar' means inside and 'Bahya' means outside. In this way breath is stopped or retained in between inhaling and exhaling for some time or it can be said that inhaling and exhaling are stopped for some time in between and regulated.

Tasmiṇ sati (vāasapra) vāasayōrgati vicchliēdaḥ Prāaṇāayāamaḥ । Yog Darshan 2/4', after sitting in the prescribed manner controlling the speed of inhaling and exhaling is called Pranayam. Pranayam is the science of respiration. It is the axis around which the entire life-cycle revolves. Chapter 2, shloka 16 of Hath Yog Pradipika says that as a lion, elephant and tiger is tamed/ controlled by carefully handling them, in the same way Pran or life energy can also be controlled gradually depending on the capacity of the body. Otherwise it can be fatal. The age of a Yogi is not counted in days but in number of breaths. The Yogi, therefore, adopts rhythmic pattern of breathing slowly and deeply. This rhythmic breathing calms down the nervous system, strengthens the respiratory system and reduces the desires. As the desires and aspirations reduce, the mind becomes free from tension conditions and thus becomes the best source/tool for deep concentration. Incorrect practice of breathing can lead to several diseases like hiccups, vata related diseases, asthma, cough, cold, head, eyes and ear related problems and irritability. It takes time to learn the correct method of rhytmic breathing by taking deep, slow and stable breaths. Retainning the breath (before practising Kumbhak) one should practice deep and rhythmic breathing thoroughly. As when ash is removed by wind, fire comes out, in the same way regular practice of Pranayam removes all kinds of vices or lusts and a divine light shows up with total strength. Removing all kinds of illusions and confusions from mind is pure Rechak. The experience of 'I am the soul' is correct Poorak and stabilizing the mind with this strong determination is Kumbhak in real sense. This is the refined Pranayam as explained by Shankaracharya.

Every individual unknowingly says 'Soham' with every breath, where Sa – he, Aham – I; which means "I am that avinashi purush" – In the same way every individual breaths out 'Aham sah', which means "I am he". This mantra goes on throughout the lifetime of an individual. A Yogi experiences the importance of this mantra and therefore gets out of all sorts of bonds that restrict him. He sacrifices his breath and dedicates it to God and imbibes the virtues of life in the form of blessings from Supreme soul. Pran shakti existing in the soul of the body is a part of cosmic life energy. With the practice of Pranayam one can attempt to bring equality between the life energy existing in the body of the human being with the divine life energy (cosmic energy) existing in the universe.

A philosopher mystic of the 17th century Ekkan says, "If you want to inspire your calm nature, intelligence of the soul then you have to first regulate your breathing process. The reason being that when breathing is under control only then your heart will also be calm. When breathing is irregular then it is harmful. Therefore before doing any work you have to regulate the breathing, so that you have a mild behaviour and quiet/peaceful disposition".

Mind, intelligence and ego are like a chariot, which move with the help of powerful horses. One of the horses is Pran or life energy and the second is lust. Whichever is more powerful the chariot of mind will move in that direction. If the breathing process is in our control and is strong then desires will also be under our control; the person having total control on his sensory organs and mind remains stable. If lust is predominant then breathing is irregular, the mind is disturbed and depressed. Therefore Yogi who has a thorough knowledge and command over the science of respiration controls the mind by controlling the respiration and thereby the mind. He always tries to control the playfulness of mind. While practicsing Pranayam the eyes shoud remain closed so that our mind remains stable at one place. When Pran and mind are united then we realize inexplicable happiness/ecstasy.

Emotions influence the speed of breathing, and in turn a controlled respiration controls the anxious and emotional mind. The main objective of Yog is to control the mind and keep it stable. A Yogi practises Pranayam in order to control his breathing. He becomes capable of controlling his sensory organs, which helps him in reaching the stage of restraining the sensory organs. Only then the mind is prepared for meditation.

The mind is considered to be in two stages – pure and impure. The mind is pure when it is free of lusts and impure when it is full of lusts. When the mind is calm, stable and free of laziness, confusions and obstructions then it reaches the stage of tranquillity. This is the highest stage of meditation. This stage is not the stage of ignorance or lunacy. But it is the conscious state of mind when it is free of all sorts of thoughts and lusts. On one side we have a person whose mind is full of lusts and on the other side we have a Yogi who is in the state of tranquillity.

There is a lot of difference between the two, the first person is careless and the second tries to be free of worries. This is a union of respiration and mind and it is also the dedication of all stages of thoughts and presence of sensory organs, which has been termed as Yog.

Life energy or Pran

Air is one of the minute forms of energy of universe or cosmic energy (in reality carrier of cosmic energy). It is an energy , which is present in the human body as well. The important tasks to be completed with the help of this energy/strength have been classified into five types according to the principles of Hath Yog. These are known as air and its five costituents. These are: 1. Pran, which is used to denote the air that circulates in the chest area and controls the respiration, 2. Apana or wind that is evacuated from anus and which controls the evacuation of urine, 3. Samana or the air that is helpful in the digestion process and provides fuel to food,4. Udana, which is circulated in the pores of chest and controls the entry points of food and windpipe and 5. Vyana that is spread all over the body and divides the energy/strength obtained from food and respiration. There are five other secondary Prans namely, Naga which controls the movement of eyelids to stop the entry of air at the time of giving pressure on stomach, Krikal which stops anything going above the nose or below the throat in case of cough or sneezing, Devdutt which refills Pran or life energy when it is lost due to yawning indicating that the body is tired or wants to sleep. The last is Dhananjay, which remains in the body even after death and sometimes swells up the dead body.

According to Yog Darshan, there are four types of Pranayam. They are:

Bahya Vritti, Abhyantarvritti, Stambhavritti and Bahyantar Vishayapeskshi

Bāaḥyāabhyantara ṣṭambhava (ttirdē) kāala saṇkhyāabhih parida (ṇritō dēerghasōokṣmaḥ)
(Yog 2/50)

Bāaḥyāabhyantara Vyāa kṣēpēe) chaturṭhaḥ   (Yog 2/51)

Bahyavritti

- Sit in Padmasana or Sidhasana and exhale completely all at once with full force.
- Exhale and perform Mool, Uddiyan and Jalandhar bandh and hold the breath outside for as long as possible.
- When you feel like breathing air, remove all the three bandhs and inhale slowly.
- Inhale and without retaining it inside breathe out completely as before. Repeat this 3-21 times.

This is totally harmless and overcomes playfulness of the mind. It increases the digestive fire and is beneficial in stomach diseases. It makes the mind sharp and active. It strengthens semen and helps in improving condition of Sawapna Dosha, early ejaculation and other sexual diseases.

Abhyantar vritti Pranayam

- Sit in a meditative pose, exhale completely and inhale as much as you can. The chest should be full of air and the lower abdomen should be contracted in. Inhale and do Moolbandh and Jalandhar bandh.
- Retain the breath inside as long as possible and remove the bandhs when you want to breathe out. Breathe out as slowly as possible.
- This is beneficial for curing all types of lung related disorders, and especially for asthma patients. It makes the body strong, bright and gives natural glow.

Stambhavritti

As the name implies, this is a self-suspended Pranayam or total control of mind on breath. With perfection of this Pranayam, the breath becomes so minute as if it is stopped. Although breathing goes on but it goes so easily that we become totally introvert, desireless, peaceful and totally balanced personality. This is highest state of spirituality. In other words, we experience deep and precise awareness of cosmic life energy and oneness with the Almighty. The following are steps for this Pranayam:

- sit in a suitable right posture and note the natural process of breathing in and breathing out. If breath is going in or has gone in fully stop it where it is and keep it retained as long as easily possible. Chanting OM will be very useful
- Similarly, if breath is going out or has gone out fully, stop it where it is and keep it retained as long as easily possible. Introducing bandhas in this greatly accelerates the progress in this Pranayam. With practice, one can reach such a rhythm of breathing wherein mind at will can control it. As the mind becomes progressively calmer in this Pranayam, the breathing becomes very minute.

Bahyantar vishayakshepi

When you exhale, stop the breath outside for some time and when you inhale then stop it inside for some time. In other words when life energy is being exhaled then try to block it with the help of Apana Vayu and when Apana Vayu tries to come in then the Pran Vayu should block its entry. In this way, both the air block each other, this helps in controlling the mind and sensory organs. This helps us in understanding very complex and minute details of a subject very easily. The body gets strength and becomes stable, courageous and wins over the sensory organs. Such person is able to understand all the classic, complex and very difficult subjects/sciences/creative arts within a short time and present it in the required form. The mind becomes pure and stable. The women should also practise Yog in the same manner (Third chapter of book Satyartha Prakash authored by Swami Dayanand).

We can understand it better in this manner. Let us bring Pran from above and Apana from below and make them fight in the nostril, in other words try to stabilize the air in between the eyebrows that has the tendency to remain in the chest area and go out by making it enter from above; try to stabilize the Apana air in the nostrils which has the tendency to remain below the navel and tries to come in from outside by making it enter the nostrils from outside. Now push the airs against each other, in other words do not allow the Pran to go out and do not allow Apana to enter inside. In this way the opposite action will help you in controlling the Pran or vital life energy. Concentrate the mind between the eyebrows while practicsing this Pranayam (Second chapter – Dhyan Yog Prakash). The same thing has been written in Bhagwadgita about this Pranayam

Sparśāan kritwāa bahirbāahyāanśchakṣuh chāivāantare bhruvōh ।
Prāaṇāapāanāu kritwāa nāasāabhyāamantara chāariṇāu ॥

Try to concentrate the mind on the subject and forget about the surroundings, form, taste, smell etc. Focus the mind in between the eyebrows. Try to bring Pran and Apana on the same level in other words first bring them in opposition and then try to stabilize them at equal levels. The person who is always focused, controls his sensory organs and mind. He/She always proceeds on the path of salvation, is free of desires, anger and fear, and is truly liberated

Yatēndriya manōbudhirmōkṣaparāayaṇah
Vigatēchehhayakrōdhō yah sadāa mukta āiva sah ॥

(Bhagwadgita, 5/27)

The same thing has been explained in the following verse:

Apāanē juhvati prāanamprāanam tathāaśpare)
Prāanaēpāauagatēe ruddhawāa prāanāam parāayaṇāah ।
Aparēniyatēa hāarāah prāanam juhvati ।
Sarvēśpyētē yaggyavidō yaggya kṣayita kalmāah ॥

(Bhagwadgita 4/ 29-30)

'Apane Jahuti Pranm'- it means: conjoining/coception of Apana with Pran/ vital life energy is Bhastrika. Conjoining/conception of Pran (life force) with Apana is Kapalbhati Pranayam. This is because in Kapalbhati Pranayam we forcefully conjoin the Apana residing below navel with Pran (vital life force). Blocking the movement of Pran outside is Bahya Pranayam; breathing in and stopping the breath inside is 'Bahyantar' Pranayam. Conjoining/conception of Pran engaged in basic metabolism of digestion with Pran (life force) is Sthambhavritti Pranayam. Practising Pranayam in this manner accomplishes all the goals of life and the tendency to commit sins ends. We can see that there is similarity between Lord Shri Krishna and Saint Patanjali with respect to Pranayam. They have expressed the same thing in different ways.

'Abhyantar' Kumbhak taught by Saint Patanjali and Lord Shri Krishna has been divided into eight parts in Hath Yog Pradipika as Suryabedhanmujjayi, Sitkari, Shitali, Bhastrika, Brahmari, Moorcha, Plavinitishthya and Kumbhak.

Pranayam in Vedas and Upanishads

Controlling the vital life energy or Pran is Pranayam. All the actions carried out on by our body have direct or indirect relation with Pran. The inseparable relation between life and death of an individual is also due to the Pran. In Sanskrit, the word 'life' is made from humours that contains life energy and the word 'death' is made from sacrificing life. Life means holding life force and death is withdrawing/ sacrificing life force. Our Vedas and Upanishads talk about unending glory of Pran or vital life energy. Atharvaveda says : Prāaṇāapāanāu mrityōrmāa pāatam swāahāa, in other words Pran and Apana should protect us from death. Manu says the following about Pran.

Dahyaṇtē dhmāayamāanāanaam dhāatunāam liyathāa malāah) ।
Tathēṇdriyāaṇāam dahyaṃtē dāamh prāaṇasya nigrahāat ॥ (Manu 6/71)

It means when gold and other metals burn in fire, the dirt and faults are removed. In the same way when the sensory organs and mind are under control, the conditions and ill feelings present within are removed automatically. Hath Yog Pradipika says:

Prāaṇāayāamāirēva sarvē prāapruyaṇti matāa iti ।
Āachāryāaṇāantu kāanchidanyat karma nasammatam ॥

(Hatha Pradipika 2/38)

According to 'Goraksha Shatak' a Yogi should remove his passions with the help of proper posture, be free of sins with Pranayam and mental conditions with the help of resistance towards passions.

Āasanēna-gō haṇti prāaṇāayāamēna pāatakam ।
Vikāaram māanasam yogēe prat yāahāarēna sarvadāa ॥

Pran and mind are closely related to each other. Regular practice of Pranayam helps in concentration of mind.

Chalē vāatē chalaṃ niśchalē niśchalaterṃ bhavēt ।

Practice of Pranayam removes ignorance, anger present in the form of anguish and lies. The refined mind is able to concentrate automatically and with the help of concentration the mind reaches the stage of deep meditation.

Yog Asanas are helpful in getting rid of the problems of the body. Whereas, Pranayam is more effective on both internal body and outer or physical body. Lungs, heart and brain are important parts of our body and all the three are closely related to each other from the health point of view.

Broadly speaking Pranayam is the method of rhythmic breathing, which strengthens the lungs, increases blood circulation, cures all the diseases and increases longevity.

According to medical science through breathing we fill up lungs with air (which contains oxygen - Pran vayu). This oxygen is transferred to all the blood capilaries spread over the lungs and the carbon dioxide from these capilaries is transferred to lungs. The oxygenated blood carried by the blood circulation system supplies oxygen to each and every cell of the body and the carbon dioxide generated in the cells is taken back in the blood.

Generally people are not habituated to take deep breaths and therefore only one-fourth part of the lungs work and rest is left idle. The lungs resemble the honeycomb and have around 7,00,30,000 spongy pores. When we breathe normally Pran or life energy is circulated in only two crore pores and the remaining are idle without any work. As a result they become stiff and foreign particles are accumulated on it. This leads to tuberculosis, cough, bronchitis and other serious diseases.

In this way, the partial functioning of lungs affects the purification of blood. The heart becomes weak and as a result the person dies prematurely. In this condition, Pranayam gives long life to the person. Controlling the Pran or life energy can cure different diseases. The person can lead a happy and disease-free life with the knowledge of Pranayam and also inspire others to lead a healthy life. This is the reason that every religion, considers Pranayam to be an important aspect of all religious activities and functions.

Pranayam can provide an easy solution for all anguishes, worries, anger, disappointment, fear and lust, and other mental conditions. It increases the mental capacity, memory power, sharpness, understanding, foresight, investigating power, grasping, wisdom, intelligence and other mental qualities. The person can enjoy a long happy life with regular practice of Pranayam.

Regular practice of Pranayam teaches the art of deep respiration automatically. God has gifted us with body and the numbers of breaths are limited. The person gets a new birth depending on his deeds in previous birth.

Sati mōolē taḍvipāakō jāatyāayurbhōgāaḥ (Yog darśan) ।

(Yog Darshan 2/13)

One gets the life in the form of man, bird, animal, insect etc. depending on his good and bad deeds and enjoys birth, longevity and pleasures in life. A person who practices Pranayam uses lesser breaths to a limited extent and hence he lives longer. The creatures, which breathe slowly live longer. (see Table below)

Number of Breaths taken by each Creature Per Minute			
Pigeon	34	Bird	30
Duck	22	Monkey	30
Dog	28	Pig	36
Horse	26	Goat	24
Cat	24	Snake	19
Elephant	22	Human being	15
Tortoise	5		

The creature gets lifespan depending on the pace of respiration. We can see it in our surroundings. A tortoise can live up to 400 years. A person who practises Yog breathes eight times in the beginning and then slowly reduces it to four per minute. Hence a yogi can live up to 400 years.

Mechanical Analysis of Yogic Activities or Pranayam as Popularised by Swami Ramdevji

Respiration

The respiration includes two processes in our body at blood cell level and at tissue cell level. We perform both these processes while breathing, perform respiration systematically in a balanced way in Pranayam. Most apparent benefits of Pranayam are increased oxygenation of blood and increased blood circulation. These benefits can also be derived from aerobic exercises. However, there is a fundamental difference in them. Whereas aerobic exercises are catabolic (energy spending) in nature, Pranayam is anabolic (energy generating) in nature. Apart from giving benefits of higher oxygen up take and improved blood circulation, Pranayam smoothens the working of endocrine glands which makes it possible to eliminate serious health problems such as hypertension, diabetes, depression, coronary blockages, Alzheimer disease, Parkinsonism, insomnia and host of diseases that occur due to malfunctioning of endocrine gland system. We shall discuss this later.(See Table below)

The differences in catabolic and anabolic processes

Catabolic Processes	Anabolic Processes
• Halt in synthesis of protein, fat and carbohydrates.	• Increased synthesis of protein fat and carbohydrate (growth)
• Increased breakdown of above for energy mobilization.	• Decreased breakdown of above (growth and energy storage)
• Elevated blood levels of glucose, free fatty acids, loading of immune system.	• Increased production of cells for immune system.
• Increased production of RBC and liver enzyme for energy.	• Increased WBC of thymus and bone marrow.
• Decreased bone repair and growth.	• Increased bone repair and growth.
• Decreased production of cells for immune system. Thymus shrinks and circulating WBC decrease.	• Increase in cellular, hormonal and psychological process.
• Increased BP and cardiac output.	• Smoothens Heart Rate, lowers BP optimises cardiac output.
Jogging, brisk walk, aerobics.	Pranayam

Respiratory System

Primary function of respiratory system is to ensure oxygen for the use of cells & eliminate carbon dioxide produced by the cells. It is important to know that a certain minimum level of CO_2 is required in blood stream. In respiratory system following six parts play significant role :

1. nasal cavities or oral cavity; 2. Pharynx; 3. Trachea; 4. Primary bronchi; 5. Secondary Bronchi; 6. Bronchiols; 7. Tertiary bronchi; 8. Alveoli (site of gas exchange).

Alveoli is micro unit of respiratory system. There are about 300 million alveolies in the lung structure. Their total surface area is nearly 75-100 square meters. Exchange of O_2 and

CO_2 with blood takes place at alveoli by diffusion. The O_2 diffuses to blood from alveoli and CO_2 diffuses from blood to alveoli which are very tiny grape like structures. There are more than 300 million alveoli surrounded by blood capillaries. Diaphragm is one of most important muscles in the human

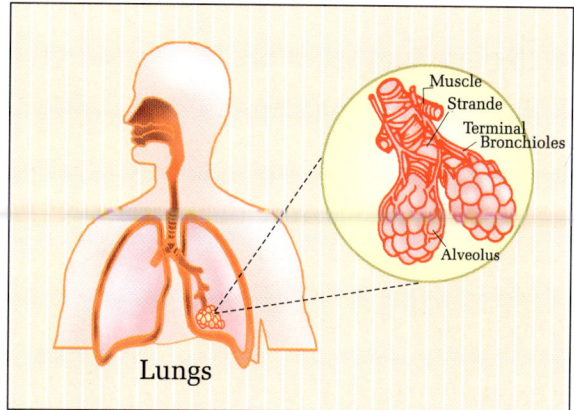

Human lungs and constitution of Alveoli

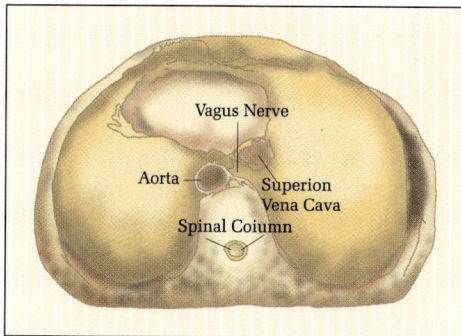

Structure of diaphragm muscle

respiratory system.

Inhalation: Contraction of external intercostals muscles leads to elevation of ribs and sternum, increased front to back dimension of thoracic cavity, lowering of the pressure in the lungs. This allows fresh O_2 laden air to enter the lungs.

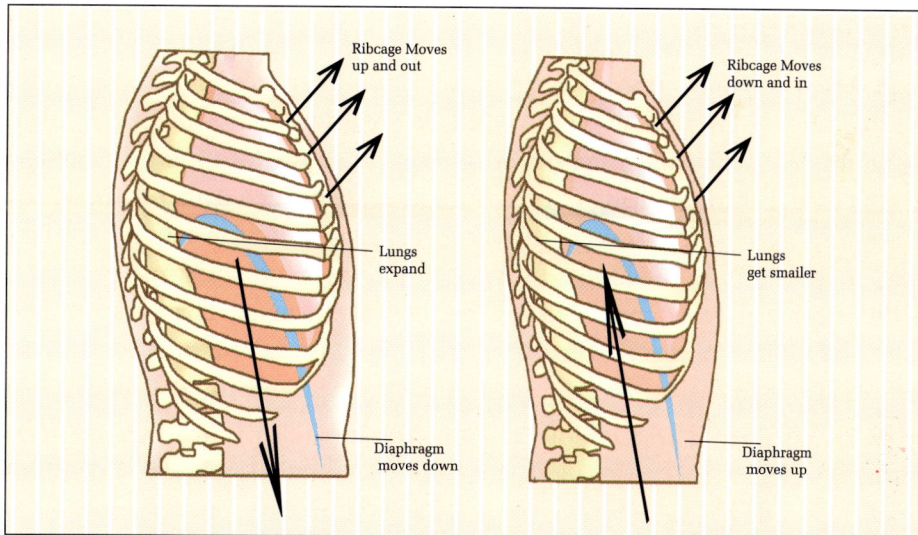

The movement in chest cavity during the process of respiration

Contraction of diaphragm results in lowering of the diaphragm resulting in increased vertical dimension and reduction of pressure in the lungs. This also allows fresh O_2 laden air to enter the lungs. The involvement of diaphragm in the process of inhalation greatly increases the air moving to lungs. Thus, with more air we get higher level of blood oxygenation. In majority of the cases, people use only chest muscles which can be considered as incomplete breathing.

Physiological Effects of Pranayam

The three major areas of physiological mechanisms initiated and enhanced by Yog /Pranayam practices are:

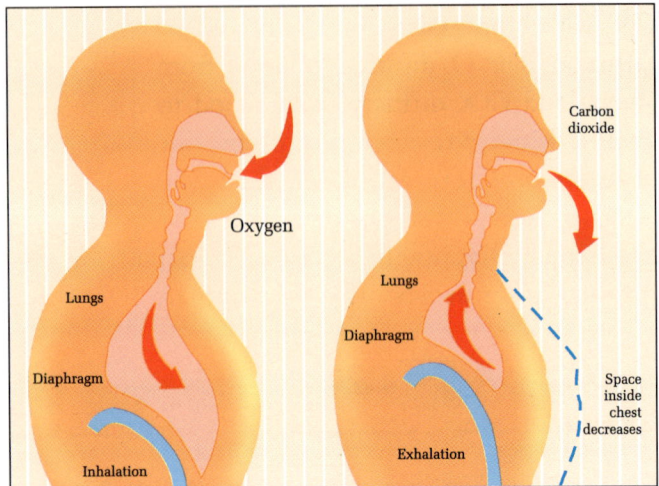

The Mechanism of breathing

- Oxygen metabolism
- Lymph system
- Brain and nervous system

Oxygen Metabolism

The human system begins to disorganize and die within minutes without oxygen. Therefore it is quite logical to think that altering oxygen metabolism might be curative for diseases that have an oxygen deficiency component to their etiology. Both moderate and vigorous body movement and accompanying muscle work increase oxygen demand in cells. Evidence from research in exercise physiology demonstrates that muscular activity accelerates the rate of oxygen uptake from the blood. It has been shown that training and practice increase ventilitory threshold, anabolic threshold and mechanical efficiency. This suggests that regular body movement with increased breath activity supports adaptation toward increased functional efficiency in the uptake and utilization of oxygen from the blood.

Recently there has been a tremendous amount of activity in both research and clinical practice which suggests that many deficiency disorders and degenerative diseases are, at least partially, attributable to defective oxygen metabolism, oxygen deficiency or hypoxia.

The practice of Pranayam – Yog increases oxygen availability which potentially:

- supports energy (ATP, AMP, and ADP) generation.
- generates water as a byproduct of energy metabolism which contributes a major portion to the lymph supply.

Energy Generation

It has been well-established that the energy necessary for cell work and body heat regulation is supplied through the reaction of oxygen and glucose to form high energy phosphate bonds. There is a direct relationship between oxygen demand, impulse to breathe and basal metabolic rate (BMR, the rate at which the cells in the body consume oxygen and glucose to produce water, carbon dioxide and energy).

Hydrolysis of adenosine triposphate (ATP) is accompanied by the release of chemical energy for cellular and muscular activity.

The food consumed by us gets converted into glucose. The oxygen received by the cell is utilized to generate the basic energy, pure water and the carbon dioxide as given by the following representative formula :

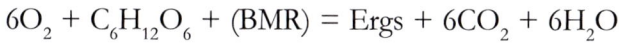

$$6O_2 + C_6H_{12}O_6 + (BMR) = Ergs + 6CO_2 + 6H_2O$$

Air + Food + (BMR) = Energy + carbon dioxide + water

Water Production

A second critical benefit of increased oxygen metabolism generated through the practice of Pranayam is linked to the lymph system. Besides the production of energy, in the phosphorylization cycle, there is also the generation of pure water as a waste product or byproduct.

This water is dramatically and directly increased when oxygen consumption is increased in the cell. Because this water becomes involved with the internal cleansing performed by the lymph it is a major link between the breath and lymphatic system function.

Immune Function

The ATP drives the activity of every cell. Therefore, immune function as well as the production of immune resources (white blood cells, lymphocytes, T-cells, natural killer cells, etc.) are indirectly dependent on oxygen consumption.

Free Radical Balance

There are multiple factors that modify oxygen demand and uptake besides the cell work of body movement and organ function. Such factors include the effects of chemical and environmental stress caused by foods, water and air-borne pollution. Emotional, relational or career stress, the stress of injury and the stress of infection also affects the body's ability to absorb and utilize oxygen. Accumulation of these effects can negatively impact on oxygen metabolism and precipitate functional imbalances in the human system.

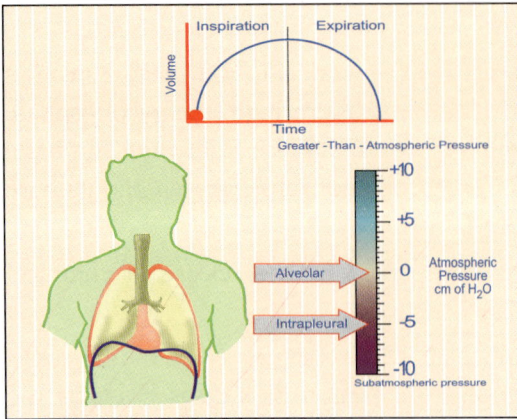

The alveolar pressure during state of relaxation

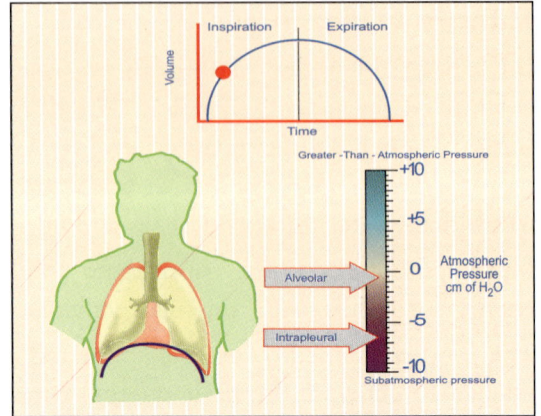

The alveolar pressure during Bhastrika breathing

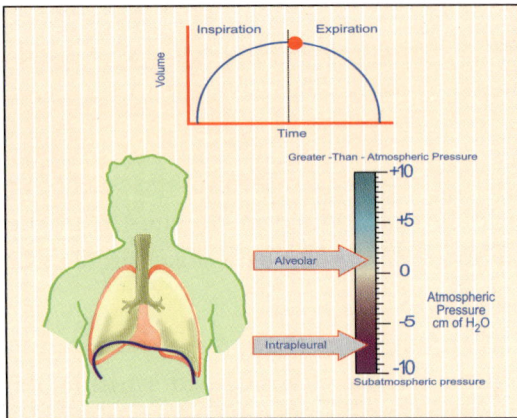

The alveolar pressure during state of inhalation

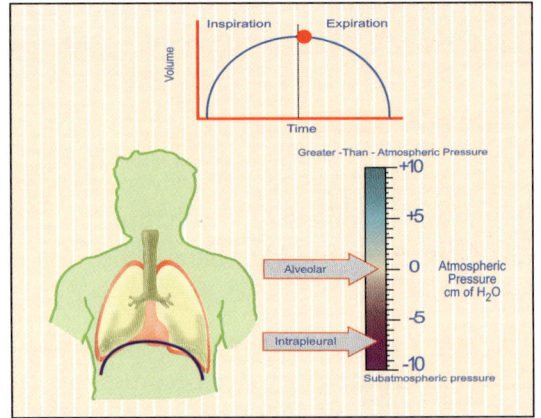

The alveolar pressure during final stage of inhalation

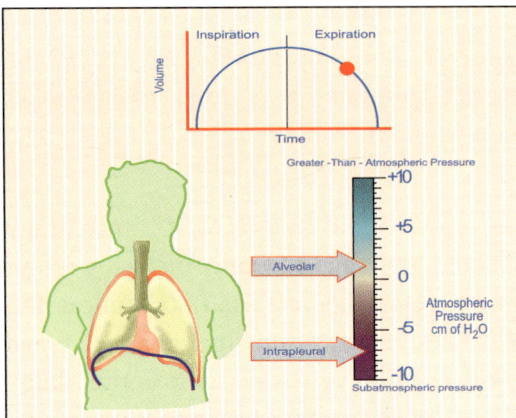

The alveolar pressure during exhalation

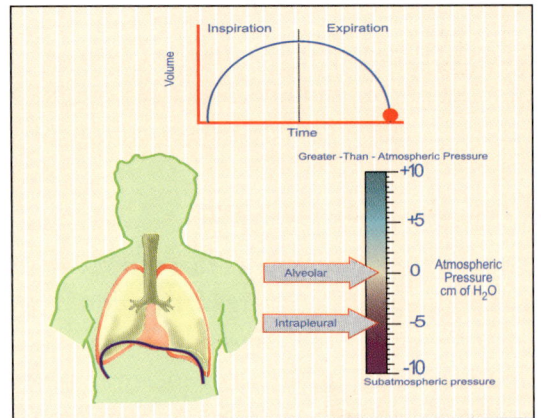

The alveolar pressure during final stage of exhalation

The normal activity of energy metabolism creates a certain number of byproducts. These molecules are called free radicals. With the impact of the above mentioned stressors greater amounts of free radicals are produced. All normal molecules have paired electrons in their outer electron orbits. Free radicals are unstable molecules with an unpaired electron in their outermost electron orbit. In an effort to return to a stable state these renegade molecules steal electrons from healthy molecules causing tissue damage and aging. The body produces a number of antioxidant enzymes, super oxide dismutase, catalase, glutathione peroxidase and methione reductase, whose job is to neutralize the free radicals produced in normal energy metabolism. However, in an imbalanced or unwell system demand for antioxidant enzymes is high and natural productivity, due to pathology, may be low.

When slow, deep breathing and moderate body motion is activated as in Yogic exercises there is an increased demand for oxygen molecules which are taken up from the blood. The potential for free radicals to bond with this available oxygen, neutralizing the free radical population, can be greatly accelerated when regular Yogic exercise/Pranayam is included in a person's daily health routine.

There are a number of strategies for resolution of oxygen deficiency disease (ODD). These include the use of antioxidant nutrients (vitamins A, C, E and selenium), antioxidant enzymes, coenzyme Q10 etc.). There is, however, nothing more, inexpensive than oxygen itself taken in maximum daily doses through Yogic exercises/Pranayam.

Lymph

The lymph fluid is actually part cellular water and part blood plasma. The lymphatic system has remained rather neglected in most Western scientific traditions. Compared to the heart, for example, the lymph is relatively unexplored.

In general, the lymphatic system is a network of organs, tissues, vessels, nodes and flow potentials. It collects interstitial fluid, infused with the by products of cellular activity, and transports it centrally where it rejoins the blood system.

Bhastrika Breathing

Figure shows the pressure levels in one typical alveolus and the pleura. At the beginning of the inhalation process, the alveolar pressure is atmospheric while pleural pressure is about - 5 cm of water column. At this stage, contraction of intercostals muscles start and the ribs as well as sternum start to rise. Front to back dimensions of the thoracic cavity start increasing and vacuum starts building up and O_2 laden fresh air starts flowing to lungs. When the diaphragm is used, its downward travel further increases the vacuum in the lung space and more airflow starts.

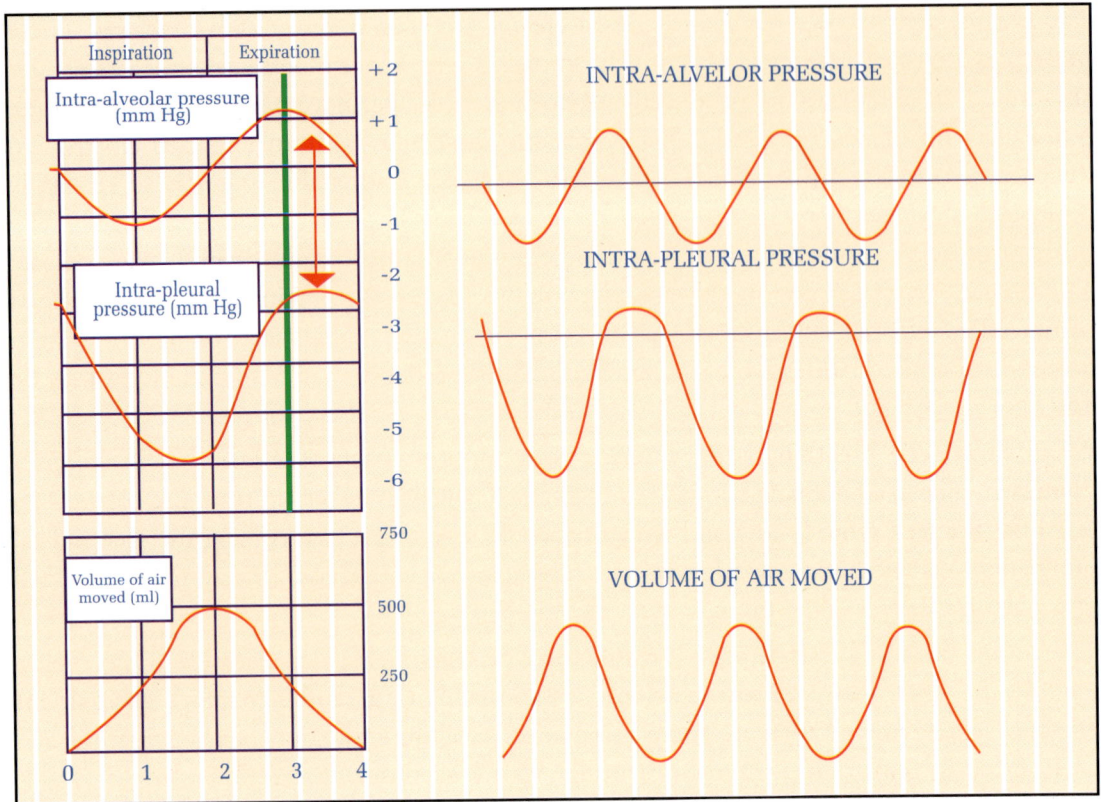

Pressure and flow variation in one breathing cycle

Pressure & flow variation with deeper inhalation and forceful exhalation in Bhastrika Pranayam

During Inhalation

The alveolar pressure has changed from initial atmospheric, to vacuum and the intrapleural pressure has become more negative. The dotted line in figure shows the position of diaphragm at the beginning of the inhalation process.

The pressure distribution at the end of inhalation part and immediate start of exhalation process and pressure history midway the exhalation part of the breathing cycle are shown in Figures given earlier. At the end of exhalation, the pressure distribution will be the same.

Since we are considering equal times for both inhalation (inspiration) and exhalation (expiration), the pressure time history in one breathing cycle is as shown in figure.

The figure shows pressure and mass flow variation in one cycle of breathing spanning 4 seconds. Thus, the breathing rate in quiet Bhastrika breathing is 15 breaths per minute and entire respiratory system and organs below the diaphragm are subjected to pulsations/ oscillations.

It is obvious that the pressure pulsations and air mass flow rates can be drastically increased if the depth of inhalation and force of exhalation are increased. This will help the respiratory system, abdominal system below the diaphragm and encased blood circulation system to vibrations/oscillation with great benefits. Firstly, the oxygen uptake and carbon dioxide evacuation in the blood gets greatly improved with more improvement in blood circulation.

Normal quiet breathing

At this stage, it is necessary to bring out the difference between Bhastrika breathing and normal quiet breathing. In quiet breathing, one takes about 1 second for inspiration/ inhalation and 3 seconds are taken to carry out the exhalation/expiration phase as shown in figure. In quiet, non-Pranayam breathing, inhale is of 1 second duration, while exhalation is for 3 seconds – 15 breaths per minute.

One of the key factors in Pranayam is deep breathing. The human chest has capacity to

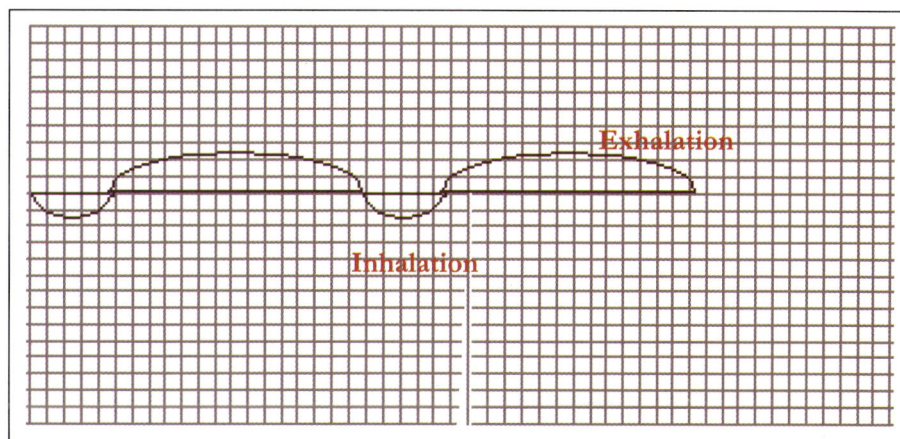

Quiet breathing

accommodate much more air than what we inhale in normal quiet breathing. Experiments have shown that in normal/quiet breathing, approximately 500 ml of air is inhaled. Out of this, only 350 ml is useful air. This is because the lungs have dead pockets (where no gas exchange takes place) of the size of approximately 150 ml. This quantity (350ml) as well as the mode of breathing may be sufficient for our daily routine life but cannot meet the requirements of improved blood circulation and smooth functioning of our nervous system including the endocrine gland system.

Kapalbhati Pranayam

This Pranayam is claimed to be one of the best detoxification exercises. With every forced

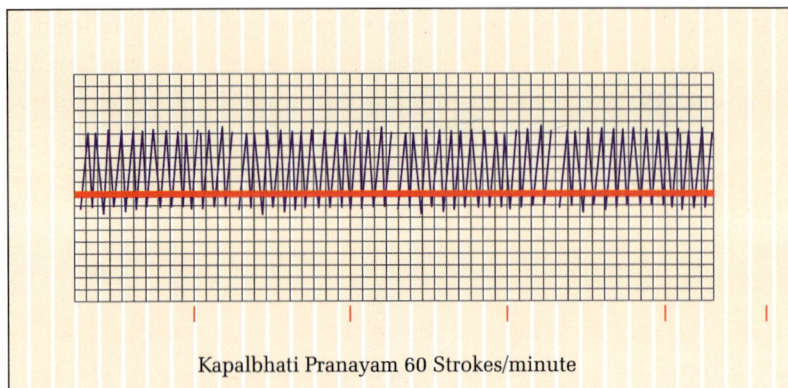

Kapalbhati Pranayam 60 Strokes/minute

The speed of respiration during Kapalbhati Pranayam

expiration, the body ejects congestants as well as other toxins in the respiratory system. With this Pranayam also, as with Bhastrika, the respiratory system as well as the organs below the diaphragm and the encased blood circulation system experience pulsations. The pressure on abdominal viscera from diaphragmatic motion during Kapalbhati (and also in Bhastrika Pranayam to a somewhat lesser extent) contributes to strong venous blood return to heart. The pressure pulsations as well as vibrations of the system also cause removal of blockages in the circulation system. The mechanism associated with removal of blockages in the circulation system is similar to the controlling mechanism in "Enhanced External Counter Pulsation" (EECP) technique which is claimed to be a very strong alternative to balloon angioplasty and coronary bypass surgeries. In EECP also, the pressurized cuff mounted on lower legs and pelvis press on the arteries/blood vessels only when the blood is returning to heart, the entire action is computer controlled. The EECP is OPD procedure and is totally non-invasive. The medical literature contains a lot of success stories of EECP. One can now see that in Kapalbhati as well as in Bhastrika Pranayam the blockages in the circulation system get removed in addition to detoxification and availability of larger quantity of O_2.

Life force in Pranayam, is called Pran

As there are different power places and powers in the universe, we too have a 'life force' (Pran) in our bodies which is connected with our respiratory system. The imbalance in this system causes diseases. Thus, we get 'chaitanya' (ever pervading energy field) from respiration. Balance in life is achieved by pairing Pran (ever pervading energy field, also called "Chaitannya") and Udana, which is nothing but the manifestation of "Chaitannya". These correspond to inhalation and exhalation of breath. Without Udana, Pran has no meaning since Pran is the energy potential (source of energy if we consider it in the thermodynamics context) and Udana signifies that the inhaled energy has been utilized (sink in thermodynamics context). This indeed is a great concept. Pran itself comprises of five elements called the Panch Pran. These are: Pran, Udana, Samana, Apana, Vyana.

Pran which is ever pervading energy field, Chaitannya , enables inhalation of cosmic energy.

Breathing and Brain

The most desirable route of breathing is through the nasal cavity. The nasal cavity provides filtering and conditioning of air meant for breathing.

As mentioned earlier, the breath is the only Channel through which we draw the life force (derived from universal life force/energy) for our body. Since the life sustaining and regulating system is located in the brain, the brain must "breathe" properly. Of course this "breathing" is different from the breathing air through the respiratory system as there is no gas exchange in brain breathing.

With every breath, we draw not only air (comprising nitrogen, oxygen etc.) but packets of life energy. The nasal cavity which performs this duty is the part of the skull which also provides hermetical sealing for brain. The nasal cavity has some features which enable the brain to "breathe". These features are like modem in the computer which enables computer to access the internet. The failure of universal life receptor in our brain results in death. The Indian sages, several thousand years ago, had discovered this and also that brain breathes, pulsates in the skull.

The diffusion of atmospheric air with the circulating cerebrospinal fluid (CSF) takes place at this place. The bathing of the brain and the spinal cord is done much the same way as ventilation of the lungs takes place by inhalation and the exhalation. The life energy taken through the breath is transferred to CSF which keeps the brain and its contents alive. The cerebrospinal fluid keeps on circulating between the brain and the spinal cord as shown in figure. Thus, to and fro translocation of CSF between brain and the spinal cord occurs at a certain periodicity which plays an

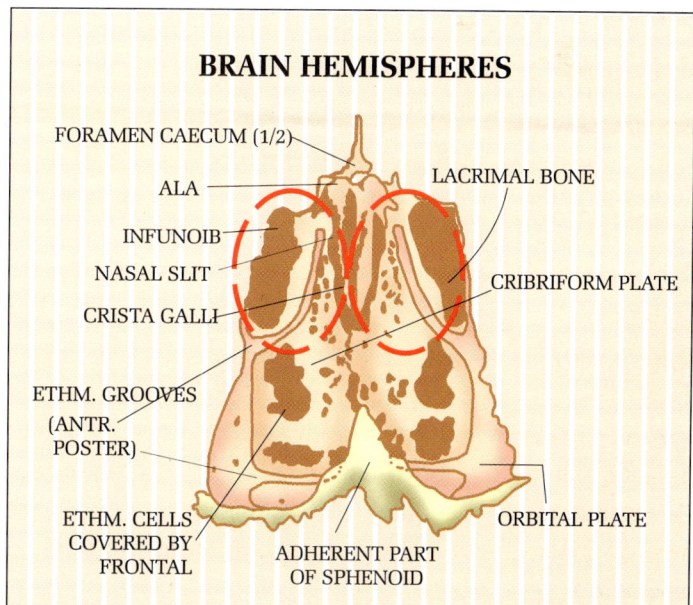

BRAIN HEMISPHERES

FORAMEN CAECUM (1/2)
ALA
INFUNOIB
NASAL SLIT
CRISTA GALLI
LACRIMAL BONE
CRIBRIFORM PLATE
ETHM. GROOVES (ANTR. POSTER)
ETHM. CELLS COVERED BY FRONTAL
ADHERENT PART OF SPHENOID
ORBITAL PLATE

extremely important role in our physical as well as mental health.

Cerebrospinal fluid

The cerebrospinal fluid (CSF) is a clear, colourless body fluid similar in composition to blood plasma and sea water. It protects brain and the spinal cord. A brain weighing about 1.5 kg in air weighs only 50 grams in CSF. The fluid on account of its sodium and the potassium content has excellent electrolytic properties. This makes it as the most suitable medium of flow of energy and information. The electrolytes (sodium and potassium) present in CSF maintain an electrical balance that controls functioning of the nervous system.

A cross-section of the brain : Remembering the position of the two hemispheres of the brain above the ethmoid bone we can now visualize how the dura mater of the brain receives a very small portion of the breath through the perforated cribriform plate

The CSF supplies nutrients and eliminate waste products in the nervous system. Several types of neuropeptides exist in CSF (about 100 known so far). These neuropeptides are nerve proteins mostly produced in the brain. Some of most outstanding features of the neuropeptides are:

Neuropeptides in CSF are called the "messenger molecules" who distribute information throughout the body and coordinate practically all life processes on cellular basis. Neuropeptides also coordinate body functions on emotional level since they are concentrated in the limbic system – seat of emotion. Neuropeptides are essential body chemicals that bind selectively to a specific receptor site on the surface of the cell. Each human cell has hundreds of thousand sites for neuropeptides and the nerve cells have millions.

Neuropeptides coordinate body functions such as metabolism, respiration etc. on cellular level. The cellular processes in turn bring about dramatic functional changes in the tissues, glands, organs and the entire body system. Thus, by processes which bring the neuropeptides in action, it is possible to cure even dreaded diseases such as cancers without resorting to chemotherapy and surgery. The circulation of CSF, which contains a large quantities of neuropeptides, is thus most important from the point of view of the health of the body and mind.

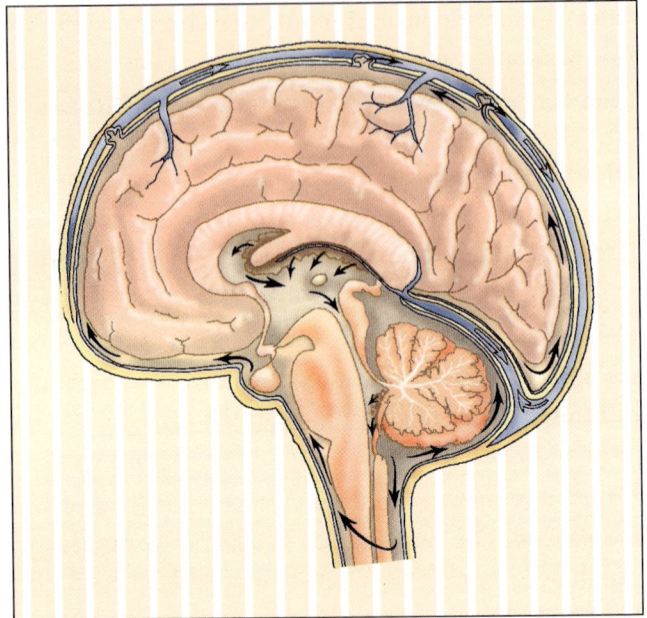

Circulation of CSF is done by two pumping mechanisms; one at the top (cranium) and one at the bottom (sacrum). It is very important to note that the sacral pump at the bottom of spine gets properly activated only when breathing involves diaphragm. During inhalation, the diaphragm muscle contracts down on the sacrum pumping CSF up the spinal cord into the brain. During exhalation, CSF moves from brain to spine. The forceful exhalation in Kapalbhati Pranayam ensures travel of neuropeptides laden CSF to spine and thus the important endocrine glands are properly fed with life energy via nerve fibers located on both sides of spine. Kapalbhati is thus a very important Pranayam which brings about dramatic cures of several complex diseases.

The flow of CSF to and fro brain causes pressure pulsations in the cranium. These pulsations can be monitored using EEG techniques. These measurements including pathological tests done on CSF drawn through lumber puncture are very useful in diagnosing various malfunctions in the brain.

Pranayam strongly recommends a deep slow, rhythmic breathing involving diaphragm since only this ensures proper circulation of CSF in brain and the spinal cord. This in turn feeds the life energy to all the endocrine glands that control the visceral function of the body This essentially is the major reason that majority of serious ailments can be cured/eradicated by practising Pranayam, Yogasanas and taking healthy diet. The recent research also shows that when the flow of CSF is optimum, it enables awakening of higher levels of consciousness.

Anulom – Vilom Pranayam and CSF circulation

This is one of the most important Pranayam that helps us to bring balance between the dominances of left and right hemispheres of the human brain. The Indian sages, several thousands years ago, discovered the phenomenon of alternating cerebral balance of the right and the left brain hemispheres, its relationship to nasal flow cycle and need to balance them. They discovered that during the entire day, dominance of left and right hemispheres of the brain keep alternating at a certain periodicity. They found that when the right hemisphere of the brain dominates, the left nostril is clear and the air flow takes place through the left nostril. When the left hemisphere of the brain is dominating, the right nostril is clear. When the two hemispheres of the brain are balanced, both the nostrils are open for air flow. Practice of Anulom – vilom Pranayam enables this.

The respiration, whether normal or Pranayam breathing, results into oxygenation of blood and removal of CO_2. However, a certain minimum level of CO_2 in blood is required as excess O_2 in blood can be very dangerous.

Third Eye

According to yogic science, Nadis are the Channels or circuits that carry the human resonating energy fields (responsible for physical, mental and spiritual life). There are more than 72,000 Nadis; however amongst them most important are three Nadis. They are "Ida", "Pingala" And "Susushumna". The Nadis are the nerve currents on either side of spinal cord (Ida and Pingala) and through the hollow canal in the spinal cord (Sushumna). Normally the either of the Ida or Pingala nerve currents will be active. Sushumna is usually dormant. Everytime we breathe, air carrying with it the packets of life energy travels either through Ida Nadi or Pingala Nadi and after circulating up and down passes out of the nostril. Ida Nadi begins at the left nostril, at the root of the nose just where left nostril converges into the right. It then passes through cerebellum and medulla oblongata and runs along the left side of the spinal cord and ends at the lower end. Similarly, Pingala Nadi begins from right nostril passes through cerebellum and medulla oblongata and runs through right side of the spine. It ends at the base of spine. Sushumna Nadi, though not directly connected with either of the nostrils begins at the base of brain or the medulla oblongata, runs down the central cavity of the spinal column and ends at coccyx where all the three Nadis (Ida, Pingala and Sushumna) are connected. Within the root of the nose where two nostrils converge (junction of the cribriform plate and the Crista Galli) and where Ida/Pingala Nadis begin is one of the most vital spots in the body. In yogic science, it is called Adnya Chakra (the third eye) and is said to be giving extra ordinary capabilities/intelligence to the person who has been able to activate by certain spiritual attainments.

Stressed State

❖   in the stressed state, the predominant autonomic nervous system is sympathetic. In this state our breathing is rapid and mostly using chest muscles only.

❖   with no or very little participation of diaphragm muscle in breathing, the flow of CSF is rapid and irregular. continued state of stress therfore seriosly affects the health both in mind and the body.

❖   in extreme case of "fight" or "fleight", our heart rate, breathing rate and blood pressure rises.

❖   this is an open invitation for proliferation of number of diseases or syndromes including hyper tension (BP), pain, depression, diabetes etc. this is called stressed state.

❖   the only way this can be corrected almost instantaneously is by performing slow, deep and rhythmic breathing.

Heart Rate Variability

Heart rate variability is variation of beat to beat duration. As mentioned before, during inhalation the heart beat tends to increase since inhalation is the action phase. The heart beat tends decrease during exhalation since exhalation is the relaxation phase. Thus if the relaxation is complete the heart rate will be significantly lower in exhalation than that during inhalation.

Higher is the heart rate variability, better is the health of the heart. One of the parameters cardiologists check during the stress/tread mill test is the time taken by the person undergoing this test to reach the normal heart beat rate. In healthy people, heart drops fast with termination of rigorous exercise done during the stress test. If the heart beat does not drop sufficiently, it indicates possibility of coronary blockages.

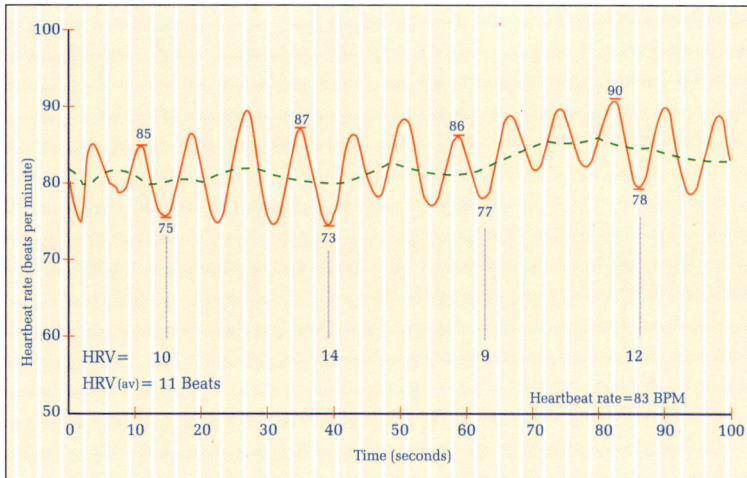

Steady Heart Rate Variability during Pranayam

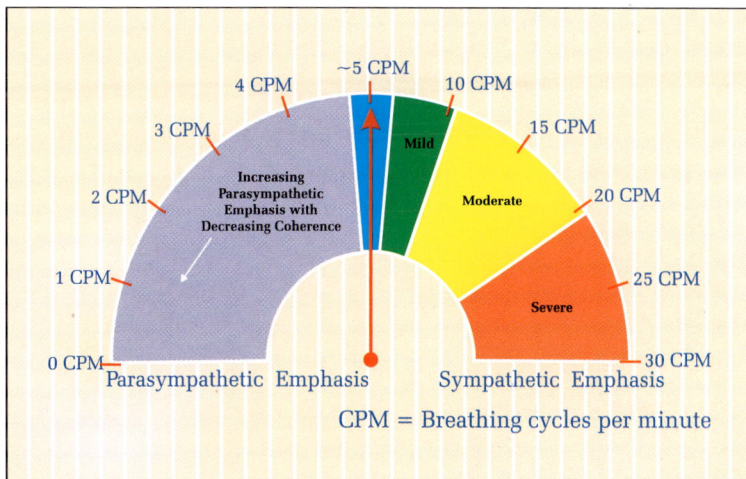

Breathing rythm for a person during the Mild, Moderate and Severe stages of work

Heart rate is triggered by the sympathetic and Parasympathetic activities of the autonomic nervous system. Heart beat naturally varies with breathing cycle. This phenomenon is called "respiratory arrhythmia"

Conclusions

The following important conclusions are drawn from the discussion in previous sections.

- The present work aims at explaining the reasons for the success of Pranayam in overcoming complex health disorders. Of late, there has been a tremendous patronage given to Pranayam. However, Pranayam does overcome several complex health disorders only when it is done correctly. For this purpose it is necessary to understand the basic/fundamental physiological processes occurring in our body vis-a-vis the breathing process we follow.

- In Pranayam, which is nothing but organized breathing process, the rhythm and depth of breathing plays a major role. The present work may guide the individual to adopt this suiting to his body.

- We have shown that Pranayam is an anabolic exercise which greatly improves blood circulation.

- Pranayam breathing requires involvement of the diaphragm muscle. This results in creating favouruable vibrations in the respiratory organs as well as in the abdominal contents.

- Pranayams such as Kapalbhati and deep Bhastrika, if practised regularly, help not only in removal of coronary blockages but also prevent their formations in future. Diaphragm is also mediator of all biological and emotional rhythm of our body including autonomic nervous system. This is one of the principal reasons behind effectiveness of Kapalbhati Pranayam.

- The biggest beneficiaries of Pranayam are the autonomic nervous system including the endocrine glands in the brain and the body. This requires efficient "breathing" of the brain. The nervous system (somatic as well as autonomic nervous systems) originates in the brain which also houses most important endocrine glands (hypothalamus, pineal, pituitary etc.) of the body. These glands in turn control other glands in the body.

- The 'nostrils' of the brain is the perforated cribriform plate in the ethmoid bone which is a part of the skull. There are slits on either side ofcrista galli (which divides cribriform plate in two parts). These slits are occluded by dura mater of the brain. The two hemispheres of the brain are located in this region.

- The brain floats in the sea of cerebrospinal fluid contained in the covering of the brain.

The cerebrospinal fluid continuously circulates from brain to spine and spine to brain. The rate of this circulation closely matches with rate of breathing. The cerebrospinal fluid comprises of neuropeptides which are messenger molecules and control physiological processes at the cellular level. The life energy inhaled with breath is transferred to cerebrospinal fluid through the dura mater of the brain hemispheres resting on either sides of crista galli. The cerebrospinal fluid, through its circulation, in turn distributes it to the nervous system and the glands throughout the body.

■ The two hemispheres of the brain have alternating dominance throughout the day. The rhythm of the cerebral cycle is tightly coupled with nasal cycle. When the left brain is more active, right nostril is free and the left nostril is relatively congested and vice versa. This phenomenon was known to Yogic science several thousands years ago. The yogic science has given the concept of Nadis. Important amongst them are Ida, Pingala and Sushumna.

■ The concept of Nadis help us understand how alternate breathing Pranayam, called Anulom - vilom is exceedingly beneficial as it helps body to balance the cerebral dominance (or Nadis).

■ There is strong co-relationship between breathing rhythm, heart beat rate variability and the rhythm of autonomic nervous system. At lower breathing rates such as 5-6 breaths per minute a high degree of synchrony in all these rhythms occurs. These result in total tranquility, lower heart rate, reduced blood pressure, low blood sugar level and many such benefits. Pranayam is the cheapest and simple method for spiritual growth and for maintaining good health.

Some Rules for Practising Pranayam

● Pranayam should be practised in a calm, peaceful and clean place, if possible near water.

● In cities the surroundings are polluted hence before doing Pranayam burn Ghrita or Guggul and fill the place with fragrance. If possible light a lamp with clarified butter.

● Sidhasana, Vajrasana or Padmasana are suitable for practising Pranayam. The mat or seat used for Pranayam should be bad conductor of heat, use blanket or Kusha etc.

● Always breathe through nostrils. This will filter the air and maintain the body temperature through Ida, Pingla nerves and the foreign particles are blocked outside only.

● Pranayam should be done after four or five hours of taking meals. After waking up in the morning finish the morning chores and then practise Pranayam as this is the best time.

- In the beginning practise it for five or 10 minutes and then slowly increase the duration and take it up to half or one hour. Always practise in fixed numbers, not less or more. If stomach does not get cleared in the morning then take Harad or Triphala churna with hot water at bed time. Kapalbhati Pranayam is also beneficial for clearing stomach.

- The mind should be happy and calm while practising Pranayam. Pranayam also makes the mind calm, happy and focused.

- Pranayam should be practised according to the season and body constitution. Some Pranayam increase the body temperature, some give coolness, whereas some are normal.

- If Pranayam causes tiredness then take five or six normal breaths and rest for sometime.

- Pregnant women should not practise Kapalbhati, Bahya Pranayam and Agnisar. They should practise rest of the Pranayam slowly. Practising Pranayam will help in giving birth to healthy and intelligent progeny.

- Eat pious, simple and non-oily food, milk, fruits, and *ghee*, vegetables, sprouted grains, Coarse grains like porridge.

- Do not stop breath forcibly while practising Pranayam. Inhaling is known as Poorak, stopping it inside is called Kumbhak, exhaling is known as Rechak, controlling the breath outside is called Bahya Kumbhak.

- Pranayam does not mean only Poorak, Kumbhak and Rechak but it is controlling and balancing the speed of breath and Pran and also concentrating the mind on one particular subject.

- Before practising Pranayam chant loud and deep 'Om' and sing devotional songs. This will give peace of mind and concentration. It is very necessary to have peace of mind which is free of thoughts while practising Pranayam. Chant Gayatri mantra, Om to get spiritual strength.

- Keep the eyes, mouth, nose and other organs in their natural state while practising Pranayam. Be calm, tension free and practise it in simple manner. The neck, spine, chest and hips should be absolutely straight while practising Pranayam. This is beneficial and gives good results.

- For some reasons if you are unable to sit on the floor, you can do Pranayam sitting on a chair, couch or bed. Make sure that you sit straight and seat should not be too soft. If you can not sit at all, you can do Pranayam lying down as well.

- It should be done slowly and steadily without any kind of hastiness.

Yathāa siṃhō gagō vyāaghrō bhavēd Vaṣayaḥ Śanāiḥ Śanāiḥ ।

Tathāiva vaśyatē vāayuḥ aṇyathāa haṇti sāadhakaṃ ॥

- It is just like controlling the wild animals such as like tiger, lion, elephant etc. When we show hastiness the animals can attack us in self-defense. In the same way Pranayam should also be done slowly and duration should be increased gradually.

- It should be done after taking bath and doing of prayar etc. If you want to take bath after practising Pranayam then wait for 15 - 20 minutes. Practise Pranayam under guidance from a teacher and learn how to do Asana, Pranayam, Mudras etc. A sick person should give due attention to precautions as advised.

- Memorize the following verse and chant in mind while practising all types of Pranayam in order to get the complete benefits.

Yuktāahāaravihāarasya yukta chēśya karmasu ।
Yukta swapnāa vabōdhasya yōgō bhavati dukhahāat ।

Useful Bandhs in Pranayam

The generation of power in our body with the practice of Yog, asana, Pranayam and bandh is controlled and taken in. 'Bandh' means stopping or tying. The bandhs are extremely important in case of Pranayam and it is incomplete without it. Yog Asana, Pranayam and bandh circulate life energy in our body and make us introspective.

The bandhs have been mentioned underneath.

Jalandhar bandh

Sit in Padmasana or Sidhasana and inhale. Both the hands should be kept on knees and bend the chin slightly downward so that it touches the upper chest area. This is known as Jalandhar bandh. The eyes should be focused in between the eyebrows. The chest should be straight; this bandh holds the network of nerves in the neck area.

- It makes the voice sweet, melodious and attractive.

- It blocks Ida and Pingla nerves and therefore life energy enters the Sushmana nerve.

- It is beneficial for all the throat related diseases. It should be practised in diseases like tonsillitis, thyroid etc.

- It arouses the Vishudhi chakra.

Uddiyan bandh

The action, which helps the Pran to move up and enter the Sushmana nerve, is called Uddiyan bandh. Exhale and relax the stomach area. Then contract the stomach as if you are trying to touch the back (internally). Do Jalandhar bandh and lift the chest slightly upwards. Let the stomach touch the back. Do it as much as possible, inhale and repeat as above. Begin with three repetitions and increase gradually.

In the same way stand straight, place both the hands on knees to perform the bandh.

It cures stomach related problems, it is beneficial in diabetes, gastric trouble, constipation and hernia problems.

It arouses Pran and purifies Manipur chakra.

Moolbandh

Sit in Padmasana or Sidhasana and do Bahya or Abhyantar Kumbhak, contract the rectum, urinary bladder. In this bandh the lower abdomen gets stiff. It is easy to do this along with Bahya Kumbhak. The experts can easily perform it for several hours. It should be practised for long duration under an expert's guidance.

- This bandh arouses the Mooladhar chakra and helps in arousing of Kundalini.
- It cures constipation and piles, increases digestive fire.
- It strengthes the semen and is important for practising celibacy.

Maha bandh

Sit in Padmasana or any other meditative pose and perform all the three bandhs together, this is called Maha bandh. The benefits are same as mentioned above. While doing Kumbhak all the three bandhs are performed.

- The Pran moves upwards.
- Purifies and strengthens the semen
- It helps in the confluence of Ida, Pingla and Sushmana

Right posture for Pranayam

The spine should be absolutely straight for practising Pranayam. Sit in any meditative pose like Padmasana, Sukhasan, and Vajrasana. A chair can be used if it is uncomfortable to sit on floor but the spine should be straight. Nowadays people practise Nadi Shodhan and other Pranayam while walking, this is wrong practice and can be very harmful. Pranayam increases the vital life energy and arouses the chakra attached with the spine. Therefore, it is necessary to sit straight. Practising Pranayam in correct posture on the floor or chair helps in concentration of the mind.

Seven Techniques/Processes of Pranayam as Popularized by Swami Ramdevji Maharaj

The seven types of Pranayam are mentioned in different texts but every Pranayam has its own importance. A person cannot practise all the seven types daily, therefore Swamiji has formulated a scientific method and spiritual process of all the seven steps of Pranayam with the help of his Guru's blessings and own personal experience. This whole process takes around 20 minutes and the benefits are as mentioned below:

- It maintains the equilibrium of vata, pitta and kapha.
- It improves the digestion system and cures all the stomach-related diseases.
- It cures the diseases related to the heart, lungs and brain.
- It is beneficial in case of obesity, diabetes, cholesterol, constipation, gastric trouble, acidity, respiratory problem, allergy, migraine, blood pressure, kidney diseases, sexual diseases and even incurable diseases like cancer etc.
- It develops the immunity.
- It can protect a person from hereditary diseases or person to fight diseases such as high blood pressure, diabetes and heart disease.
- It controls hair loss, premature graying of hairs, wrinkles, eyesight, loss of memory power, ageing and increases longevity.
- It gives natural glow, brightness and shining on the face.
- It helps in purification, arousal of chakra thus providing spiritual strength (arousal of Kundalini).
- The mind remains stable, calm, happy and enthusiastic, it prevents mental diseases and depression etc.
- The person is able to reach the stage of meditation automatically and develops the capability to meditate for several hours.
- It cures all the physical and mental diseases and removes negative thoughts like lust, anger, greed, attachment, pride and others.
- It removes all the foreign particles, tonsils and other disorders.
- Negative thoughts are removed and the person practising Pranayam is always happy, optimistic and full of enthusiasm.
- Samaṭwaṃ yōga uchyatē yogaḥ karmasu kāuśalam ꠰ The regular practice of Pranayam balances the mind and body and develops the physical, mental, spiritual and intellectual abilities.
- Pranayam increases the positive attitude, qualities, productivity and creativity.
- Pranayam develops a healthy and sensitive person. A person possessing healthy mind and body can never indulge in violence, crime, corruption, suicide, bribery, dacoity, theft, indiscipline, prostitution, duping etc. Therefore Pranayam and Dhayana are the only solutions to fight out negative energies like violence, crime, indiscipline, treachery, irresponsible, insensitive and unreliable behaviour.

Bhastrika Pranayam

Sit in any comfortable posture and inhale till diaphragm is full and exhale with full force. This is known as Bhastrika Pranayam and should be done according to individual capacity in three different ways, slow, medium and fast. Those who have a weak heart and lungs should do Rechak and Poorak at slow pace. A healthy person and a trained person should try to increase the speed gradually and first do it at medium speed and then at fast pace. This Pranayam should be practised for three to five minutes. While practising Bhastrika Pranayam we should think that the divine strength, energy, purity, calmness and happiness prevailing in the universe is positive and that vital life energy is entering inside our body. In this way, Pranayam done with auspicious and positive thoughts is very effective.

- Patients of high blood pressure and heart disease should practise it slowly.
- When you inhale contract the stomach and fill the air till the diaphragm. This will prevent the air entering the stomach and will remain in chest and ribs.
- In summer season this Pranayam should be practiced for lesser duration.
- In case of excess kapha and sinus problem which results nose being blocked then close the right nostril and do Rechak and Poorak from left nostril. Then close the left nostril and do Rechak and Poorak with right nostril at slow, medium and fast pace. Then finish Rechak and Poorak with both the nostrils and practice Bhastrika Pranayam.
- The eyes should be closed and chant Om in mind with each breath.
- It cures cold, catarrh, allergy, respiratory problem, asthma, sinuses and other diseases. It strengthens the lungs, heart and brain as they get pure energy.
- It cures tonsils, thyroid and other diseases of the throat.
- It brings the tridoshas in equilibrium and the toxic, foreign substances are evacuated from the body.
- It stabilizes the mind and Pran or vital life energy. It is helpful in arousal of Kundalini.

Kapalbhati Pranayam

Kapal means brain and Bhati means light, brightness, shine, glow etc. The Pranayam, which brings glow, light, shine on the forehead is called Kapalbhati. This is slightly different from Bhastrika Pranayam. In the latter inhaling, exhaling is done with the same speed but in Kapalbhati focus is laid on exhaling with full force. We do not try to inhale but air enters automatically while exhaling. The person should exhale with full concentration. The stomach contracts and expands automatically and force is exerted on Mooladhar, Swadhisthan and Manipur chakra. This should be practised at least for five minutes daily. While practising this Pranayam we should think that air that we are breathing out is taking away with it all the diseases present in the body. The person suffering with a particular disease should think in this manner and remove the negative feelings present in his mind like anger, lust, greed, attachment, jealousy, hatred, etc. If we think that our body is getting rid of the diseases and positive energy is entering then it has positive impact.

This Pranayam should be practised for at least three minutes and then increased up to 15-20 minutes. In case of tiredness take rest in between after regular practice. It can be done nonstop for five minutes. This is the maximum duration for Kapalbhati. In the beginning the person might experience back and stomach pain but it disappears after some time. In summer the person predominant with pitta nature should practice it only for two or three minutes.

- It increases the glow, brightness and beauty of the face.
- It is beneficial in phlegm related diseases like asthma, allergy, respiratory problems, sinuses etc.
- It cures diseases related to lungs, heart and brain.
- It is extremely beneficial in case of obesity, diabetes, gas, constipation, acidity, kidney and prostrate problems.
- Regular practice of Kapalbhati for five minutes cures constipation, diabetes without any medicines. It reduces extra fat on stomach and back by four to eight kilos within one month and it also removes the blockage from arteries.
- The mind remains stable, calm and happy. The negative thoughts are kept at bay and the person is free from depression and other mental diseases.
- It circulates divine strength in all chakras or centers and purifies them.
- This Pranayam is very beneficial and has a positive impact on stomach, pancreas, liver, spleen, intestines, prostrate and kidney. This Pranayam is alone capable of giving all the benefits for stomach, which cannot even be obtained from asana. It strengthens the weak intestines.

Bahya Pranayam (with tribandh)

- Sit in Padmasana or Sidhasana and exhale all at once completely and with full force.
- Do Moolbandh, Uddiyan and Jalandhar bandh and control the breath outside for as long as possible.
- When you feel like breathing in then remove all the three bandhs and breathe normally.
- Inhale and repeat the Pranayam without stopping it. Repeat this 3-21 times according to capacity.

One should always think positive while doing this Pranayam and think that all the diseases and dosha present in the body are going away and the body is being filled with fresh new positive energy. This type of auspicious and positive attitude gives beneficial results.

This is totally harmless Pranayam. It controls the playfulness of the mind, increases the digestive fire, it is beneficial in stomach diseases. It makes the mind sharp and intelligent. It purifies the body, cures early ejaculation and humours related problems. Bahya Pranayam strengthens the stomach organs and in the beginning the practitioner might complain of pain in the diseased or weak part of the stomach. Therefore, give rest in the beginning and do all the three bandhs while doing this Pranayam.

Anulom-vilom Pranayam

Press the right nostril with right thumb and breathe in completely from left nostril then close the left nostril with middle and ring finger and exhale completely from right nostril. Then inhale from right nostril and exhale from left nostril.

Ida or left nostril indicates moon, moon power or calmness, therefore this Pranayam should be started from left nostril for Nadi Shodhan. The pace of breathing should be increased first to medium and then fast. Inhale with full strength and breathe out in the same manner. Rechak and Poorak done at fast speed increases the sound of the vital energy. This completes one cycle. This rhythmic breathing should be repeated, viz. inhale from left nostril and exhale from right nostril and vice-versa. Initially it causes tiredness within two or three minutes of practice. Take rest and repeat it after sometime. It can be done from 5 to 25 minutes. Regular practice for some days will increase the strength and within one month the practitioner can practise it for five minutes minimum. Every person should practice it for at least five minutes. In summer it should be done for five to 15 minutes. Five minutes of Anulom vilom Pranayam arouses the Mooladhar chakra. This is known as Urdhvaretas in Veda and in modern Yog parlance it is known as arousal of Kundalini. While practising this Pranayam we should think of 'Om' mentally. This increases the concentration and the mind reaches the higher stage. While practising this Pranayam one should think mentally that Sushmana Nadi is getting aroused. A divine light is glowing in all the chakras. The person should think that the whole body is glowing with a divine light. The divine light, should be experienced both externally and internally. Think that this divine light, strength of God is spreading in all directions. The Almighty God is enlightening the whole world with this divine light. Enjoy the light and increase the knowledge. The knowledge attained when the Kundalini is awakened opens the six wheels in the way of Sushmana Nadi. Guru is just the source of inspiration for this power, he associates us with divine compassions. This real knowledge is attained from the strength of God. Anulom-vilom Pranayam practised with this divine knowledge and feelings is beneficial for physical, mental and spiritual strength. A divine light arises from Mooladhar chakra, arouses Kundalini and the mind moves upwards and the person attains the real knowledge.

- This Pranayam purifies 72 crore 72 lakh 10 thousand and 210 nerves. When the nerves get purified the body becomes healthy, strong and bright.

- It is beneficial in case of joint pain, dysentery, gout, Parkinson's disease, nervous weakness, vata, urinary problem, humours loss, low sperm count, acidity, pitta, cold, catarrh, sinuses, asthma, cough, tonsils and other diseases. It balances all the three dosha.

- It opens the blockages in the heart arteries. Regular practice of this Pranayam is capable of opening 30 - 40 percent blockages within three to four months. We have experienced this after testing it on several patients.

- It cures the irregularities in cholesterol, triglycerides, HDL, LDL etc.

- It overcomes negative thinking and increases positive thoughts. It gives happiness, enthusiasm and courage.

- This Pranayam purifies mind, body, thoughts and values. It cures all the diseases of the body. The mind is engrossed in Omkar.

- Practising this Pranayam for 250 - 500 times arouses Kundalini.

Brahmari Pranayam

Inhale and press the nostrils with the tips of middle fingers and concentrate on Agya chakra, in between the eyebrows. Close both the ears with thumbs and make a sound like bee and chant Om. Repeat it once again and do at least three times and up to 11 - 21 times maximum. This Pranayam should be done with full concentration and deep devotion towards God. We should think mentally that God is bestowing his grace, happiness and peace on us. The God appears in the form of a divine light and will take away all the ignorance present in the mind and make me wise. In this way, the Pranayam should be done with pure feelings and the practitioner will be able to meditate automatically. This stabilizes the playful and wavering mind. It is beneficial in case of mental tension, anxiety, high blood pressure, heart disease etc. and is highly useful in Dhayana.

Udgeet Pranayam

After doing all the above-mentioned Pranayam concentrate on breathing and chant Om. The shape of our eyebrows resembles the letter Om. The whole body and universe is filled with Om. It is not a person or a shape; it is a divine power, which manages the entire universe. The breathing speed should be so low that we should not be able to feel it. It should be so mild that a piece of cotton kept in front of the nose should not move. Slowly increase the duration up to one minute. Try to experience the breath from within. In the beginning you will experience it in the tip of the nose but slowly you will experience it deep within and the practitioner will reach the stage of deep meditation. One should practise it while going to bed as this will help in getting sound sleep and in getting rid of bad dreams.

Pranv Pranayam

This is the highest stage of Pranayam. It can also be called as the stage of Dhayana. Practically speaking concentration is the result of Pranayam. Practice of this Pranayam controls the mind and sensory organs and the practitioners get into the depth of concentration. Saint Patanjali has descried this stage as **Taṭra praṭyayāikaṭāanāṭāa ḍhyāanaṃ** ।

Concentration is the even flow of knowledge of unity in between eyebrows, navel and heart. Do not think of anything else except of Almighty God at the time of practising. Being engrossed in the thought of omnipotent, bright and quite form of God is Pranv Pranayam.

Dhyana (concentration) is associated with us every moment. According to the Indian culture it completes every process. Therefore, today also whenever our elders or parents advice us, they ask us to do every work with concentration, study with concentration etc. But what is concentration? Nobody bothers to ponder on this issue. We see that this word is associated with us in every work of life and therefore should understand that concentration is inevitable in life. Human being is incomplete without concentration. Success cannot be guaranteed in attaining any material or spiritual goal in its absence. Concentration leads to happiness and peace of mind.

We can find the importance of meaningful chanting of Omkar for attaining concentration. God has created all parts like eyebrows, eyes, nose, lips, ears, heart and chest in the shape of Om.

In this way the practitioner chants Om and experiences the presence of omnipresent, omnipotent, unending and Almighty God and engrosses in his divine form. Omkar is not an individual or shape, it is a divine light, which is controlling this entire universe. The followers of different religions, communities, sects call it by different names and worship it. The soul is invisible in this body, but all the tasks inside the body are carried on under its supervision, in the same way we cannot see the divine strength present in the universe in the form of Om but it is controlling the whole universe.

The mind is concentrated on respiration and Udgeet is worshipped with Pran. All the sensory organs are full of faults, because our eyes can see both good and bad scenes. The ears listen to both vulgar and decent language. Similarly the nose can smell both fragrance and odour, the tongue can speak both lies and truth. The taste takes in both edible and inedible things, the good and bad thoughts arise in our mind. Therefore, nothing is perfect.

Pran is completely faultless and uniform. Therefore we should take the shelter of faultless Pran in order to realize the faultless divine and uniform consciousness. Whenever you get time, try to introspect, inhale and exhale at both fast and slow pace.

Practise Pranv Pranayam with every breath. See that pace of breath should be so soft that the sound should not be heard even to self. Try to take one respiration in one minute. Try to see the respiration from within. Initially you will experience the touch of respiration only in the tip of the nose. Slowly you can experience the breath deep within. Practise meaningful chanting of Omkar along with respiration as it will help in attaining concentration. The practitioner is able to engross in the divine form of Almighty God with regular practice of this Pranayam. He attains priceless divine happiness suitable for meditation. The practitioner should concentrate in this manner at the time of sleeping.

This will help in enjoying sound sleep. Internal negative power transforms into positive power, diseases get cured and life is filled with positive energy, chastity, and good health.

Pranayam Beneficial in Treatment of Diseases

Surya Bhedi Pranayam

Sit in meditative pose and do poorak with right nostril then do Kumbhak with Jalandhar and Moolbandh and do Rechak with left nostril. Increase the duration of Antar Kumbhak gradually. Increase the repetitions in odd numbers and take it up to 10. While doing Kumbhak the focus should be on the brightness of the Sun. In summer reduce the duration of practice and repetitions as it increases the temperature and pitta in the body. It cures the diseases caused due to vata, kapha, blood impurities, skin problems, stomach worms, leprosy, syphilis, contagious diseases, indigestion, and gynecological problems. It is helpful in arousal of Kundalini. It controls ageing and should be done after Anulom-vilom. Doing this Pranayam with Kumbhak improves heart function, activates the body and reduces weight. Repeat 27 cycles twice daily.

Chandra Bhedi Pranayam

Do poorak with left nostril and then do Antar Kumbhak. It is best to practise this Pranayam with Jalandhar and Mool Bandh. In this Pranayam poorak is always done with left nostril and Rechak with right nostril. It is just opposite to Surya Bhedi, while doing Kumbhak think about the bright shining Moon. Reduce the practice in winter.

It brings down the body temperature, overcomes fatigue and decreases heat. It controls the anxiety of mind and controls the burning sensation caused due to pitta.

Ujjayi Pranayam

Contract the throat and inhale while doing this Pranayam. Sound similar to snoring is made while contracting the throat. Sit in meditative pose and inhale from both the nostrils. Contract the throat and you will feel the touch of air in the throat. The air should not touch inside the nose. When the air touches the throat a peculiar sound is produced. In the beginning do not do Kumbhak, practise only Poorak and Rechak. After Poorak practise Kumbhak for same duration and then double its duration (1:2). If Kumbhak is to be practised for more than 10 seconds then you should do Jalandhar and Moolbandh also. In this Pranayam close the right nostril and do Rechak with left nostril. It is beneficial for those who suffer from chronic cold, cough, dysentery, indigestion, liver problem, phlegm, fever, spleen and other diseases throughout the year. Regular practice makes the voice sweet and melodious. It is the best Pranayam for arousing Kundalini, meditation, and concentration. It also cures lisping in children.

Karna Rogantak Pranayam

Do Poorak with both the nostrils and then close the mouth, both nostrils and throw out the Poorak air from both the ears. Push the air upwards four to five times and then do Rechak with both nostrils. Repeat it two to three times. It is beneficial for ear diseases and improves hearing power.

Shitali Pranayam

Sit in meditative pose and keep the hands on knees. Fold the tongue and open the mouth and do Poorak with mouth. Inhale from tongue and fill the air in lungs. Control the breath for some time and close the mouth and do Rechak with both the nostrils. Then fold the tongue and do Poorak with mouth and Rechak with nose. Repeat it 8 - 10 times. Reduce the practice during winters.

You can also do Jalandhar Bandh with Kumbhak. People suffering from kapha, tonsillitis should not practice Shitali and Sitkari Pranayam.

- It is beneficial in diseases related to tongue, mouth and throat. It cures the diseases of spleen, fever, indigestion etc.
- The practitioner is able to control thirst and hunger with regular practice. This has been mentioned in Yog books.
- It controls high blood pressure, is beneficial in case of pitta related diseases and purifies blood.

Sitkari Pranayam

Sit in meditative pose and try to touch the tongue upwards and join the upper and lower

Comment: Read Swami Ramdev Baba's 'Pranayam Rahasya' for complete information regarding Pranayam, types, method of practice and its effects.

row of teeth and open the lips. Now make see-see sound, inhale from mouth and fill the air in lungs. Do Jalandhar bandh and remain in this position for as long as possible. Close the mouth and do Rechak with nose. Repeat at least 8 to 10 times. In winters reduce the practice. This can also be done without Jalandhar and Kumbhak Bandh. While doing Poorak the teeth and tongue should be stable at their position.

- The qualities and benefits are similar to Shitali Pranayam.
- It cures dental problems like pyorrhea, diseases of throat, mouth, nose, tongue etc.
- It reduces sleep and controls the body temperature.
- The patients of high blood pressure should practise it 50 - 60 times for benefit.

Nadi Shodhan Pranayam

In the beginning this Pranayam should be done like Anulom-vilom. Inhale from left nostril and exhale from right nostril. After inhaling stop the breath and do Moolbandh and Jalandhar Bandh. Then remove Jalandhar Bandh and exhale slowly with right nostril. After exhaling completely inhale and do Kumbhak, control the breath inside and then exhale from left nostril at slow pace. This completes one cycle of Nadi Shodhan. If this Pranayam is done without using fingers and on the basis of concentration then it is even more beneficial. This helps in concentrating the mind on the Pran and mind becomes stable. We should not make any sound while inhaling and exhaling. This should be done at least one to three times or more if possible. In Nadi Shodhan Pranayam the ratio of Poorak, Antar Kumbhak and Rechak should be 1:2:2, this means, Poorak for 10 seconds, Antar Kumbhak for 20 seconds and Rechak for 20 seconds. Later the ratio should be 1:4:2. Not only that you can join Bahya Kumbhak as well in other words do poorak, antar Kumbhak, Rechak and Bahya Kumbhak in the ratio of 1:4:2:2. This Pranayam should be done at a very slow pace. Do not bother about number of repetitions and do according to body capacity. Long, deep Pranayam done at slow pace is very beneficial. The actual result is derived with proper rhythmic breathing and breath control. There is no need to take rest in between. While doing Poorak, Kumbhak, Rechak chant Gayatri mantra and Om mentally. Be optimistic and practise it with devotion. The benefits are similar to Anulom-vilom Pranayam.

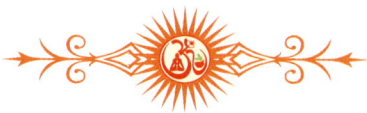

Chapter 4

WORLD TAKES TO YOG WITH SWAMI RAMDEV

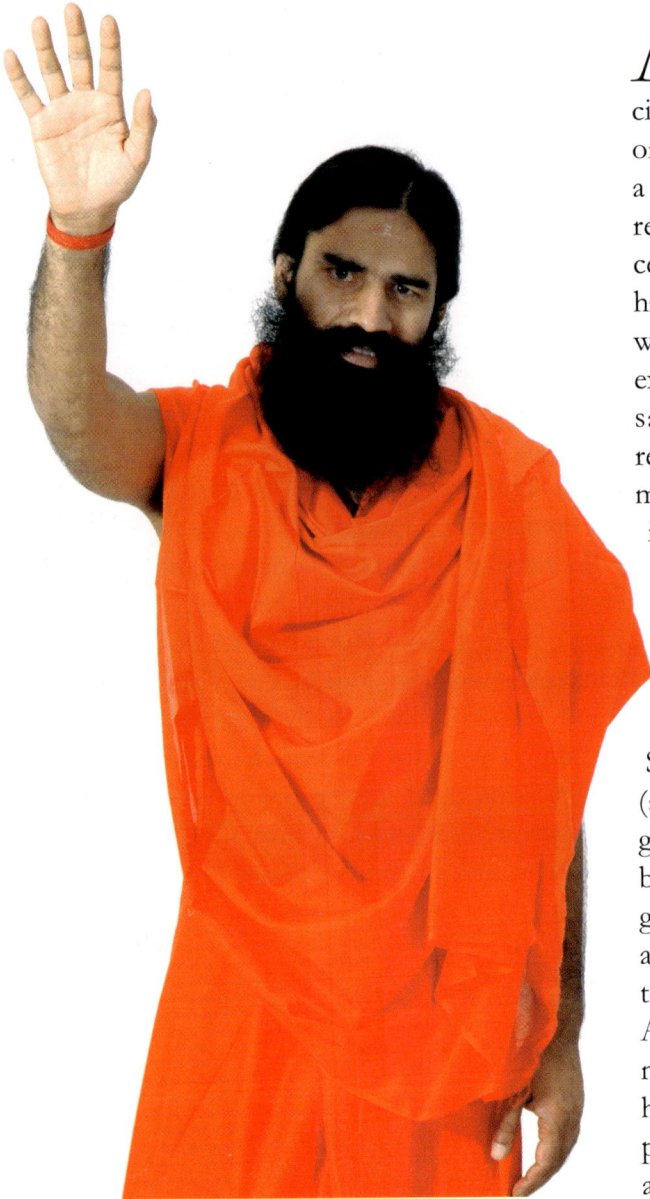

Adopting a particular knowledge, education, tradition, culture or civilization in one's life-style is not an ordinary situation. The public accepts a tradition after repeated experiments, research, study, and usage for several centuries. Innumerable learned people have contributed in the field of Yog and we owe this knowledge to them. We express deep gratitude towards all those sages. However, this knowledge remained more of a secret during the medieval period. Some people practised it just to improve flexibility, enhance beauty and to achieve a good figure. People didnot pay much attention to ground rules of Sadhna for maintaining good health and Pranayam for achieving Dhayana and Samadhi. By doing physical excercise (asana) people were able to achieve good figures and their bodies also became more flexible leading to the generally held perception that Yog was all about asanas. Such a perception was too narrow and inapt for Yog vidya. Also truth is that practising asanas did not relieve one of difficult diseases like heart blockage, cancer, high blood pressure, diabetes, hepatitis, asthma and arthritis.

21st Century Rediscovers Yog/Pranayam

Efforts made by Pantjali Yogpeeth led to the wider acceptance of Yog as countless people realized that their serious ailments were getting cured with the practice of Pranayam. Today people of every age, segment, caste and religion have made Yog part of their daily routine. Indeed it is an incredible phenomenon when people from all walks of life have accepted culture and tradition of Yog. It is also true that till such time Yog is fully backed by clinically controlled trial, some selfish, prejudiced people will continue to indulge in the politics of allegations and counter allegations. However, such controversies indirectly help in promoting Yog. Whatever experiments we have done till now, prove that Yog can be a solution for all the problems of the world. Experiment followed by results constitute the process of reaching truth. We are committed to establish Yog and Ayurved as evidence based medicine on international platform.

Besides commoners, senior politicians, administrators, senior judges, media and management professionals have learned Yog directly from Swami Ramdevji Maharaj. Many states have made Yog education compulsory in educational institutions. Defense personnel, police officers, and people associated with this field have learnt Pranayam and are making efforts to introduce it in their system. Swamiji has been instrumental integrating world's spiritual and divine strengths.

A big mission is being carried on to give Yog an international platform. Trained Yog teachers of Patanjali Yogpeeth are giving free Yog education in several countries including UK and USA. In almost every district of the country, Patanjali Yog training committees are fulfilling their responsibilities with complete dedication and devotion. Around five to 10 lakh main and assistant Yog teachers will be ready to take charge by the end of 2007 and 2008. We can together achieve the goal of building a healthy India and world. Daily practice of Yog not only gives good health but also develops healthy thoughts, attitude, positive mind and develops good qualities. We believe that Yog would become a part of international culture very soon and the whole world will accept Indian philosophy of life supported by scientific evidence. We Indians should take pride in the fact that wider acceptance will also strengthen the path of world peace and welfare. Yog will help in creating a healthy, sensitive society, nation and world. A healthy and sensitive mind and body will be free from all kinds of violence, casteism, regionalism, communal differences and gradually there shall be more of harmony, love, peace, humaneness, sense of service, empathy and tolerance in this world. There will be heaven on earth. The integration of science with spiritualism will reduce the negative impact of development.

Swamiji is carrying on his Yog revolution guided by the principle of – Sarvey Bhavantu Sukhinah Sarvey Santu Niramaya that is to make all the people happy and disease-free. Nobody should feel insecure or be poor. Swamiji is executing this mission through Yog camps, so far more than hundred camps have been organized in India and abroad. The main objective of these camps is to make the whole mankind healthy, free of pain, suffering and diseases. Swamiji has a dream that is to see India regaining its old status of a world mentor and to guide people in recognizing their ultimate goal and in realizing their full potential. There is nothing hum an in conquering the world with muscle and money power. The main thought behind the concept of a world mentor is that India should continue its work to propagate human values and should lead and protect the people who are oppressed and suffering because of all sorts of reasons.

There could be no other sublime objective than the objective of building a 'Healthy India and Healthy World'? Swamiji is working tirelessly towards the aim of taking Yog to the last person in this world which is not only a difficult but almost next to impossible task. Though print and electronic media have played a major role in propagating knowledge of Yog and establishing it all over the world, it also promotes negative aspects of life like violence, lust and crime intentionally or unintentionally. However it is heartening to point out that media in general has displayed a very positive approach in extending Yog to each and every individual.

Swamiji through Yog is committed to the welfare of not only Indians but for the people of the whole world and has made a great progress in his mission of making 'Healthy India, Healthy World.' His in-depth discourses on issues relevant to today's life and knowledge on how to lead an ideal life based on Vedic principles and how to develop one's life in totality - are a source of inspiration and motivation for the general public. He is a yogi, an ascetic who has selected the path of Yog to relieve the mankind from suffering, depression and tension. His approach is not about aiming for profits like multinational companies which only aim for profits and he is not acting out of selfish interests to mislead or confuse people. Revered Swamiji has organized Yog camps in almost all the big cities of India and also overseas in UK and USA. Besides Swamiji has addressed and trained thousands in various Yog camps organized in schools, colleges, jails and as part of social and spiritual programmes. In the next few months Swamiji Maharaj plans to hold Yog camps in UK, USA, Canada, Thailand (Bangkok), Dubai (UAE), Indonesia, Mauritious, Holland, Kenya, Uganda, Yogoslavia, Tanzania and Nepal. Swamiji's Yog revolution has reached almost all the nations of the world through electronic media, various magazines and newspapers and through his own publications.

Yog, A Ray of Hope for People in Despair

Since ancient times, sages have been saying: Sharirmadhyam Khaludharam Sadhnam, i.e. for doing work and for enjoying life, healthy body is the only instrument required. Modern medical science also considers prevention to be the primary step. It is necessary to make

Yog a part of daily routine. It is true that some may have the means to benefit from the big hospitals and be able to afford the huge cost. But 65 percent of Indian population and a large number of people in other countries who cannot even think of seeking expensive medical treatment, have been blessed with life-saving medicine in the form of Yog. It is also a blessing for those who are well off but are almost dead as they suffer from diseases which are taken as incurable. They have the resources but donot know what treatment to take. Yog and Pranayam have prevented people from falling into the deep dark ditch of diseases. Yog is the support for people filled with dejection and hopelessness as Yog opens a new path when all other paths are closed.

Just walk in into any Yog camps of Swami Ramdevji and you can experience the unity in diversity of this country. The people gathered might be wearing different clothes but the hearts feel the same, features could be different but the minds think the same, interests can be different but creativity is the same. You can see people of all ages, religions, community, caste, and class mingling together and striving for one common goal of achieving good health through Yog. It will be difficult to experience such a fascinating sight anywhere else except at Swamiji's Yog camp.

Rich and poor, men and women, young and old all come in huge numbers to gain some knowledge from Swamiji. People start queuing up in front of the venue in the wee hours, they start arriving very early to secure a place in Yog camps. When it is usually time to go to sleep, people start getting ready to reach the camp and strive to get to the camps on time. The enthusiasm, the curiosity is worth seeing. You can see a little girl holding her grandmother's hand and a grandfather could be seen carrying his grandson on the shoulders to the Yog camp. These are just a few instances to give you a feel of our camps. If you get into a traffic jam even on a usually desolated road, it must be that a large number of people could be rushing to a Yog camp or coming back from it. Even in a country like England, where people wake up late in the morning, thousands of cars and vehicles can be seen stranded on the roads in the wee hours, it is a sure sign that Swamiji's camp must be on somewhere nearby.

These incidences cannot be expressed in words, nor captured in pictures. However, we are presenting a few pictures here where you can see the presence of millions of people who come to listen and catch the glimpses of a saint.

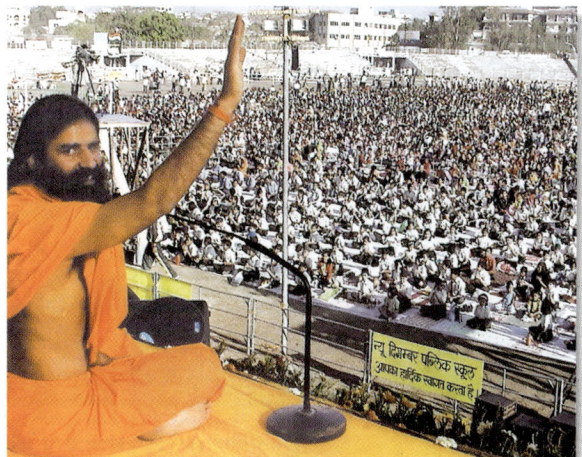

Glimpses of Yog camps organized at different places

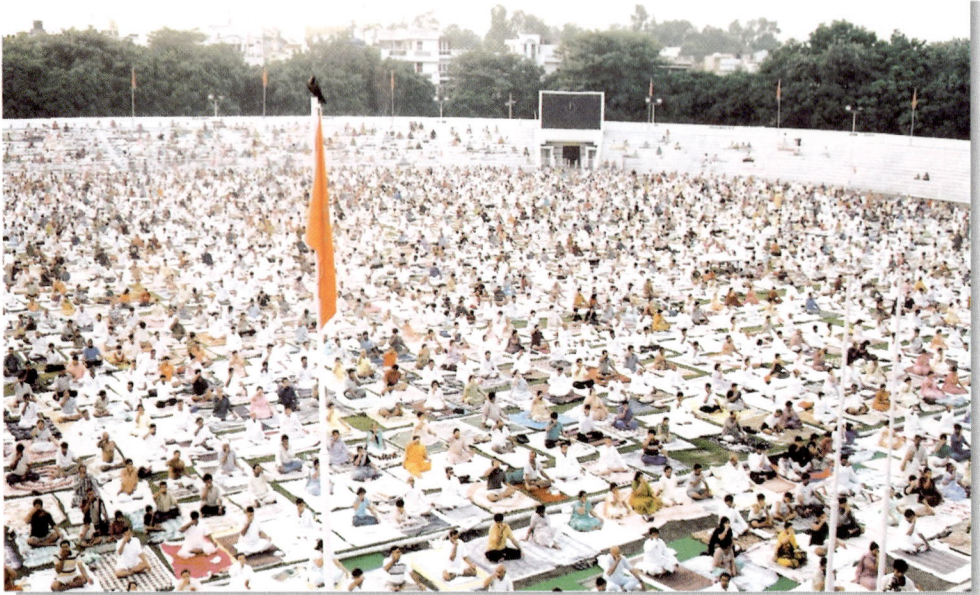

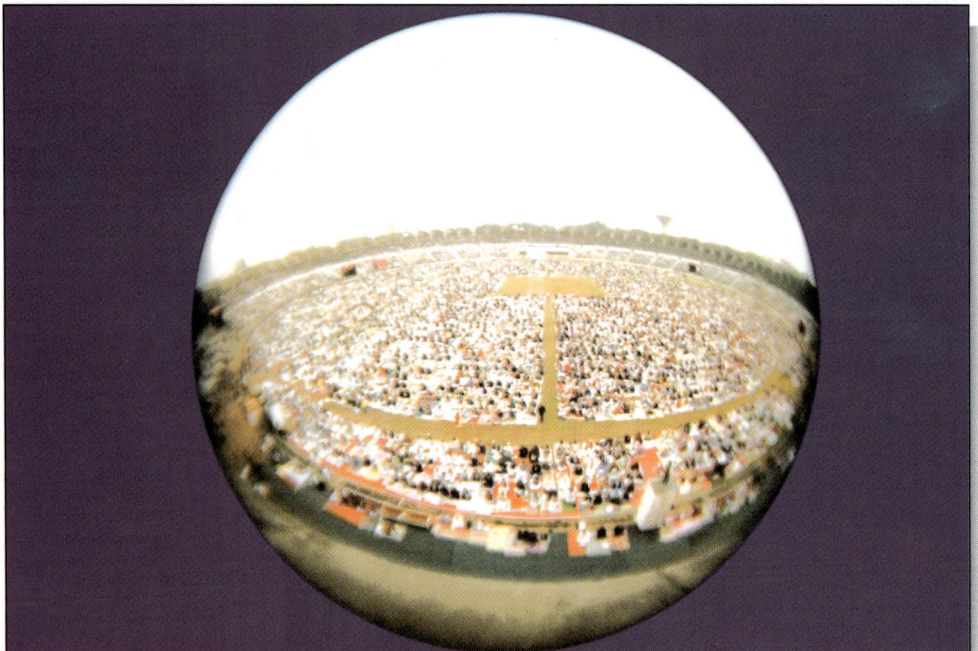

Millions have attended the Yog camps globally

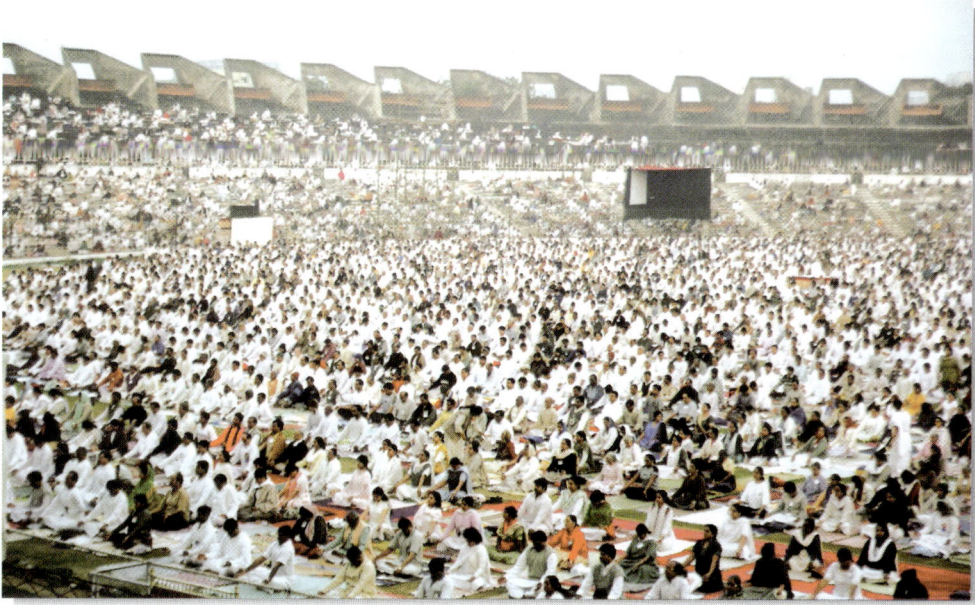

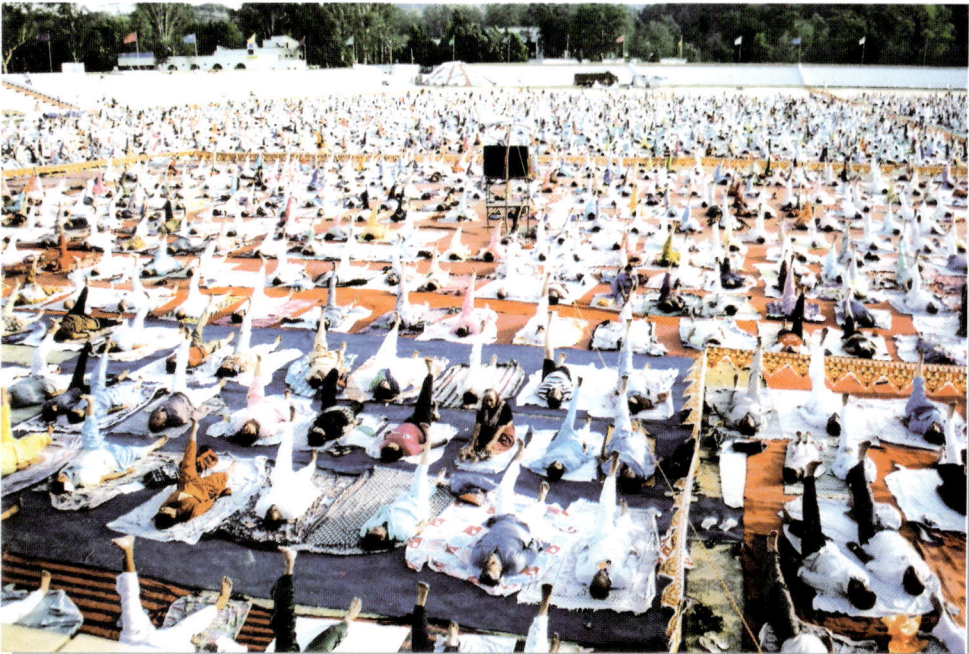

Millions of people practise Yog and Pranayam daily all over the world

High Profile People of World from all Walks of Life Find a Common Platform in Yog

Some of the top personalities of the world whether social workers or intellectuals, actors or actresses, industrialists or conglomerates, bureaucrats or political leaders, ruling party or opposition party, if they have come together at one common platform leaving behind their competition and differences then it is none other than the platform of Yog. Whenever Swamiji's Yog camps are organized the very important persons of the that particular city are always present at the venue. If they have not been able to attend the camp due to some unavoidable reasons then they have contacted Swamiji and learnt Yog in the privacy of their homes.

Swamiji's efforts have attracted the famous personalities of not only India but also the world. It is only because of his worldwide Yog movement that today various international organizations are inviting him for various projects. Many top personalities of the nation and abroad including First citizen of India, honourable President, Dr A.P.J. Abdul Kalam, Vice-President Bhairon Singh Shekhawat, Noble Prize Winner Harry Croto, Britain Health Minister, Patricia Hewitt have discussed Yog in detail with Swamiji. UNESCO has invited Swamiji to participate in poverty-eradication programs

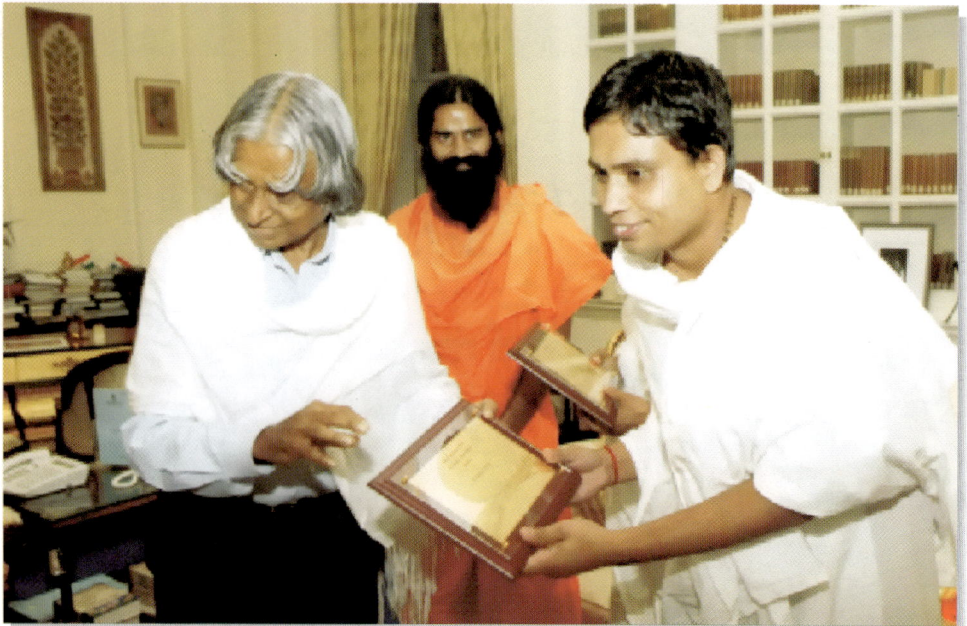

Acharya Balkrishnaji receiving a special momento from
President A.P.J. Abdul Kalam in presence of Swamiji

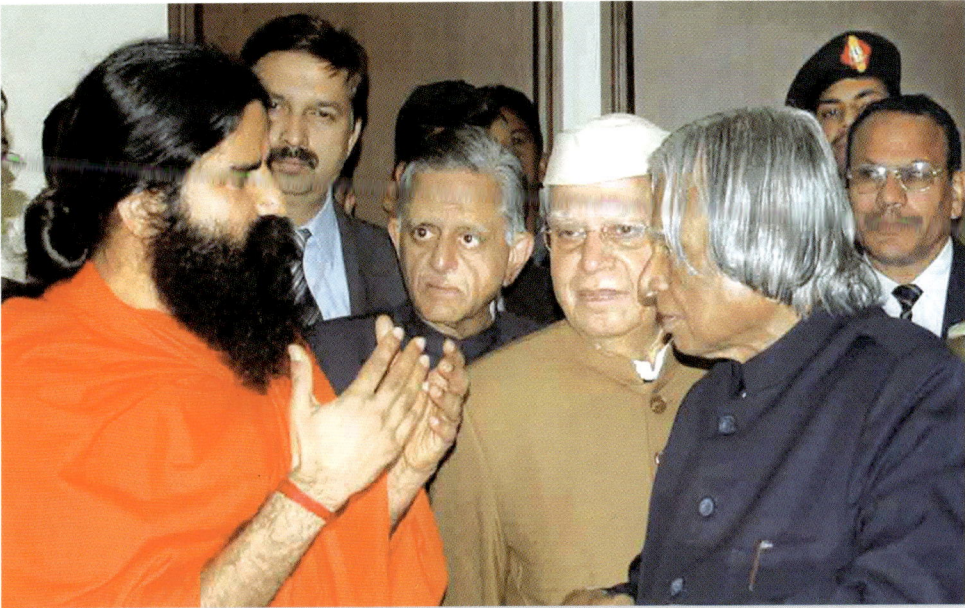

President A.P.J. Abdul Kalam disscussing Patanjali Yogpeeth's role in his Vision 2020 programme with Swami Ramdevji in presence of Governor Shri Sudarshan Agarwal and then Chief Minister Shri N.D. Tiwari of Uttarakhand

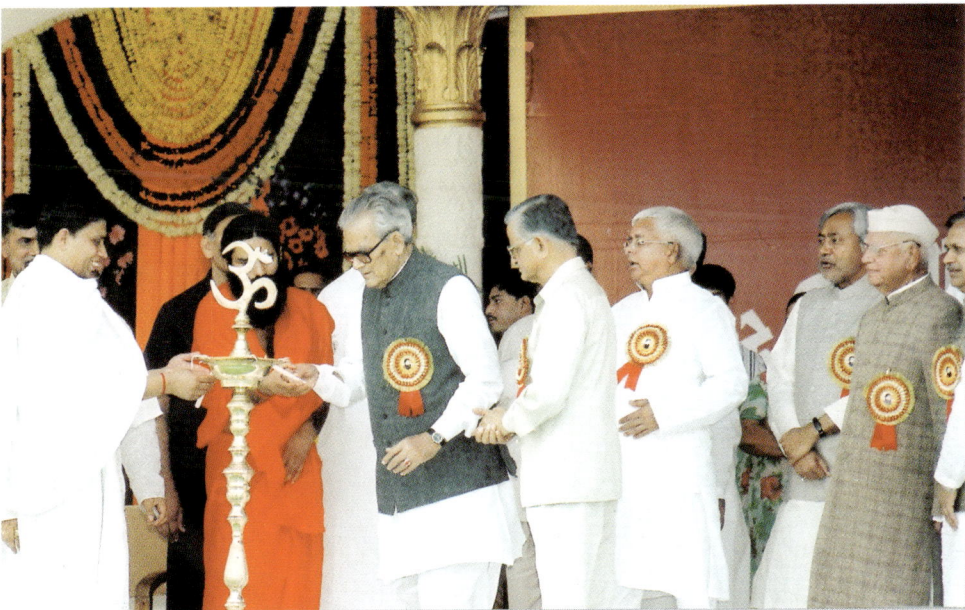

Vice-President Bhairon Singh Shekhawat inagurating the first stage of Patanjali Yogpeeth

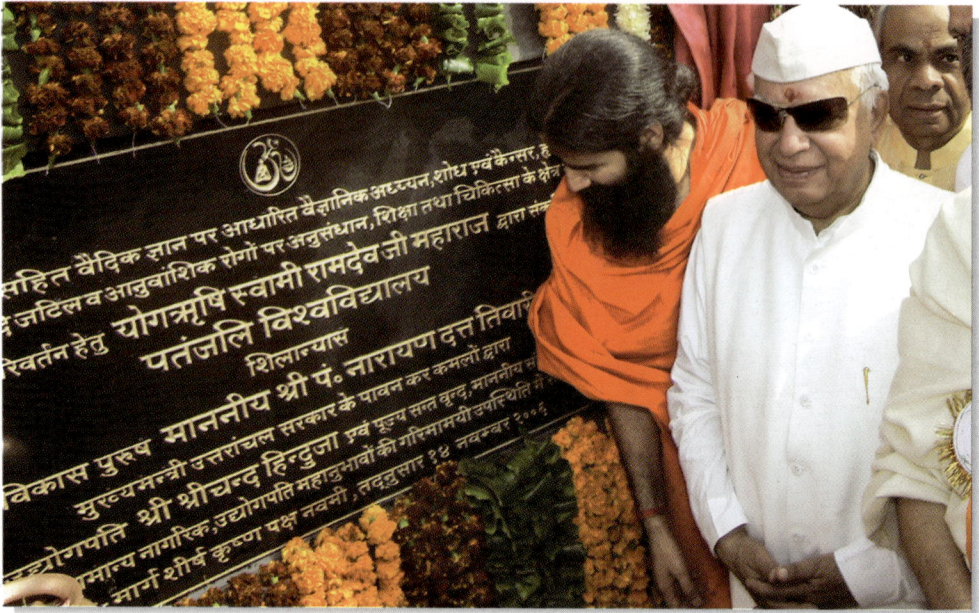

Shri N.D.Tiwari, Former Chief Minister of Uttarakhand, laying the
foundation stone for Patanjali University at Hardwar

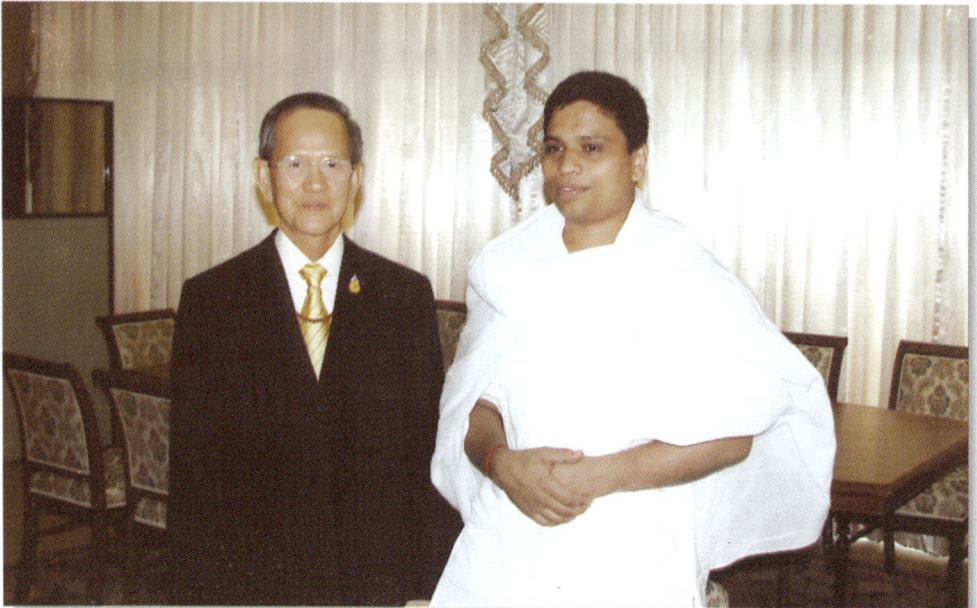

Acharya Balkrishna ji with Thailand's Defence Minister Boonat Somtat

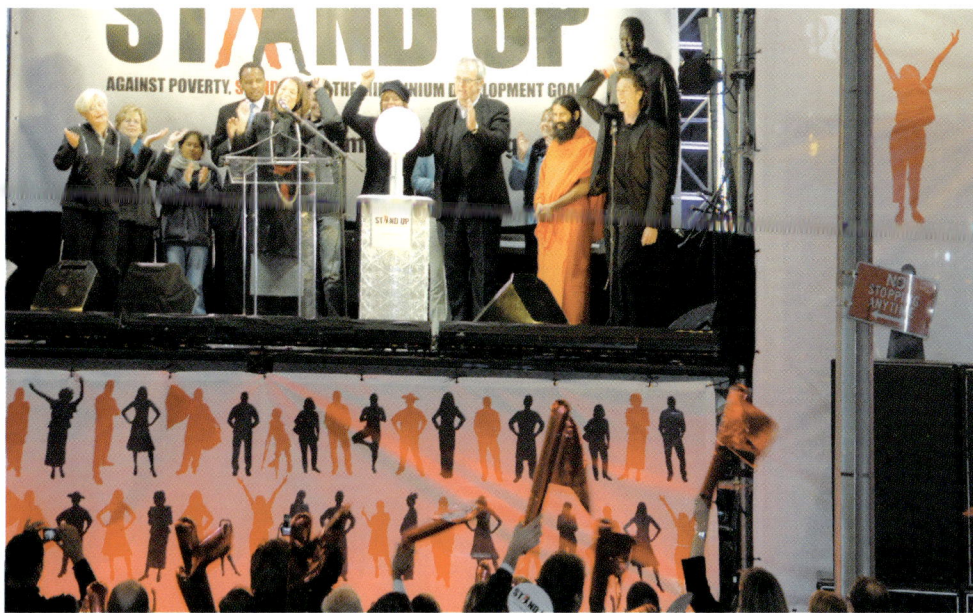

Swami Ramdevji representing India at 'Stand Up Appeal Against Poverty' organised by UN at Times Square, New York

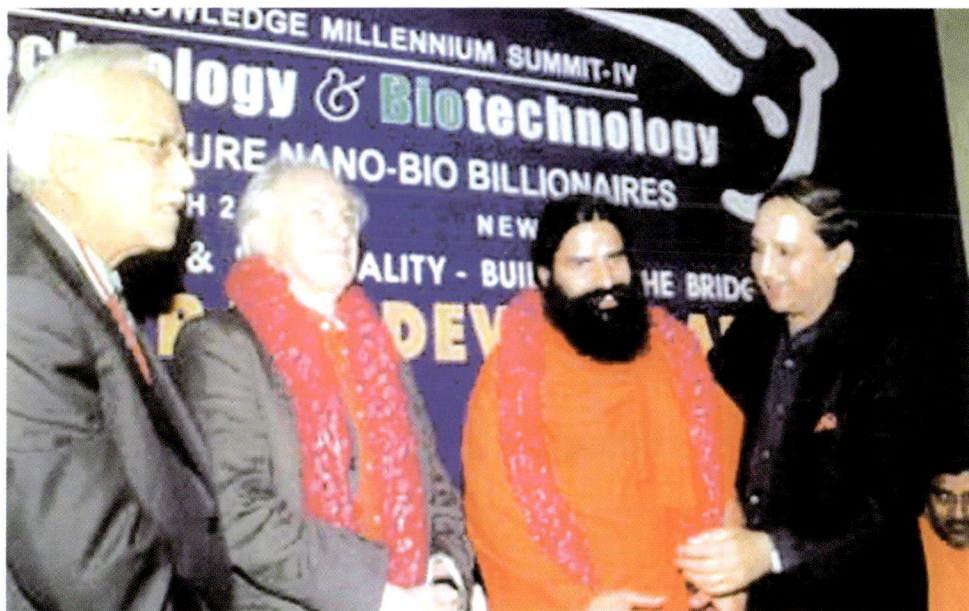

Swami Ramdevji with Nobel Prize Winner Prof. Hary Croto at a 'Live Scientific Dialogue' organized by ASSOCHEM

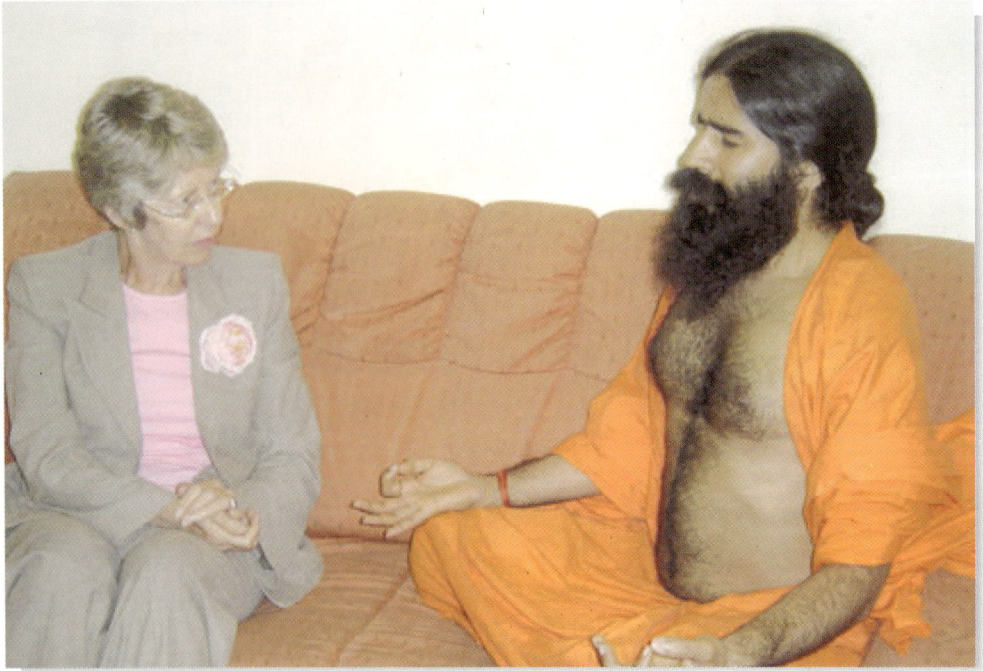

Swami Ramdevji enlightening Health Minister of UK, Ms Patricia Hewitt
about Pranayam

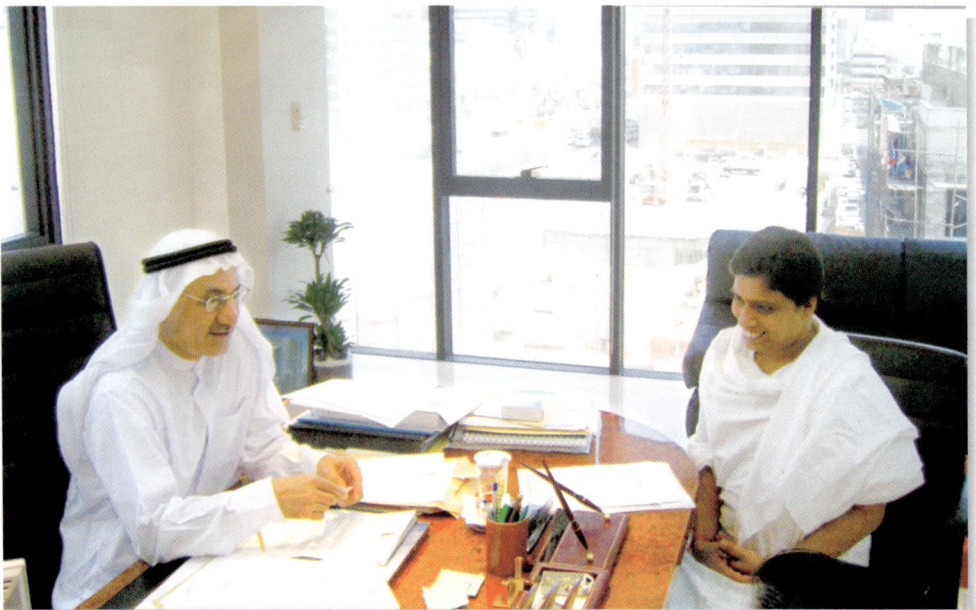

Acharya Balkrishnaji in dialogue with Dubai's Health Minister
Mohammad al Kutami about Yog

Children are the Future of the Nation

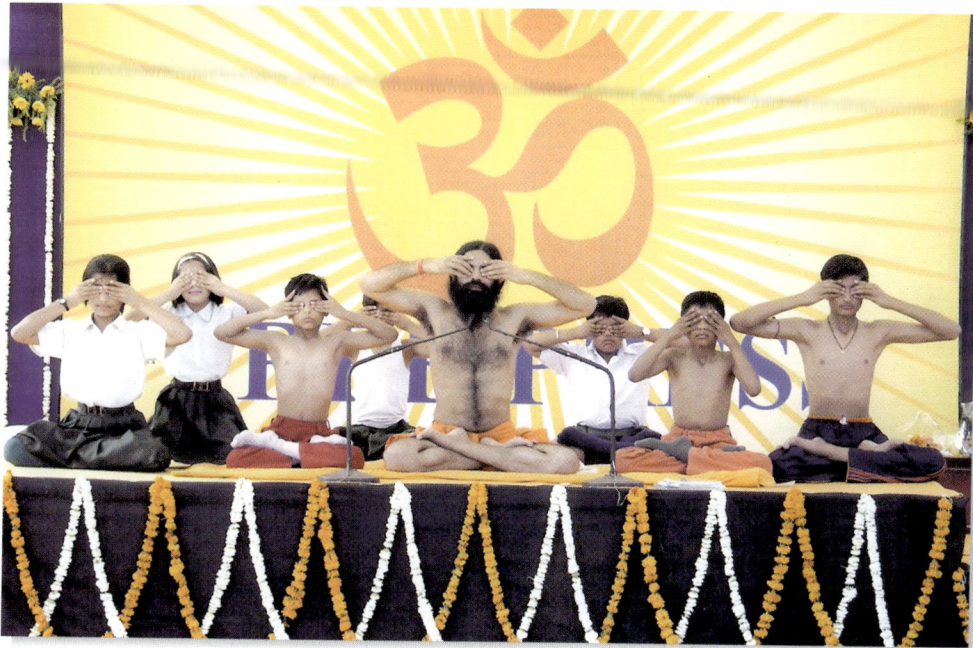

Children performing Yog with Swami Remdevji in a Yog Camp

Children are the future of the nation, they are the backbone of our nation, if we inculcate good values and virtues in them from a young age then we can certainly reach great heights. They should be taught about our rich culture, and we should teach them the harmful effects of addiction like alcohol, drugs, fast food, junk food, cold drinks and how the nation's wealth can be saved. If children are healthy, the nation will also be healthy. Swamiji organizes special camps for children with this objective in mind. The presence of children in these camps has been between 25 thousand to 1.25 lakh in 100 camps organized at different places, which has given direct benefit to more than 50-60 thousand lakh children. This develops the confidence that if children practise Yog along with their grandparents, then nobody can stop India from getting back its status of the World Mentor. Today several millions of children are learning Yog from Swamiji. We are presenting a few pictures here to show the overwhelming response received from children. Swamiji's efforts have inspired children towards patriotism, culture and balanced diet. They will definitely be able to control the temptation for junk food and cold drinks.

Yog is equally necessary for children

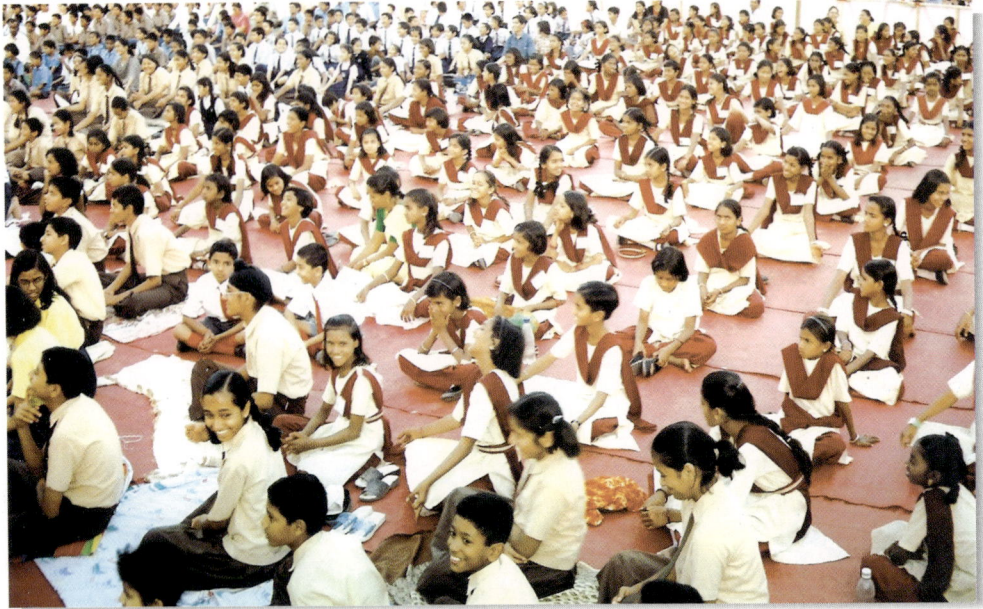

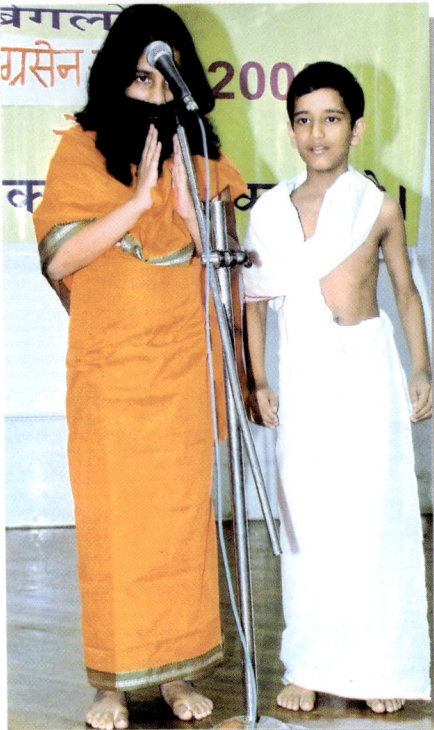

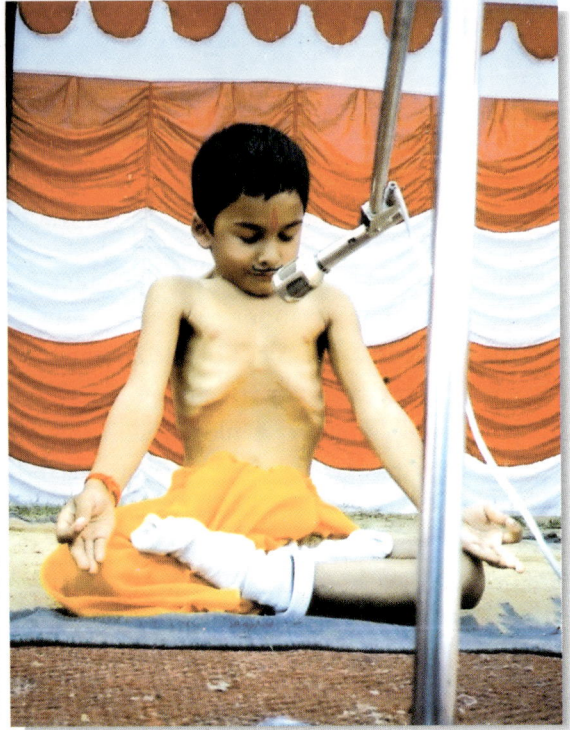

New generation takes on to the path of Yog and Pranayam

Yog for Defence Personnel

Soldiers guard the borders of our nation and work for more than 16 hours a day. They are supposed to be alert and vigilant all the time and have to brave tough weather conditions. Moreover, they do not see their families for several months together and yet they are committed to protect the motherland. They are indeed fortunate as they have the chance to serve the motherland. But it is also true that incidences of irresponsibility are increasing whether it is police, defense force or any other system associated with security of the nation. They are dividing themselves internally due to severe pressure and they are also making their families orphans. The personnel who are supposed to make the society free of terror and war, are in the whirlpool of fear, insecurity and depression today. The only resource to change the heart, attitude of these people is Yog. Swamiji has organized Yog camps in different institutions associated with police and defense. He has aroused the feelings of patriotism and tried to relieve defence personnel from mental tension and physical ailments. Today, thousands of army personnel are associated with this noble mission. Here are a few glimpses.

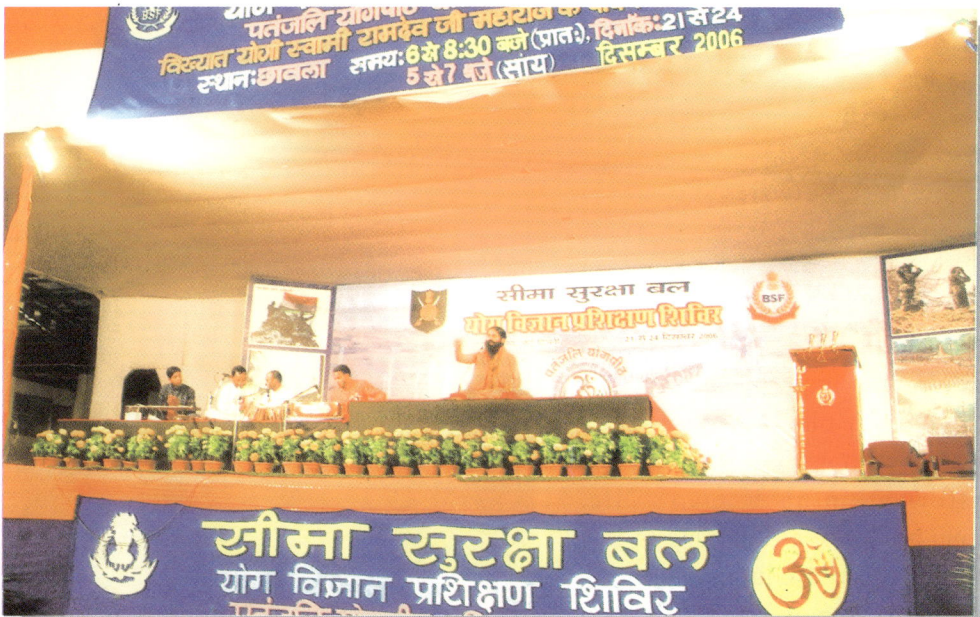

Swami Ramdevji teaching Yog to the Border Security Force personnel

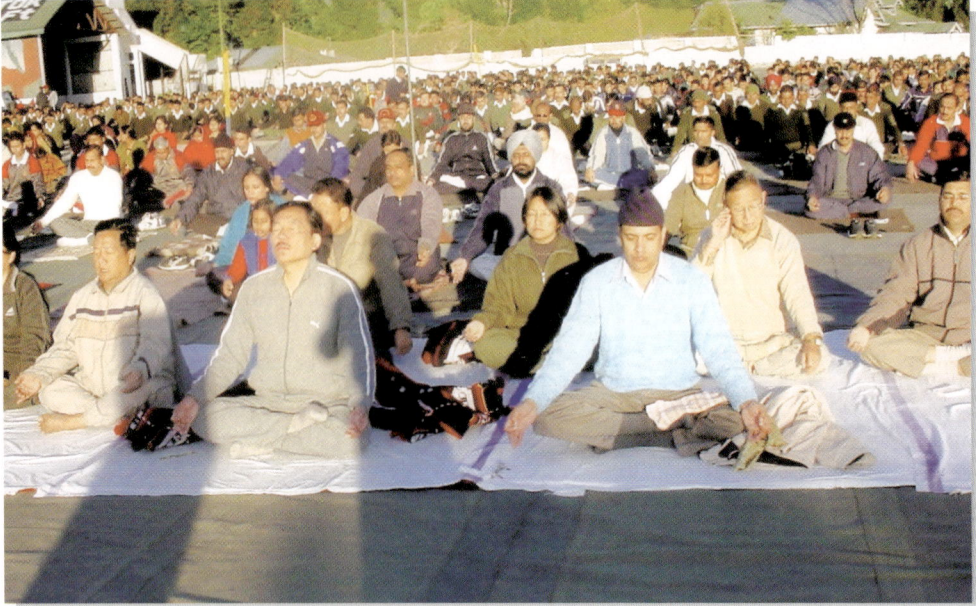

Prisoners performing Yog (above and below)

Yog in Prisons: Transforming the Criminal

If a person commits crime knowingly or unknowingly he or she is imprisoned, but if the person's inner consciousness motivates him to do some good work for the society, human being, nation then probably this would be the biggest gift for the mankind. The main objective of punishment is improvement. If this process takes place through self-realization then it will bring complete transformation in a man's life. Swamiji has made a beginning in this direction. When a criminal will look within in the light of Yog, it is sure to bring about positive change in their

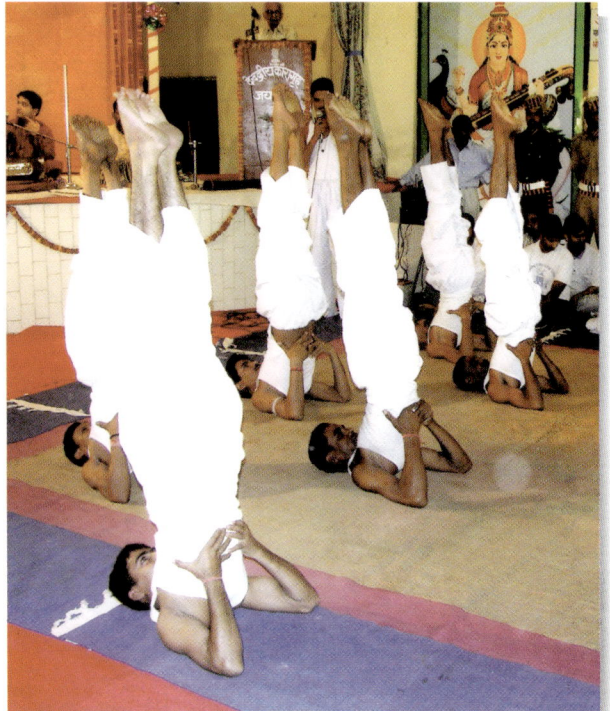

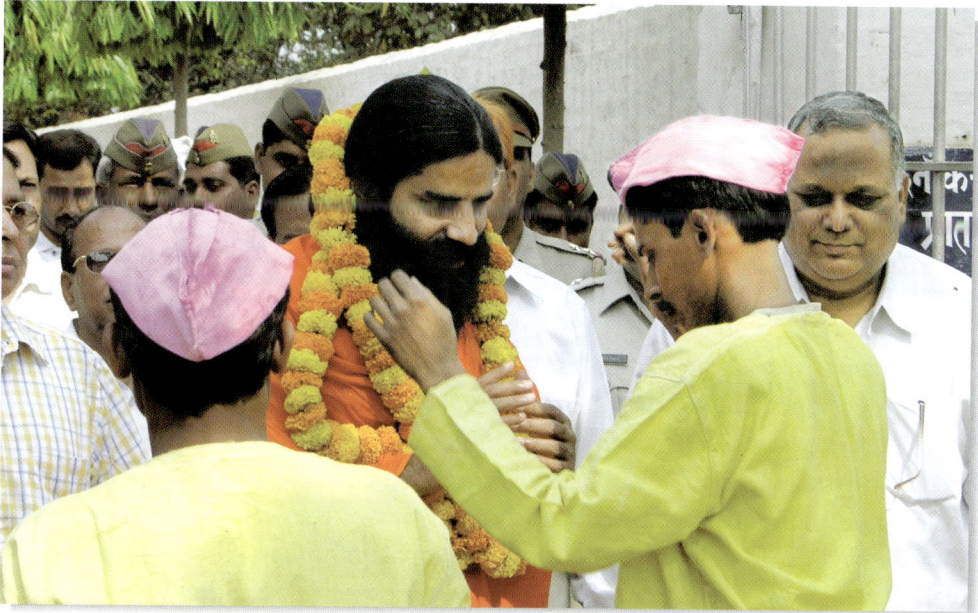

Prisoners welcome Swami Ramdevji at Tihar Central Jail in New Delhi

attitude towards life. Swamiji believes that it is necessary to look at negative aspects of a criminal humanely in order to establish peaceful society. When the society and individual will be free from criminal attitude then problems like terrorism, robbery, dacoity, murders, kidnapping will reduce. Swami Ramdevji Maharaj has organized Yog camps in different prisons including Tihar Central Jail, New Delhi. He has brought terrorists and criminals on the platform of Yog and aroused the feeling of patriotism in their hearts. The result being that today the prisoners are giving Yog training to their fellow inmates.

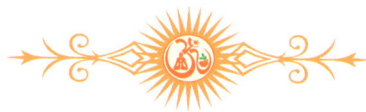

Chapter 5

A BOLD INITIATIVE IN SCIENTIFIC RESEARCH ON YOG

Yog is intrinsic part of Indian culture and spiritual knowledge which has been existing since time immemorial. Thousands of sages and seers have contributed to the field of Yog over ages. These sages and seers, apart from development of deep concentration/ meditation, developed a total health-building system comprising Pranayams, Mudras and Asanas to cure any disease, how so ever complexless, in body and mind. Regular practice of this health-building system keeps the diseases of body and mind away. It is very diffi-cult to imagine the kind of experiments carried out in the development of Pranayama (breathing) exercises to determine the process for respiration, its form, time, duration, and benefits derived from these practices and other intricacies. Similarly, while developing asanas, they must have deeply researched into each asana for several years because the principle : Asanani Chatavanti Yavantyo Jeevjataya (Dhyan Vindopanishad) holds good. They observed the shapes and movements of different creatures living in water, land and air, and developed the methods of asanas. It is interesting to note that the shape of not only the living beings but also all the visible things available in the nature were adopted in Yog, for example, plough (used in Halasana), mountain (used in Parvatasana), tree (used in Vrikshasana) etc.

When we look at the asanas from a scientific perspective, we wonder as to why did the sages adopt the shapes of birds, animals and other things of this world in their lives? For example, Mandookasana (frog), Bhujangasana (snake), Garudasan (eagle), Ushtrasana (camel) etc. were developed based on obsevations about animals. If we scientifically analyse the postures in each of the asanas, we will clearly see that they tone up body muscles, diaphragm, spine, abdomen, neck etc. For instance, Pavan Muktasana greatly helps in evacuation of polluted air/gas accumulated in the stomach, Sarvangasana tones up the thyroid glands and also gives energy/nourishment to the whole body. Similarly in case of Pranayam, Kapalbhati Pranayam was developed to purify the body through detoxification of respiratorty and digestive systems. This gives a kind of glow to the forehead (Kapal) or head. When we critically analyse the asanas and Pranayam in Yog, we realize and appreciate the fact that a very strong scientific basis was behind every component of Yog. Unfortu-nately, with the passage of time, only the methods were available while the scientific analysis of effect of Yog was forgotten and disappeared. It is this basis that requires an accomplished person to analyse these effects on scientific basis and present it to the world.

Scientifically speaking, we need the contribution of a scientist sage who is capable of testing and proving the concepts of Yog as per the modern medical parameters. One such person is Swami Ramdevji who has studied modern medical science in depth along with Yog and has proved the facts that Yog cures meet modern medical parameters. He very confidently and courageously invited international scientists to work together to evaluate and prove scientific basis of Yog. This is the first ever such attempt in the history of the world when somebody has given an open invitation to prove every step of Yog as per scientific standards and worked on it. Swamiji humbly sums this up in these words, "I have just tried to prefix the letter 'Pra' in Yog, which means scientific experiment." Yog, Pranayam, asana and other kriyas are age old. Swamiji first selected some of the simple and easy Pranayam and Yog asanas from the ocean of Yog, which can be practised by people of any age group and any health condition without difficulty. This was indeed a very complicated and taxing job. Selecting a few asanas from the deep ocean of Yog, which could be suitable for all people, preventing diseases, controlling recurrence of diseases, curing serious diseases permanently, arousing individual talents, generating positive, creative, qualitative and productive qualities, providing external beauty along with curing internal diseases and reach the ultimate destination of spiritual journey in order to realize the ultimate truth was indeed complicated. Swamiji, however, achieved all these.

Experimenting with Yog, which could make the people disease-free and take them to the highest peak of meditation was a very challenging task. Today, the whole world is familiar with the efforts made by revered Swamiji who put in his divine talents, devotion, austerity, practical utility knowledge of Yog, logical ability, scientific attitude with a pious feeling of welfare of mankind.

The results of Yog experiment have been declared and now the top scientists from medical world are analyzing these results. The results of Yog experiments prove that Yog is a complete health-building solution. Yog, Pranayam were available only in the old classics, some saintly people and yogi practised it and tested it to some extent, but it was limited to three to five minutes of daily practice. This practice was used in order to control the playful mind, but revered Swamiji tested and proved the life-saving benefits of Pranayam and complete health benefits. Swamiji presented it to millions of people through various Yog camps and through electronic media. The common man was unwilling to practise complex asana like Shirshasana, Paschimottasana or Chakrasana etc. Realizing this, Swamiji (unveiling the deep hidden secrets of Yog) devised alternative simple/easy asanas which could be performed by all people and demonstared their effectiveness to masses who also followed them with great results. He, thus, accomplished the first stage of his great mission 'Healthy India, Healthy World.' We, in the forthcoming sections are presenting the results of his scientific experiments on Yog supplimented with the relevant statistical data. These reults will certainly prove to be an eye opener for all those who are resistant, ignorant, suspicious and doubtful about effectiveness of Yog. We are confident that people by and large would definitely be able to accept Yog as the most scientific tool for achieving best health of the body and mind available on this globe. What we are presenting is our first attempt. This work of scientific research and documentation will continue till we complete the task of studying and proving the effects of Yog in the treatment of   all diseases through clinicaly controlled trials and genetic research as per the requirements of modern medical science. We are confident that one day Swamiji's dream, that nobody should die prematurely, will be realized. We would be definitely able to accomplish our mission with the genuine support of all the citizens of the world.

Pran – Nanotechnology in Medical Science

Nanotechnology is the synthesis and application of ideas from science and engineering for the conceptualization and production of novel materials and devices of extremely small sizes. The prefix nano means one billionth (10^{-9}) and nanotechnology deals with sizes of nanometer (nm), usually less than 100 nm. The smallest part in the human body is a blood cell which is approximately 2000 nm in length, although bacteria are around 200 nm. So from a physical point of view it may seem that this technology has nothing to do with human body and medical science. But the body is not merely physical, it has non-physical aspects like consciousness and mind that all depend on the vital force – Pran; life cannot exist without it. Pran is synonymous with breathing which requires oxygen and in that sense oxygen and Pran can be considered equivalent. Oxygen is a physical quantity and the dimensions of its molecule are in the range covered by nanotechnology. It is a component of air that plays an essential role in all chemical and metabolic processes in the body. Thus, oxygen can be used as a nano element in regulating the processes going on in the body.

This is exactly what Swami Ramdevji has done and actively used Pran at nano level through exercise like Prannyam. The nanotechnology approach is far more effective and it has been even used for making artificial bones that are as strong as steel and much lighter. This is done by manipulating molecules on surfaces. It has been found that if through different Pranayams oxygen intake into the body is manipulated, serious diseases such as heart ailments, angina, rheumatism, and many others can be successfully treated. This process has also helped in maintaining excellent overall health.

The entire universe has been created by a combination of the basic elements-earth, fire, air, water and space; but there is one another element that is present in all these five (and hence everywhere) and that is oxygen. Earth contains oxygen, nitrogen, carbon and hydrogen; fire – oxygen and carbon; air – oxygen, nitrogen, and carbon dioxide; water – oxygen and hydrogen. Space is the container for the mobility of all air elements along with oxygen. Oxygen has an important role in creation and structure of every cell and every part of the human body. The five basic constituents of the body (panchadhatu) are blood, flesh, bone, marrow, and semen; they all contain oxygen which is also the main element in hormones and various chemicals in the body. In fact, it is the element that sustains life in all living organisms in the universe.

Science led to the Green Revolution by discovering the role of nitrogen. Hydrogen, carbon and other elements are being used to make various devices including bombs. In medical science, oxygen has been used for emergency treatment. It is not far fetched to believe that soon we will be using Pran element for treating all diseases. Semen and egg (from ovaries) are the main entities for the initiation of the body formation; oxygen is the main element that gives mobility to sperms and nourishes the egg. In Upanishads, the physical body is called annamaya kosh or the food sheath. Anna (grain) stands for food and again oxygen is present in it along with other constituents. The main things in bread, vegetables, fruits, milk etc. that provide nourishment to the body are carbohydrates, proteins, fats, minerals and vitamins. Although in the universe as well as the human body, there are other elements like carbon, nitrogen, and hydrogen, in the body made of five elements mentioned above (panchdhatu) the vital force and consciousness comes only due to oxygen. The smallest unit in the body is a cell; its nucleus is its brain and mitochondria are where energy is generated. In both of these the motion and its propelling force come from oxygen. The life yagya that is going on in the body and is called metabolism, is fueled only by oxygen. The generation of energy in every cell of the body occurs because of oxygen and glucose. If in the mitochondria of the cell the process of energy generation is not concluded successfully, the body does not function properly internally as well as externally. Oxygen is the main contributor in the creation and decay of the cells and for the storage of energy in them.

Oxygen plays the main role in preventing the destructive processes in the body and enhancing constructive and acquisitional processes. Today, the serious conflicts occurring in the body because of lack of exercise, stress, improper diet, irregular routine and unrestrained life give rise to imbalance of the three humours (vata - wind, pitta - bile, and cough) which is called metabolic syndrome in medical terms and occurs because of improper functioning of anabolism. Vata is anabolism, pitta is metabolism, and cough -the result of these two is catabolism. This imbalance causes depression which leads to high blood pressure, diabetes, obesity, heart ailments, indigestion, insomnia, and even cancer.

The inequity of the humours, improper functioning of the digestive process, imbalance of the basic body elements (panchdhatu), accumulation of excrement, and unhappiness of the mind and soul have become the cause of our unhealthiness. This has caused the imbalance of hormones and chemicals that makes us dependent on various medicines.

Each and every cell of our body is our prototype and has the capability of producing our own double. Experiments with Pranayam on millions of people done so far lead to the conclusion that it is possible to be disease-free by providing an optimum amount of oxygen to the body parts ranging from the cells to organs through these exercises accompanied by positive thinking. Pranayam is nothing but oxygenating blood, internal exercise, and positive life-style. We provide optimum oxygen to the blood cells through bhastrika and anulom-vilom Pranayams; kapalbhati is a scientific way of giving mobility and energy flow to the internal parts of the body; with bhramari and udgeeth we begin to have a healthy and worry-free life by awakening feelings of reverential faith, surrender, trust, and an urge for positive thinking.

In this presumption, oxygen is the basis for all the processes. Curiously, at birth itself we took a deep breath in the guise of crying that initiated all the internal functions with the awakening of our mind; in effect nature made us do Pranayam even at the time of birth by making us cry. The oxygen inhaled through Pranayam and all internal exercises scientifically accomplished by it act as self-healer for the body. Pranayam is self-medicine and self-treatment that do away with the need for surgical intervention for joints and spine problems, and even for heart diseases. We then realize that Pranayam is a unique science. It keeps the level of anabolism high and that of catabolism low in the body; this retards the aging process preventing untimely old age and giving a prolonged life. On the basis of scientific results of Pranayam experiments we can say that when Pran, i.e. oxygen element is fed into the body by certain methods at a definite time in a definite amount with proper thinking, positive changes occur automatically and Pran starts acting like a complete medicine. This is the essence of Yog science and of perfect health; this is the basis of a healthy, prosperous, and sensitive life of an individual and even of a nation.

We find basically the same evidence of pranic science in the Vedas also. For example:

Āavāatahibhāaṇja vivāatayāahi yad rōopaḥ ।

Twahi vivuabhāaṇyo dēvanāam dōota iyasē ॥   Rigved

Pran, i.e. oxygen is a medicine. It enters and flows in the body in various ways. It is not just a medicine but complete and universal medicine. This Pran is the carrier of all grandeurs of the universe. It is a holistic treatment and the basis for perfect health. The emotional changes that come as a result of Yog practice, i.e. from regulating Pran by different methods are as authentic and scientific as the bodily changes; our scriptures have authentic and scientific evidence of this. In Chhandogya Upanishad we find:

Prāaṇa pitāa prāaṇaḥ māatāa prāaṇaḥ bhrāatāa ।
Prāaṇa ṣwasāa Prāaṇaḥ āachāaryaḥ prāaṇa brāahmaṇa ॥

To a person afflicted by terrible mental diseases like depression and schizophrenia the sages of Yog tradition say:

Do not panic, do not lose courage, and do not be nervous. Do not live in isolation and insecurity. There is no need to get disheartened. Take refuge in Pran and do Pranayam. This

Pran is father, it is mother, and it is brother and mother-in-law. It is also preceptor and brahman. Here Pran is described in a flowery language using similes. The sages point out to the emotional effects of Pran by using different similes. One who protects is father; one who serves with affection, love, compassion, austerity, sacrifice, patience, and courage is mother; one who provides sustenance is brother; one who refines conduct, speech, disposition, and thinking is preceptor; and one who guides to Brahm is brahman. Pran enters our heart as mother and makes the physical heart healthy. We have proved this even with scientific evidence; what is more, Pranayam creates in our heart maternal love, affection, compassion, and sensitivity. With the practice of Pranayam we develop feelings of patience, courage, sacrifice, and surrender; despondent with the miseries of life a person forgets his despondency and begins to enjoy a happy life again. Pran becomes the brother providing physical and emotional sustenance and becoming the preceptor it refines our conduct and life itself.

Pran affects our thoughts directly. When thoughts become pure with Pranayam our diets and disposition also become pure. Therefore, a person practising Pranayam forsakes violence, crime, dishonesty, and other evil conducts; he proceeds on the path of self-restraint and morality, and becomes a sensitive individual. This is the most desirable need in today's conditions. Pranayam is the remedy for ever-increasing dishonesty, distrust, immorality, violence, crime and corruption. Making life pure it takes us to God and makes us realize truth and bliss; removing all maladies it leads us to detachment, stable mental equilibrium and thereby to self-realization and nirvana.

Prāaṇaṣyēda vāi sarva yaṭ ṭridivi pratiṣṭhitaṃ ।

Māateva puṭrāan rakṣaṣwa śrēeścha pragjyāaṃ cha vidhēhi naḥ iti ॥ Upaniṣada i.e. The entire universe is under Pran. O Pran, protect us sons like mother; lead us to prosperity and consciousness.

Pranayam is the bedrock of material growth and spiritual progress. The twenty-first century is one of confluence of science and spirituality, and the great mantra of this century is Pranayam. There are extensive proofs of the power of Pran in the scriptures:

Prāaṇāaḥ vāava vasavaḥ ।
Prāaṇāaḥ vāava rudrāaḥ ।
Prāaṇāaḥ vāava āadiṭyāaḥ ।

i.e. Pran is Vasu meaning it is the basis for building life, it is Rudra for getting rid of diseases, and is Aditya for preventing life from disintegration.

In this book, we have also given scientific documentation of the emotional effects of Pranayam. On the basis of the traditional Vedic knowledge of Pranayam and scientific investigations based on that knowledge now we can say that in today's world, when nanotechnology is making its way into every field of science, Pran is the nanotechnological element of medical science.

Swami Ramdevji is truly a sage and great thinker with austerity, knowledge, and endeavour as marvelous as those of ancient sages. His thinking and viewpoints are so clear and at the same time so extensive that he knows what the society wants today, what it thinks, what it should get, and what it is actually getting. He also knows how to give what it deserves. In all of this he has kept in view today's environment and conditions. He started his work with the welfare of the society and humanity as the main objective. In order to enlighten the general public about Yog, for the past few years he has started organizing large-scale Yog training or Yog science camps all over the country and abroad because he knows very well that in order to take Yog to the common man it is necessary to go beyond the confines of currently existing centres. At the same time using the satellite TV channels he is telling people all over the world to make Yog an essential part of their life-style. Thus, he is helping the world experience the bliss of healthy life and is doing that by boldly proclaiming Yog's scientific basis. In his camps, there is an entire team of doctors and scientists who examine the effects of Yog using international standards.

For the participants of the camp an extensive report is prepared to see the effects of Yog practice on them. The team assembled for investigating these effects in accordance with the standards of modern medical science includes prominent doctors. Apart from these doctors, pathology technicians from various hospitals are also included in the team. This high-level team examined the effect of Yog at every level. The reports give detailed analysis of the effects.

These test reports will be available in this book in appropriate places as per context and one can easily infer from them the excellent and effective power of Yog. In course of these tests many incurable diseases like obesity, blood pressure, heart ailments, cancer, kidney problems, arthritis, spondylitis, cirrhosis, and various stomach related diseases have also been examined. Many other required tests are performed to see to what extent Yog contributes to the treatment. The tests are done once before starting Yog exercises to determine the existing state of the person. Then after practising Yog for a predetermined period the tests are done again to see the effect of Yog and to determine to what extent the exercises have helped the person.

Yog and Parameters of Modern Science

Since the ancient times, Yog has been the successful path for devotion, worship, good health and life-style. It is on the basis of Yog sadhna that our sages and seers enjoyed longevity and have propagated the art of disease-free life-style. Life became complex over centuries and new dangerous and serious diseases began to spread. The modern medical science has been trying to diagnose these new diseases but has not been able to find the cure so far. Today cancer, AIDS, diabetes, hepatitis, high blood pressure, heart disease, respiratory trouble etc. are increasing at a fast rate. Crores of rupees are being spent on research but complete cure is still a dream to come true. As far as treatment for improving the health is concerned modern medical science has failed till date. What we need presently is a complete medical system, which can protect our health, so that the person does not fall ill at all. If the person falls ill due to some reason then he should be cured with minimum physical and monetary loss. It is certain that Yog medical science and other medical systems can be combined to develop such a system. In order to achieve this the medical professionals should leave behind all types of inhibitions and come forward for the sake of human welfare. Yog is not only a method of physical exercise but it is a complete medical science. Today, everybody understands the medical affects of Yog as per the directions and appeal of revered Swami Ramdevji Maharaj. Explaining any subject or knowledge in scientific manner has become the need of the hour. It is very necessary to analyze the impact of disease on the body and different organs in scientific manner. Yog is the gift of ancient sages and seers, which can fulfill the concept of complete health independently and with the combination of other medical sciences. Pranayam is the most important, easy and simple process of Ashtang Yog as propounded by Saint Patanjali.

Today, revered Swami Ramdevji has a prominent place in the area of Yog training. Thousands of people of all ages, gender and communities attend his camps and are reaping the benefits of Yog. Today majority of the people are suffering from physical and mental diseases. People are getting benefits from asana and Pranayam and they are becoming devotees of Swamiji. The doctors are not able to believe that Yog can cure the diseases and give miraculous results.

(i)   Yog camps organized for the first time to face the challenge

Six challenging scientific Yog camps were organized between 1 August and 26 October 2005 under the guidance of Swami Ramdevji in order to fulfill the mission of 'Healthy India, Healthy World'. People suffering from different diseases took part in these camps. The participants were mainly patients of obesity, diabetes, high blood pressure, cancer, heart disease, renal disorders, arthritis, spondylitis and other diseases. The first camp was organized during 1-6 August 2005 for the patients of obesity. The second camp was organized during 11-18 August 2005 for the patients of diabetes. The third camp was organized 21-28 August 2005 for the patients of hypertension. Patients of heart disease, kidney dysfunction, arthritis and spondylitis attended the camp organized during 31 August 4 September 2005. Another camp was organized for the patients of obesity during 10-17 September 2005. The final camp was organized during 18-26 October 2005 in which patients of heart disease, kidney dysfunction, arthritis and spondylitis took part. The Yog residential camps were organized in the premises of Patanjali Yogpeeth (Trust), Hardwar. The main highlights of the camps were that many people from India and abroad participated in these camps.

(ii) Parameters used in Yog camps and Introduction of Medical Practitioners

As mentioned earlier, Swami Ramdev has stressed on proving his efforts on scientific basis. Everything is as per the standards of modern science so that people are free of myths. Benefits of Yog were tested with latest scientific methods and the results were made open to the people so that Yog's actual benefits could be recognized. Therefore, latest and up-to-date machines were used for the purpose. Here some special parameters which were used during the Yog camps are mentioned.

- Haemoglobin
- MCV
- TLC
- Hepatitis B
- Hepatitis C
- Platelets
- MCH
- DLC
- Hemotocrit
- HIV
- Alpha feto protein – indicator for liver cancer
- Prostrate specific antigen – prostrate gland –indicator for liver cancer
- Ovarian and uterus cancer indicator – C A 125 ovarian and uterus cancer indicator

Biochemistry Test

- Blood sugar
- LDL – bad cholesterol
- Serum creatinine
- VLDL– bad cholesterol
- HDL – good cholesterol
- Tryglycerides – bad fat

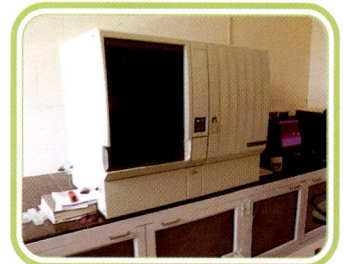

Triturates

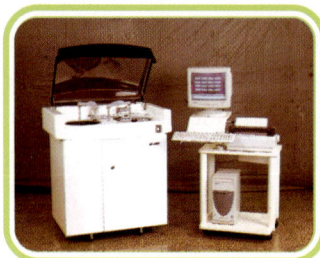

XL Axle 300

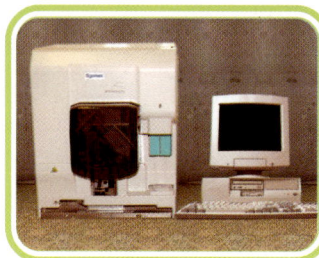

XT 2000I

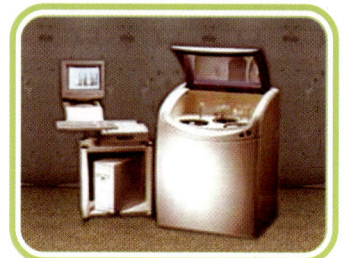

XL – Axle 600

Machines and Tools used for various tests

Medical Team for Tests

An introduction of the medical practitioners who contributed their valuable time for medical tests of people in the Yog camps

Dr H.P.Kumar

Director, Medical Health

Sahara India Medical Institute Limited

Former D G M H, Uttar Pradesh Government

Dr R.P Singh

C.M.O, Hardwar

Dr R.K.Gupta

MD, Pathology, HOD, Pathology Department

SGPGI, Lucknow

Dr S. N.Khan

Pathology,

Hardwar

Dr R.K.Mishra

DM, Cardiologist,

Uttar Pradesh Health Service

Dr P.Lal,

Senior Physician

Dr Niraj Arya

MD, Pathology

Patanjali Yogpeeth Hardwar

Dr Ajay Mohan

Senior Physician

Dr Rakesh Mohan

Senior Physician

In addition, many other doctors and pathology professionals from various hospitals have taken part in these camps and contributed in this noble mission.

(iii) Details of participants

All the registered members attending the camps were given the facility of accommodation and food. Besides the patients were advised to discontinue the medicines, which they were taking although the patients who were having very severe disorders were asked to continue the medicines. The main purpose of discontinuing the medicines was to see the impact of Yog on different diseases. All the patients had to undergo medical check up before and after beginning Yog. Former Director of Sanjay Gandhi Post Graduate Institute, Lucknow, and senior doctors of Uttar Pradesh and Uttarakhand Government conducted the medical check ups. Latest and up-to-date machines manufactured by Trans Asia Biomedical and other prestigious companies were used for the purpose. The details of patients who reaped the benefits of Yog are given below.

1-6 August 2005	
Males	989
Females	879
Total	**1,868**

11-18 August 2005	
Males	721
Females	386
Total	**1,107**

21-28 August 2005	
Males	1,098
Females	498
Total	**1,596**

31 August-9 September 2005	
Males	664
Females	640
Total	**1,304**

10-17 September 2005	
Males	930
Females	694
Total	**1,624**

9-26 October 2005	
Males	904
Females	720
Total	**1,624**

Effect of Yog on Different Diseases

The effect of Yog on different diseases as per the scientific tests during the camps has been compiled underneath.

(i) Effect of Pranayam on Respiratory System and Related Diseases

Swami Ramdevji Maharaj organized six residential camps of seven-day duration each in order to prove Yog on scientific basis. More than 10,000 patients had undergone various medical tests. The results had surprised the scientific/medical specialists and also gave a new momentum to Yog revolution. The whole respiratory system is involved in the process of Pranayam. Nose, mouth, pharynx, trachea, bronchi, lungs and thorax are mainly involved in this process. All these parts get purified and activated, and supply sufficient amount of oxygen. In the same way at the end of normal inhalation process around one-and-a-half litre of air can be taken in. The amount of air breathed in and breathed out can be increased from half to three-and-a-half litres to four-and-a-half liters depending upon the depth of breathing. This depth can be obtained by doing Pranayam breathing. Since the air we breath contains about 21 per cent oxygen, the amount of Pran vayu (oxygen) supplied to the respiratory system significantly increases in the Pranayam breathing. The air that we breathe in while inhaling contains around 79 per cent of nitrogen, 20-21 per cent oxygen, 0.04 per cent carbon dioxide and other vaporous gases. The amount of air exhaled through the process of oxygenation includes 79 per cent nitrogen, around 16 per cent oxygen, four per cent carbon dioxide and other gases. As the amount of nitrogen is same while we breath in and breath out, conversion to four per cent carbon dioxide (in exhalation) and reduction in oxygen level by equal amount is a significant change. This is known as oxygenation.

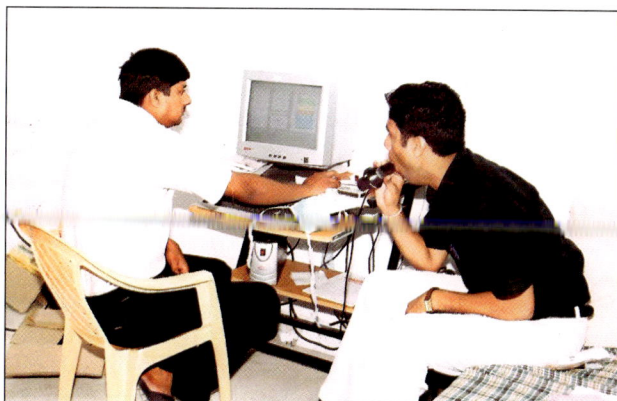

With the process of Pranayam we can increase the normal volume of ventilation by 10 times without any physical labour or muscular exercise. When we increase physical labour the body demands more oxygen, whereas in the process of Pranayam the amount of oxygen increases, which purifies blood and every cell gets required amount of oxygen. The cells get nutrition with the help of energy created by the process of ATP (Adenosine Tri-Phosphate). In this way, Pranayam controls the degeneration of cells caused by necrosis. We can therefore call Pranayam as the best antioxidant.

With regular practice of Pranayam like Kapalbhati, Anulom-vilom, Bhastrika, Nasabhitti etc., the waste materials can be removed from the body and respiratory diseases like tuberculosis, cough, asthma etc. can be cured. The effects of Yog and Pranayam on various parts of respiratory system were studied as per the directions of revered Swami Ramdevji Maharaj. As per the modern medical standards the participants of residential camps were tested for pulmonary function (PFT) before and after the camps with the help of latest spirometry machines in order to prove the authenticity of Pranayam. The participants were made to practise Yog and Pranayam for two hours in the morning and evening where in they were made to practise Bhastrika, Kapalbhati, Bahya Pranayam, Anulom-vilom, Brahmari, Udgeet, Ujjayi and other asanas. This study showed immediate positive improvement in forced vital capacity (FVC), maximum voluntary ventilation (MVC) and peak expiratory flow rate (PEFR).

Results of Pulmonary Function Test (PFT)

First residential camp

- Number of patients tested for PFT before the camp – **345**
- Number of patients with irregular PFT rate before the camp – **95**

◆ Number of patients tested for PFT after the camp – **125**

	No. of people with irregular PFT	No. of people with irregular PFT after the camp	Patients benefited	Significant improvement
PFT	95	40	55	57.8

Second residential camp

◆ Number of patients tested for PFT before the camp – **1144**

◆ Number of patients with irregular PFT rate before the camp – **132**

	No. of people with irregular PFT before the camp	No. of people with irregular PFT after the camp	Patients benefited	Significant improvement
PFT	132	51	81	61.36

◆ Number of patients tested for PFT after the camp – **149**

Third residential camp

The third residential camp organized under the guidance of revered Swami Ramdevji Maharaj from 31 July to 7 August 2005 had the participation of around 730 people who were tested for spirometry test (PFT). Out of these, around 230 people were detected with irregular PFT. After the camp the patients with irregular PFT were tested again. The study done on the basis of international standards showed significant improvement in 150 patients, whereas 80 patients did not show much improvement although they also got some benefits but were not included in this category.

◆ Number of patients tested for PFT before the camp – 730

◆ Number of patients with irregular PFT rate before the camp – 275

	No. of people with irregular PFT before the camp	No. of people with irregular PFT after the camp	Patients benefited	Significant improvement
PFT	230	80	150	65.22

◆ Number of patients tested for PFT after the camp – 230

◆ 65.22 per cent patients with irregular PFT before the camp showed significant improvement after the camp.

Fourth residential camp

◆ Number of patients tested for PFT before the camp – 728

	No. of people with irregular PFT before the camp	No. of people with irregular PFT after the camp	Patients benefited	Significant improvement
PFT	235	93	142	60.43

◆ Number of patients with irregular PFT rate before the camp – 269

◆ Number of patients tested for PFT after the camp–235

Fifth residential camp

- Number of patients tested for PFT before the camp – 630
- Number of patients with irregular PFT rate before the camp – 245

	No. of people with irregular PFT before the camp	No. of people with irregular PFT before the camp	Patients benefited	Significant improvement
PFT	207	86	121	58.45

- Number of patients tested for PFT after the camp – 207

Sixth residential camp

- Number of patients tested for PFT before the camp – 112
- Number of patients with irregular PFT rate before the camp – 75

	No. of people with irregular PFT before the camp	No. of people with irregular PFT after the camp	Patients benefited	Significant improvement
PFT	71	27	44	61.97

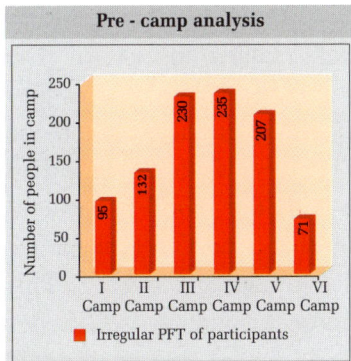

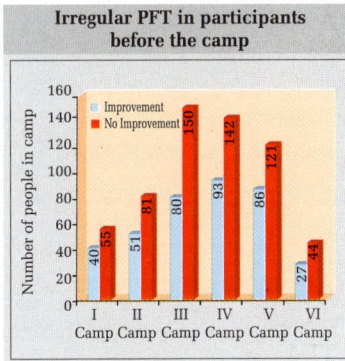

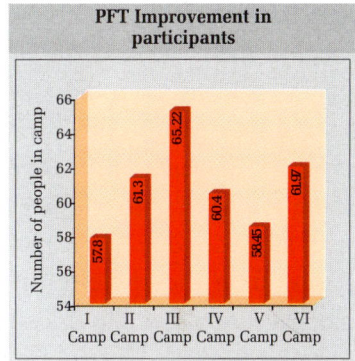

- Number of patients tested for PFT after the camp – 71

(i) Effects of Pranayam on Blood Circulation System (Cardio-pulmonary System)

Heart is the most important part of our body. Around 500 ml blood is thrown out every time the heart beats. This means that over period of one day (more than 1 lakh beats), the amount of blood sent to various organs of the body will be of the order of five lakh cubic inch. This oxygenated blood supplies blood to various parts of the body. This strength of the heart is equal to lifting one tonne weight up to a height of 41 feet. In this way, the heart functions round the clock. The heart works harder than a normal machine and hence needs maximum amount of *Pran vayu* or oxygen. The heart gets one-fourth amount of blood that is circulated in the whole body in every heart beat or minute.

The heart nerves begin from the cardiac plexus, which is made from both the branches of sympathetic and Vegas nerves. The sympathetic nerves spread and reach the stellate ganglia, which simulate the heart or sino atrial node or atrio ventricular node. The Vegas nerves that end in the ganglion cells and spread there are important for the heart. These nerves spread in the HIS bundle and arteries, heart and muscle walls. Pranayam regulates the sympathetic and Vegas nerves and other processes. It helps in the smooth functioning of heart.

Heart diseases are caused due to improper functioning of heart. Excessive excitement of involuntary nervous system due to various reasons causes palpitation/trachycardia; less excitement/bradycardia, heart contraction due to various reasons causes heart weakness, low pulse rate when blood does not properly reach the artery. The ECG helps in diagnosing this disease. Such heart beats are called Ectopic beats.

In the same manner, low functioning of heart is caused by blockage in heart arteries, coronary artery disease. Heart attack/heart disorder usually results in chest pain, high blood pressure, stiffness of arteries and other diseases. The number of heart patients are increasing every year due to blockage in arteries, coronary thrombosis etc. According to modern medical point of view the cause of this problem is high level of cholesterol. The fluid generated from digestion of food and reaches the blood and from there it goes into liver and converts into dicacids like, glycocolic, taurocholic etc. These acids reach the stomach and help in the digestion of fat present in the food. They get absorbed and then reach the liver with the help of intrahepatic circulation. However, the blood cholesterol level increases due to irregular life-style and eating habits. When this condition remains for a long time the cholesterol gets accumulated in the arteries and causes blockage. This blockage increases the risk of heart attack. This disease can also occur due to insufficieney of enzymes and deficiency of vitamin C.

Regular practice of Pranayam and taking bottle gourd juice helps in controlling heart disease. Pranayam is helpful in supplying oxygen. The oxygenated blood supplies oxygen to various parts of the body which secret adrenaline hormone, glucose, fat, fatty acids and thereby builds energy. This is very beneficial in diseases like coronary heart disease, blockage in heart arteries, thrombosis etc. Heart is the centre of blood circulatory system, which weighs around 342 gm and is made up of empty muscles. It beats more than one lakh times in a day and pumps blood into the arteries that is equal to running a distance of 60,000 miles. If any problem or disorder occurs in the heart then different diseases arise in the body and is known as heart disease.

The heart disease is of the following types

+ Herediatary/congenital

+ Functional (Coronary heart disease and Pulmonary heart disease)

The functional disorder can be cured soon, whereas the genetic disorder is cured slowly or generally cannot be cured.

When there is some blockage in coronary artery or any of its branch or when fat accumulates then the muscles do not get nutrition and this reduces functioning of heart, leading to heart disease, palpitation, chest pressure, pain and disorder of heart arteries. Nowadays this disease has become common due to wrong eating habits and irregular life-style. Many a times the patients die due to heart attack.

First residential camp

The patients (1,044) coming to the residential camps were tested for ECG and complete lipid profile before and after the camps in order to check authenticity of Pranayam. It was automatically proved that Yog is undoubtedly beneficial in heart diseases.

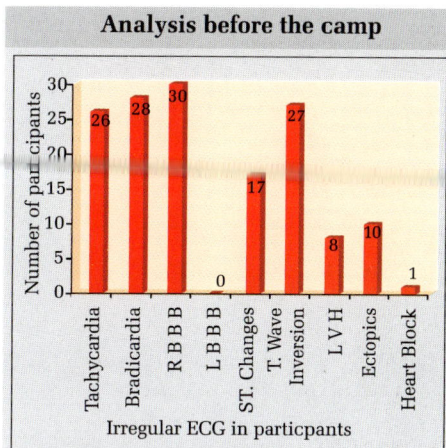

Analysis before the camp

Irregular ECG in participants

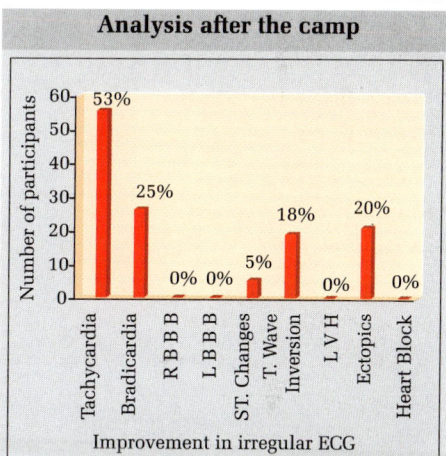

Analysis after the camp

Improvement in irregular ECG

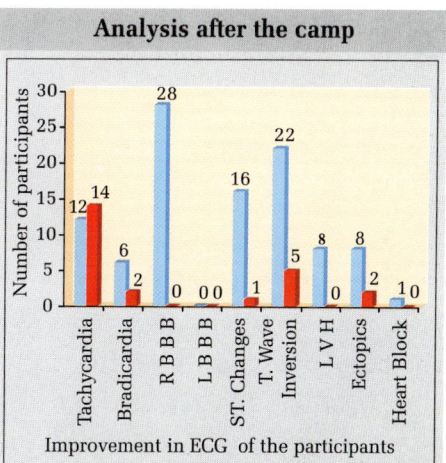

Analysis after the camp

Improvement in ECG of the participants

Ailment	No. of people before camp	No. of people after camp	Difference (ECG)	Gain (per cent
Tachycardia	26	12	14	53.85
Bradicardia	8	6	2	25
LAD 5	5	0	0	
RBBB28	28	0	0	
LBBB0	0	0	0	
Inferior Infraction	6	6	0	0
Anetrior Infraction	1	1	0	0
Anteroseptal Infraction	3	3	0	0
ST changes	17	16	1	5.88
Twave Inversion	27	22	5	18.52
LVH 8	8	0	0	
RVH 0	0	0	0	
Ectopics	10	8	2	20
Atrial Fibrillation	1	1	0	0
Heart Block	1	1	0	0

- Number of patients tested for ECG before the camp – 1,044
- Number of patients with irregular ECG before the camp – 71

Around 71 people were found to be having irregular ECG before the camp and were tested again after the camp. Positive change was seen in 14 patients as per the international standards and 20 per cent of patients got favourable results.

Second residential camp

- Number of patients tested for ECG before the camp – 1,144
- Number of patients with irregular ECG before the camp –141

Third Residential camp

- Number of patients tested for ECG before the third residential camp – 730
- Number of patients with irregular ECG before the camp–169

Around 169 people were

Ailment/disease	No. of people before camp	No. of people after camp	Difference (ECG) camp	Gain (per cent)
Tachycardia	27	10	17	62.96
Bradicardia	9	5	4	44.44
LAD	11	11	0	0
RBBB	12	8	4	33.33
LBBB	12	12	0	0
Inferior Infraction	4	4	0	0
Anetrior Infraction	2	2	0	0
Anteroseptal Infraction	2	2	0	0
ST changes	23	21	2	8.7
T Wave Inversion	40	37	3	7.5
LVH	10	10	0	0
RVH	4	4	0	0
Ectopics	9	2	7	77.78
Atrial Fibrillation	0	0	0	0
Heart Block	4	3	1	25

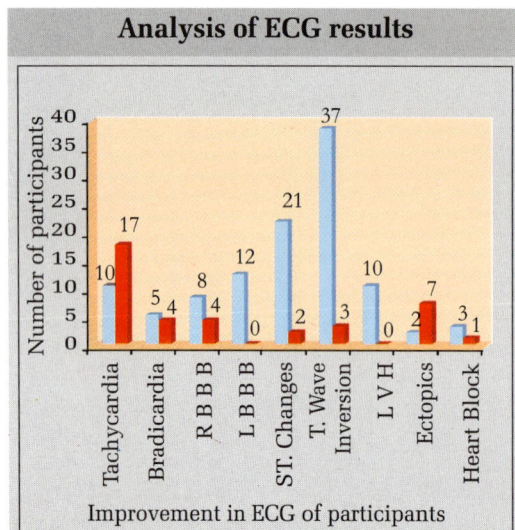

Analysis of ECG results

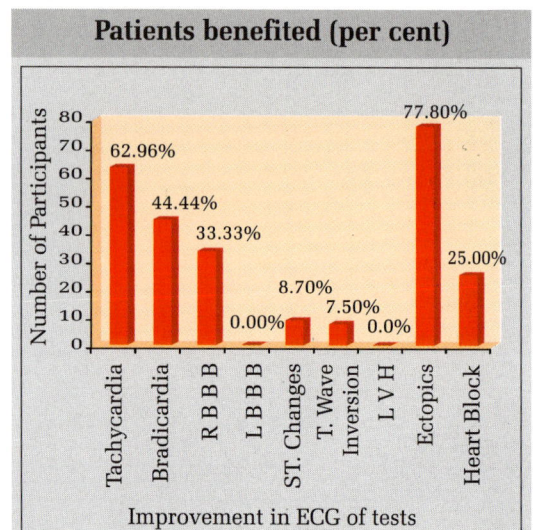

Patients benefited (per cent)

found to be having irregular ECG before the camp and were tested again after the camp. Positive improvement was seen in 37 patients as per the international standards and 21.85 per cent of patients got favourable results.

Fourth residential camp

* Number of patients tested for ECG before the camp – 792
* Number of patients with irregular ECG before the camp – 161

Around 161 people were found to be having irregular ECG before the camp and were tested again after the camp. Positive improvement was seen in 40 patients as per the international standards and 24.84 per cent of patients got favourable results.

Ailment/disease	No. of people before camp	No. of people after camp	Difference	Gain (per cent)
Tachycardia	18	7	11	61.11
Bradicardia	8	4	4	50
LAD	11	11	0	0
RBBB	9	8	1	11.11
LBBB	7	6	1	14.29
Inferior Infraction	0	0	0	0
Anetrior Infraction	0	0	0	0
Anteroseptal Infraction	0	0	0	0
ST changes	31	27	4	12.90
T wave Inversion	51	40	11	21.57
LVH	11	10	1	9.09
RVH	2	2	0	0
Ectopics	9	3	6	66.67
Atrial Fibrillation	0	0	0	0
Heart Block	4	3	1	25

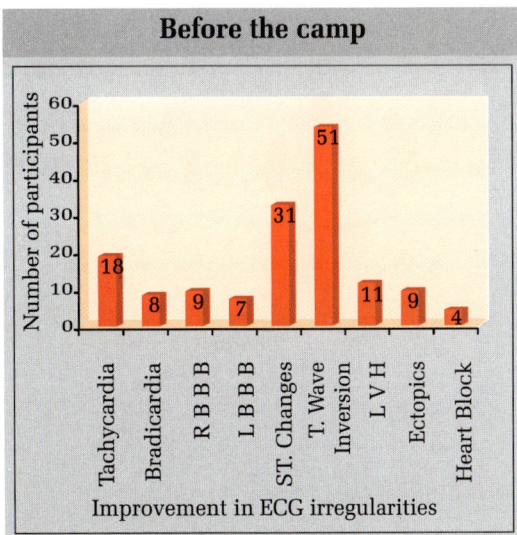

Before the camp

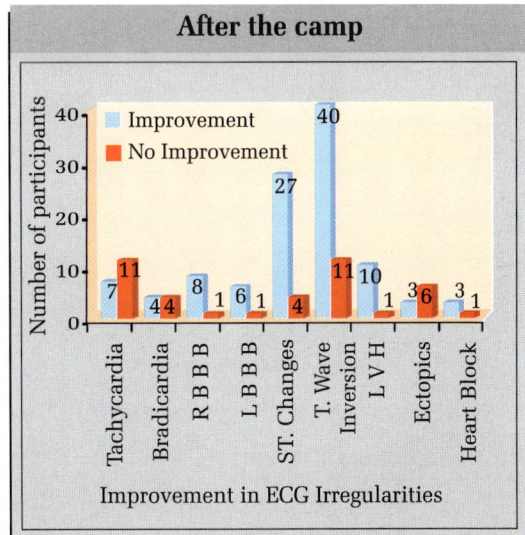

After the camp

Fifth residential camp

- ◆ Number of patients tested for ECG before the less camp – 807
- ◆ Number of patients with irregular ECG before the less camp – 89

Around 89 people were found to be having irregular ECG before the camp and were tested again after the camp. Positive improvement was seen in 20 patients as per the international standards and 22.47 per cent of patients got favourable results.

Ailment/disease	No. of People before camp	No. of People after camp	Difference (ECG)	Gain (per cent)
Tachycardia	12	7	5	41.67
Bradicardia	2	2	0	0
LAD	1	1	0	0
RBBB	28	26	2	7.14
LBBB	7	7	0	0
Inferior Infraction	0	0	0	0
Anetrior Infraction	13	13	0	0
Antroceptal Infarction	2	2	0	0
S.T. changes	0	0	0	0
T. Wave Inversion	11	5	6	54.55
LVH	3	3	0	0
RVH	0	0	0	0
Ectopics	8	2	6	75
Atrial Fibrillation	1	0	1	100
Heart Block	1	1	0	0

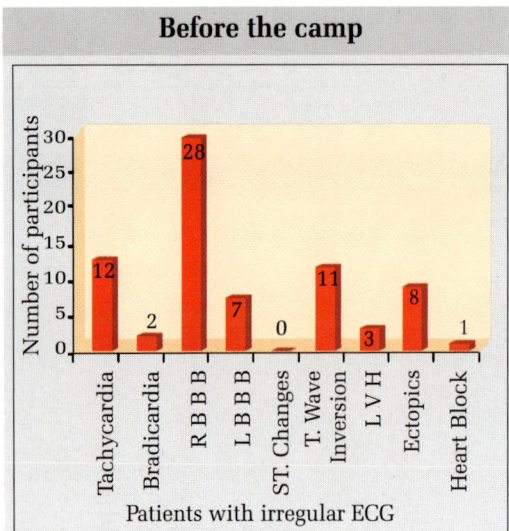

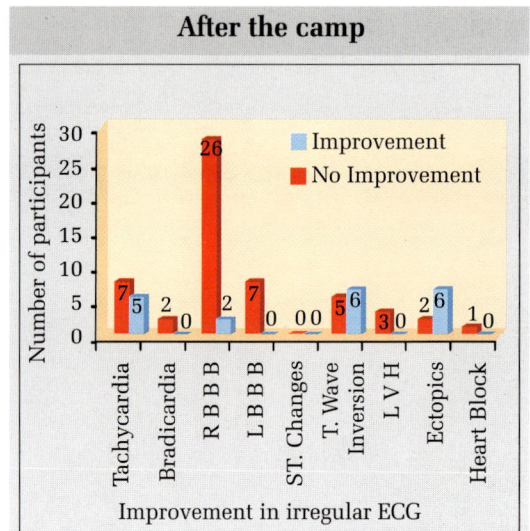

Before the camp

After the camp

Sixth residential camp

- ◆ Number of patients tested for ECG before the less camp – 1144

◆   Number of patients with irregular ECG before the camp – 141

Around 141 people were detected with irregular ECG before the camp and were tested again after the camp. Positive improvement was seen in 40 patients as per the international standards and 22.84 per cent of patients got favourable results.

The parameters included total cholesterol, HDL cholesterol, LDL cholesterol, VLDL cholesterol and triglycerides. The participants were also tested for complete lipid profile under different parameters. In this the tests for total cholesterol, LDL cholesterol, HDL cholesterol, VLDL cholesterol and triglycerides were also included. The tests done in various camps showed surprising results.

Ailment/disease	No. of people before camp	No. of people after camp	Difference (ECG)	Gain (per cent)
Tachycardia	36	26	10	27.78
Bradicardia	28	22	6	21.43
LAD	1	1	0	0
RBBB	5	5	0	0
LBBB	7	7	0	0
Inferior Infraction	5	3	2	40
Anetrior Infraction	7	6	1	14.29
Antroceptal Infraction	0	0	0	0
S.T. changes	0	0	0	0
T Wave Inversion	38	28	10	26.32
LVH	2	1	1	50
RVH	0	0	0	0
Ectopics	38	31	7	18.42
Atrial Fibrillation	1	1	0	0
Heart Block	1	1	0	0

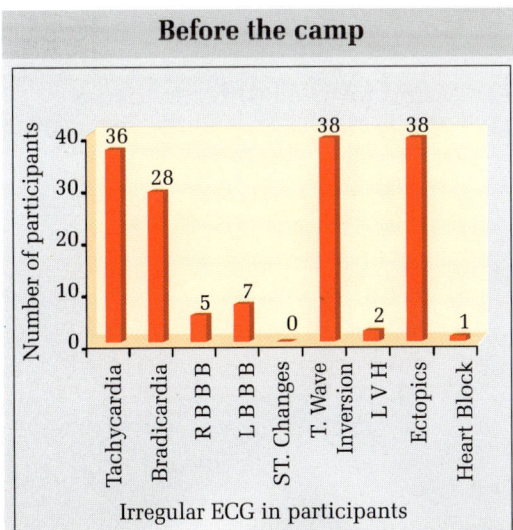

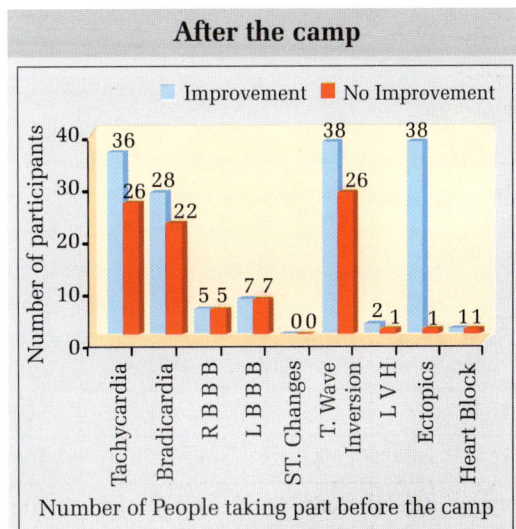

Before the camp

Number of participants — Irregular ECG in participants

After the camp

■ Improvement ■ No Improvement

Number of participants — Number of People taking part before the camp

Lipid Profile test before camp

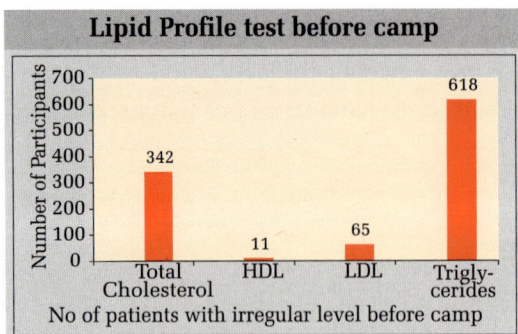

No of patients with irregular level before camp

Parameter	No. of people with irregular level before the camp	No. of people with irregular level after the camp	Improvement	
			No	%
Total cholesterol	342	12	330	96.49
HDL	11	13	-2	-18.18
LDL	65	0	65	100
Triglycerides	618	0	618	100

Lipid profile before camp

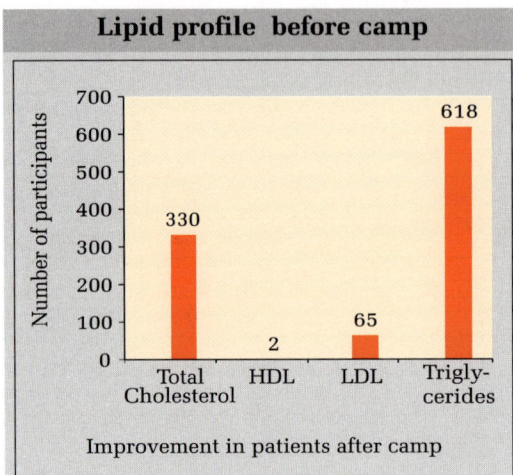

Improvement in patients after camp

Lipid profile test before camp

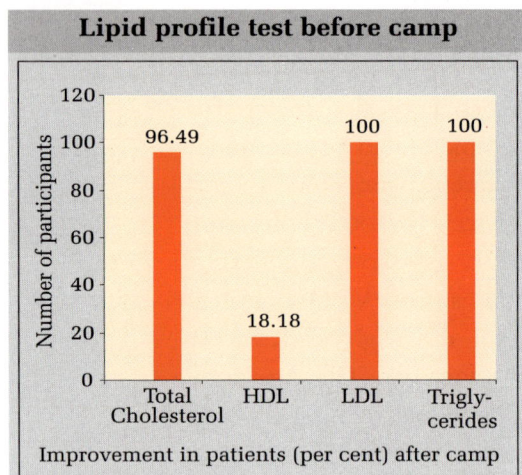

Improvement in patients (per cent) after camp

The Yog camp organized from 31 August to 6 September 2005 had 1,377 patients in all and blood samples were collected for complete lipid profile. The results have been given in the table underneath.

Parameter	No. of people with irregular level before camp	No. of people with irregular level after camp	Impro-vement	
			No	%
Total Cholesterol	261	10	251	96.17
HDL	23	8	15	65.22
LDL	41	0	41	100.00
Triglycerides	409	0	409	100.00

Lipid profile test before camp

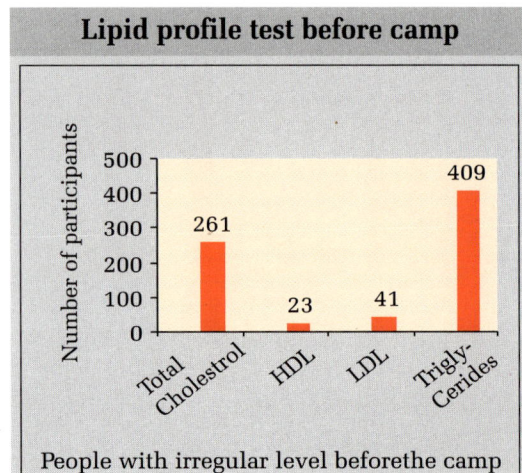

People with irregular level beforethe camp

Lipid profile test after camp

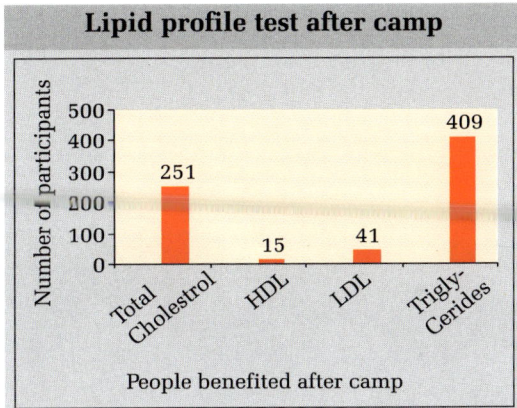

People benefited after camp

Patients benefited (per cent)

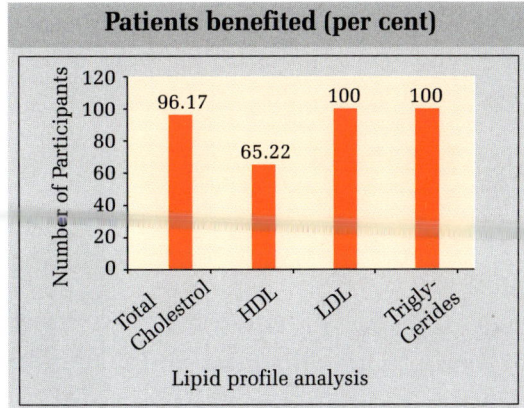

Lipid profile analysis

About 1,186 patients participated in the Yog camp organized from 12 to 27 August 2005 and the blood samples were collected for lipid profile. The results are presented underneath.

Parameter	No. of people with irregular level before camp	No. of people with irregular level after camp	Improvement	
			No	%
Total cholesterol	186	113	73	39.25
HDL	32	12	20	62.50
LDL	50	21	29	58
Triglycerides	393	223	170	43.26

Analysis of lipid profile

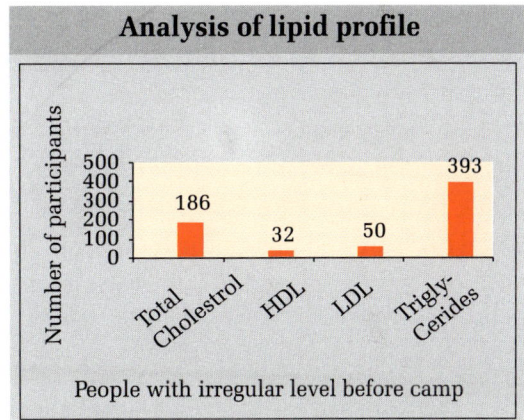

People with irregular level before camp

Analysis of lipid profile after camp

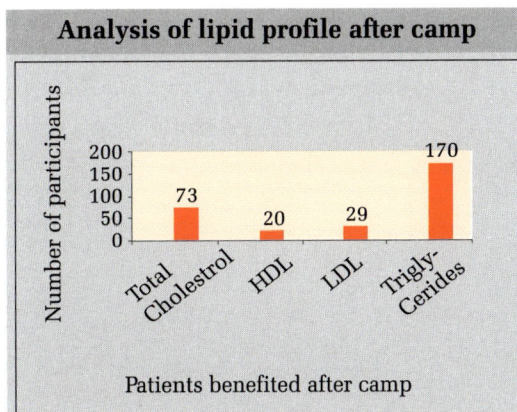

Patients benefited after camp

Analysis of lipid profile after camp

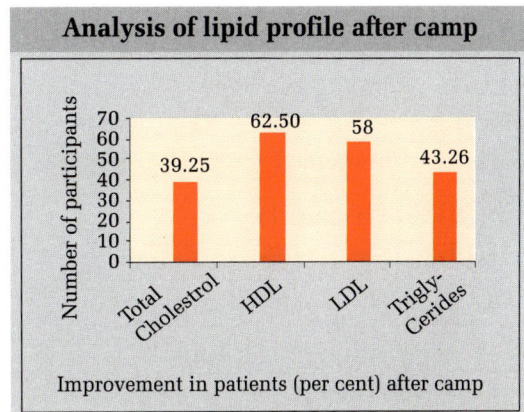

Improvement in patients (per cent) after camp

Around 1,399 patients participated in the Yog camp organized from 10 to 17 September 2005 and the blood samples were collected for lipid profile and their results are also mentioned in the table underneath.

(iii) Effects of Pranayam on Blood Pressure

The pressure exerted on the walls of arteries due to blood circulation in different parts of the body by the heart is called blood pressure. The thickness and density of blood and the resistance by the walls of the arteries determines blood pressure.

Generally an autonomic nervous system (ANS) controls the blood pressure. The different parts of body like hypothalamus, thyroid, parathyroid, sympathetic, parasympathetic nervous system, adrenaline, secreted through adrenaline and noradrenaline hormones are controlled through ANS. The left side of the heart throws the blood towards the arteries with full force and is called the systolic blood pressure and during the rest period the main flexible arteries come back to the normal position with force and the pressure that is exerted on the artery walls is called diastolic blood pressure.

Around 15-20 per cent of the total heart patients and 10 per cent normal persons suffer from high blood pressure. This disease is increasing at a very fast rate in the whole world due to stress and competitive life.

Regular practice of Pranayam and Shavasana controls the blood pressure completely. The patients attending the camp were tested for blood pressure before and after the camps. Surprising results were noticed within seven days of the camp. The high blood pressure patients were divided into five categories to study the affects. They were:

1. >180/110 mm Hg;
2. 160 /110 to 180 /110 mm;
3. 130/ 90 to 160/100 mm;
4. < 120/80 mm Hg; and
5. 130/90 to 120/80 mm Hg.

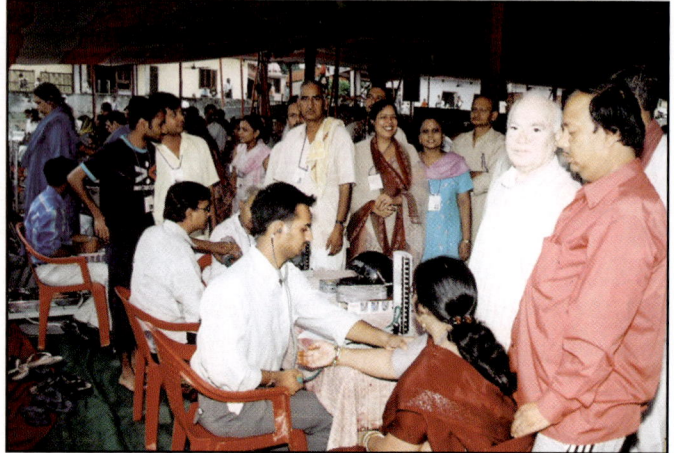

The patients of blood pressure show the symptoms of insomnia, headache, depression, confusion, restlessness, nausea etc.

Yog camp organized from (11 to 17 August 2005)

Before the camps around 965 patients were tested for high blood pressure and 806 were having blood pressure above the normal level. On the last day of the camp 895 patients were tested again for blood pressure. The study is being presented in a tabular form underneath. During the camp nobody was given medicines to control blood pressure. In the following table data of only those patients is being given who were tested for high blood pressure before and after the camps.

Range (mm Hg)	No. of people before camp	No. of people after camp	Difference
>180/110	25	7	18
160/100 to 180/110	37	23	14
130/90 to 160/100	299	113	186
120/80 to 130/90	145	188	-43
<120/80	120	295	-175

Analysis of blood pressure before camp

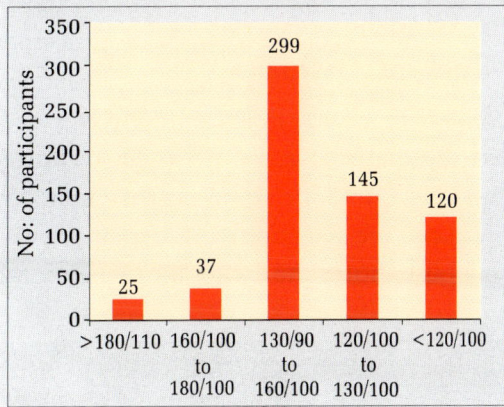

Analysis of blood pressure after camp

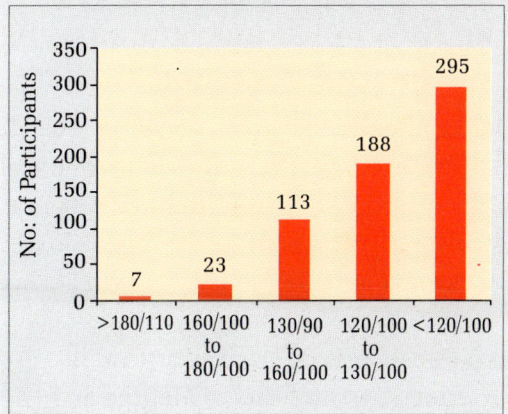

Yog camp organized from 1 to 7 September 2005

Before the camp around 812 patients were tested for high blood pressure and 361 were

Range (mm Hg)	No. of people before camp	No. of people after camp	Difference
160/100 to 180/100	41	18	23
130/90 to 160/100	338	60	278
120/80 to 130/90	427	53	374
<120/80	159	675	-516

Analysis of blood pressure before camp

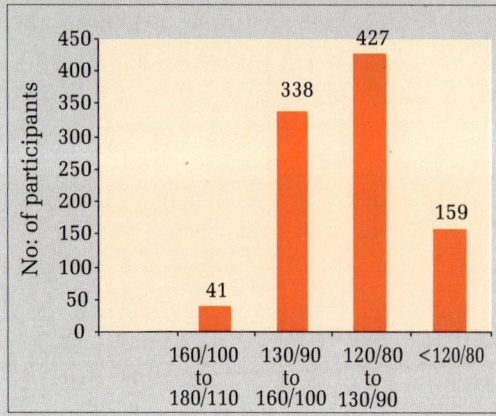

Analysis of blood pressure after camp

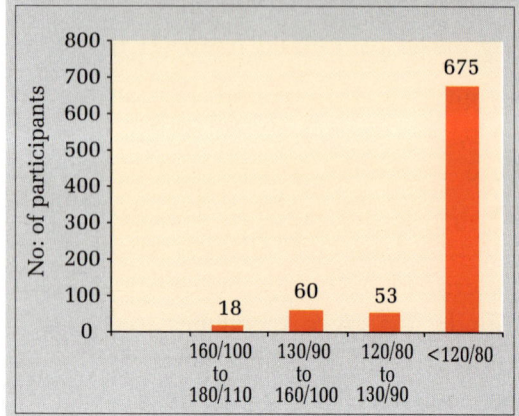

having blood pressure above the normal level. On the last day of the camp 626 patients were tested again for blood pressure (see table). During the camp, nobody was given medicines to control blood pressure. In the adjacent table, data of only those patients has been included who were tested for high blood pressure before and after the camps.

(iv) Effect of Pranayam on Endocrine Glands (Internal Secretion Glands) and Related Diseases

On the basis of study conducted on several lakh patients practising Pranayam we concluded that Pranayam activates the endocrine glands and the equilibrium of these glands cures different diseases. The hormones generated from some glands or some organs enter the blood directly and activate the digestion of food or excite the secretion of different organs. For example anterior pituitary growth hormone metabolism hormone excites the metabolism.

It activates the pancreas to convert sugar into glycogen. Secretion is produced from the phlegmatic substance, duodenum and activates the digestive juices of pancreas. Similarly, sex hormones like androgen in males and estrogen in females are produced in the age group of 12-14 years. These hormones are responsible for physical and mental changes. The physical and mental behaviour, chest development, shoulders, pelvis, voice, growth of hairs, attraction towards

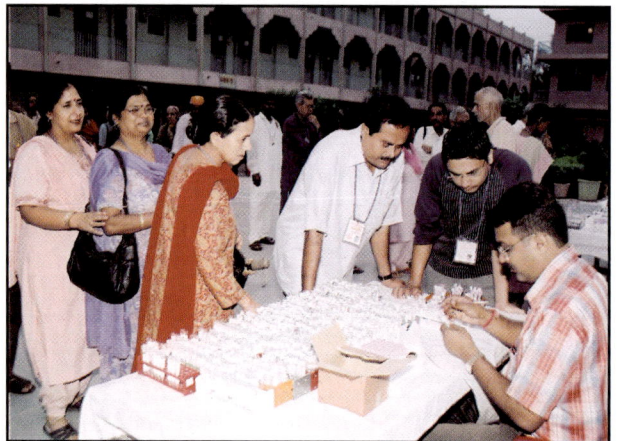

each other are all controlled with these hormones. Tri-ido thyronine (T_3) and thyroxin (T_4) hormones are secreted through thyroid glands. These hormones are important for the proportionate development of the body. The growth of skeleton is also dependent on the secretion of these hormones. This gland controls the metabolism. The mental and sexual growth is dependent on this gland.

Ujjayi Pranayam practised along with deep and mild Kumbhak maintains the adrino medullary hormonal level. The thyroid hormones are helpful in oxidation that takes place in bones, flesh, brain and other organs. Burning of glucose in body organs, production of glucose from glycogen in liver, digestion of fat and cholesterol in blood, digestion of proteins in body, evacuation of nitrogen and phosphorous, heart function are all dependent on it. Hyperthyroidism leads to lean body, fast heart beats, tremors, whereas hypothyroidism causes swelling of the body, increases cholesterol level and affects the metabolism in the body. The participants were tested from T_3, T_4, TSH level before and after the camp. All the patients with irregular levels showed cent per cent improvement.

(v) Effects of Pranayam on Patients of Diabetes

Presently diabetes has taken the form of a very serious disease. Out of 20 life-style disorders mentioned in Ayurveda, diabetes is the most dreadful one. Madhava Nidan mentions:

> Āasyāasukham ṣwapnasukhaṃ dadhēeni, grāamyāuḍakāanōoparasāaḥ payāaṇsi ।
> Navāaṇnapāanaṃ gurvāikṛitaṃ cha, Pramēha hētuḥ kaphakṛichcha saṛvaṃ ॥

In other words sitting comfortably, sleeping on soft bed, excess consumption of milk, fat, curd, eating meat of aquatic animals and those living on land, like fish, tortoise etc. eating new rice, sugar candy and things which are sweet in taste and aggravate *kapha* causes diabetes. If the loss of humour is not treated on time then it converts into diabetes.

In case of diabetes the sugar level increases due to reduced insulin generation in the pancreas. This causes inefficient assimilation of carbohydrates.

According to modern science there are four types of diabetes

* Insulin dependent diabetes
* Non-insulin dependent diabetes
* Pregnancy (gestational) related diabetes
* Diabetes of young.

The first type of diabetes is seen in the youth below the age of 25 years and the patient is dependent on insulin throughout life.

The second type of diabetes begins after the age of 25 years and is the common type of disease. It is also caused due to hereditary reasons.

Third type of diabetes is seen generally in 10-15 age group and patients need to take regular Insulin. This kind of diabetes is not hereditary.

The fourth type of diabetes is seen in the age group of 20–30 years because of anorexia

Practice of Kapalbhati, Bhastrika, Mandookasan, Yog Mudrasan and other asanas activate the pancreas and helps in proper secretion of insulin. As a result the blood sugar level remains at normal position. The insulin dependent patients also get positive results with the practice of Yog and Pranayam.

The patients coming to the camp were tested for blood sugar level before and after the camp in order to prove the authenticity of this fact.

Positive changes were seen even in the common symptoms of diabetes like polyurea, polyphagia, polydysia, weakness and painful discharge. This proves that Pranayam and Yog are beneficial in case of diabetes.

Results of fasting blood sugar in Yog camp organized from 21 to 27 August 2005

Tests for sugar level in camps

Parameter	Total samples	People with irregular level before camp	People with irregular level after camp	Improvement	Improvement (per cent)
Fasting Glucose	928	859	557	302	35.16

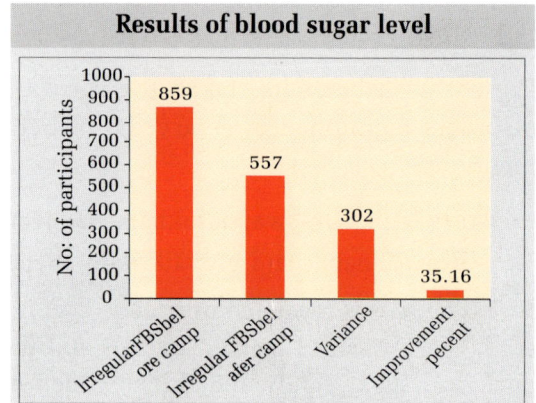

Results of blood sugar level

Results of fasting blood sugar in Yog camp organized from 31 August to 6 September 2005

Tests for sugar level in camps

Parameter	Total samples	People with irregular level before camp	People with irregular level after camp	Improvement	Improvement (per cent)
Fasting Glucose	886	643	212	431	67.03

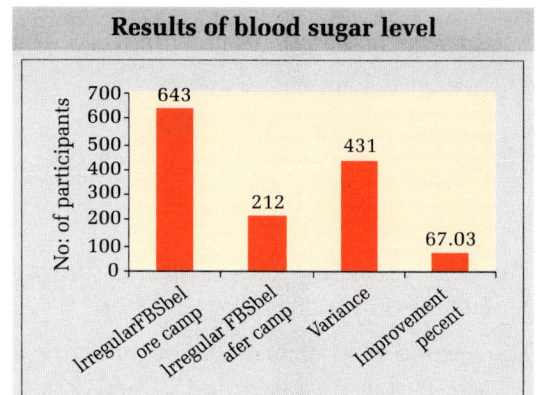

Results of blood sugar level

Results of fasting blood sugar in Yog camp organized from 10 to 17 September 2005

Tests for sugar level in camp

Parameter	Total samples	People with irregular level before camp	People with irregular level after camp	Improvement	Improvement (per cent)
Fasting Glucose	1071	738	593	145	19.65

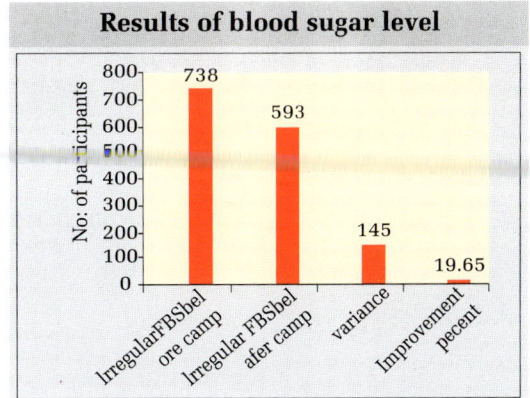

Results of blood sugar level

(vi) Effect of Pranayam on Obesity

Accumulation of fat in body leads to obesity. Fat is the fourth humour of our body and when its formation is excess in comparison to other humours it leads to obesity. This disease is common in developed countries and affluent families. Irregularity in internal secretion glands also becomes one of the reasons for this problem. According to Sage Charak it could be hereditary as well. Normally fat deposits on stomach, hips, thighs and waist area. Besides the obese people perspire a lot, which emits a lot of odour. The obese person has the urge to eat at short intervals. The palpitation increases with slightest exertion. The analysis of over weight and obese people is being presented here with the help of bar graph. It is evident that majority of the patients reduced 5-10 kg weight within one week.

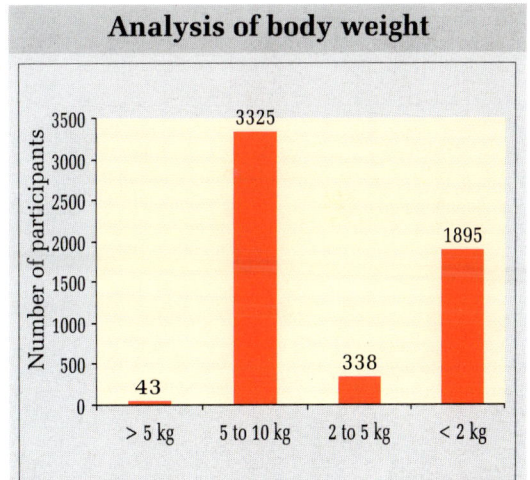

Analysis of body weight

(vii) Effect of Pranayam on Kidney Diseases

Kidney is one of the most active organ of our body. It is bean shaped organ weighing around five gram each. The kidneys control the water level in our body. They excrete the waste material produced in our body. Kidneys are also helpful in controlling the high blood pressure level in the body. In case kidneys fail to function normally our body becomes diseased.

Kidney dysfunction is of two types :

Acute renal failure (severe kidney inactivity) : It is caused due to infection, malaria, eating contrary food, enlargement of prostrate glands and dehydration in body.

Chronic renal failure (kidney degeneration): Following are the reasons for this disease.

* Diabetes – 34 %
* High blood pressure – 30 %
* Glomerulonephritis (improper discharge of urine) - 36% (In this disease, the nephrons degenerate gradually)

Results of creatinine level in Yog camp (21-27 August 2005)

Standard	Total samples	People with irregular level before camps	People with irregular level after camps	Improvement	Improvement (per cent)
Serum creatinine	1267	52	5	47	90.38

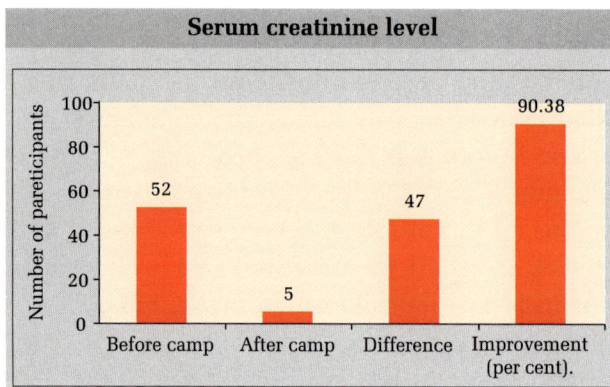

Serum creatinine level

Results of creatinine level in Yog camp (31 August to 6 September 2005)

Standard	Total samples	People with irregular level before camps	People with irregular level after camps	Improvement	Improvement (per cent)
Serum creatinine	920	14	3	11	78.57

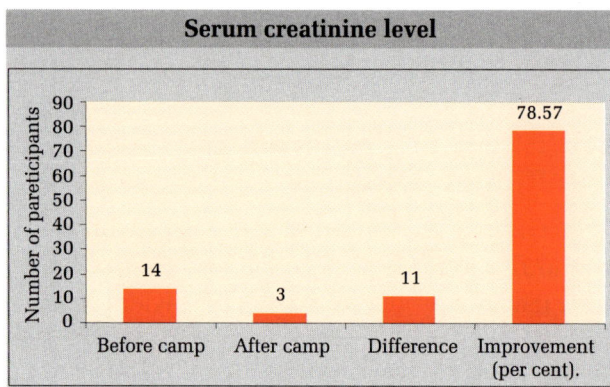

Serum creatinine level

Analysis of different diseases and physical irregularities in different participants of Yog camps

Ratio (per cent)

Sex	Age group	Obesity	Diabetes	Hypertension	Heart disease	Arthritis	Asthma	Kidney diseases	Spondylitis	Thyroid	Prostate	Cancer	Depression	Hepatitis
Females	Up to 35 years	34.95	22.95	6.00	7.43	6.67	1.90	1.33	0.57	11.71	4.76	0.40	0.06	0.30
	35–50 years	31.33	20.00	11.33	8.00	7.90	2.57	0.76	0.86	12.48	3.62	0.29	0.67	0.19
	Above 50 years	16.04	22.13	14.69	12.12	10.78	2.76	0.77	1.54	14.30	4.23	0.51	0.13-	0.00
Yog	(A)	25.85	21.75	11.23	9.59	8.77	2.46	0.93	1.07	13.04	4.21	0.44	0.49	0.16
Males	Up to 35 years	29.58	29.26	10.64	8.06	3.99	1.56	1.41	1.49	4.85	5.95	0.78	1.17	1.25
	35– 50 years	26.49	28.88	15.75	5.48	4.79	3.24	1.62	1.54	5.87	4.40	0.46	0.46	1.00
	Above 50 years	14.14	29.05	16.29	14.49	5.93	2.63	0.75	1.54	6.09	6.90	0.35	0.09	0.09
Yog	(B)	21.50	29.44	14.66	10.30	5.11	51	1.15	1.53	6.08	6.02	0.49	0.47	0.64
Total participants		23.37	26.13	13.10	10.05	6.69	2.49	1.06	1.33	9.07	5.24	0.47	0.40	0.43

Ratio (per cent) of patients of male and female particpaints depending on diseases

		Obesity	Diabetes	Hypertension	Heart disease	Arthritis	Asthma	Kidney diseases	Spondylitis	Thyroid	Prostate	Cancer	Depression	Hepatitis
Females		47.56	35.79	36.63	41.06	56.41	42.25	37.78	34.51	61.79	34.53	40.00	43.90	16.22
Males		52.44	64.21	63.37	58.56	43.59	57.55	62.22	65.49	38.21	65.47	60.00	56.10	83.78

A particpant could be suffering from one or more diseases

Analysis of tests done in camps

Total number of male and female participants registered in the camps

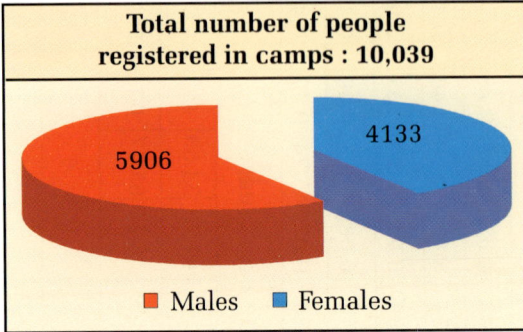

Total number of people registered in camps : 10,039

5906

4133

■ Males ■ Females

Total number of Indians and foreigners registered in the camps

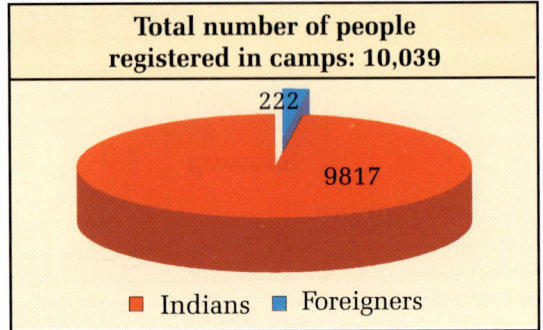

Total number of people registered in camps: 10,039

222

9817

■ Indians ■ Foreigners

Tests done to reduce obesity

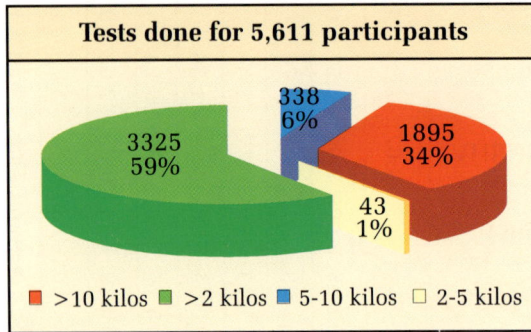

Tests done for 5,611 participants

338
6%

1895
34%

3325
59%

43
1%

■ >10 kilos ■ >2 kilos ■ 5-10 kilos □ 2-5 kilos

Tests done to reduce diabetes

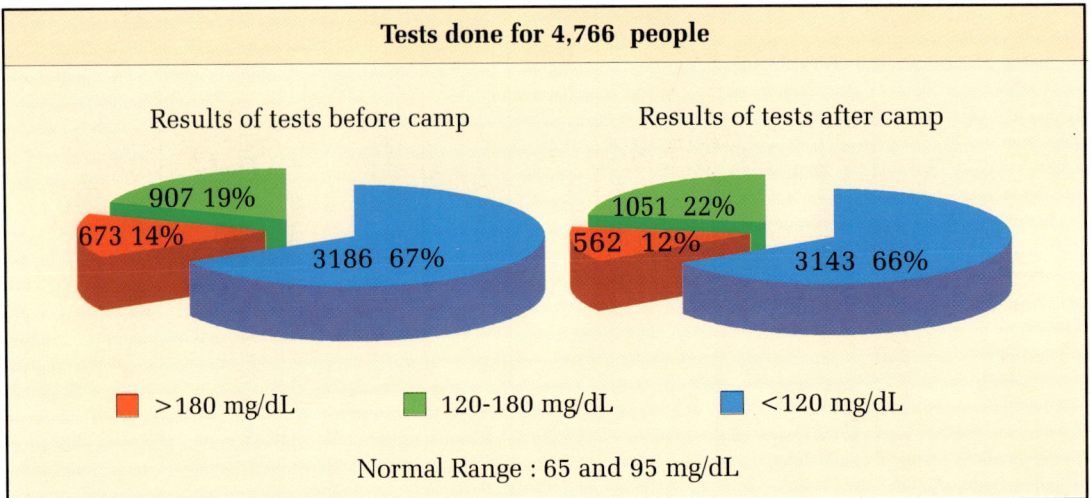

Tests done for 4,766 people

Results of tests before camp

907 19%

673 14%

3186 67%

Results of tests after camp

1051 22%

562 12%

3143 66%

■ >180 mg/dL   ■ 120-180 mg/dL   ■ <120 mg/dL

Normal Range : 65 and 95 mg/dL

Tests done for high blood pressure
Ideal blood pressure range 120 / 80 mmHg

Tests done for 2,724 people

Result of tests done before the camp

Result of tests done after the camp

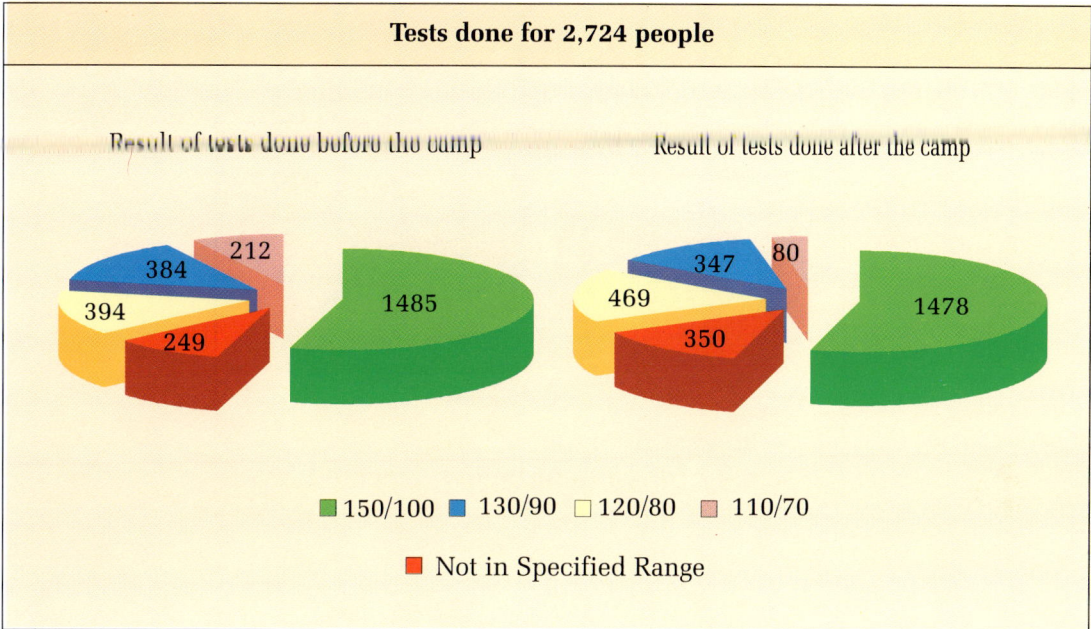

212 384 394 249 1485

347 80 469 350 1478

■ 150/100 ■ 130/90 □ 120/80 ■ 110/70

■ Not in Specified Range

Tests done for cholesterol level
Ideal blood pressure range 120 / 80 mmHg

Tests done for 5,486 people

Results of tests before camp

Results of tests after camp

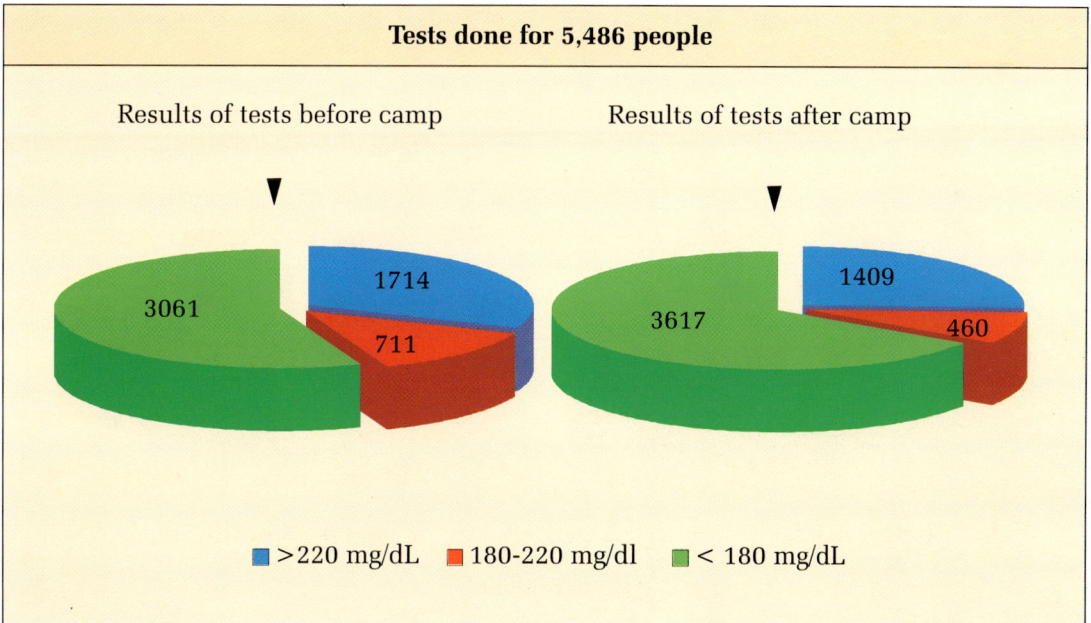

3061 1714 711

3617 1409 460

■ >220 mg/dL ■ 180-220 mg/dl ■ < 180 mg/dL

Tests done for renal/kidney function

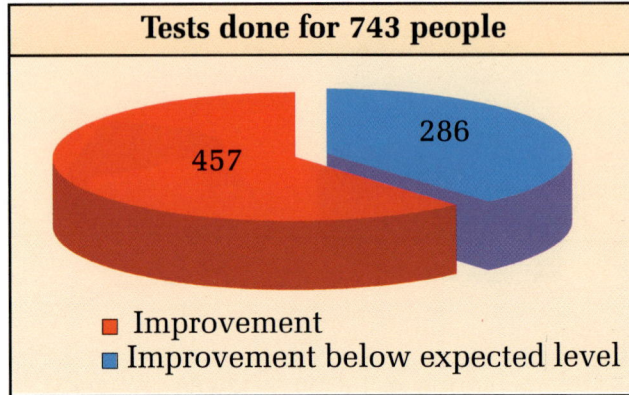

Tests done for 743 people

457

286

- Improvement
- Improvement below expected level

Tests done for serum creatinine
Normal range 0.5-1.50 mg/dl

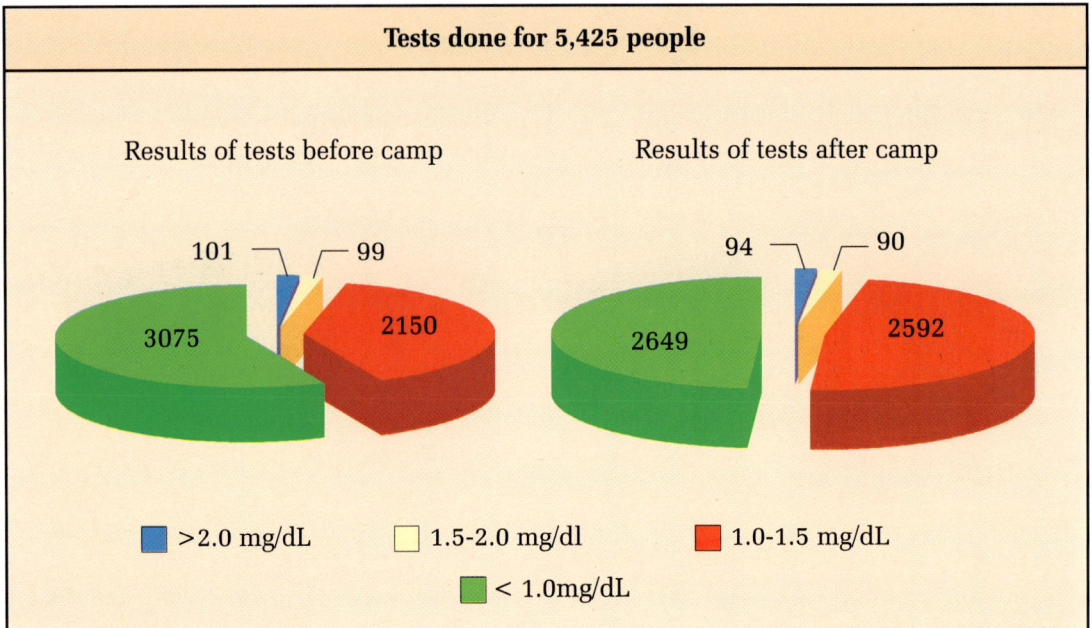

Tests done for 5,425 people

Results of tests before camp

101   99

3075   2150

Results of tests after camp

94   90

2649   2592

- >2.0 mg/dL
- 1.5-2.0 mg/dl
- 1.0-1.5 mg/dL
- < 1.0mg/dL

Yog camps organized specially for clinical trial

Two residential Yog camps were organized in the premises of Patanjali Yogpeeth under the guidance of Swami Ramdevji Maharaj for clinical trial of effects of Yog and Pranayam. The first camp was organized from 2-10 October 2006 and the second camp was held from 27 October to 4 November 2006. The effects of Yog and Pranayam on weight, blood pressure, pulmonary function test (PFT), electrocardiogram (ECG), thyroid profile, blood sugar level, lipid profile, kidney profile, liver function test, RA factor, uric acid and various cancer tests (AFP, PSA, CA-125) were studied. Patients were divided into various groups for the purpose. The patients were classified on the basis of diseases, viz. obesity, high blood pressure, respiratory disorder, heart disease, thyroid dysfunction (hypo and hyper thyroidism), diabetes, liver disorder, kidney disorder, arthritis and cancer.

The weight and lipid profile was measured in case of obese patients before and after the camp. The patients of high blood pressure and heart disease were tested for lipid profile and electrocardiogram, blood pressure. Fasting blood sugar test was done for patients of diabetes. The patients of respiratory diseases underwent pulmonary function test. Thyroid function test (T_3, T_4 and TSH) was done for thyroid patients. Haemoglobin test was done for patients of anaemia. Patients of liver disorder were tested for liver function test and kidney patients were tested for kidney function test (serum creatinine, serum urea and haemoglobin level).

The cancer patients were tested for AFP, PSA, CA-125, whereas arthritis profile consisting of RA factor, uric acid and haemoglobin was done for arthritis patients. Written consent was taken from all the patients before these medical tests. Every participant was informed about each and every detail of medical study conducted. The patients were given simple and light food during the medical tests. Swamiji made all the patients practice Yog and Pranayam for two hours in the morning and evening.

The patients were not allowed to take any medicine during the medical test, which were being taken earlier. The medical results obtained before and after the camp were analyzed on different parameters under this open level clinical trial.

Results

(i) Effect of Yog and Pranayam on body weight : 500 patients were selected to study the effect of Yog and Pranayam on body

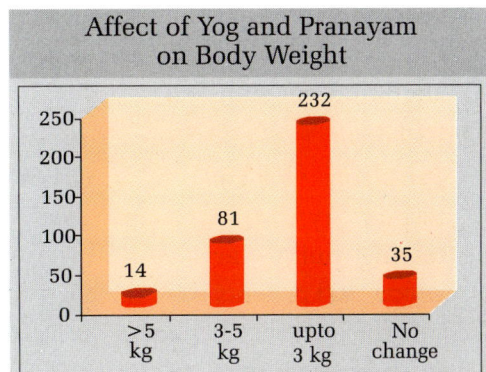

Affect of Yog and Pranayam on Body Weight

weight in Yog camps. Out of which, 362 patients were selected for analysis of results. Whereas other participants were kept out of the analysis due to technical reasons.

Yog and Pranayam increase the basal metabolic rate and causes oxidation of excess fat, which controls body weight. The above result makes it clear that regular practice of Yog and Pranayam controls body weight.

(ii) Effect of Yog and Pranayam on high blood pressure : 500 patients of high blood pressure were selected to study the effect of Pranayam on blood pressure. The blood pressure was measured before and after the camp. Out of which, 203 patients were selected for analysis of results and the rest were excluded due to technical reasons. A graphic representation of the results of study is being given here.

(iii) Effect of Yog and Pranayam on heart patients (ECG test) : 110 patients were tested for ECG before beginning Yog treatment. Out of which, 50 patients were abnormal, which were tested again after the camp. Of them, 35 patients were selected for analysis of results and the rest were excluded due to technical reasons. The results of tests show that there was significant improvement in bradicardia, tachycardia, ST changes and arrhythmia level. The electrocardiogram of LBH, RBBB and LBBB did not show any improvement.

(iv) Effect of Yog and Pranayam on lung function (PFT) : 500 patients of respiratory problem were selected for testing pulmonary function. Out of which, 300 patients were included for the study. The selected patients were tested for pulmonary function test (PFT) before

Affect of Yog and Pranayam on patients of Blood Pressure

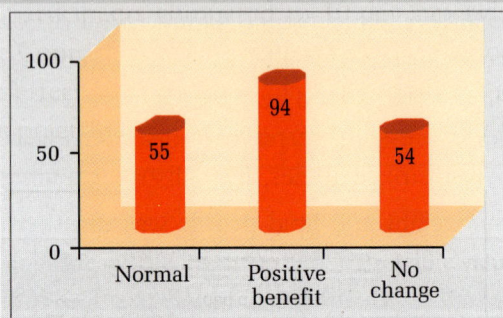

Normal: 55, Positive benefit: 94, No change: 54

Affect of Pranayam on ECG test

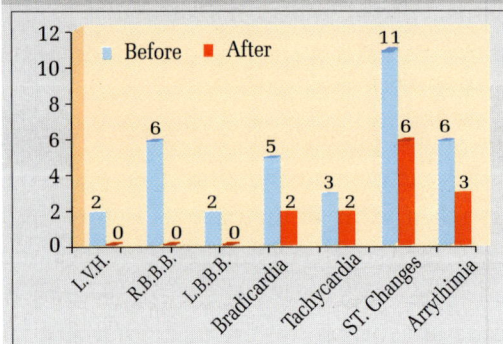

Before / After —
L.V.H.: 2 / 0; R.B.B.B.: 6 / 0; L.B.B.B.: 2 / 0; Bradicardia: 5 / 2; Tachycardia: 3 / 2; ST. Changes: 11 / 6; Arrythimia: 6 / 3

Affect of Yog and Pranayam on PFT

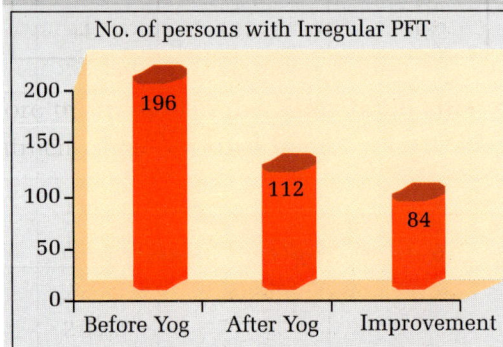

No. of persons with Irregular PFT

Before Yog: 196, After Yog: 112, Improvement: 84

and after the camp to study effect on lung function. The PFT levels of 196 patients were abnormal and were tested again. The analysis of results showed that 42.9% patients showed significant improvement in PFT level as per international standards.

(v) Effect of Yog and Pranayam on thyroid function : 140 patients were tested for thyroid hormone test before the camp. Out of which, 20 patients were detected with hypothyroidism, 112 with hyperthyroidism and remaining 8 patients had normal hormone profile. The analysis of results showed that 55 per cent of patients with lower level before camp were having normal hormone level after the camp. About 76 per cent of the patients had normal hormone level. The patients with higher level also showed considerable improvement.

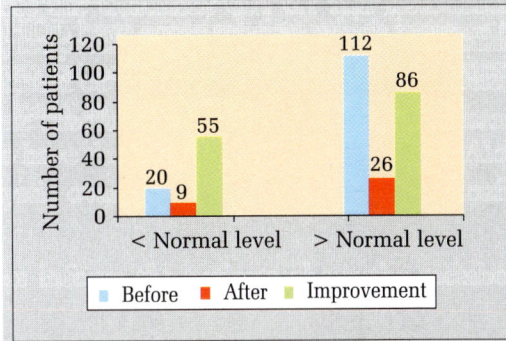

Effect of Pranayam on Thyroid Functioning

(vi) Effect of Yog and Pranayam on arthritis profile : 110 patients were selected and tested for haemoglobin, RA factor, and uric acid before and after the camp. The analysis of results showed that patients of arthritis had significant improvement with Yog and Pranayam as per international standards. The patients showed 45, 46 and 55 per cent improvement in haemoglobin, RA factor and uric acid respectivly.

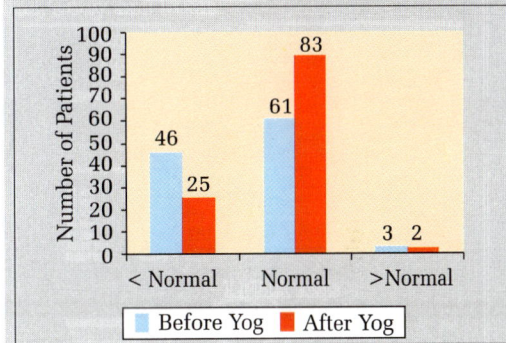

Effect of Pranayam on Haemoglobin

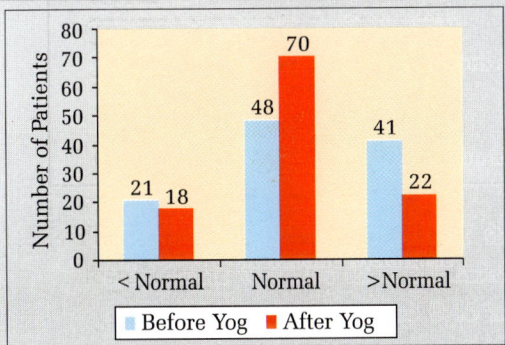

Effect of Pranayam on level of RA factor

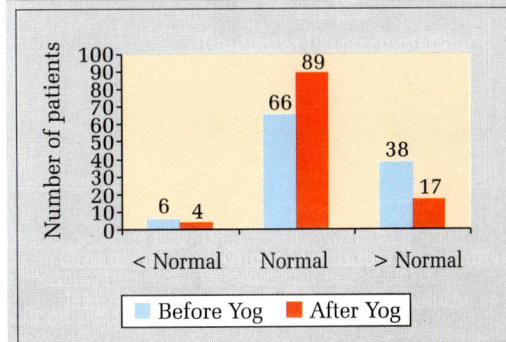

Effect of Pranayam on level of Uric acid

(vii) Effect of Yog and Pranayam on cancer patients : Twelve cancer patients were selected before the camp for the test. The clinical and physical tests were conducted before the camp and related tests like AFP, PFA, and CA-125 were also done for these patients. The analysis of results after the camp showed more than 50 per cent clinical improvement.

Effect of Pranayam on AFP level

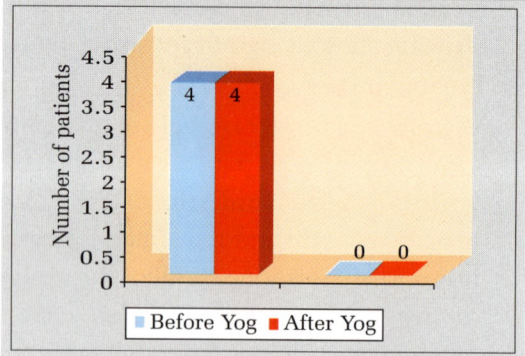

Effect of Pranayam on PSA level

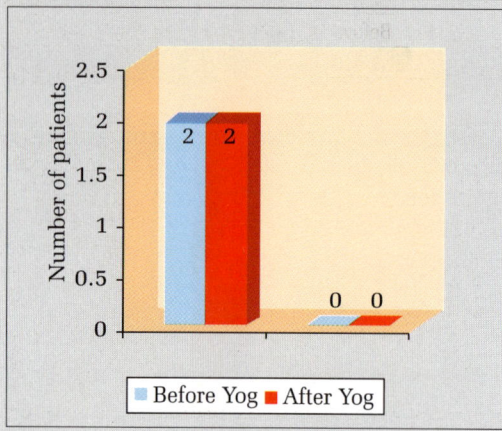

Effect of Pranayam on CA - 125 level

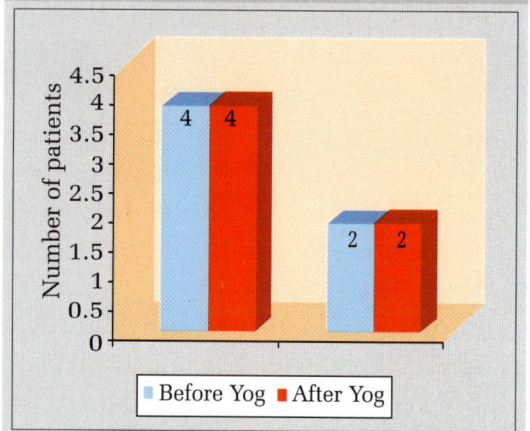

(viii) Effect of Yog and Pranayam on anaemia : Twenty five anaemic patients were selected before the camp. The haemoglobin level was tested before and after the camp. Six patients showed normal level, while remaining ones showed improvement.

Effect of Pranayam on Haemoglobin

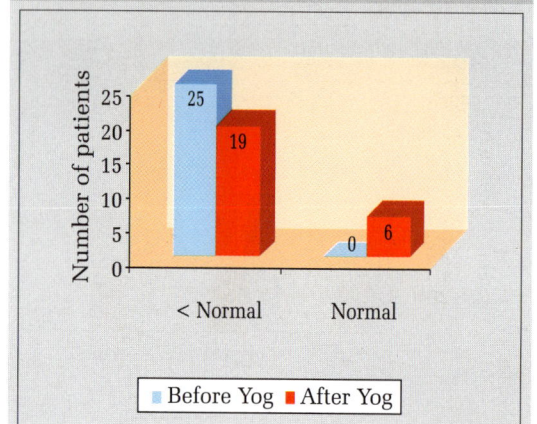

(ix) Effect of Yog and Pranayam on patients of diabetes : 1,080 patients were selected for studying the effect of Yog and Pranayam on blood sugar level. The blood sugar level was tested before and after the camp. About 54 per cent showed considerable improvement. All the patients were asked to stop medication before the beginning of study.

Effect of Pranayam on Blood Sugar

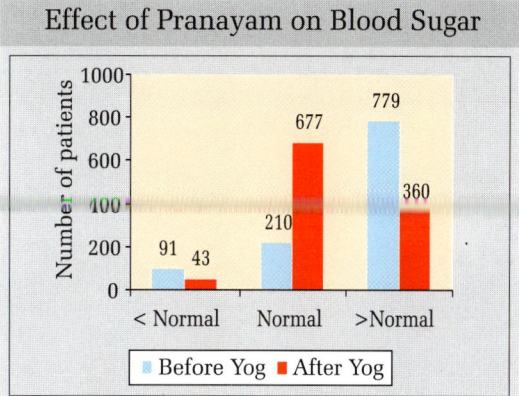

(x) Effect of Yog and Pranayam on lipid profile : 1,080 patients were selected to study the lipid profile. The tests for total cholesterol, HDL, LDL, VLDL and triglycerides were done before and after the camp. As per international standards, the total cholesterol, HDL, LDL, VLD, and triglycerides showed 62, 65, 54, 39 and 62 per cent improvement respectively.

Effect of Pranayam on Cholesterol Level

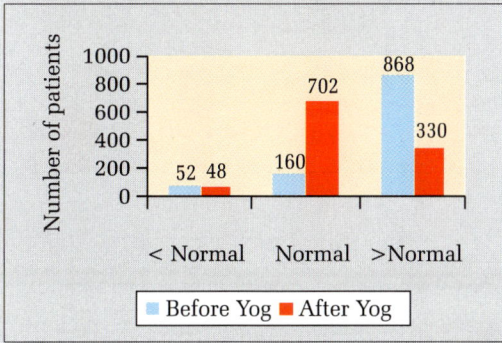

Effect of Pranayam on HDL Cholesterol Level

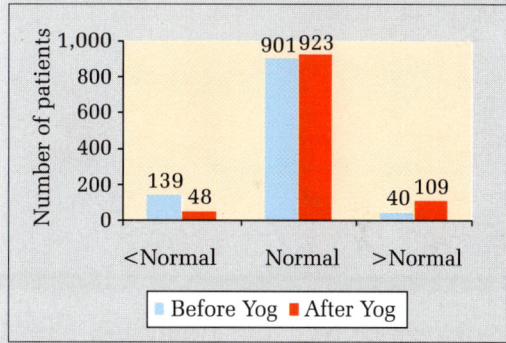

Effect of Pranayam on Triglyceride Level

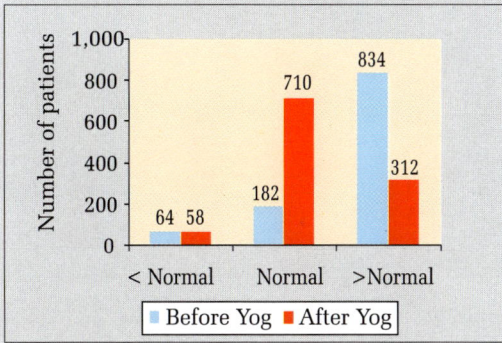

Effect of Pranayam on VLDL Cholesterol Level

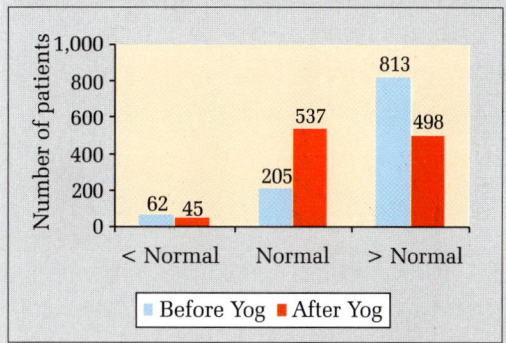

(xi) Effect of Yog and Pranayam on liver function : 1,080 patients were selected before the camp to study the liver function. The tests for total cholesterol, ALP, SGPT and SGOT were done on patients before and after the camp. As per international standards total Bilirubin, ALP, SGPT and SGOT showed 50, 67, 56 and 64 per cent respectively.

Effect of Pranayam on Total Bilirubin Level

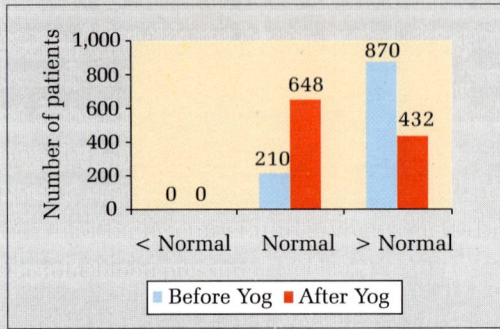

Effect of Pranayam on ALP level

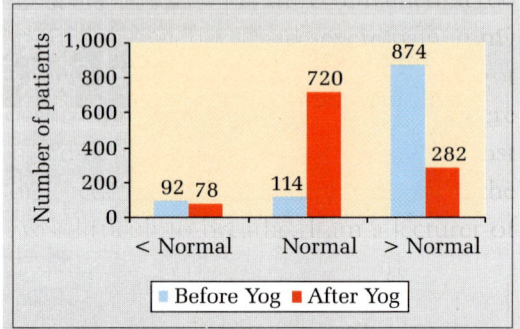

Effect of Pranayam on SGOT level

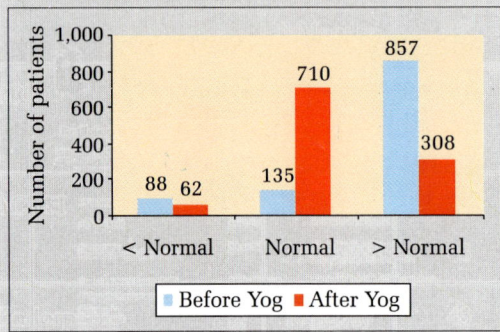

Effect of Pranayam on SGPT level

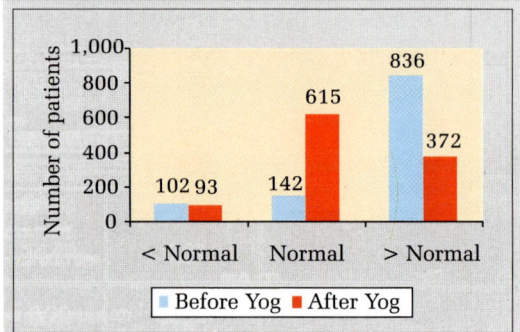

(xii) Effect of Yog and Pranayam on renal function : 1,080 patients were selected for renal function study. The patients were tested for serum urea and serum creatinine

Effect of Pranayam on Serum Urea Level

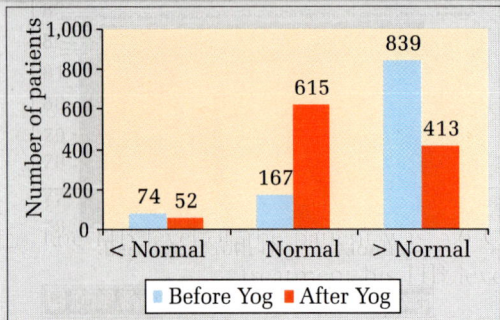

Effect of Pranayam on Serum Creatinine Level

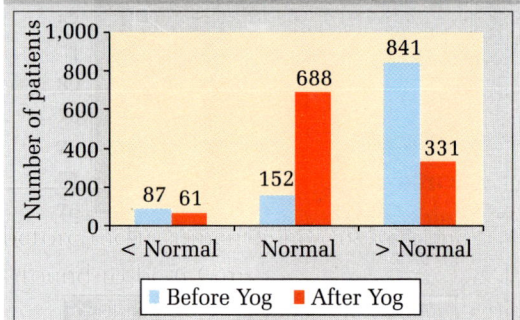

level. There was 51 per cent improvement in urea level, whereas creatinine level showed more improvement (61 per cent).

Conclusion

Clinical trial under the guidance of Swami Ramdevji Maharaj has been initiated in order to establish Yog, Pranayam and other ancient Indian medical systems scientifically. The main objective of these studies is to present the authenticity of Yog as per the scientific standards. Yog, Pranayam and other traditional medical systems do not need any evidence. But we are living in scientific age and modern science has progressed to a considerable extent in the recent past. Therefore, it is necessary to analyze as to how can we adopt our systems as per modern scientific parameters and establish the same at the international level. The present analysis of medical tests proves that Yog and Pranayam are capable of curing normal diseases along with serious and chronic diseases. There is a need to practise Yog and Pranayam in a systematic and rhythmic manner. Swamiji made the patients follow all the rules with strictness during the clinical trial. The Yog practitioners reap psychological, intellectual and spiritual benefits along with physical benefits. The participants were uncertain whether to discontinue diabetes medicine or insulin. Patients learnt how to lead a healthy life with regular practice of Yog and diet control and how to maintain normal blood pressure level without taking medicines. Yog and Pranayam work on receptors like medicines. This miracle is hidden in the strength of Yog and Pranayam. Swamiji has analyzed the medical gain of Yog and Pranayam on a large scale with the help of Yog camps. Indian medical team of specialists worked on these tests along with modern science scholars. The present study has shown significant improvement in body weight, high blood pressure, pulmonary function, electrocardiogram, blood sugar level, lipid profile, liver profile, renal profile, arthritis profile etc. There is a need for a long-term study on the effects of Yog and Pranayam.

Effect of Yog and Pranayam on Bone Mineral Density

An open level clinical study

Bones are significant in the constitution of human body and give a frame to the body. Malfunctioning in the development of bones leads to different kinds of diseases. Osteoporosis, osteopenia, scoliosis and osteomelasia are the main bone related diseases. The prevention of bone degeneration is the best cure for these diseases. Timely medical attention along with Yog and Pranayam can be helpful in prevention of bone degeneration. In some diseases bone density increases, while in other cases it depreciates. Weakness is caused in both conditions. Bone density increases in the following conditions:

- Osteoporosis: This is a hereditary condition, where calcification in bones increases and the chances of fragility increases.

- Osteopoikilosis: This is also a hereditary condition in which calcification spots appear at different places on the body.

- Secondary accumulation: Deposition of calcium due to some primary cause is seen in this condition.

- Myloseclerosis: The spine becomes stiff in this condition.

- Renal osteodystrophy: kidneys fail to maintain the proper levels of calcium and phosphorous in blood.

- Fluorosis: Drinking water containing high amount of fluoride increases bone density.

- Paget's disease: This is an old age disease, in which the bones swell, increase in size. Sometimes the big bones bend like bows and this condition could be fatal.

Depreciation of bone density is generally seen in the following conditions :

- Osteomalacia

- Deficiency of vitamins in food

- Stetorrhoea: Excessive secretion of sebaceous glands

- Poor kidney functioning

- Diseases of liver or pancreas

- Osteomalacia caused due to deficiency of vitamin D

- Deficiency of calcium in food.

A special test is done in order to detect the internal condition of bones. This is known as bone mineral density test. Different types of machines are used for this purpose. The central machine tests the hipbone, spine and bones of entire body to find out the bone mineral density. Peripheral machine detects the bone density in fingers, wrists, knees, calf bone, and ankle bone. This machine is considered to be effective and can measure the bone density of all the bones in the body. This is a simple test done with the X-rays technique. Wherein the body is subjected to mild radiation, which is not harmful. This test is done with bone densimeter machine, which operates on Dexa technique. WHO has recognized only Dexa technique for this purpose. The problem is detected through X-ray only after 30 per cent degeneration takes place.

The information obtained from bone density is useful for the physician to detect bone capacity. This test provides information about fragility of bones. Normal or low bone density increases the chances of bone degeneration. This information will be useful in preventing bone degeneration.

Bone mineral density test is also a simple, quick, painless and totally safe process. It reveals the calcium content in bones and also the factors endangering the bone degeneration. This test should be done in the following conditions:

- Those who have been detected with osteopenia or osteoporosis through X-ray.
- Menopause in women before 45 years and regular intake of estrogen hormone.
- Women in the age of 65 years or above.
- In case of bone degeneration after menopause.
- Family history of osteoporosis.
- People habituated to regular intake of steroids.
- Patients of excessive secretion of salivary glands, diabetes, liver and kidney diseases, joint pain, and arthritis.
- Vertebral disorder in spinal cord.

Prevention is the best treatment for diseases caused due to disorder of bone constitution. Calcium, vitamin D rich food, sunlight or sunbathing, Yog-Pranayam and exercise can be helpful in preventing bone related problems. These remedies are followed in the treatment as well. The importance of calcium and vitamin D cannot be explained exactly but it has been proved that Yog and Pranayam are very helpful in increasing bone mineral density and strengthening the bones.

Regular practice of Yog, and Pranayam are beneficial in increasing the bone mineral density and strengthening them. Clinical trial was conducted in the premises of Patanjali Yogpeeth under the guidance of Swami Ramdevji Maharaj and Orthopedic surgeon, Dr Akhilesh Gumasta of National Hospital (Orthopedic Department), Jabalpur.

Selection of patients

The patients of osteoporosis and osteopenia visiting the Out Patient Department of the hospital were screened for the purpose of studying the effect of Yog on bone mineral density. The patients were informed about all the aspects of the trial.

After the completion of different formalities, 128 patients were selected for the medical research. Out of which, 50 patients (18 males and 35 females) of osteoporosis and 78 patients (43 males and 35 females) of osteopenia were selected. Only non-Yog practitioners were selected for this purpose.

Treatment: All the selected patients were made to practise the complete package of seven asanas and Pranayam as popularised by revered Swami Ramdevji Maharaj. During Yog practice the patients were given a simple diet. The practise was carried on in the premises of Patanjali Yogpeeth under the guidance of qualified Yog teachers.

Classification of Patients on the basis of disease

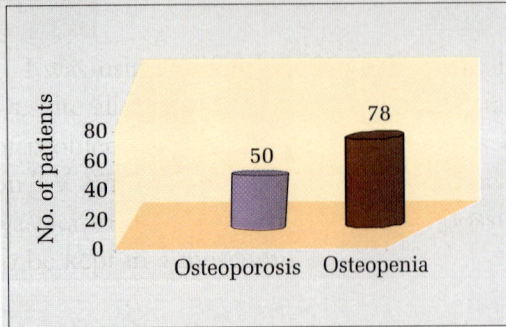

Classification of Patients on the basis of sex

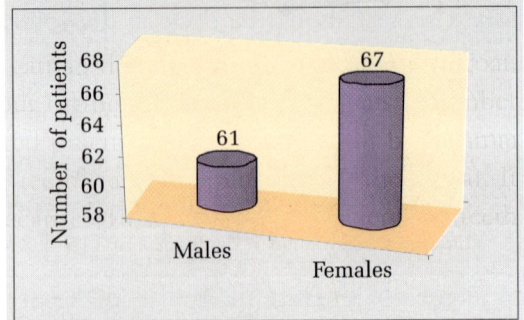

Classification of osteoporosis patients on the basis of sex

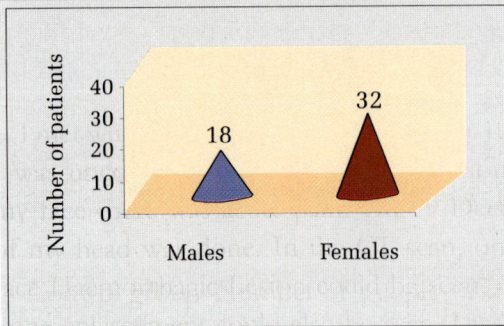

Classification of osteopenia patients according to sex

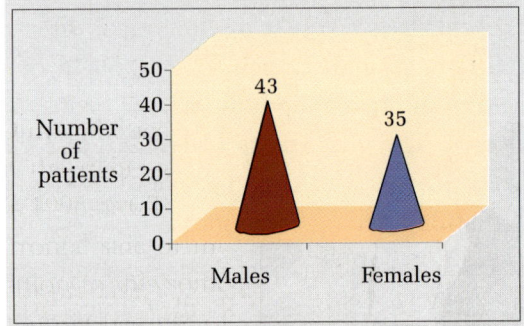

Tests: The bone mineral density was tested with the help of densimeter at the Bone and Skeleton Department of the hospital on 15 October, 2006 before beginning Yog treatment. The test was repeated after 40 days of Yog.

Classification of patients			Efficiency level	Confidence level
Osteoporosis	Males	18	4.240'	99.73
	Females	32	4.017'	99.73
Osteopenia	Males	43	4.67'	99.73
	Females	35	3.66'	99.73
Total		**128**	**5.77'**	**99.73**

Results : The data of bone mineral density test collected before and after Yog practice was analyzed statistically. The results were drawn with the theory of sign of nope-parametric test and efficiency level and confidence level of patients is being presented here in tabular form.

The efficiency and confidence level in (men) osteoporosis patients was 4.24 and 99.73 per cent respectively. The figures in case of women of the same disease were 4.017 and 99.73 per cent respectively. In the same way patients of osteopenia (men) showed efficiency and confidence level of 4.67 and 99.73 per cent, whereas the women showed of 3.66 and 99.73 per cent, respectively.

This research makes it clear that the T-score of bone mineral density shows considerable improvement along with increasing the strength of bone after 40 days of Yog practice.

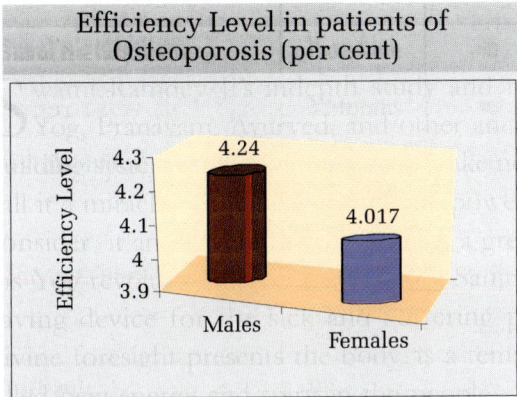

Efficiency Level in patients of Osteoporosis (per cent)

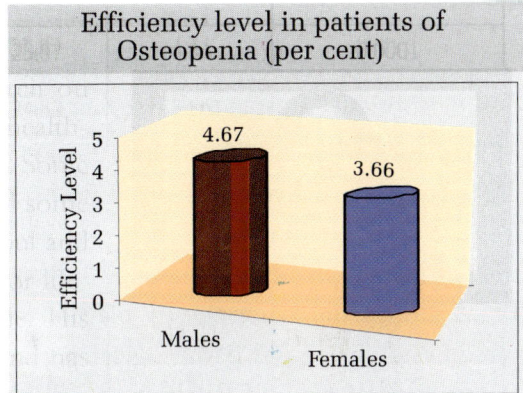

Efficiency level in patients of Osteopenia (per cent)

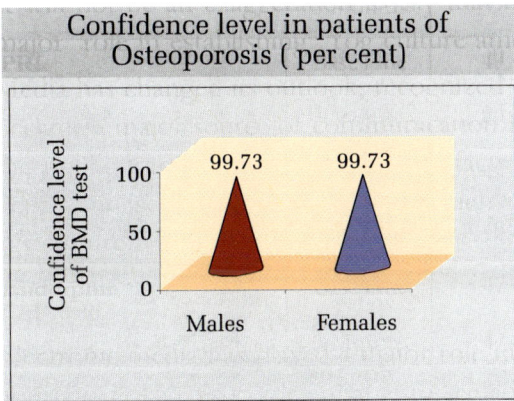

Confidence level in patients of Osteoporosis (per cent)

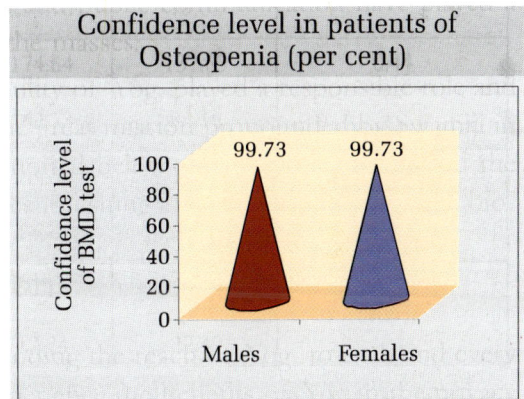

Confidence level in patients of Osteopenia (per cent)

Cautions: The number of osteoporosis, osteopenia and bone degeneration patients is increasing day-by-day. If these diseases are not treated on time they could lead to fracture. The women are more prone to this risk compared to men. Some of the reasons for these problems are irregular daily routine, lack of physical exercise, hormonal imbalance or excessive consumption of hormonal tablets, degeneration of bone cells or fragility. The present study has proved that Yog and Pranayam can prevent these diseases and also cure them. There is a need to prove the authenticity of Yog with continuous research and tests. There is no doubt about the fact that Yog and Pranayam are capable of curing different diseases.

Effect of Yog on Sports Medicine

The condition of Indian sports is not very encouraging excluding cricket. There are many reasons – lack of proper training, lack of self-confidence and unwillingness from government. Swami Ramdevji Maharaj looking into the discouraging condition of football has appealed the Indian Football Federation to send the junior players to his Ashram. Swamiji invited junior football team of Mohan Bagan athletic club as a part of this effort so that they can be trained in Yog and Pranayam. After the training the team played World Cup (junior football) during the first week of August at Manchester, UK. This team represented India and its performance was encouraging.

The players were given in-depth training in Yog and Pranayam for seven days at Patanjali Yogpeeth for building self-confidence and complete personality development. They were trained in two sessions conducted in the morning and evening. The effect of Yog and Pranayam on the efficiency of players was studied scientifically. The test included various physiological and pathological parameters. The medical test was concluded under the rules of ICH – GCP, which included various equipments like body and fat analyzer, PFT, TMT, centrifuge automated Hematology Analyzer, Manual Hematology Analyzer, Blood Gas Analyzer, XL-600, Fully Automatic Biochemistry Analyzer etc.

Dr Vishwajeet Mukherjee, Dr. R. S. Gaur and other scientists worked in this team under the leadership of revered Swamiji and Acharya Balkrishna.

Background

When a person takes part in a sport or competition the systematic respiratory process affects the performance. Deep and long breathing helps in concentration and overcoming performance anxiety.

Yog and Pranayam controls the respiratory process. They can contribute positively in improving performance. The two ancient health-building systems can become ideal training for the players. Regular practice of Yog and Pranayam reduces stress and increases flexibility. Pranayam can play an important role in balancing exercises and almost all games. Pranayam can overcome mental and physical imbalance.

Different experiments like physical exercise, diet and regimen have proved that they control lipid content in body and generate energy and vigour. The tests done on patients of chest pain and blockage in arteries showed significant effect in lipid profile. Another test done on patients of high blood pressure showed that Yog and Pranayam are highly effective in controlling heart diseases. The same results were shown in another test. Our initial studies show positive effect on different parameters of heart and lungs functioning and bone metabolism.

Another study showed that Yog and Pranayam were effective in controlling body mass, BMI etc. Therefore, Yog and Pranayam cure diseases and also play a positive role in improving performance and efficiency level.

Objective: To study the effect of Yog and Pranayam on efficiency and performance of players along with physiological, pathological and neurological changes.

Equipment and Method:

1. **Primary and secondary parameters:** The following parameters were included in the analysis of effects on efficiency, strength and performance of players.

   - Improvement in first second in pulse rate, blood pressure, weight, BMI, TMT, fat %, FVC and FEV1.

   - Improvement in total blood profile, haemoglobin percentage, liver function test, kidney function and lipid profile.

   - Any other ill effect (if any).

2. **Type of study :** Open level trial.

3. **Methods for reducing or controlling voice**: Non-randomized observational study

4. **Selection of players:** Healthy football players below the age of 15 years were included in the study. Players habituated to smoking and alcohol were not included in the study.

5. **Practice of Yog and Pranayam:** All the participants were made to practise Yog and Pranayam from 8 to 13 July 2006. The morning session was held from 5.30 to 6.30 AM and the evening session from 6.30 to 7.30 PM. The players were given balanced food along with the practice and were made to follow regimen. They were not allowed to take any medicine during the training period to avoid serious consequence. The Yog and Pranayam training of all the participants was strictly supervised.

6. **Determination of efficiency:** The following parameters were included to determine efficiency:

Physiological parameters

- Pulse rate
- Body mass index
- FVC
- Blood pressure
- BMI
- FEV1

Pathological parameters

- Complete blood picture

- Hb %
- Blood sugar
- Lipid profile
- Renal function test
- Liver function test

7. **Determination of security:** All the parameters suitable for determining feeling of security in players were used in the study. The players were not exposed to any kind of insecurity and special care was taken with respect to diet.

8. **Statistics:** The data was presented on the basis of Mean +- SD (Standard Deviation) in order to determine the results.

Tests and results: The demographic pattern of age, height, weight of all the players is being presented in tabular form.

Positive results were seen on body weight, BMI, fat per cent, maximum pulse etc. and other parameters during the seven-day Yog and Pranayam session. There was significant improvement in FVC and FEV1 level. In the same way, there was a significant change in lipid profile parameters like total cholesterol, HDL, LDL, triglycerides, VLDL etc. The changes in parameters of liver function test are also being presented in tabular form.

Average Change in Physiological Standards

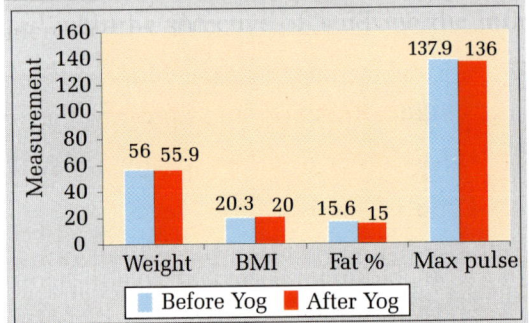

Parameter	Before Yog	After Yog
Weight	56 ± 5.4	55.53
BMI	20 ± 1.6	20 ± 1.5
Fat (per cent)	15.6 ± 4.1	15.2 ± 4
Max pulse	137.9 ± 7.3	136 ± 7.4

Physical Data taken Before Yog practice

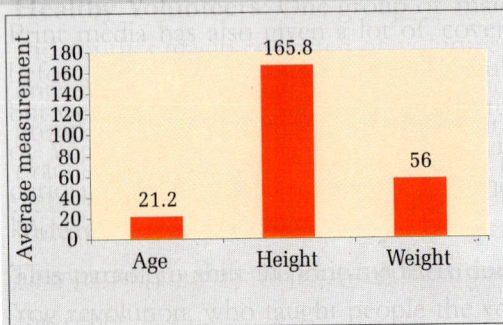

Average Change in Physiological Standards

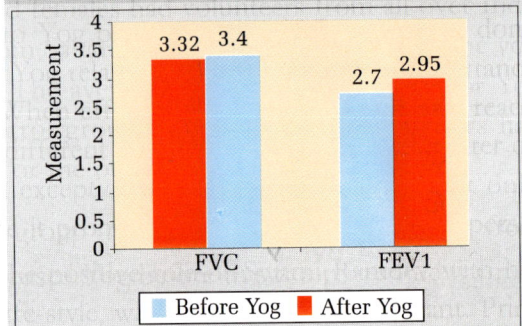

Physical data taken before Yog practice			
	Age	Height (cm)	Weight (kg)
Males (N±25)	21.2 ± 10.48	165.8 ± 3.66	56 ± 5.48

	Before Yog	After Yog
FVC	3.32 ± .4	3.35 ± .27
FCVI	2.73 ± .47	2.95 ± .3

Parameter	Before	After
Cholesterol	154.9 ± 24.2	126.8 ± 19.7
HDL	50.5 ± 8.5	46.6 ± 6.3
LDL	88.3 ± 16.9	73 ± 14
Triglycerides	129.8 ± 46.4	85.08 ± 35.31
VLDL	19.8 ± 7.1	13 ± 5.4

Average Change in Physiological Measurements

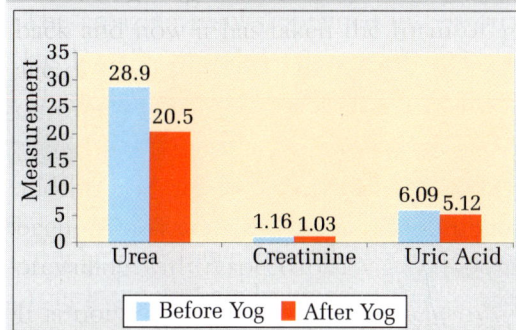

Average Changes in Pathological Standards

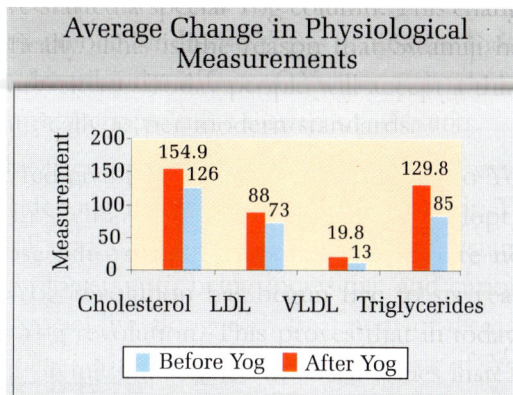

Parameter	Before Yog	After Yog
Urea	28.9 ± 5.6	20.54 ± 4.52
Creatinine	1.16 ± 0.9	1.03 ± .1
Uric acid	6.09 ± 0.8	5.12 ± .86

Parameter	Before	After
Bil-T	1.27 ± .78	1 ± .55
Bil-D	.527 ± 2.2	.486 ± .21
Bil-ID	.75 ± .53	.51 ± .35
A. Phos	183.81 ± 77.6	183.9 ± 75.1
SGOT	42.3 ± 6.51	34 ± 7
SGPT	24.94 ± 10.97	25 ± 10.6
Protein	8.678 ± .32	7.98 ± .33
Albumin	4.48 ± 1.15	4.25 ± .154
Globulin	4.22 ± .35	3.73 ± .31

Average Changes in Pathological Standards

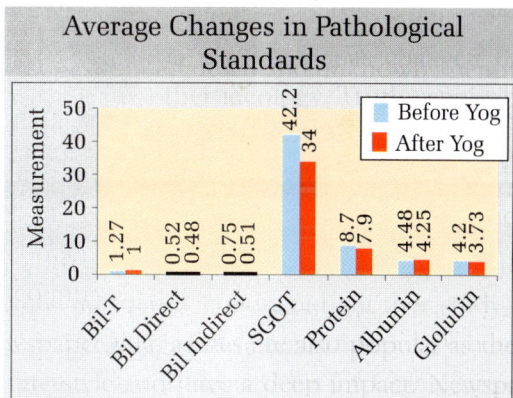

Conclusion

The positive effect of Yog, Pranayam and balanced diet on obesity, liver function, kidney function, blood lipid profile, heart arteries disorder etc. were proved. The positive effect of Yog and Pranayam on weight, body mass index, fat percent, maximum pulse, pulmonary function test, lipid profile, renal function test and liver function test in the present study can be clearly seen.

The present study has proved that Yog and Pranayam: (i) are significant for improving efficiency, strength and performance of players; (ii) are capable of curing obesity and related diseases; (iii) contribute in improving pulmonary function, which controls diseases related to respiratory system completely; (iv) Are helpful in controlling blood cholesterol, triglycerides and other levels, which cures heart and related diseases; (v) increase the liver function, which cures digestion and liver diseases; and (vi) are helpful in controlling renal function test parameters like blood urea, creatinine and uric acid level, which proves that Yog and Pranayam are helpful in the treatment of kidney, urinary disease and gout.

Hence Yog and Pranayam can be used in different ways.

Revered Swami Ramdevji Maharaj presented the health kit to Indian junior football team in the form of Yog and Pranayam. Children below the age of 15 years were trained for a brief Yog and Pranayam course for proper physical, mental and spiritual development. The players were given balanced and simple food during the training period. The performance chart was prepared for each student under the directions of experienced Yog teachers, medical practitioners and scientists.

Complete physical and pathological check-up was done before and after the Yog training. The results were very encouraging. Divya Yog Mandir Trust has started a mission to relieve physical and mental stresses through Yog and Pranayam instead of stress killers that are generally used by international teams. This will take us forward on the path of establishing Indian culture and science at the international level. We have been able to develop concentration, energy and vigour in players through regular practice of Yog and Pranayam.

Yog Science Camps in UK

Millions of people from all over the world are supporting Swami Ramdevji Maharaj whole-heartedly in his mission for establishing Indian scientific based systems and moral values at international level. They are extending full support and are determined to accomplish the mission. Thousands of people are contributing in this multidimensional Yog revolution from not only India but also abroad. Swamiji is proving the scientific basis of Yog at various levels. This mission caught momentum when the scientific analysis of Yog was conducted during Swamiji's session in England. This was the first instance when a Yog session was organized outside country as a part of mission of 'Healthy World'. Non-resident Indians, Britishers and people from other countries belonging to different castes, religions and communities came in large numbers to participate in the sessions organized at Elembridge, Lester, Bolton and Middlesex (London) and reaped the benefits of Yog. The participants took a resolution to adopt Indian food, practise Yog and teach Yog to others. The seven-day sessions organized in different cities also offered facilities for medical

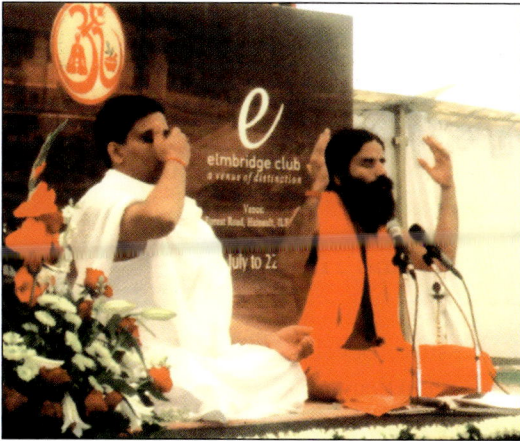

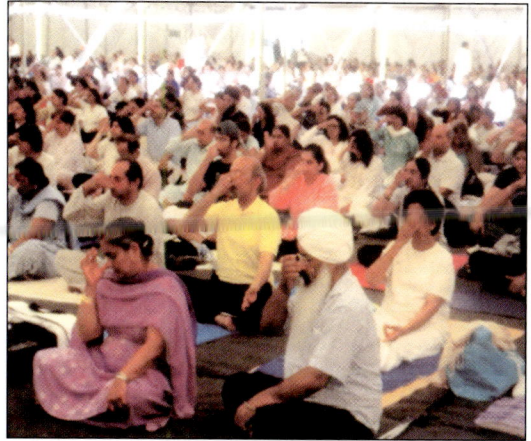

Acharya Balkrishnaji along with Swami Ramdevji Maharaj training the practitioners in a Yog session in UK

check-ups. Positive results were obtained in the tests conducted for blood pressure, sugar level, cholesterol etc. before and after the camp.

Members of Medical Advisory Team (UK)

A medical advisory team was appointed in August 2006 under the guidance of Swami Ramdevji and Acharya Balkrishna Ji. This team studied the effect of Yog and Pranayam on main diseases like hypertension, obesity, blood sugar, asthma and different types of allergies. The report of the study was published in different reputed medical journals. The team consisted of the following members:

- Dr Raman Gokul, MBCHB, MD, FRCFASN (Chairman)

- Consultant Nephrologist and Prof. Medicine University, Manchester, UK

- Dr Nilesh Samani, BSc, MD, FRCPFCC, FMED, MCI, BHF

- Prof. Cardiology and Main Department, Cardiovascular Science Department, Leicester University, U.K

- Dr Pratibha Dutta, MBBS, MPH, MSc, FFPHM
  Director, Public Health, Red Bridge Primary Care Trust, Alfred Essex, UK

- Srishti Damari, SRN

- Clinical Nurse Specialist Palliative and Cancer Care
  Nurse Manager, Mary Curie Palliative Care Unit, London, UK

  ◆   Dr Hemant Kumar, MBBS, MBE
      General Practitioner, Bharani Medical Center, Slog, UK

In UK some of the main health problems are :

Obesity, diabetes, high blood pressure, heart disease, respiratory and related diseases, depression, stress, mental tension, cancer, Arthritis etc.

Yog camps conducted at Alford, Leicester, Bolton and Horo in United Kingdom adopted following medical standards:

Various medical tests for diabetes, high blood pressure, obesity and, lipid profile were done after taking written consent from the volunteers participating in Yog science session.

Different tests were done before the Yog session and after 6-7 days of session.

Body weight, height, blood pressure, blood sugar and serum cholesterol of 428 volunteers suffering from above mentioned diseases were tested before and after the Yog session. Around 510 volunteers took part in   the beginning of the session, out of which 82 people did not turn out for second test.

Average Weight of all the Volunteers Before and After 6-7 days of Yog Sessions

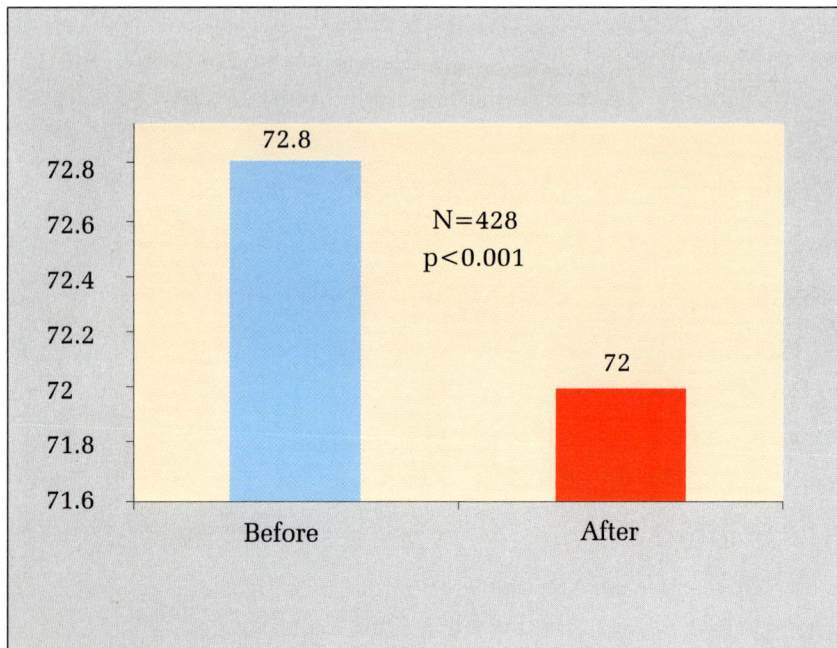

Bar chart showing average weight Before = 72.8 and After = 72, with N=428, p<0.001. Y-axis labelled from 71.6 to 72.8.

Average Body Mass of all Volunteers Before Camp and After 6-7 days of Yog Sessions

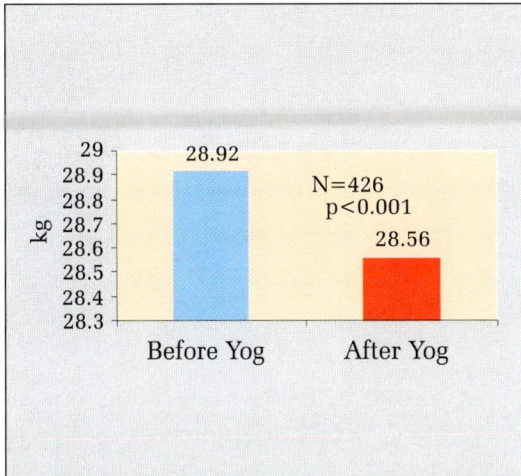

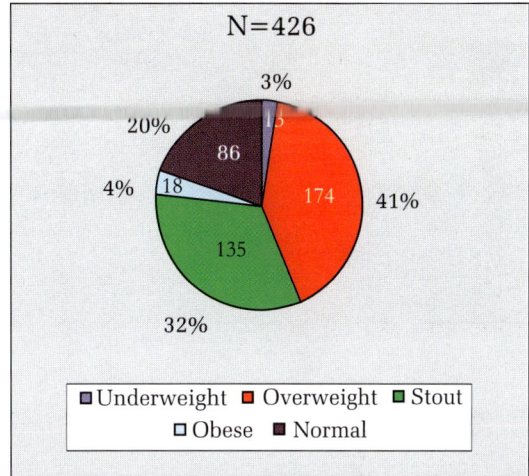

Average Body Mass (Standard Deviation) of all volunteers Before Camp and After 6-7 days of Yog Sessions

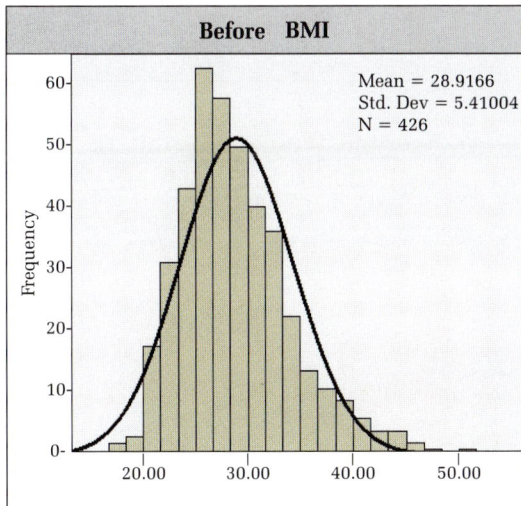

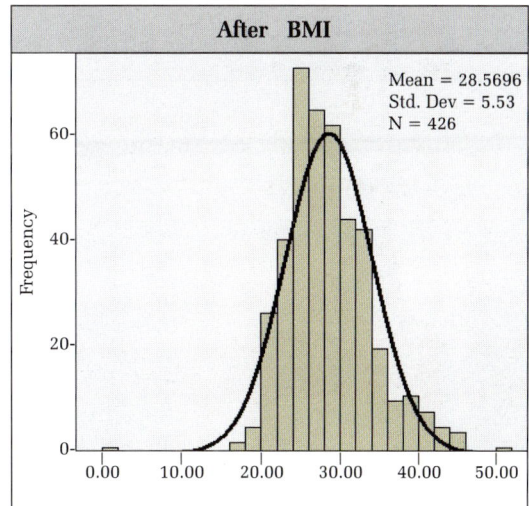

Change in Average Body Mass Index in various groups after 6-7 days of camp

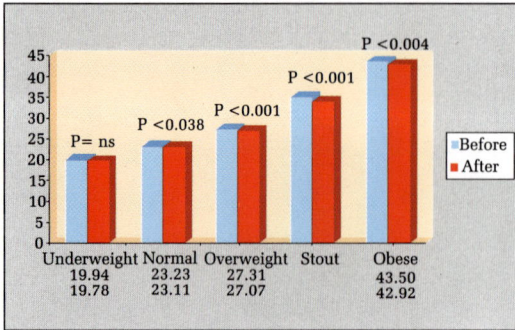

Change in Body Mass Index– Underweight Standards

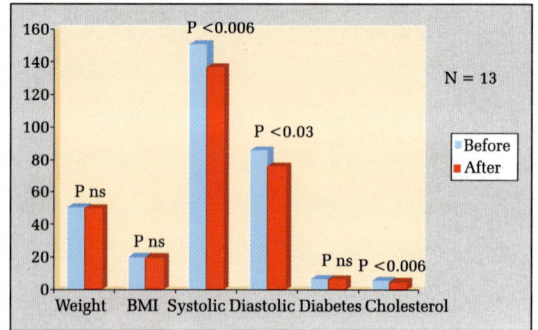

Change in Body Mass Index– Normal Standards

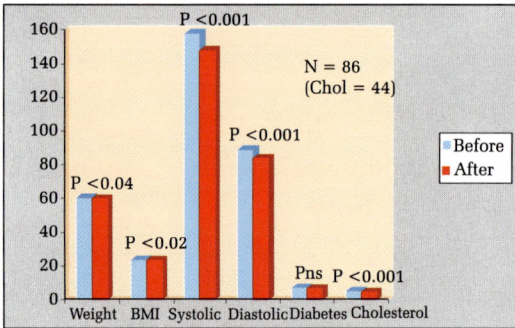

Change in Body Mass Index– Stout Standards

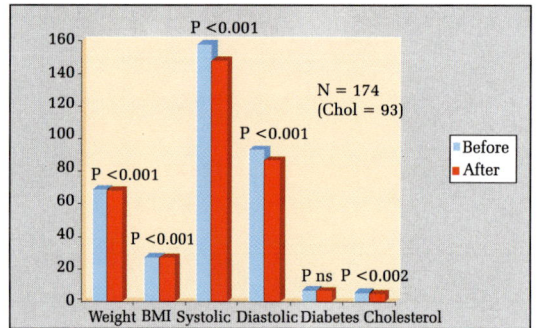

Change in Body Mass Index– Overweight Standards

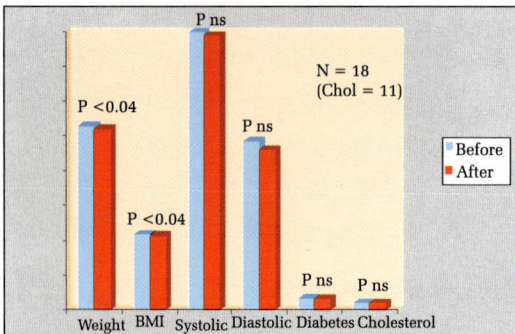

Average Weight Loss in all participants After the camp

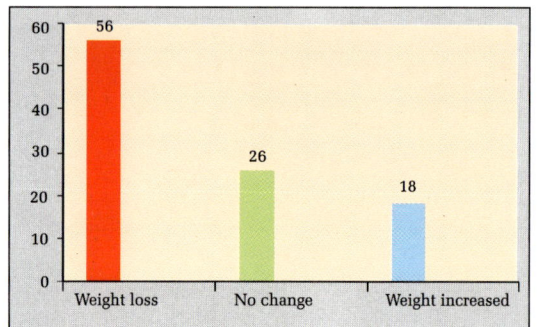

42% lost >2kg (100 out of 238),
Maximum weight loss = 9.5 kg

Avergare Blood Pressure in all participants during 6-7days of Yog Practice

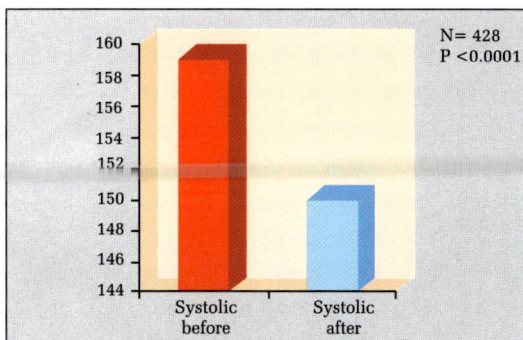

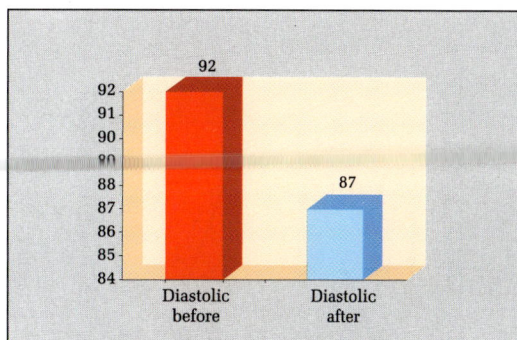

Average change in Sugar Level in all participants during 6-7 days of Yog Practice

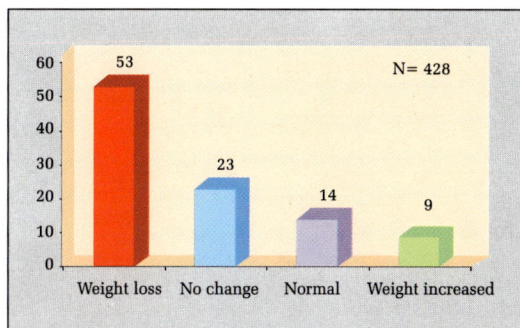

Average Blood Pressure (Standard Deviation) in all participants during 6-7 days of Yog practice

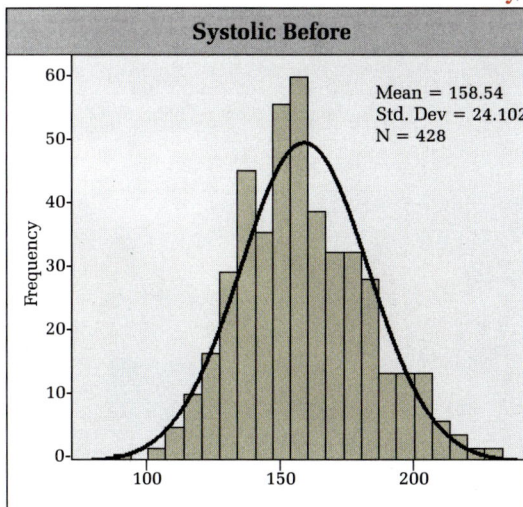

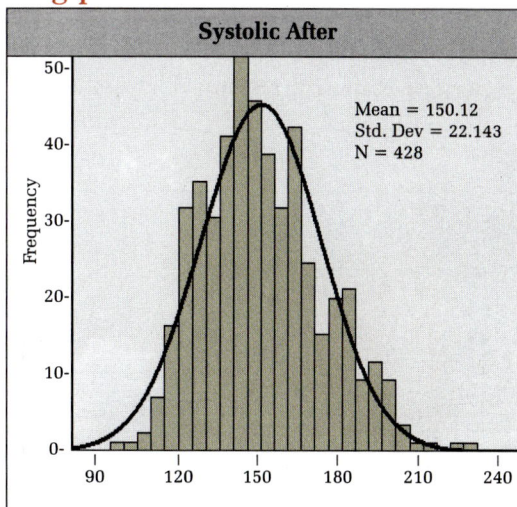

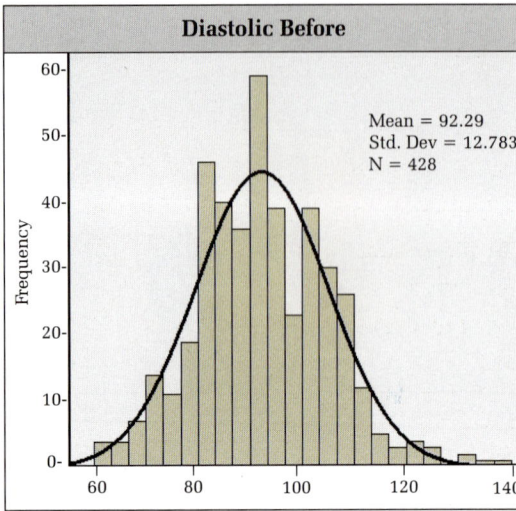

Diastolic Before

Mean = 92.29
Std. Dev = 12.783
N = 428

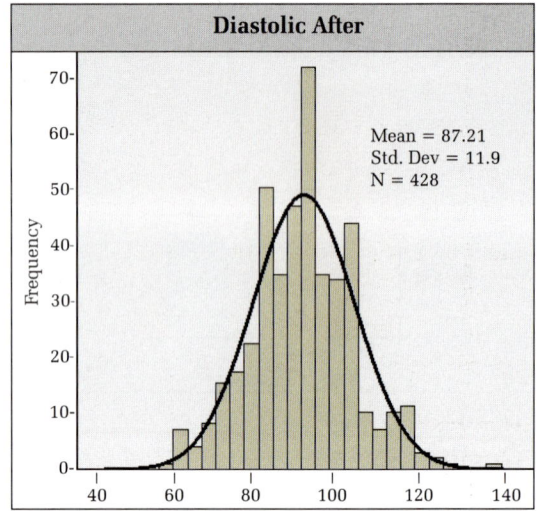

Diastolic After

Mean = 87.21
Std. Dev = 11.9
N = 428

Average Changes in Sugar Level of all participants during 6-7 days of Yog practice

Average Sugar Level in all participants during 6-7 days of Yog Practice

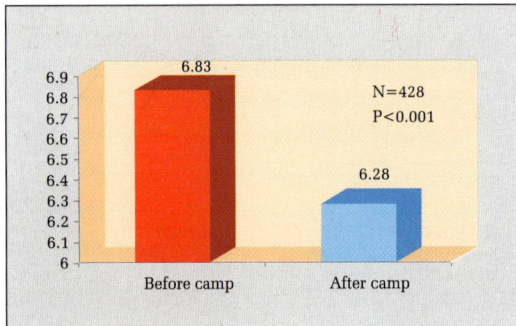

6.83   N=428
          P<0.001
6.28

Before camp   After camp

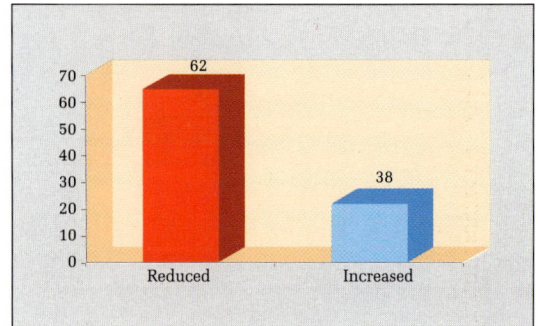

62
          38

Reduced   Increased

Average change in blood cholesterol level in all participants during 6-7 days of Yog practice

Average blood cholesterol level in all participants during 6-7 days of Yog practice

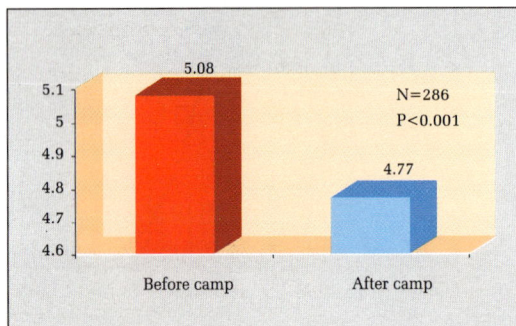

5.08   N=286
          P<0.001
4.77

Before camp   After camp

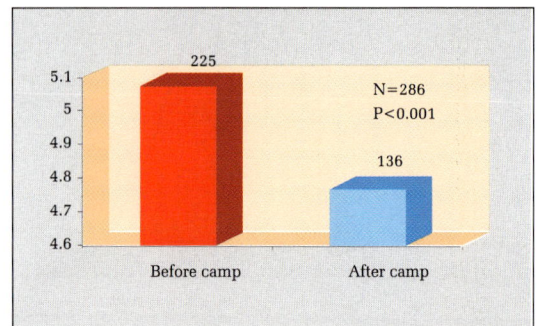

225   N=286
          P<0.001
136

Before camp   After camp

Study of Psychosomatic effects of Yog/Pranayam on Participants in Yog science Camps in UK

A large-scale public survey was conducted in UK to study the psychosomatic effect of Yog and Pranayam in people. People of all age groups, castes, communities, class and religion gave overwhelming response. All the participants were given a questionnaire and data was compiled on the basis of feedback given pertaining to general perceptions about Yog and Pranayam. This survey made it clear that Yog and Pranayam are the need of the hour. The participants reaped benefits with the practice of Yog and Pranayam. They got mental, spiritual, intellectual, personal and general benefits along with physical benefits.

The classification of participants on the basis of sex, education, age group, occupation, life-style and economic status has been described below through pie chart.

Pie chart representing Yog awareness and practice

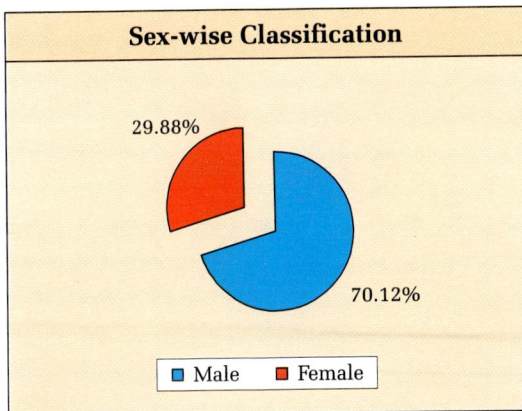

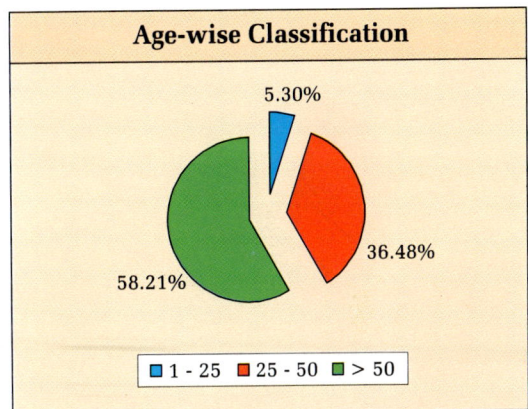

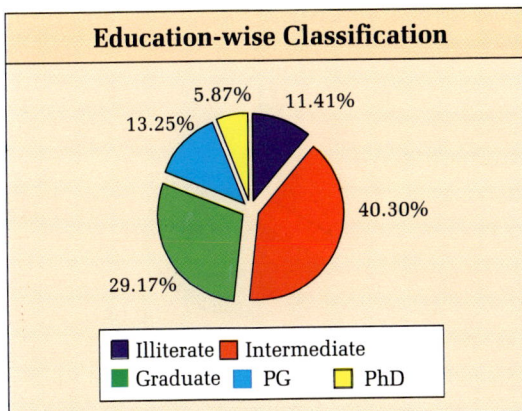

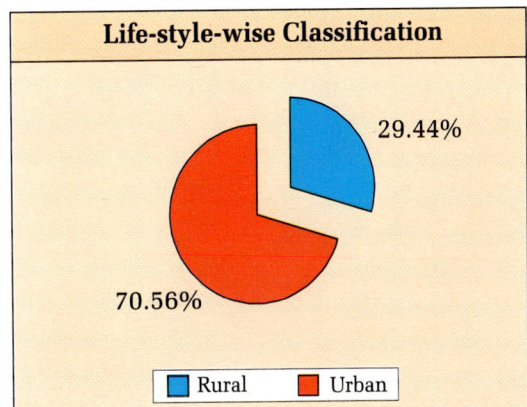

Sex-wise Classification

29.88%

70.12%

■ Male   ■ Female

Age-wise Classification

5.30%

36.48%

58.21%

■ 1 - 25   ■ 25 - 50   ■ > 50

Education-wise Classification

5.87%   11.41%

13.25%

40.30%

29.17%

■ Illiterate ■ Intermediate
■ Graduate ■ PG ■ PhD

Life-style-wise Classification

29.44%

70.56%

■ Rural   ■ Urban

Income- based Classification

5.64%

36.82%

57.55%

Legend: High | Medium | Low

Yog Awareness

9.39%   2.15%

25.24%

50.17%

13.05%

Legend: Not told | TV | Residential Camps | Non Residential Camps | Other

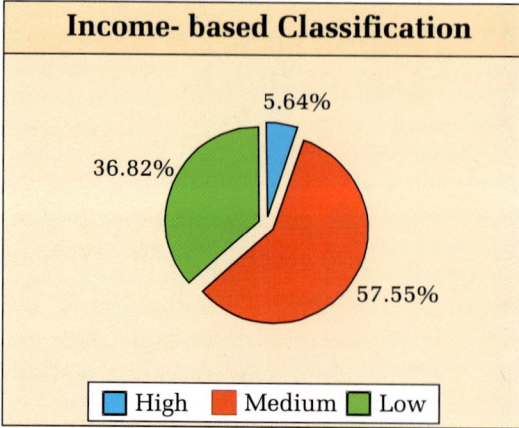

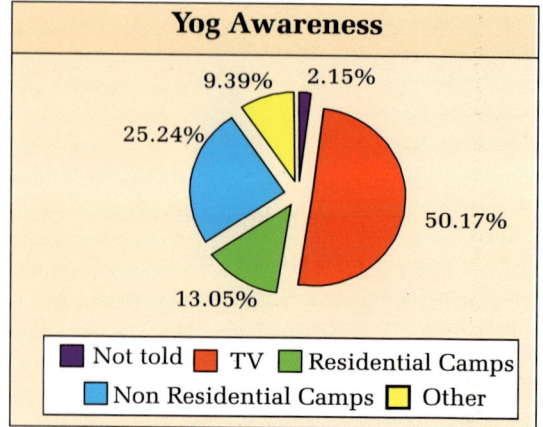

Survey indicates that the participants gained considerably in weight, blood pressure, joint pain, diabetes, liver disorder, heart disease, asthma and other problems. The pie chart representation shows the percentage gain in various diseases.

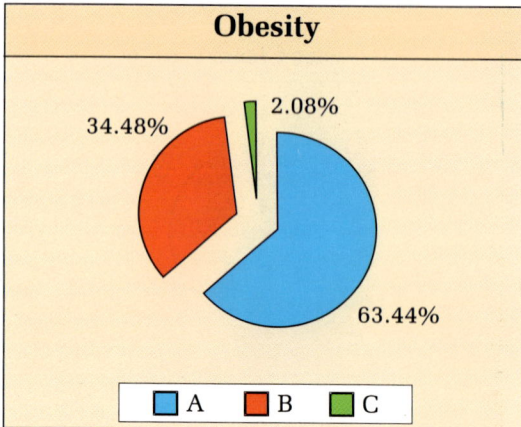

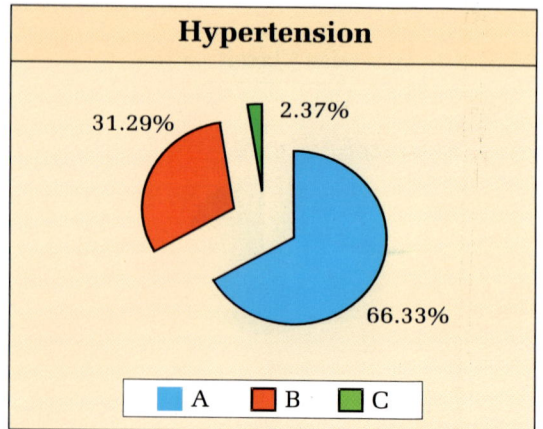

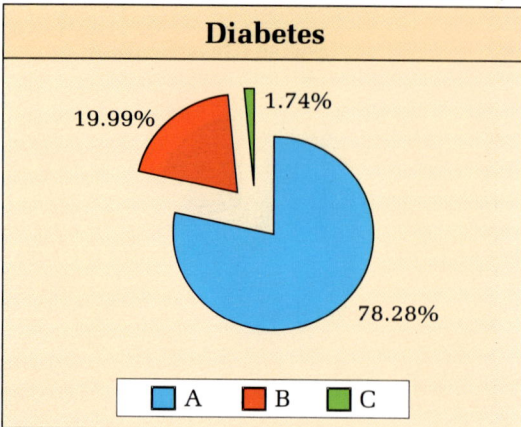

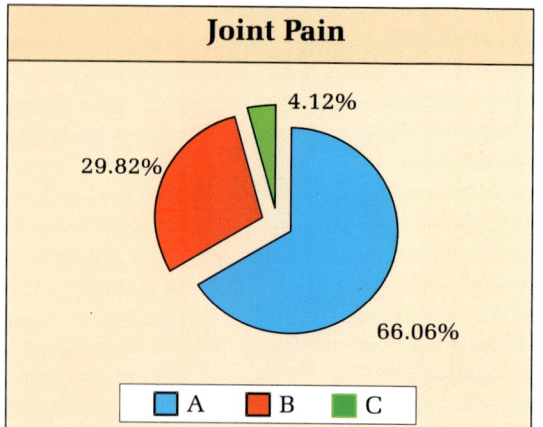

Obesity

2.08%

34.48%

63.44%

Legend: A | B | C

Hypertension

2.37%

31.29%

66.33%

Legend: A | B | C

Diabetes

1.74%

19.99%

78.28%

Legend: A | B | C

Joint Pain

4.12%

29.82%

66.06%

Legend: A | B | C

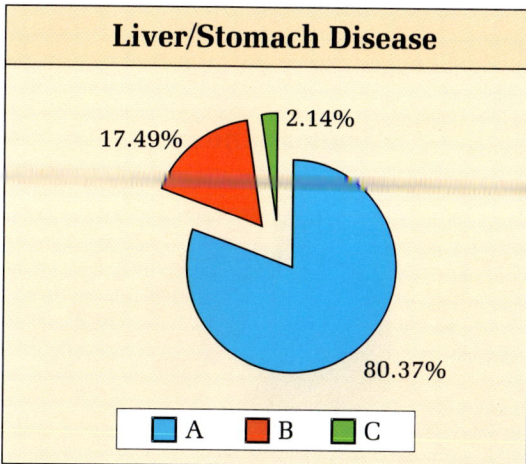

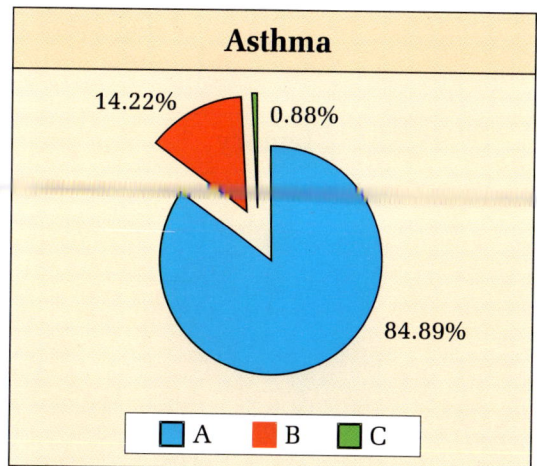

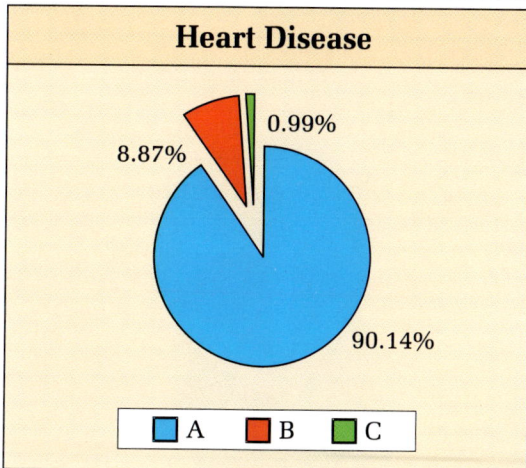

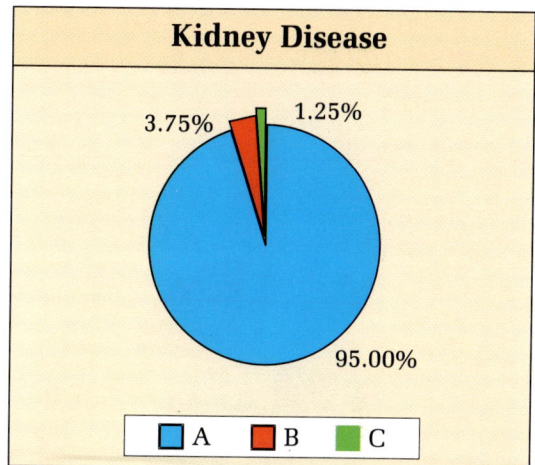

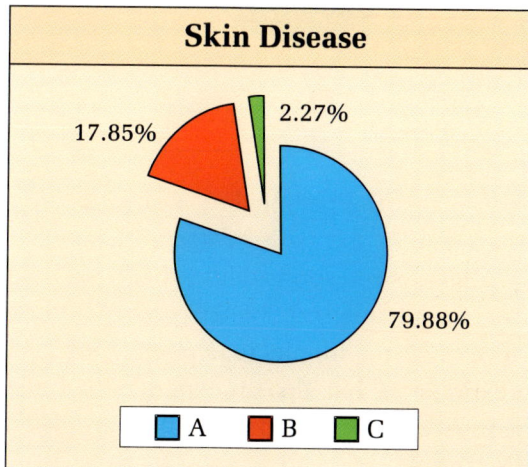

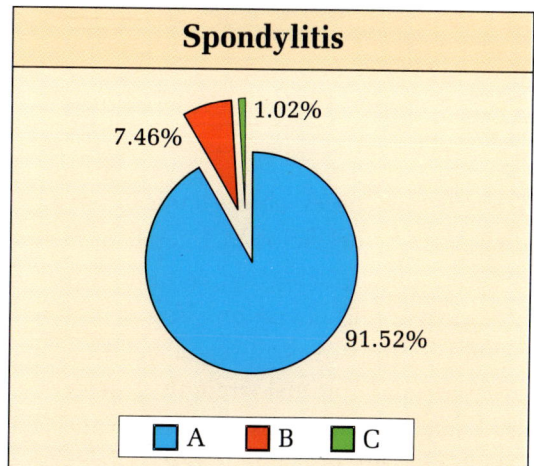

Liver/Stomach Disease

17.49% 2.14%

80.37%

A B C

Asthma

14.22% 0.88%

84.89%

A B C

Heart Disease

8.87% 0.99%

90.14%

A B C

Kidney Disease

3.75% 1.25%

95.00%

A B C

Skin Disease

17.85% 2.27%

79.88%

A B C

Spondylitis

7.46% 1.02%

91.52%

A B C

A : No disease   **B : Improvement / Totally cured**   **C : Increased**

Significant change in mental stress, memory, attitude, social relations, respect to elders and others along with physical gain in participants

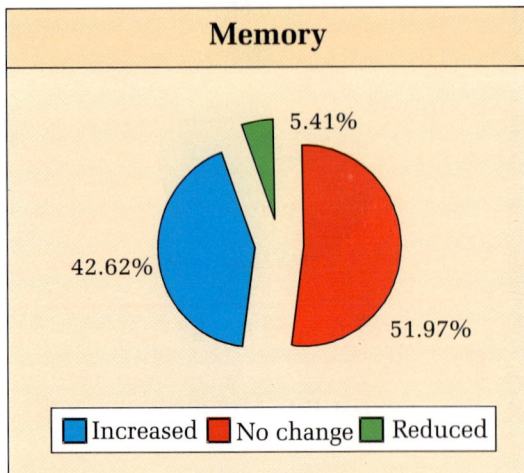

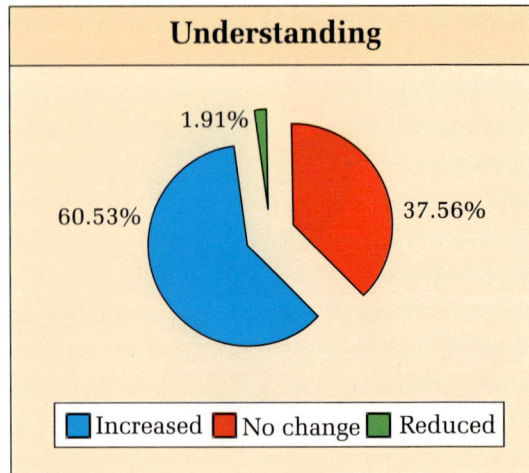

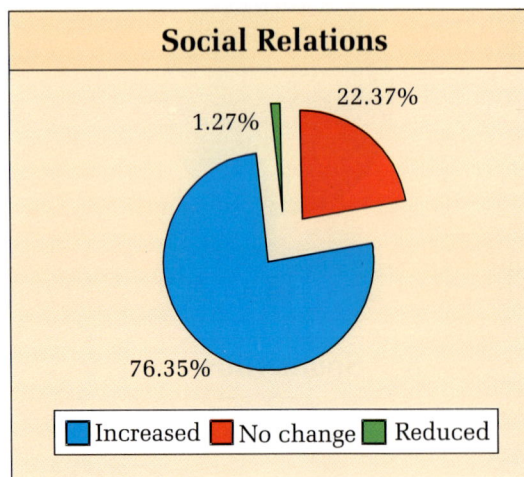

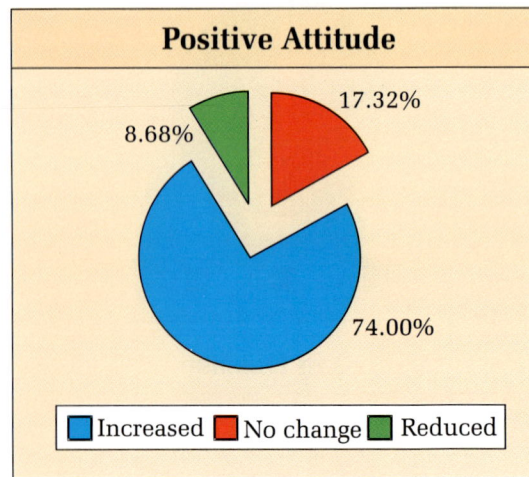

Memory

5.41%
42.62%
51.97%

Increased | No change | Reduced

Understanding

1.91%
60.53%
37.56%

Increased | No change | Reduced

Social Relations

22.37%
1.27%
76.35%

Increased | No change | Reduced

Positive Attitude

17.32%
8.68%
74.00%

Increased | No change | Reduced

The present survey clearly indicates that Yog rejuvenates the personality, it acts like life-saving medicine, helps in overall development, guides on the path of accomplishment, fulfilling duties, achieving economic progress, fulfilling the responsibilities of household life and gaining liberation. Yog is a holistic science and fully capable of giving desired results. It improves physical health, mental development, intellectual power, internal progress, and spiritual strength. It is not just an expression, but also an experience of life, as shared by thousands of participants. The scientists and medical practitioners are taken aback with the miraculous results of Yog and Pranayam.

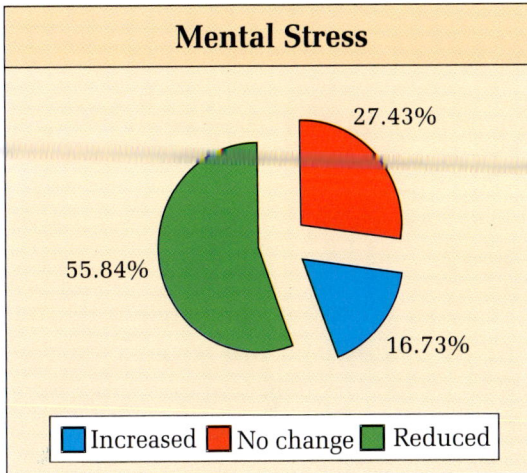

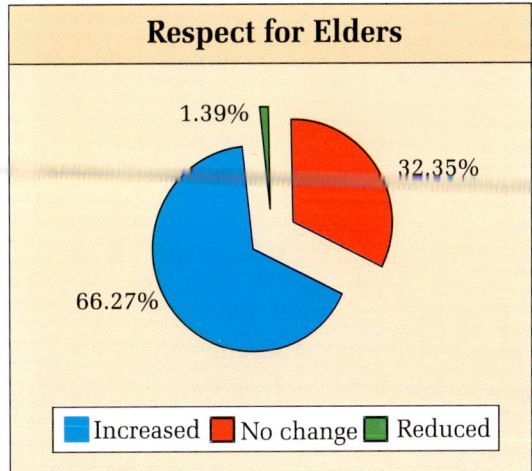

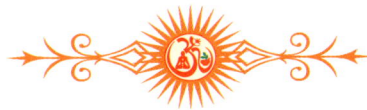

Chapter 6

STRESS : ORIGIN, CAUSE AND EFFECT

Stress the Main Cause of All Diseases

The post-industrial revolution period in India and abroad has brought along with it lot of social and economic changes at a very fast rate. Before industrial revolution a large percentage of the population used to live in rural areas and was dependent on agriculture. In those days, joint families was a tradition that was followed by all the people and they had their own legal system and social structure to lead that kind of life-style. Industrial revolution was brought in by the West and it took around a century to reach India. However, this change had some negative impact as well, which could be clearly seen on the social and economic structure of the society. The small rural areas converted into suburban areas and cities and major cities turned into metropolitan cities. The poor and unskilled rural folk took shelter in big cities and joined the labour workforce. They did not have any other alternative and were forced to do so for the sake of livelihood. Their economic condition was extremely weak with additional responsibilities often in the form of loans. They migrated to cities and worked in mills and factories and began to contribute as the major workforce of India. The migration from rural to urban areas became the order of the day and this also reduced the size of family. The joint family system was disappearing gradually. It paved way for small or nuclear family concept, which consisted of parents and their children.

This social change caused due to industrial revolution is the main reason for stress because living in a nuclear family in the city was very different than living in free environment in villages. The family members lacked the moral and economic support, which they used to get in joint families despite its disadvantages. The emotional security vanished completely amidst busy city life. Whenever the family member suffered from some emotional crisis it did not have the security and shield of joint family. Besides emotional insecurity the industrial revolution also saw the impact of increasing diseases due to fast rate of population growth. The resources were limited but the population was increasing. In the absence of resources and urbanization people were forced to live in unhygienic and dirty places. Many members of the family were forced to live in small dwellings leading to emotional suffocation. All these negative conditions gave rise to insecurity and people started getting into vices and addictions.

If we look back through the pages of Indian history we see that our country was under the foreign rule for more than 500 years and has not been able to come out of its clutches till now. All these factors had serious impact on Indian traditions, its culture and heritage. The stronger side of its life, the spiritual approach to life was neglected and people were cut off from their roots. Indian religious traditions and its spritual strength was very effective in tackling with the personal, economic and emotional problems. The later half of the 19th century saw the spiritual renaissance when Swami Dayanand, Swami Vivekananda Ji and others brought in social and cultural revolution and aroused spirituality among the people. Other sages and seers moved the revolution forward in the first half of the 20th century. However, it took time to show the real impact.

On one hand the common Indian felt insecure and weak due to the destruction of ancient social and economic structures, desire to lead luxurious life, industrial revolution, preference for micro or nuclear family system and migration of rural population to urban areas. On the other hand the deficiency of spiritual strength, complexities of societies and lack of economic and emotional support led to mental stress. In the 19th and 20th centuries, larger number of deaths were caused due to infections and in the later half of the 20th century this number reduced owing to advances made during industrial revolution.Now in the 20th century greater number of people are suffering from stress-related diseases such as:

- ◆ Hypertension
- ◆ Diabetes
- ◆ Obesity
- ◆ Heart disease
- ◆ Stomach problems
- ◆ Irregularities in cholesterol level

A Brief Description of Nervous System and Brain

The human brain is different from other creatures due to its thinking and reasoning power. The human brain does a lot of creative work and stress is a part of thinking process. Why does stress take place? Before understanding the reason it is necessary to understand the constitution of human nervous system, brain and it's functioning. The human brain has many parts, some of which are directly related to stress. They are as follows:

Cerebral cortex

This part of the brain performs the functions of logical analysis, thinking and imagination.

Limbic System

Limbic system is a group of complex structures and systems, which is situated on both sides of the thalamus and below the cerebrum. Hypothalamus, hippocampus, amygdala and other systems are attached with the brain. This is primarily important for our emotional nature and plays an important role in retaining our memory. The figure shows one half of the brain, but the brain stem is joined with it. The limbic system is the part, which is lying on the left side of the thalamus, and thalamus is in turn situated in front of the hypothalamus.

Hypothalamus

It is a small part of the brain, which is situated on both sides of the third ventricle of thalamus. It is situated in ventricles of cerebrum, which is full of cerebrospinal fluid. This is attached with fluid of spine and is just above the pituitary gland and in the middle of optic nerves. Hypothalamus is the most active part of the brain and is related to h o m e o s t a s i s . Homeostasis is the process of sending back something to a fixed point. It works like a thermostat. For example, when our room gets over cooled, the thermostat informs the furnace and it starts heating the room and when the room becomes hot and crosses a particular temperature, then the thermostat sends signals to furnace to stop the function of the furnace.

A Cross-sectional view of the brain, ventricles, spinal cord and meninges

Hypothalamus is responsible for hunger, thirst, reaction for pain, happiness and other desires like sex, anger or aggressiveness etc. It also controls the sympathetic and parasympathetic nervous system, which means it regulates pulse rate, blood pressure, respiration and emotional reactions.

It gets inputs from different sources and Vagas nerve gives information regarding swelling of stomach and blood pressure. It gets information of rising body temperature from brain stem due to reticular formation. It gets information about darkness and light from the nerve. Innumerable neurons spread in ventricles give the information about important elements of cerebrospinal fluids or toxins, which are responsible for vomiting. It also gets messages from limbic system and from other parts of olfactory nervous systems, which control hunger and lust.

Hypothalamus contains certain receptors, which give information about blood temperature.

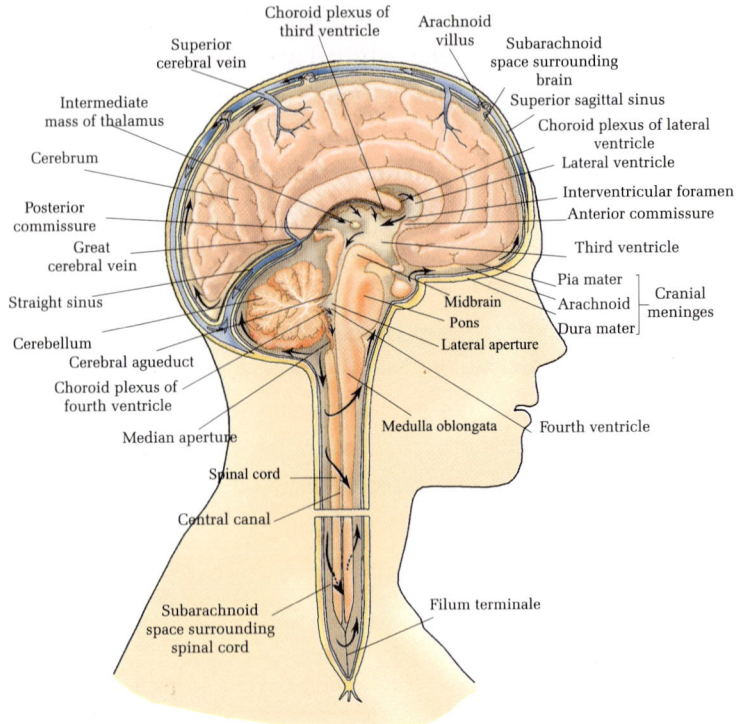

According to a recent invention, it was found that lepton protein is produced from lepton fat cell. When we eat in excess, hypothalamus recognises different aspects of hypothalamus blood and makes it active. Lepton reduces our hunger. In some people this secretion is more due to genetic reasons and the hypothalamus does not get the information that they are eating more. Whereas in many obese people this change is not seen, therefore, a lot of research needs to be done in this area.

Hypothalamus sends information to other parts of the body in two ways; they are automatic nervous system and pituitary gland. The former gives permission to hypothalamus to control and regulate blood pressure, heart rate, respiration, digestion, perspiration and other functions of sympathetic and parasympathetic system.

The latter controls the hypothalamus. It is attached with the pituitary gland through nerves and other chemicals, which arouse the hormones. As we all are aware pituitary is considered to be the master gland and regulates all the hormone development and metabolism.

Stress + Negative Thinking
Stimulates Limbic - Hypothalamus System in brain
↑ Stress + Negative Thinking
Symptoms of Disease
Change in Stress with Yog, Pranayam, Meditation, Diet
Stress + with Yog and Pranayam
Regulates Limbic Hypothalamus System LPHA Normalizes
↓ Stress Hormones
HOMEOSTATIS (All the body functions revert to normal state)

Hippocampus

Hippocampus has two types of hormones, which extend till amygdala and turns back. It is very useful in converting data or information present in the brain, which helps us in retaining the required information for a longer time. When this part gets damaged the human being cannot remember anything and lives in his own world. Whatever he experiences in the new life remains like a blurred vision and does not remember anything that has happened before the damage. This is very painful situation.

Amydgala

It is two groups of neurons of almond shape, which is situated below the hippocampus and both sides of thalamus. When electricity is passed through it, anxiety is the outcome.

If it is removed then the person becomes just like a pet animal and incapable of giving any reactions, which used to arouse anger. But it includes more than the emotion of anger, when it is removed the animal also reacts differently on the partner, which probably inspires their reactions of sex and anger.

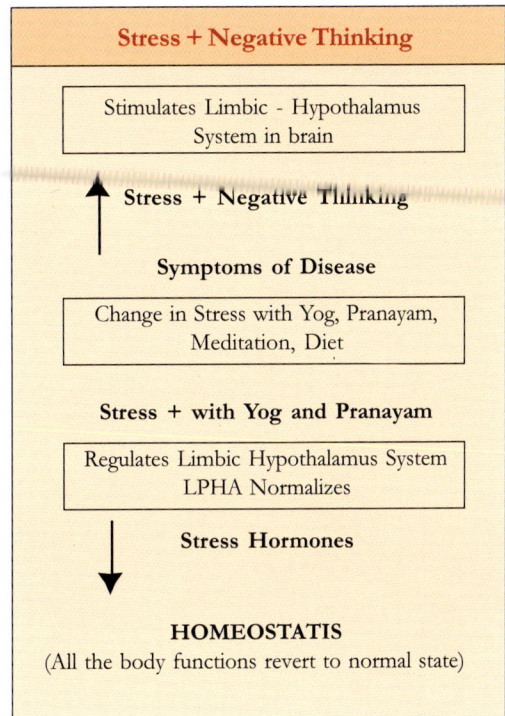

```
┌─────────────────────────────────┐   ┌─────────────────────────────────┐
│      Mind, Brain and Body       │   │      Mind, Brain and Body       │
│               ↓                 │   │               ↓                 │
│             Stress              │   │   Stress ✚ Practice of Pranayam │
│               ↓                 │   │            & Yog                │
│  Stimulates Limbic-Hypothalamus │   │               ↓                 │
│  Pituitary Adrenalin Axis       │   │  ┌───────────────────────────┐  │
│               ↓                 │   │  │    Regulates Limbic       │  │
│ Stress System and Resistance    │   │  │  Hypothalamus System      │  │
│          Power                  │   │  └───────────────────────────┘  │
│               ↓                 │   │               ↓                 │
│    Cortisol and Adrenalin       │   │    Improves Stress Hormone      │
│               ↓                 │   │     and  Immune System          │
│ Infection and Condition of      │   │               ↓                 │
│          Arteries               │   │   Increases Disease Fighting    │
│               ↓                 │   │          Capacity               │
│        Unhealthy Body           │   │               ↓                 │
│                                 │   │   Better Mind, Brain and Body   │
└─────────────────────────────────┘   └─────────────────────────────────┘
```

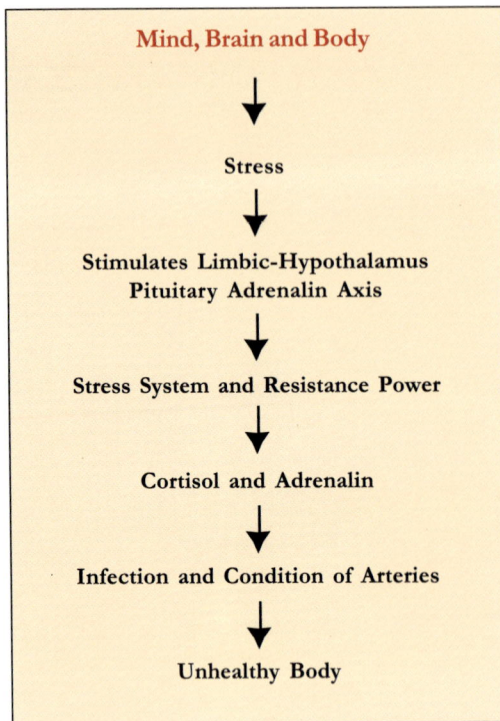

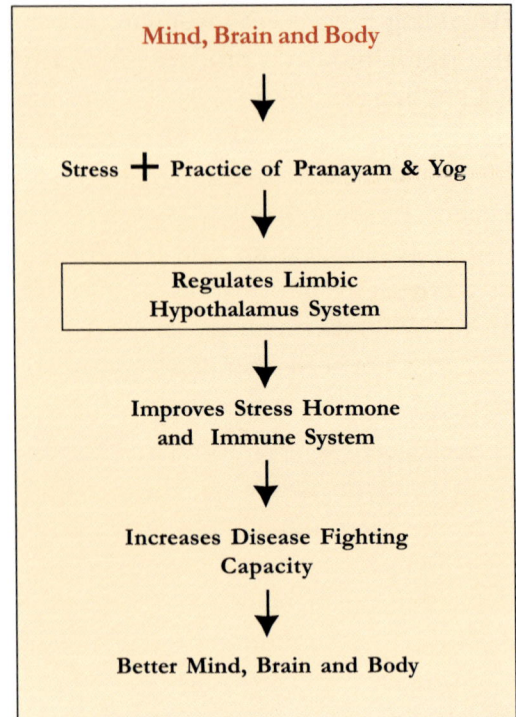

Related Places

Besides hypothalamus, hippocampus and amygdala there are certain other components near limbic system which are completely joined with it. Cingulate gyrus is a part of cerebrum, which is just above the corpus callosum and near limbic system. It makes the path from thalamus to hippocampus and appears as if this emotional work is responsible for concentration, which combines memories with pain and smell.

The ventral tegmental area of brain stem is made of dopamine paths, which are responsible for satisfaction. The person having damaged ventral tegmental area experiences great difficulty in getting satisfaction and they generally fall into the trap of drinking alcohol, drugs, sweets or gambling etc.

Ganglia vessel lies above the limbic system and on both corners. It is tightly attached to the cortex lying just above it. It is responsible for repeating a particular thing, experiencing the happiness of winning prize and concentration.

Frontal cortex is the part of frontal lobe, which is found in front of motor area and is closely attached to limbic system. It quickly thinks about future and gets involved in making plans and expressing reactions. It appears as if it is included in paths of dopamine and plays a major role in showing happiness and habits.

Automatic Nervous System

The second part of nervous system plays a major role in our emotional side of life, this is known as automatic nervous system. It is divided into two parts; the primary function is to work against each other. The sympathetic nervous system begins from spinal cord and passes through various parts of the body. Its work appears as if it is preparing the body to fight against powerful processes. For example saving our life in case of some danger or preparing for some fight.

Activating sympathetic nervous system has following effects

- Dilation of pupils
- Opening eyelids
- Arousing sweat glands
- Expansion of blood vessels
- Contracting blood vessels in other parts of the body
- Increasing heart rate
- Opening of bronchial tubes in lungs and slow evacuation process in digestive system.

Limbic and hypothalamus system

Emotions take birth in this part of the brain, for instance anger, lust, desire, the power of smelling, recognizing the smell, memory etc. Here the organs of action and senses collect the information and distribute it to different parts of the brain based on the functions. In case of an emergency where there is a danger to life, risk of losing a dear one; the reflexes of the brain react sharply and necessary action is taken. This action takes place from the motor of the brain, which sends messages to different muscles and body parts. This condition is known as acute stress but some processes in which mental depression, absence of emotional support, economic constraints, social crime, losing status in life etc. Such messages travel from organs of actions and senses to limbic and hypothalamus system and reach the cerebral cortex. These messages are then analyzed and accordingly sent back to the limbic and hypothalamus system. During this entire process, there is a constant mental stress which has an instant effect on the motor system. This involves hiding the emotions, shamelessness etc. The human being hides such emotions and stores them in the brain and this constant stress or tension are sent to the pituitary gland through limbic and hypothalamus system. From this part stress hormones are secreted. One part of the brain is autonomic nervous system, which has two parts – sympathetic and parasympathetic nervous system. Due to continuous stress sympathetic nervous system becomes dominating, increased secretion of adrenaline or noradrenaline takes place making parasympathetic nervous system becomes inactive.

With the regular practice of Yog and Pranayam the unwanted or negative thoughts are discarded by the brain. As a result the secretion of stress hormones starts slowly and secretion of adrenaline and infusing hormones starts increasing. The parasympathetic nervous system becomes active again and releases body of stress. Storing of energy starts. This condition relievs body from negative effects of excess release of stress hormones. Yog and devotion of God helps in removing negative thoughts from cerebral cortex and brings in positive changes.

These two organs receive and send the messages. The power of thinking, analyzing and remembering important information is carried on with the help of these two organs and thoughts are generated in the brain.

The minutest part of the nervous system is a nerve cell that performs the important function of sending messages to brain and receiving back. Let us imagine that all the information and memory gets converted into chemical information and gets accumulated, which proves to be useful for future. When we experience something we correlate that incident or person with the information present in the memory.

For instance the computer stores input in its memory. The input is converted into data in the form of electricity in computers and electromagnetic signals in case of human beings.

Spinal Cord

The part of brain, which generates feelings, emotions, anger, the power to smell, hunger, sexual desire is called limbic and hypothalamus system. This part is present in the animals as well. Human brain alone has the reasoning capacity besides thinking and analyzing the information and this power is present in the cortex of the brain. The cortex blocks those information which are not correct. However, it so happens that the human being controls emotions being part of cultured society, which actually needs to be expressed. This leads to mental stress. Hormones are secreted from pituitary gland in order to generate the emotions. There are two systems in the brain that act like messengers:

♦ Autonomic nervous system
♦ Motor and sensory system.

Autonomic nervous system is not in our control and affects every part of the body. It is again classified into two parts: sympathetic system and parasympathetic system.

Both these systems are balanced with the help of Pranayam, which has a positive impact on the body. When we are under stress the sympathetic system gets excited and becomes the cause of physical stress and stress related hormones like adrenaline, noradrenaline and cortisol are secreted. Pranayam works like purifier of the nervous system and balances it. According to Ayurved, the messages from the organs of action and sensory organs reach the brain and they are analyzed, correlated and investigated in the cortex. The messages which are unimportant or not suitable for the society, health and body are separated in the cortex and the person performs good work, leads a happy and contended life and sets an example in the society.

Pranayam helps in the secretion of endorphin and encephalin hormones. These two hormones are the subjects of medical research these days. It is said that disequilibria in serotinin, dopamine and noradrenaline hormones leads to mental depression and disappointment that can be balanced with the help of Pranayam, Yog, meditation and *satsang* or mass prayers. The person can lead a happy and healthy life and contribute positively for his family, society and nation at large.

Brain and Stress

Stress is a gift of modern society. The desire to achieve more and enjoy all the material happiness is causing a lot of physical and mental stress and the consequences are too evident. Stress has a direct impact on brain, because emotions, thoughts, anxiety and dreams generate from the brain. When the brain has to work beyond its capacity, it leads to mental stress. In this condition hormones and nervous system play a major role and we need to understand it so that we can reduce the stress level and lead a healthy and contented life. When we are under stress the hormones secrete in excess and irregular manner and we fall into the trap of diseases. Before understanding mental stress and its causes, it is necessary to understand the structure of brain.

Reasons and Factors of Stress

Imbalance between cerebral cortex and emotional cortex leads to stress but following are the main reasons for it:

External Factors : Daily routine of a person, working style depends on the surroundings to a great extent.

Internal Factors : It is combined impact of genetic and various factors of environment. Genetic factors are not in our control but it is very necessary for our psychological health. It gives a final shape to our thoughts, desires, behaviour and expectations.

External Factors : The external factors of stress are in our surroundings and working conditions. For example:

♦ **Society and family :** Lacking expected cooperation or support from family members, lack of communication or discussion among the family members, difference of opinion etc.

♦ **Work place :** Various reasons for stress at the work place, for instance lack of clarity in role or responsibilities, not getting appreciation, dissatisfaction due to some rules etc.

- **Climatic (psychological) :** Lack of cleanliness, high temperature, lack of suitable resources office politics, insecurity, conspiracy, back biting can lead to psychological stress.

- **Basic beliefs and social changes:** The young generation differs from old generation with respect to following some rituals and traditions or old practices. Apart from that technological and economic progress has also brought about a lot of changes in the general life-style. In densely populated cities, with a large number of vehicles, fast life is exploiting people and is also one of the major factors for rising crime graph.

- **Economic :** Financial constraints and economic changes like lack of money, savings, government policies etc. cause stress.

- **Politics :** Politics within an institution, of the nation has direct impact on the service class and professionals living in that country. This is one of the biggest reasons for stress in general.

- **Environment :** Different aspects pertaining to environment like increasing population, pollution, temperature, deforestation, epidemics etc.

- **Beliefs, priorities and expressions :** These are some hard facts which are prevailing from our birth and have a direct impact on us, for example, food habits, dress codes etc.

- **Principles and moral values :** These are important to fulfill our social responsibilities.

- **Priorities :** We need to prioritize as our priorities change in different stages of our life. Our priorities also depend on our beliefs and principles.

- **Social expectations :** Good position in service or establishing good business. Expecting good status in the society, name and fame, sometimes living in joint families influences our expectations and becomes the cause of stress.

- **Perfection in work and responsibilities :** How best can we fulfill our responsibilities towards our family, friends and society, this is also one of the reasons for stress.

- **Balanced communication :** The way we express ourselves in front of others depends to a great extent on the family circumstances, working style and general surroundings.

- **Comforts :** We understand the importance of money since our childhood and is extremely important in order to fulfill our desires and develop our personality.

- **Self-respect :** It depends on the social and family atmosphere where we are born and brought up.

Internal Factors: Internal factors define our behavioural pattern and some of the examples are as follows:

- **Parents :** Behaviour of our parents, their experiences and their personal relations, leave a long-lasting impression on children and influences their behaviour and nature.

- **Family :** Other members of the family like grandparents, brothers, sisters, uncle, aunt etc. their mutual relations have a deep impact on our lives.

- **Society :** Social structure, basic beliefs and expectations have a deep impact on our behaviour and life-style.

- **Educational institutions :** School, college and teachers play a very important role in overall personality development and grooming.

- **Friends and colleagues :** We live in close proximity with friends and colleagues and the mutual relations have an impact on our interpersonal behaviour.

- **Religious and spiritual environment :** Religious and spiritual environment are the foundation for our discipline and faith. We get inspiration from our religious atmosphere prevailing in our surroundings and perform good deeds.

- **Physical constitution :** Our physical looks, body constitution has a deep impact on the senstivity and feeling of security.

- **Literature and media :** These two are the main deciding factors for human behaviour, social expectations etc.

- **Financial resources :** A person's financial condition denotes his or her status and feeling of security but at the same time a rich person has to face a lot of mental stress in order to keep his cash safe and maintain the social status.

- **Personal experiences :** During education period our mental development takes place on the basis of our behaviour, thinking, loss, profit, desires, disappointment and achievements. The same experiences become the basis for fulfilling our actions and reactions in future.

Excess of information

Today, we can get any kind of information at the click of a mouse. Internet, television channels, newspapers and magazines are full of different kinds of information. The common man is under stress due to excess of information obtained from various sources.

High standard of living: Today the general standard of living has improved. People are able to buy consumer durables like television, fridge, computers, cars and whatever they want. People are working for longer hours and beyond their capacity in order to procure these comforts, which ultimately leads to stress.

Physical health: The increasing desires have a negative impact on our health. We tend to get habituated to different kinds of vices for the sake of fulfilling our desires. Today people are having poor health due to irregular routine and changing life-style. People complain of poor eyesight, headache, diabetes, high blood pressure etc. These diseases can lead to heart diseases and even paralysis in future.

Balanced routine: It is necessary to control the stress level before it reaches the saturation point and we can avoid stress to a great extent.

Finance: It is said that money is the root cause for all problems. It creates different types of stresses. Need for money arises at every stage in our life, for example, daily needs, accommodation, food, entertainment, comforts and sources of luxury. Financial mismanagement and imprudent investments give birth to stress.

Work and vacation: For majority of the people work is the main cause of stress. Many people work for 16–18 hours and

Limbic System

Hippocampus

Arcuate Nucleus

Hypothalamus

amygdala

Pituitary
Gland

Functions of Limbic System
Sexual desires
Anger
Food tendencies
Depression
Happiness, satisfaction
Emotions
Secretion of hormones
Dopamine
Serotonin
Nonadrenoline

Nonadrenoline

are happy while working. The main reason for stress due to work is dissatisfaction with work. We should always be happy to reduce our stress level and be satisfied with the results. We need to be disciplined to perform well and feel satisfied.

Family

Family plays an important role in deciding the stress level. Some people complain that when they are working they are fine but feel stressed after coming back home. Family should help the person to reduce stress because family is the first social institution, which gives security and affection to people and thinks for welfare of the person.

Emotional support: Lack of emotional support is also one of the reasons for increasing stress level. The person gets inspiration from relatives, wife, children and reliable friends and colleagues. He undergoes stress in the absence of moral support or encouragement. Family is the foundation for belief. We should be selfless and supportive in every sense.

Egotism: Majority of the people possess a lot of wealth, good position, good family and are always helpful to others but undergo stress in order to portray themselves as unique and different from others. A person should avoid this.

Social and community life: Man is a social animal and possesses a lot of knowledge.

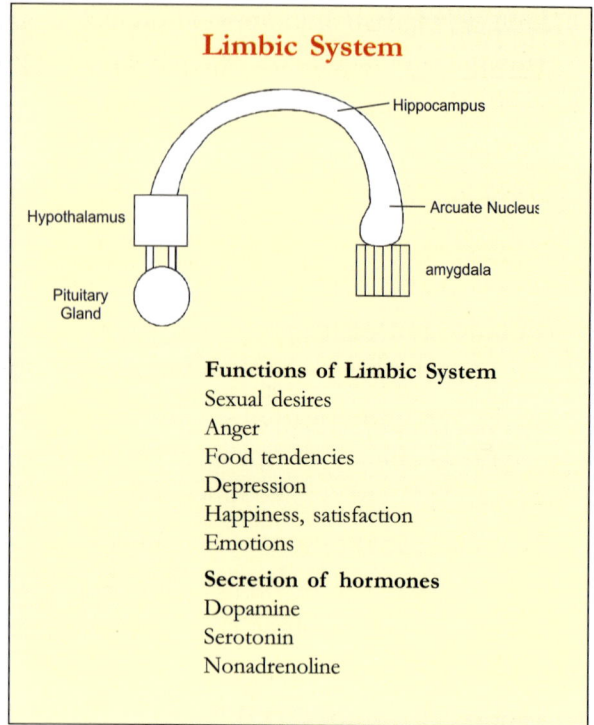

Health and social atmosphere are all necessary for a person. He also requires friends, neighbours and family in new environment and the people who give a lot of social security and affection.

Spirituality: Chastity, morality and spiritual life are the main factors for life, which provide stability, humanity and peace to individuals. It is the feeling to have faith in Almighty God and lead a life as per his directions and rules. A balanced person fulfills his social responsibilities and leads a happy life.

Recognizing Social Stress

Today the world has progressed scientifically but it is very difficult to understand mental stress and probably there would be no unit developed to measure it. A person who is under mental stress is unable to avoid the dangers arising from it and cannot measure the symptoms. They are as follows:

- **Behaviour :** Stress attracts the person towards wrong habits or vices like tobacco, alcohol and slowly the person gets into the trap. Biting nails and shaking legs are all signs of mental stress.
- **Sensitivity:** People become restless and lose patience.
- **Emotional:** Irritable nature, lack of patience or extremely volatile, sleeplessness and bad dreams or depression are symptoms of emotional stress.
- **Physical symptoms:** Tension in muscles, back or neck pain, irregular breathing, perspiration and dryness of mouth are symptoms of physical stress.

The above-mentioned symptoms are just examples and not actual symptoms. They will give us simple knowledge to recognize mental stress.

Psychological Aspects of Stress and its Effect on Body

We analyzed several cases and found that people following irregular life-style are generally under stress. An attempt has been made to study such cases and find out the factors responsible for increasing stress so that it can be reduced with proper balancing techniques. Some people over react in simple issues and that itself becomes the cause of stress. This happens due to typical characteristics. The person with such characteristics comes under Group A.

The qualities of tolerance, competition, attack and violence are predominant in such individuals. Such people are very punctual and always try to achieve perfection in every work. They are extremely hard-working and are busy to complete work on time. They are very ambitious and maintain authority and control. However, they are not good listeners and always disturb the conversation between two people. They are self-centered and are extremely sensitive. Such people generally have sympathy towards others and embarrass others.

Group A people honk on a busy road and try to prove that they should reach first before others. Such person gets irritated if the lift or such other source of transport moves very slowly. He or she tries to complete all types of work at one time. He behaves ruthlessly at work place due to his high ambitions. Even in social occasions he wants to get importance, get prefered seat in the cinema hall etc.

Following factors are taken into consideration to recognize Group A persons:

- Hard-working
- Competitiveness
- Dynamism
- Proactiveness
- Punctuality
- Effectiveness
- Lack of time
- Efficiency
- Short tempered
- Lack of patience
- Desire to talk about self or boasting
- Does not show interest in discussing irrelevant issues
- Very hard-working
- They think that discussions are being made unnecessarily
- Think that time is always lacking
- Irritable nature
- Disturbing others' conversation
- Always trying to correct others.

These are the characteristics of a person who wants to control the situation and likes to struggle between busy schedules.

Such people like to face challenges and get accustomed in new environment very easily. They grasp new ideas very quickly despite the fact that they are getting into the trap of emotional and physical dangers. These are the symptoms of a person who is a demon. It is a mere coincidence that all these characteristics cannot be seen in one individual and on the other side it is not that all these characteristics cannot be seen in only one person.

Different reactions are expressed at different occasions because nature differs from person to person.

People who possess the above mentioned qualities in lesser degree are included in Group B. Generally they are calm and remain in the background. They are aware of their ambitions and take out time to pursue their hobbies. They are very tolerant and listen to others and believe in forgiving others.

People in this group are characterized on the basis of following qualities :

- Like to rest
- Work slowly
- Punctual
- Cooperative
- Very composed and rarely get angry
- They are not introverts and talk freely
- They neither display their achievements nor feel the need to do it
- They are straightforward and clarify others' doubts
- They accept their mistakes very quickly
- Flexible
- They do not worry about failures
- They forgive enemies and adverse conditions
- They inspire others and also appreciate
- Take proper rest when tired
- They do not get excited
- They like to know their weaknesses
- They delegate work
- They are witty at times and enjoy light moments
- They do not have ego clashes.

We adopt these qualities from our surroundings and experiences. The qualities of people belonging to 'A' group help us in understanding the stress level and change our behaviour and nature. This is a simple factor, which causes a lot of mental stress.

Effect of Stress on General Health

Our body performs certain actions when it is under some kind of stress just like the security alarm; as it rings in case of emergency. Stress has a lot of negative impact on the brain and physical health. The body shows some changes depending on the circumstances while facing some challenges. We have heard some incidents wherein people have lifted heavy weights in order to prove themselves to the society. It is unimaginable. We generally hear about such cases in sports activities, which cannot be repeated by others, it is a big challenge for the psychology of that person. We come across some moments in our life wherein people work beyond their physical capacity and it becomes the cause of stress. Such challenging moments are directly related to stress. It is directly related to maintaining cordial relations, future planning, financial worries etc. Stress is also connected with life-style and getting accustomed in a new environment. Adrenaline and cortisol hormones are secreted from body during stress, which play a major role in natural reactions. These hormones affect the heart and pulse rate. Very fast moment of blood reduces the thickness of arteries and the fast heart rate increases blood pressure. Adrenaline hormone contracts the muscles as a result consumption of oxygen increases and we react sharply at certain moments. It also affects the respiration process.

Effect of Stress on Our Body: Stress has a number of negative effects on our body like:

- Increasing heart rate
- Increasing blood pressure
- Muscular tension
- Reduces GFR
- Increases respiration
- Increases consumption of oxygen
- Change in the rate of flow of blood
- Increases cortisol
- Increases adrenaline and catacholamine
- Increases blood sugar
- Increases serum cholesterol
- Increases acidity
- Increases the chances of getting blood clots
- Saliva dries up

Besides, it increases cholesterol and acidity. They both increase the body fuel and also affect the skin colouration. Stress causes perspiration. It is the method to measure different changes taking place in the body due to stress.

Slow Excretion in Digestion Process

One of the important effects of this part is that it becomes the cause of making adrenaline glands to secrete epinephrine in the blood. Epinephrine is a powerful hormone, which becomes the cause of reactions in different parts of the body just like sympathetic nervous system. It takes long time to control its affect due to its presence in blood stream. This is the reason that when we are sad it takes long time to come back to normal position.

The sympathetic nervous system receives messages, which are generally related to pain of internal organs because the nerves, which get the information related to pain pass through that path that gets related information from surface area of the body. Many a times this information is confusing. This pain is known as referred pain and the best example is the pain experienced in hands and shoulders during heart attack.

The second part of autonomous nervous system is called parasympathetic nervous system. The roots of this system are situated in brain stem and in the lower back portion of spinal cord. The main function of this system is to bring the body to its natural position.

Its Functions include:

- Contraction of pupil in eyes
- Functioning of salivary glands
- Inspiring the stomach to evacuate waste material
- Inspiring the intestines to work properly
- Similarly activate the lungs to evacuate air
- Dilation of bronchial tubes
- Reduce the heart rate.

The parasympathetic nervous system has certain sensitive abilities. It receives messages from carbon dioxide present in the blood, blood pressure etc. Autonomic nervous system has another part - enteric nervous system, which is often not discussed much. It is one of the rigid nerves and regulates the stomach related processes. When we suffer from stomach disorders or feel some kind of discomfort we blame this particular system.

It has been noticed that regular practice of Pranayam and Yog improves the respiratory system of the body. We have seen in our camps that people practising Yog and Pranayam have shown improvement in their pulmonary function tests. This proves that Yog can cure several respiratory problems like asthma etc.

Science of Mental Stress

"We need to have practical knowledge of physical anatomy and nervous system in order to understand mental stress" – George Everley

A lot of research has been conducted on mental stress in the past half century. If we understand what is going on in our mind and body then we will be able to control the mental stress to a large extent. The science of mental stress and its theory help us to understand the methods of controlling it. On the basis of this knowledge we can understand that it is not only necessary to make us feel better but is also an effective medicine or therapy.

First and foremost we need to ponder as to when do we feel stressed? What is the purpose of complex nervous system, functioning of hormones, organs and its processes? What leads to feeling of sickness, weakness, fatigue, headache, emotional depression etc.? We need to go back in the past in order to understand this science probably some thousand years back, this will help us to understand the process of fear towards dangers arising in our body and mind.

Mental Stress and Big Bear

Just try and imagine that you are present in that time and place where none of the modern amenities are available. You do not have any kind of comfort whatsoever, house, telephone, television, electricity, car etc. Let us imagine that we are staying in some cave or hut located in some undeveloped place or forest etc.

You were enjoying your stay and suddenly you noticed that a huge bear was approaching from behind the bushes and looks at you with hunger in its eyes.

As soon as we imagine about such incidents we get the feeling of some kind of danger surrounding us, "I am in danger and I am feeling afraid. This thought will give rise to another feeling "Run, save your life". We will feel the necessity to run away from the animal. The next thought that comes in mind is that "I need to kill that animal in order to save myself, my family and my friends." This means the feeling of fight originated in our mind, which in turn gave rise to bodily reactions, we need speed to run and strength to fight. We need the combination of these two things. This is known as fight and flight reactions.

Fight and Flight Reflexes

Our mind is flooded with bodily reactions as soon this thought comes in our mind. This mental and physical condition is explained as hyper arousal. According to Harvard Physiologist, Walter Kenen, "flight reactions are such processes which are aroused in our body automatically during some danger or emergency and the stress hormones adrenaline, noradrenaline and cortisol are secreted."

Psychological Reflexes due to Mental Stress

When mental stress begins then the sudden changes activates the nervous system, which is known as autonomic nervous system. This nervous system is responsible for several bodily functions for example, digestion of food, heart rate, blood pressure and maintaining body temperature. Nervous system gives birth to different reactions, which is totally beyond the control of a person. This is completely automatic.

Automatic nervous system or ANS has two components, which are helpful in regulating fight and flight reaction on constant basis. Sympathetic nervous system is that part of nervous system, which is responsible for this flight and fight reaction. We always feel afraid and are in pain. Sympathetic nervous system proves to be helpful in controlling the fight and flight reaction from fear and pain. As mentioned earlier it is an automatic reaction and we need to understand that we are in danger and need to get rid of psychological and emotional reactions and act with speed and power.

The second branch of ANS is parasympathetic nervous system. This arouses homeostasis. Homeostasis gives birth to internal stability of physiology and emotions. Parasympathetic nervous system is the process of reducing the speed of actions. During this process, digestion, energy and circulation of blood are controlled through central organs. The heart rate and respiration are reduced. It also brings down the blood pressure and body temperature. Normally it relaxes the muscles. During the parasympathetic process we are calm and quiet. Our body gets back the energy and strength.

Automatic nervous system is controlled by hypothalamus, which is also known as master gland. It warns against danger and sends the message to the entire body through neurons or nerve cells. It passes the message to the endocrine system as well, which are helpful in the secretion of hormones. Hormones send messages to all the cells through adrenaline and cortisol. Besides, it also helps in strengthening them and increasing speed.

Adrenaline and adrenaline flow into the blood through adrenal medulla. Adrenal medulla is a part of adrenal glands, which is located in the upper part of kidney.

Cortisol is a different hormone, which is secreted from one part of adrenal gland, which is also known as adrenal cortex.

Process of Autonomic Nervous System

Following are the changes that take place due to activation of autonomic nervous system:

- Increasing the functions and actions of central nervous system
- Increasing mental functions
- Increasing the flow of adrenaline, epinephrine and cortisol, and circulating it to all cells in the body
- Increases the heart rate
- Increases the cardio output
- Increases the blood pressure

- Increases the respiration
- Increases the metabolism
- Increases the capacity of oxygen intake
- Increases the contraction of muscles and strengthens them
- Increases the blood cholesterol output
- Increases the secretion of blood sugar coming out of liver, which energizes the muscles
- It helps in the secretion and refines pituitary glands
- It dilates the pupils of eye
- Increases the brain wave process
- It helps in the secretion of sweat glands
- It increases the blood pressure due to contraction of arterioles in the skin
- Weakens the immune system
- Contracts heart muscles
- Reduces the functioning of reproductive and sexual organs
- Poor digestion
- Dryness in mouth
- The pain is not felt
- Reduces kidney functions
- Contracts gallbladder.

Effects of Mental Stress and You

In today's life day-to-day problems are the results of mental stress. Generally, your body is also affected due to fear whether it is obvious, hidden or imagined. Harvard's Cardiologist Herbert Benson says, "Having a knee-jerk response to stress and running away from struggle in life is not the right way to deal with it".

Mental stress affects our work differently and sometimes our efficiency level increases and ultimately proves to be beneficial. This type of instant energy helps us in fighting against death, unbearable pain or an emergency situation.

Chronic Stress

If mental stress condition continues for some time then it becomes necessary to get rid of it. The reason being that the result is harmful for our body and is known as continued 'sympathetic nervous system activation' or chronic stress.

You may have come across a person saying that he is in stress continuously? Now you would be able to understand this position.

Being in a state of continous uncertainity gives rise to stress. This gives us strength on one side and inspires us to become stronger and sharper on the other side if this situation continues for longer time then it affects physical health as well.

Listen to your body. Your body conveys you something just like a person who suffers from hangover when he drinks in excess or the muscles begin to pull and there is another instance when the body feels light and energetic after morning exercise. Your body tells you that drinking alcohol is bad and morning exercise is good.

It is not good to live in stress. In case of over stress our body tells us that if it is not treated on time it can affect our health. Here it needs to be mentioned that mental stress has not been included in the 10 top reasons for death in America but has been combined with many diseases. This does not mean that stress does give rise to problems but it is certain that it is the foundation for many physical and mental problems.

Practice of Yog, Pranayam and meditation reduces mental stress, stress hormones and increases the secretion of beneficial hormones like encephalins and endorphin, and balances sympathetic and parasympathetic system. This has a favourable effect on the body and the person becomes disease-free.

Sympathetic and parasympathetic systems are recognized as Surya and Chandra Nadi respectively.

Effects of Stress on Immune System

Mental stress arouses the limbic and hypothalamic axis of brain through organs of actions and sensory organs. This anxiety increases the secretion of adrenaline, noradrenaline and cortex. Continuous stress increases the level of these hormones in the blood, which has a negative effect on different parts of the body. The same type of effect is seen on immunity system or resistance power of the body. Immunity system protects us from infections, asthma, allergy and attack of other viral diseases. When this system becomes weak then the body loses the capacity to fight out these diseases and slowly the resistance power reduces. It leads to different types of problems in the body like infections, arthritis, allergy, bronchitis, asthma etc. and the body becomes a bundle of diseases. Practice of Pranayam, Yog and meditation controls the limbic hypothalamus axis. This reduces the anxiety and reduces the high level of stress hormones present in the blood. It also increases the level of beneficial hormones like adrenaline and encephalin. These two hormones have positive effect on our body and strengthen the immunity system. The body gets the ability to protect itself from diseases and does not allow the entry of infections and other contagious diseases.

Metabolic Syndrome and Insulin Resistance

Metabolic syndrome X : This is a group of diseases caused due to mental stress that can adversely affect your cardiovascular process. Insulin resistance is a main reason for metabolic resistance. There are different factors, which play a major role in causing metabolic syndrome. When we compare with ancient times we see that our body does not get accustomed to changes as quickly as it used to in olden days. We are following the same habits that are inherited from our ancestors. Our ancestors took sufficient amount of nutritious food, which contained low level of carbohydrates and their life-style included a lot of hard work and walking, which is totally absent in present life-style. In some people the insulin resistance is increased due to genetic reasons, whereas in others it is the reason for unhealthy life-style and excessive mental stress. Insulin resistance has a negative effect on glucose and insulin levels. With time, it harms the body cells due to which the body's capacity to convert glucose into energy with the help of insulin reduces. This process leads to insulin resistance, which leads to metabolic syndrome. First and foremost it decreases insulin receptor sites at a very fast rate.

A normal healthy person contains 20,000 receptors per cell. Whereas an average obese person suffers from metabolic syndrome, and the receptors are less than 5,000. If your body has very less receptor sites then the glucose touches the cell wall and returns back and does not get converted into energy. The reason being that glucose does not enter the cell, as a result glucose remains in blood, which ultimately increases blood sugar, this sugar reaches the liver where it gets converted into fat and spreads in the whole body through blood. This process increases weight and is the main reason for metabolic syndrome.

The other main reason for this is increasing level of insulin in blood, unhealthy life-style and hereditary qualities, as a result of which pancreas produces high amount of insulin, when the cells get high level of insulin it uses insulin receptor sites and reduces in order to protect itself. Due to this process our body has very less number of receptors to finish the daily activities. This in turn increases the insulin level, which is not accepted by the cells, they flow in the blood freely. This damages the cardiovascular process, which increases the risk of heart attack.

Symptoms of Metabolic Syndrome

Many people do not believe that they are suffering with this syndrome (Syndrome X); according to an estimate 20–25 per cent of the people are suffering with this syndrome. If a person is suffering from any of the three symptoms then he is said to be having metabolic syndrome:

◆   **Insulin resistance :** When the body does not absorb blood sugar or insulin properly.

- **Fat stomach :** When the waist size is more than 40 inches in men and 35 in women.
- **High level of blood sugar :** Fasting level more than 110 mg. per dl. Triglycerides more than 150 mg/dl. HDL less than 40 mg/dl. prothrombic state (presence of high level of fibrinogen and plasminogen activator in blood) of blood clotting.

Blood pressure : 130/85 or higher

Researchers have found that conditions like metabolic syndrome and others for instance obesity, high blood pressure and high level of HDL have some relation, which increase the risk of heart disease. A study reveals that when fat accumulates on the walls of arteries then metabolic syndrome and atherosclerosis leads to heart attack.

People suffering from metabolic syndrome also have the chances of type II diabetes. Along with it women have the risk of PCOS (Polycystic ovarian syndrome) and men can suffer from prostrate cancer.

On account of the above reasons the doctors inform the patients about the metabolic

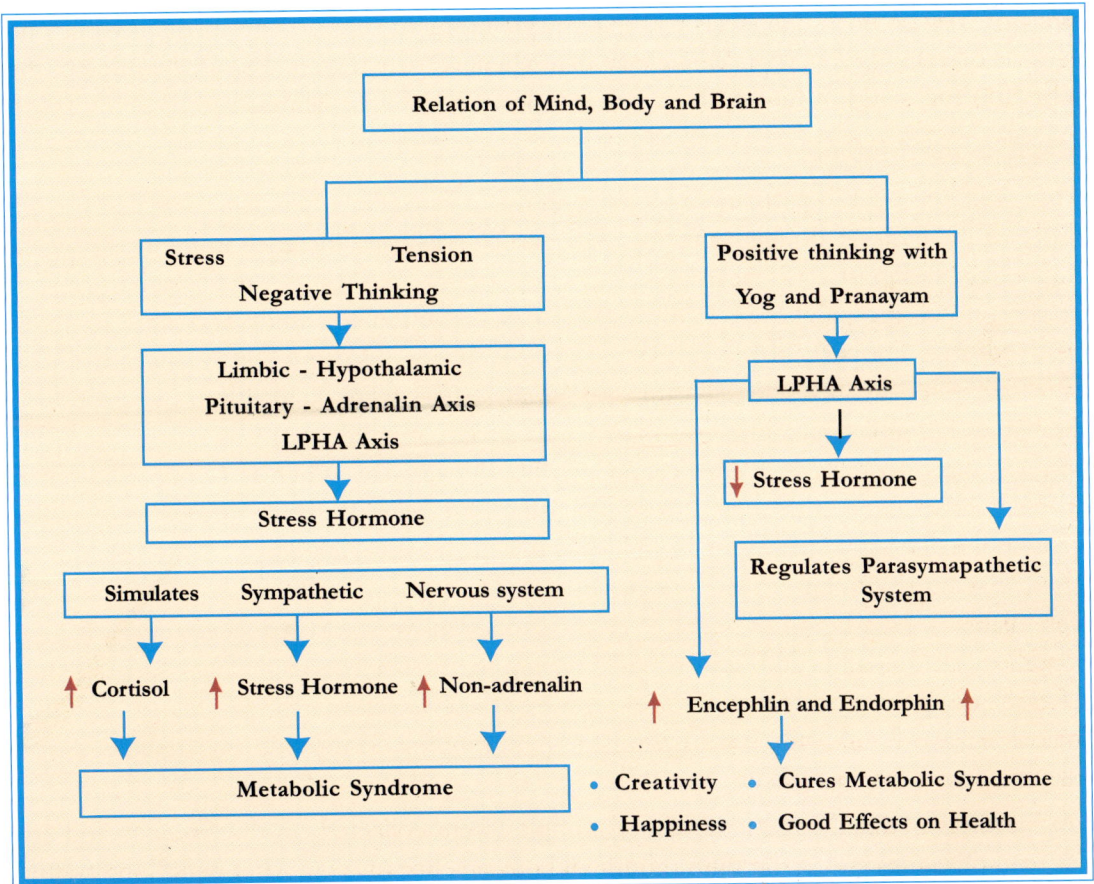

Relation of Mind, Body and Brain

Stress **Tension** **Negative Thinking**	**Positive thinking with Yog and Pranayam**
Limbic - Hypothalamic Pituitary - Adrenalin Axis LPHA Axis	**LPHA Axis**
Stress Hormone	↓ **Stress Hormone**
Simulates Sympathetic Nervous system	**Regulates Parasymapathetic System**
↑ **Cortisol** ↑ **Stress Hormone** ↑ **Non-adrenalin**	↑ **Encephlin and Endorphin** ↑
Metabolic Syndrome	• **Creativity** • **Cures Metabolic Syndrome** • **Happiness** • **Good Effects on Health**

syndrome caused due to insulin resistance and conditions responsible for it.

Presently there is no medicine available which can change the symptoms of metabolic syndrome. The modern medical science has not been able to provide suitable treatment to relieve metabolic syndrome and other mental diseases but a detailed test was conducted with resources available in order to study the effect of Pranayam on stress hormones. The main objective behind this study was to understand stress, its origin, causes from the angle of medical science and available remedies in the present conditions to overcome it.

Effect of Pranayam on Stress Hormones

(a) Control Study with Double Sampling

Senior scientists of Swami Vivekanand University, Bangalore; Sanjay Gandhi Medical Institute, Lucknow, and Sahara India Medical Institute conducted a Control study under the leadership of Swami Ramdevji Maharaj to analyze and test the psychophysical effects of stress hormones. Probably this is the first such experiment conducted to study the effect of Yog on hormone levels without any government support and made possible only because of efforts of a Yogi. We believe that whenever any research would be done in this subject in the world in future, this work will prove to be a benchmark.

Material and Method

After selection of 170 participants for the study, 119 healthy adults were selected for this study on the basis of double sampling. The participants were included in the study on the basis of age group of 20-25 years and willingness to take part. Out of the total participants, 51 had shown incapability in following the rules required for study and were excluded from the same. The participants of selected group were not practising Yog. All the participants were willing to stay in residential camp for 10 days. They were divided into two groups on the basis of double sampling. Group A (study group, number- 63) was taught Pranayam and was made to practise it for at least two hours everyday. Whereas Group B (Control group, number 56) was restricted from practising Pranayam. Both the groups were invited to listen the discourses of Swami Ramdevji and were given vegetarian food after discourses. There was no restriction on the calories intake. The parameters for exclusion from camp were diabetes, high blood pressure, liver and kidney diseases, pregnancy or breast-feeding condition, alcohol addiction, and people consuming medicines to simulate ovarian glands. After the camp the participants of Group A were asked to continue the practice of Pranayam for one or two hours daily for a period of three months. The group B participants were asked to lead a normal life.

On the basis of fixed parameters blood samples were collected on the first day and 10th day (end of camp) and in the third month without practice of Yog. After night long fasting,

Heparin was used (Sodium Heparin 400-1000 Iu / ml) and blood samples were taken to test the presence of Beta-endorphin in EDTA, whereas blood sugar from blood was collected to test the presence of fat, creatinine, nitrogen factors, SGPT, breast simulating hormone, AETH, cortisol etc. Biochemical tests were done with primary methods, whereas AETH was completed with cortisol; breast simulating hormone and Beta-endorphin was completed with Elisa or IARMA aseciras. The tests were done on the basis of selection by clinical and pathological scientists and a lot of biochemical assumptions were derived at. Independent bioanalysts did the analysis of the study.

Results

Comparison of characteristics of baseline: Around 119 healthy youth were selected. Group A (Yog group, number – 63) and Group B (Control group, number – 56) were same on the basis of weight, basal metabolism, systolic blood pressure and diastolic blood pressure.

Stress hormones: On the basis of baseline for Control and test group, there was no difference between blood cortisol, breast-simulating hormone, endorphin and AETH level.

A comparison of standards with baseline after 10 days: Comparison was done on the basis of baseline, there was a significant reduction in weight, basal metabolism, systolic blood pressure and diastolic blood pressure. The endorphin blood mean and breast-simulating hormone had reduced but the value was insignificant. The participants of Control group showed significant changes in weight, basal metabolism, systolic blood pressure, and diastolic blood pressure. Although there was non-significant change in four hormone standards compared to Yog group.

Comparison of standards after 3 months with 10 days: Around 49 participants from Yog group and 45 from Control group were present for final samples after three months. All the participants were asked questions relating to Yog practice. This was to make sure that Control group does not practising Yog; all the participants were given the same questionnaire. Three participants from this group were practising Yog and hence they were excluded from the test. The average duration of Yog practice for participants of Yog group was 7.61 hours per week. Whereas extension was 1- 2.5 hours per week. The weight, basal metabolism, systolic blood pressure and diastolic blood pressure had no significant change in participants of the Control group. There was no change in the mean of breast simulator, endorphin and cortisol, whereas there was a significant change in AETH.

The participants of Yog group showed significant drop in weight, basal metabolism, systolic blood pressure, and diastolic blood pressure. There was a significant change in mean of breast simulator, endorphin and cortisol after three months. This showed significant drop in weight, basal metabolism, systolic and diastolic blood pressure compared to the Control group with regular practice of Yog at home.

Comparison of standards with baseline after three months: There was a significant drop in weight, basal metabolism, systolic and diastolic blood pressure in participants of Yog group after three months. There was considerable change in the levels of weight and basal metabolism, and endorphin levels in participants of the Control group.

Finding: The hormone level had reduced in participants compared to 10 day supervised short-term practice of Pranayam. Although the Control group practising Pranayam at home without supervision did not show significant effect on stress hormone level. There is a need to study the effect of supervised regular practice of Pranayam on stress.

Special features (first day) of Baseline between Yog Group and Control Group

	Group	Number	Mean	Standard Deviation	Probable value
Age	Yog Group	58	36.33	7.44	0.033
	Control Group	53	33.45	6.59	
Weight	Yog Group	63	69.52	11.83	0.57
	Control Group	56	68.33	11.33	
Height	Yog Group	62	164.83	7.07	0.63
	Control Group	56	165.58	9.83	
Systolic Blood Pressure	Yog Group	63	120.57	16.26	0.7
	Control Group	56	121.54	10.87	
Diastolic Blood Pressure	Yog Group	63	81.4	7.65	0.75
	Control Group	56	81.86	8.37	
Basal Metabolism	Yog Group	62	25.64	4.43	0.56
	Control Group	56	25.13	5.09	
Endorphin	Yog Group	61	44.71	56.62	0.32
	Control Group	51	35.25	44.99	
ACTH	Yog Group	63	26	10.73	0.16
	Control Group	54	21.39	9.61	
PRL	Yog Group	63	162.55	127.50	0.75
	Control Group	56	170.53	149.46	
Cortisol	Yog Group	63	277.83	100.23	0.79
	Control Group	56	273.63	79.27	

Comparison of parameters at Baseline with those at 10th day in Yog Group (Paired T-test)

Parameters	Group	Number	Mean	Standard Deviation	Probable Value
Weight 10th day	Baseline 58	58 67.42	69.38 11.75	12.17	0.0001
Basal metabolism	Base line 10th day	57 57	25.73 24.99	4.57 4.38	0.0001
Systolic blood pressure	Base line 10th day	59 59	120.8 113.5	16.51 15.44	0.001
Diastolic blood pressure	Base line 10th day	59 59	81.5 77.9	7.87 8.81	0.007
Cortisol	Base line 10th day	60 60	280.84 223.73	101.59 71.26	0.0001
PRL	Base line 10th day	60 60	167.18 150.68	128.86 127.39	0.06
ACTH	Base line 10th day	60 60	26.43 20.73	10.79 8.17	0.001
Endorphin	Base line 10th day	52 52	47.24 37.98	59.57 48.44	0.39

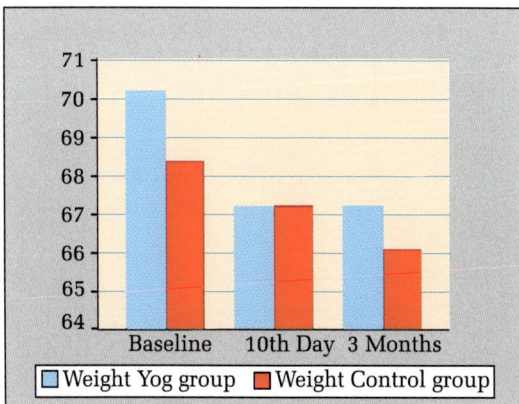

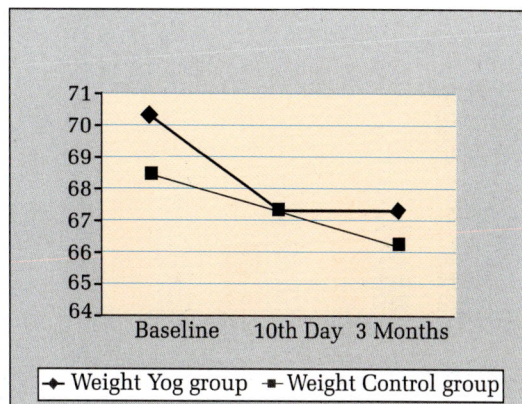

Comparision of Parameters at Baseline with those at 10th day in Control Group

	Group	Number	Mean Value	Standard Deviation	Probable Value
Weight	Baseline	55	68.33	11.44	0.0001
	10th day	55	66.62	11.13	
Basal metabolism	Baseline	55	25.13	5.14	0.0001
	10th day	55	24.48	4.88	
Systolic blood pressure	Baseline	55	121.45	10.95	0.0001
	10th day	55	113.29	9.96	
Diastolic blood pressure	Baseline	55	81.78	8.43	0.03
	10th day	55	79.49	7.24	
Cortisol	Baseline	55	275.38	78.90	0.25
	10th day	55	259.75	106.71	
PRL	Baseline	55	172.60	150.02	0.22
	10th day	55	188.78	143.92	
ACTH	Baseline	52	21.57	9.73	0.29
	10th day	52	23.59	12.03	
Endorphin	Baseline	32	23.43	37.76	0.12
	10th day	32	12.14	16.31	

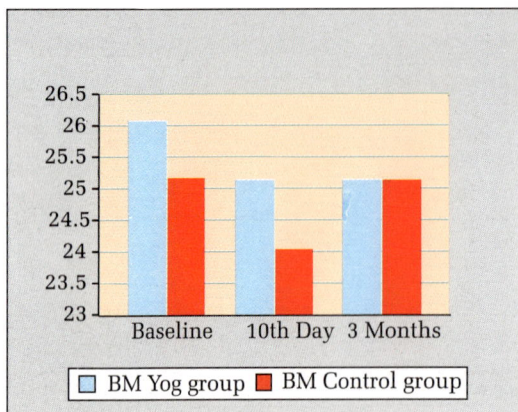

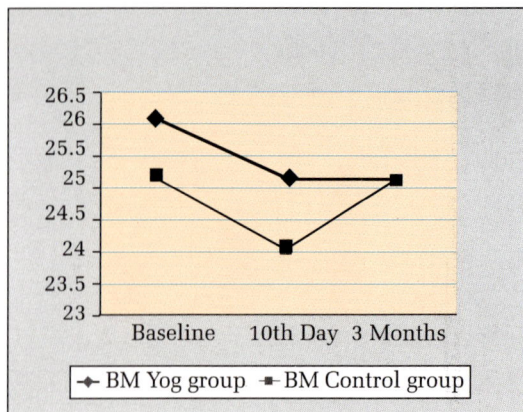

Comparison of Various Standards in Yog Group for 10 days vs 3 months

	Group	Number	Mean	Standard Deviation	Probable Value
Weight	10th day	45	60.06	12.32	0.2
	3 Months	45	67.45	11.34	
Basal metabolism	10th day	44	25.1	4.35	0.2
	3 Months	44	24.86	3.90	
Systolic blood pressure	10th day	47	113.96	16.44	0.1
	3 Months	47	116.68	16.03	
Diastolic blood pressure	10th day	47	77.91	9.06	0.9
	3 Months	47	78	10.89	
Cortisol	10th day	49	226.09	72.48	0.4
	3 Months	49	236.76	79.01	
PRL	10th day	49	157.67	136.84	0.7
	3 Months	49	162.73	85.18	
ACTH	10th day	49	20.71	8.27	.001
	3 Months	49	14.75	5.37	
Endorphin	10th day	46	36.8	46.78	0.005
	3 Months	46	15.14	29.57	

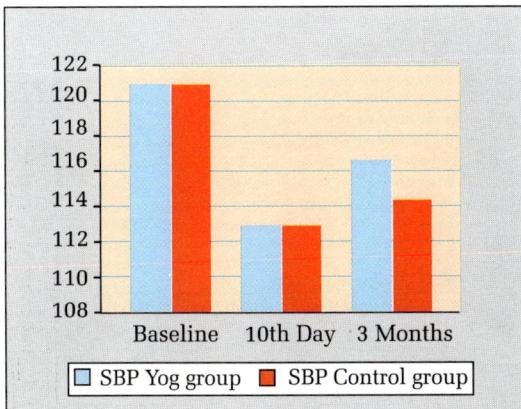

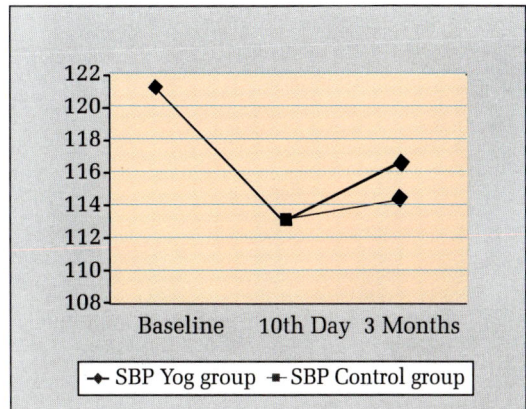

Comparison of various standards in Control Group for 10 days vs 3 months

	Group	Number	Mean	Standard Deviation	Probable Value
Weight	10th Day	45	65.87	11.36	0.3
	3 Months	45	66.18	10.46	
Basal metabolism	10th Day	45	24.49	5.07	0.3
	3 Months	45	24.62	4.95	
Systolic blood pressure	10th Day	45	112.87	9.51	0.3
	3 Months	45	114.44	10.25	
Diastolic blood pressure	10th Day	45	78.84	6.44	0.6
	3 Months	45	78.22	7.46	
Cortisol	10th Day	43	258.4	109.16	0.4
	3 Months	43	246.7	84.24	
PRL	10th Day	43	185.12	117.11	0.3
	3 Months	43	169.94	89.57	
ACTH	10th Day	43	24.43	12.87	0.0001
	3 Months	43	14.49	6.59	
Endorphin	10th Day	43	8.92	10.24	0.6
	3 Months	29	10.95	20.92	

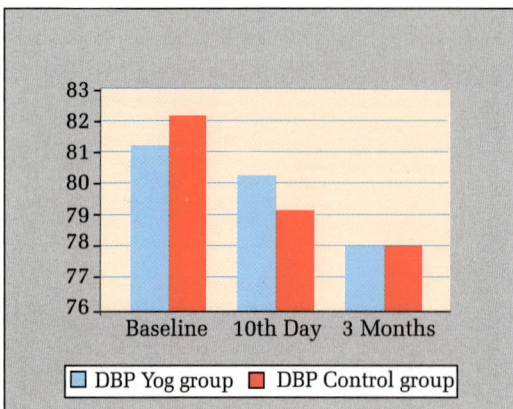

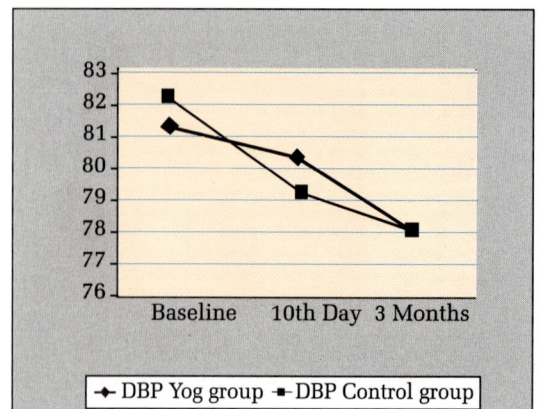

Comparison of various standards in Yog Group after 3 months

	Group	Number	Mean	Standard Deviation	Probable Value
Weight	Base Line	47	70.32	12.25	0.0001
	3 Months	47	67.58	11.36	
Basal metabolism	Base Line	46	25.87	4.34	0.0001
	3 Months	46	24.82	3.86	
Systolic blood pressure	Base Line	48	112.38	17.26	0.01
	3 Months	48	116.96	15.97	
Diastolic blood pressure	Base Line	48	81.38	80.30	0.06
	3 Months	48	78.46	11.24	
Cortisol	Base Line	49	278.91	107.03	0.007
	3 Months	49	236.76	79.01	
PRL	Base Line	49	174.64	137.65	0.44
	3 Months	49	162.73	85.18	
ACTH	Base Line	49	26.26	11.21	0.0001
	3 Months	49	14.75	5.37	
Endorphin	Base Line	47	50.15	58.72	0.0001
	3 Months	47	12.24	22.49	

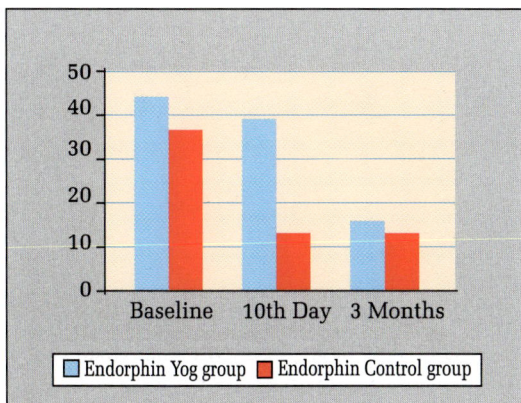

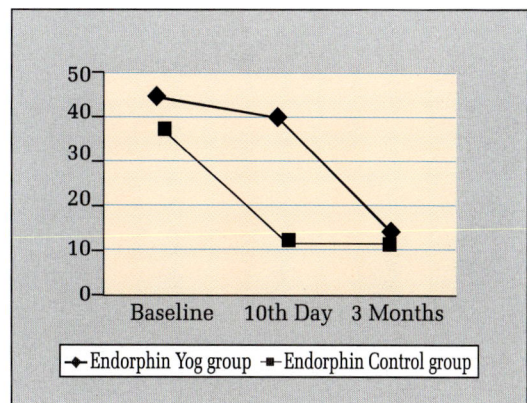

Comparison of various standards in Control Group after 3 months

	Group	Number	Mean	Standard Deviation	Probable Value
Weight	Baseline	45	67.56	11.68	0.0001
	3 Months	45	66.18	10.46	.
Basal metabolism	Baseline	45	25.14	5.33	0.0001
	3 Months	45	24.62	4.95	
Systolic blood pressure	Baseline	45	121.38	10.64	0.001
	3 Months	45	114.44	10.25	
Diastolic blood pressure	Baseline	45	81.38	7.74	0.011
	3 Months	45	78.22	7.46	
Cortisol	Baseline	43	260.84	74.35	0.3
	3 Months	43	246.70	84.24	
PRL	Baseline	43	161.24	74.33	0.3
	3 Months	43	169.94	89.57	
ACTH	Baseline	41	20.39	9.19	0.0001
	3 Months	41	14.53	6.74	
Endorphin	Baseline	38	31.59	39.70	0.005
	3 Months	38	9.79	18.43	

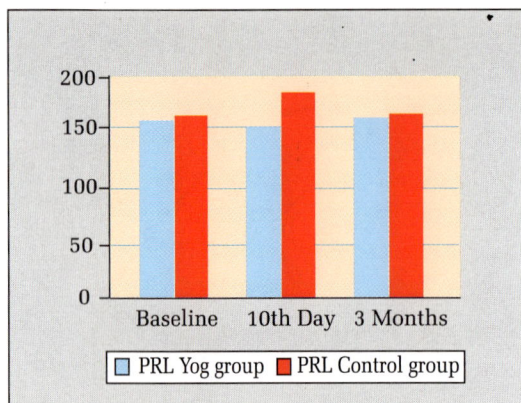

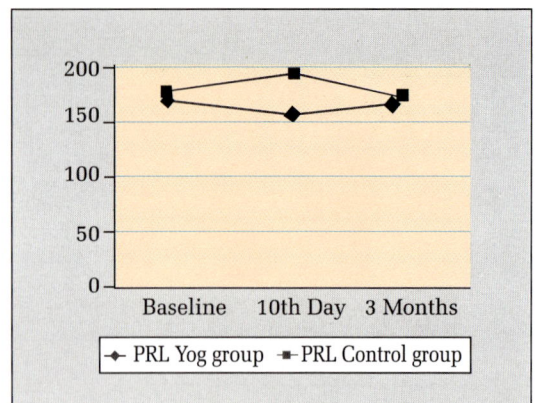

Comparison of change (per cent) in different duration in Yog and Control groups

Change %	Group	Number	Mean of change (%)	Standard Deviation	Probable Value
Cortisol- Baseline to 10 days	Yog Group	60	12.50	36.48	0.1
	Control Group	55	2.50	37.97	
Cortisol - 10 days to 3 months	Yog Group	49	+ 15.93	51.51	0.4
	Control Group	43	+ 67.64	422.69	
Cortisol - Baseline to 3 months	Yog Group	49	- 8.59	33.12	0.29
	Control Group	43	+ 0.02	43.00	
PRL - Baseline to 10 days	Yog Group	60	- 6.62	33.80	0.004
	Control Group	55	+ 20.95	59.90	
PRL - 10 days to 3 months	Yog Group	49	+ 30.72	70.35	0.38
	Control Group	43	+ 5.24	43.75	
PRL -Baseline to 3 months	Yog Group	49	+ 7.31	37.33	0.63
	Control Group	43	+ 11.13	38.45	
ACTH - Baseline to 10 days	Yog Group	60	- 10.16	48.05	0.004
	Control Group	52	+ 25.29	72.74	
ACTH - 10 Days to 3 months	Yog Group	49	- 19.05	43.11	0.06
	Control Group	43	- 33.03	26.56	
ACTH- Baseline to 3 months	Yog Group	49	- 38.15	22.01	0.003
	Control Group	41	- 19.30	33.67	

Compliance of Yog participants in Experiment Group

Yog Group practice	No:	Min	Max	Mean	Standard Deviation
Every week	48	2.00	7.00	6.0	1.35
Everyday hours	49	.25	3.50	1.23	.59
Every week hours	46	1.00	24.50	7.61	4.49

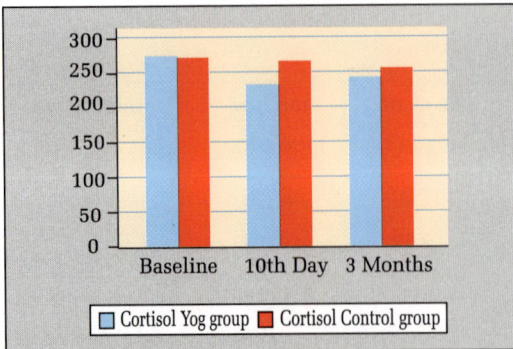

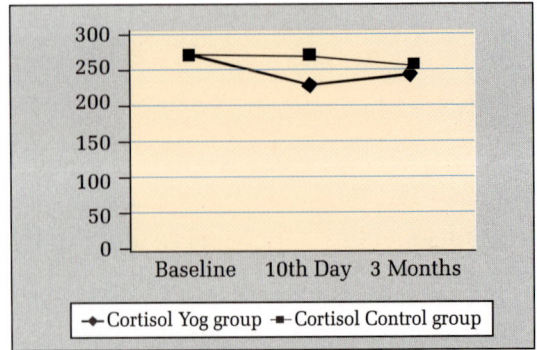

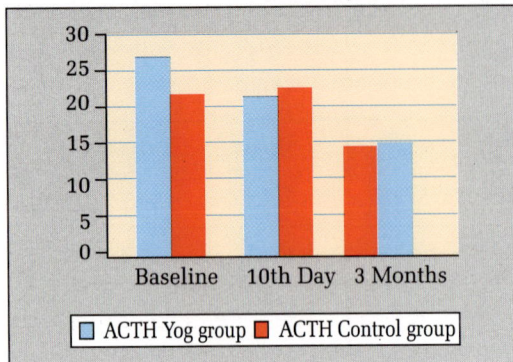

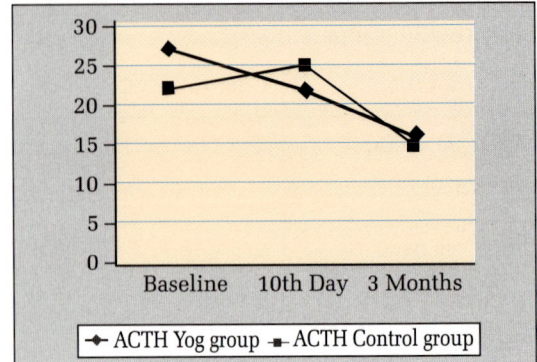

Results:

1. Control group: Number of people who did not practise Yog - 56

   No significant changes noticed on the basis of old samples.

2. Yog group: Total number of people who practised Yog - 63.

   (a) Those standards where change was noticed (10 days vs 1 day) - weight, basal metabolism, systolic pressure, diastolic pressure, cortisol, ACTH, endorphine and breast simulation hormones . These changes were not significant from biochemical point of view.

   (b) After the practice of Yog at home for 10 days to 3 months, weight, basal metabolism, systolic blood pressure, diastolic blood pressure, endorphine, breast stimulating hormones, and cortisol hormones had reduced.

Summary

1. Weight, basal metabolism, systolic blood pressure, diastolic blood pressure, endorphine, breast-stimulating hormones, cortisol hormones had reduced in Yog group.

2. There was no significant difference in Control group, which did not practice Yog.

3. It was recommended that the study should be continued for a longer duration.

Study of Psychophysiological Effects of Yog training on Healthy Volunteers and Those with Metabolic Syndrome

Scientific study was carried out to see the psychophysiological effects of eight-day Yog training on healthy volunteers and those with metabolic syndrome. Yog is an ancient Indian science and a life style. The ancient Yog texts describe the effect of Yog in a simple and sequential method. All these results are based on the personal experiences of saints.

The unmatchable effects of Yog have drawn the attention of anatomists all over the world. Yog revolution has gained momentum due to Herculean efforts of Swami Ramdevji. The results of Yog presented to the world by Swami Ramdevji have changed the initial resistance and unwilling attitude of anatomists and psychologists into being inquisitive and curious. The amazing results obtained in personal and social life along with treatment of diseases has literally forced the anatomists and psychologists to analyze the scientific basis of Yog. This has been possible only due to efforts of Swami Ramdevji. The research team of Vivekanand Yog and Research Institute, Bangalore, conducted a study on the psychophysiological effects of Yog training on healthy and those with metabolic syndrome in the premises of Patanjali Yogpeeth (Trust), Hardwar. Before knowing the results and conclusions drawn from this study and Swamiji's contribution in scientific development of Yog, it would be advantageous to know the efforts made in this direction.

General Introduction

Several people have shown inquisitiveness to understand the known and unknown scientific aspects of Yog. Many authors have understood Yog through personal experiences and mentioned its scientific results. In the beginning of 20th century, Swami Kuvalyanand and his disciple K.T. Behnan had studied the radiation effects of yogic processes and consumption of oxygen in breath Control (Pranayam) based on Yog. Later researchers like Satyanarayana and Shastri, (1958), Banger et al. (1961), Anand and Chinna, (1961) presented their conclusions pertaining to Yog. Kothari and his friends conducted another study in 1973, which presented a different type of effect of yogic processes on heart. When a person was made to sit in a deep ditch underground for 29 hours, his ECG line turned straight, which remained in the same position for five days. The electric processes of body came back to normal position around 30 minutes before digging open the ditch. The authors have however not made specific clarification about this condition.

The scientists have shown interest in understanding another yogic effect, the factor reducing the need of metabolism, this factor helps the person in staying inside a deep ditch free of atmospheric air for long time without any physical or mental pain. The study of Anand and others in 1961 and Karamabelkar in 1968 confirm this result.

Maharishi Maheshyogi popularised transcendental meditation (TM) in the sixties. This process is taught in a simple method and has scope for scientific experiment. Robert Keith Wellace (1970) has mentioned in his thesis and other research papers published later (Wellace etc.) that meditation has a definite effect on reduction in metabolic rate, change in blood chemistry, increase in galvanic skin resistance, and continuous change in EEG samples.

Several methods of meditation are prevalent in India. Yog propounders have conducted in-depth research on these methods and also propagated them. Some of these methods and research done with them are described below.

EEG on Meditation and Independent Study

Saint Mahesh propagated transcendental meditation method. It has been described as the fourth main stage of consciousness. Its practice brings about changes akin to what takes place in sleep, for example, reduction in heart rate and consumption of oxygen, and increase in the flow of skin induced electric current etc. However increase in the EEG Alpha wave and its regularity was similar to what is generally observed duing wakefulness (Wellace (1970), Vellace, Vesan, Wilson 1971). Yogic methods developed by followers of Jainism, Buddhism and devotees of other religions have also attracted people. Brahmakumari community has also developed a popular method of meditation. Acharya Rajneesh is also one of the popular names in this tradition. The list is unending if other names at regional and local levels are also included. Several scientists have published research papers on the methods of meditation developed by Brahmakumari community, transcendental meditation, Vipasana meditaton and on methods developed by Jains and Buddhists. These studies bring out interesting results related to meditation. However it is not possible to include all the results here due to lack of space.

General Research on Pranayam

Behanan (1971) said that consumption of oxygen increases by 24.5 and 18.5 per cent during Ujjayi and Bhastrika Pranayam respectively. Similarly Miles (1964) measured the consumption of oxygen during Ujjayi, Bhastrika, Kapalbhati and other Pranayam. He concluded that the consumption of oxygen during these three Pranayam increased by 32, 20 and 14 per cent respectively. The respiration rate increased by 3 breaths per minute after Ujjayi and Bhastrika Pranayam, whereas it increased by 4 breaths per minute after Kapalbhati. A person who practised Ujjayi Pranayam at different heights from the sea level found that consumption of oxygen increased by 9 per cent at an altitude of 520 meters above mean sea-level. Rao (1968) found that this rate increases by 16 per cent at an altitude of 3800 meters. The comparison was done at low altitudes as well.

Bhargav Gagot and Mascrenhas (1988) studied the breath holding rate in 20 volunteers.

The breath holding time, heart rate, systolic and diastolic blood pressure, and galvanic skin resistance were noted at different levels of respiration. All the 20 volunteers practised Nadi Shodhan Pranayam for four weeks in the initial recordings of above-mentioned parameters. The heart rate, and blood pressure (systolic and diastolic) were low and increased considerably after Pranayam. Therefore, Pranayam changes the automatic process of breath holding. Probably it takes place by increasing the voice of vagus nerve and decreasing the sympathetic rendition. Kumbhak respiration cycle is considered to be significant in Pranayam. There are two types of Kumbhak-short and long. The closed circuit method was used to study the consumption of oxygen with the help of Roth Spirometer. The respiration before, during and after Pranayam was measured. The results proved that during short Kumbhak consumption of oxygen increased by 52 per cent, whereas in case of long Kumbhak consumption of oxygen dropped by 19 per cent (Taylor and Desiraju). One person who practised Ujjayi and Bhastrika Pranayam was studied to find the mental inactivity during the practice. The study revealed that the NA waves increased widely and the inactivity reduced. The initial information of sensation and cerebrum during Pranayam were denoted in the form of change in amplification. Bud (1993) studied the positive and negative mood (condition of mind, emotional stage) and mental and physical energy in 71 normal volunteers in the age group of 21-76. He used three different methods, viz. inactivity, visualization and yogic breathing along with Pranayam. He concluded that Pranayam increases the mental, physical energy and gives a feeling of zeal more than the other two methods. Therefore, 30 minutes of yogic and respiratory practice has a special strengthening effect on mental and physical experience and increases the high positive mood.

Effect of Yog practice on higher mental processes

Motor Skills

The performance of motor skills or stiffness of hands improved to a considerable level in children after practice of Yog (1993). Improvement was also seen in adults (1994). The results show that Yog increases the skills of coordination of hands, eyes, concentration and focus. The hand grip is better in Yog practitioners compared to non-practitioners. It mentions that Yog increases motor skills in children, adults and patients of arthritis (Des et al., 2001). Yog increases the desire to learn (Manjunath and Telis, 1998) and finally Yog practice increases the tapping speed, which reduces the tiredness caused due to shaking and moving the hands.

Goals and Objectives of Study

India has produced several Yog teachers in the last century who have contributed positively in the teaching and training of Yog. Every Yog teacher has developed Yog processes depending on self practice, special processes, different ideologies and on the basis of own Yog practice. An attempt was made to prove the scientific base of useful experiences of Yog.

Swami Ramdevji has increased the popularity of Yog in the last one decade and presented it in totality. Swamiji has simplified the process of learning and training Yog.

A large number of people have shared the benefits gained with Yog practice as per Swamiji's guidance. This study was done with the main objective of health benefits and it analyzed the psychophysiological effects of an eight-day Yog training on healthy volunteers and those with metabolic syndrome.

Goals

This eight-day Yog training camp was conducted with the objective of studying the influence of this Yog module along with voluntary breath holding, autonomic balance with a shift towards parasympathetic dominance, autonomic reactions to a physical provocation like hand grip, motor functions, viz. strength of grip, speed for repetitive movement and fine motor skills, performance in a task for focused and selective attention.

Objectives

To study the autonomic and respiratory variables like heart rate, galvanic skin resistance, finger plethysmogram amplitude and respiratory rate, perceptual and motor tasks like hand grip, tapping speed performance (evacuation of additional secretions), measuring psychological variables like testing and cancellation test (number 6), and symptoms check list.

Methods

Two types of participants were included in the 10-day residential camp - healthy volunteers on the basis of medical tests and those with metabolic syndrome who were selected for the BMI test, fat line graph (line graph representing the known qualities and tests) and obesity. Each group consisted of 100 participants.

Healthy Volunteers: One group of males and females had volunteers from all over India and another group consisted of volunteers from Sahara Group of Companies. All the volunteers were in the age group of 22 and 60. The average age (SD) of volunteer for Yog group was 36.2 (7.2) and 33.3 (6.5) for Control group. Majority of the volunteers had practised Yog before this camp in some form or the other.

Volunteers with Metabolic syndrome This group included both male and female from all over the country. Majority of them had practised Yog before this camp in some form or the other.

Study Plan

For healthy volunteers : The study plan used for this included volunteers after looking into the detailed case history and medical tests on the basis of :

Volunteers coming from all over the country, who expressed the willingness to participate in the study and who were willing to practise Yog module for three months and were kept in **Yog group.**

Similarly after looking into the detailed case history and medical tests volunteers from Sahara Group of Company who expressed willingness to participate in the study were selected for **Control Group**

These volunteers were willing to be present in Yog camp in both sessions for 10 days and listen to Yog discourses of Swami Ramdevji on Yog and life-style but were not allowed to practise any method taught in camp and were willing not to practise any method taught in the context of changes in life-style for three months.

Both Yog and Control group were present in the same camp, they had common meals and followed the same daily routine. They were asked to follow self-practise and directions for the next three months.

The participants of **Control group** were analyzed on the following parameters.

- Heart rate, galvanic skin resistance, digit pulse volume and respiration
- Hand grip and tapping speeds
- Psychological factors or testing the six letter cancellation test and symptom check list.

Metabolic syndrome group : All the 100 participants practised Yog and Pranayam as per Swami Ramdevji's directions and followed the same daily routine and had common meals in the camp. They were asked to follow the fixed Yog module for a period of three months.

The participants of this group were analyzed on the following parameters:

- Motor skills
- Psychological factors
- Symptom check list.

Analysis

Autonomic and respiratory factors : (Telis, Nagratna and Nagendra, 1996), five minutes recording of figures or heart rate through EKG, galvanic skin resistance, respiration and digit pulse volume, which has been mentioned below.

This was done on first and tenth day. After five minutes of recording the blood pressure was recorded. Polygraphic recording was done using 4 channel computerized polygraphy. The EKG was recorded with standard lead -1 shape. Skin resistance was done with the help of safe electric receptors after covering it with galvanized jelly. The receptors were kept on the finger bones at a distance from the centre line below the index and middle fingers. 10 UA current was passed in the electric receptors. Respiration was recorded using volumetric stretch sensor transducer, which was placed 8 cm below the lower rib of the body as the person was seated in a straight position. This photoplethismograph was kept far from centre line of left thumb bone and then finger nerve coverage was recorded. Mercury sphygmomanometer was used for the purpose, which was kept on mid portion of shoulder and hand, the sound of artery was recorded. Lowest pressure was recorded on which the carotcoph sound was appearing to be low.

Motor Skills

O' Connor Tweezer Dexterity Test

This was determined on the basis of O' Connor Tweezer Dexterity Test (Soogi and Ukase, 1968). This tool was manufactured by Anand Agency, Pune. People were asked to lift metallic pin, small tweezers with the hand they normally work with and place them in small holes of metallic plates. The maximum speed was supposed to be used. They were told the time of commencement of test and were asked to stop after four minutes. The number of pins sucessfully placed in the plate was taken as the dexterity score. It was observed that most people used their right hand for writing, throwing ball, combing hair etc.

Hand Grip Strength

Hand grip Dynometer (Anand Agency, Pune, India) was used to test the gripping strength of both hands. The participants were asked to press the thing with maximum strength. The test was done six times, thrice with each hand at an interval of 10 seconds. They were asked to keep the hands straight, parallel to floor as mentioned earlier. The maximum value derived out of three repetitions was used for statistical analysis.

Tapping Speed

Tapping is fast and repetitive movement of front and wrist part of hand similar to the movement done at board entry. This is a test done with a pencil and paper. The participants were asked to tap on alternate circles on paper with pencil for 60 seconds. The same routine was followed on first and tenth day. The total number of tappings made on both circles were counted.

Psychological variables

Cancelation Task

A test worksheet was included for cancelation task of number 6, wherein six targets were determined, which were to be cancelled. An activity department was kept wherein the alphabets were to be arranged randomly in 22 rows and 14 columns. The participants were asked to cancel maximum number of six target letters within 90 seconds as many times as possible.

The cancelation was to be done in even, vertical line on any one of the fixed target letter. They were asked to select straight line in the present study. The total number of canceled letters and wrong cancellations were noted. The resultant figure was derived by deducting wrong cancellations from total cancellations because test was completed before and after interruption. The even worksheet was made after changing the target letters and their order (Agrawal, Kalra, Natu and Deswal, 2002) in order to avoid re-examination. This was used for experiments done after determination. The cancelation of number 6 was done with the same method as used in Indian census to obtain instant results (Natu and Agrawal 1977).

Symptom Check List

The revised symptom check list (SCL -90) was used to understand the mental level of people along with mental problems and mental stress.

Yog Sessions

Two sessions of three hour each were held for 10 days (5-8 AM and 5-8 PM). Both the groups consisted of healthy volunteers and those suffering from metabolic syndrome. Healthy volunteers took part in the control group but did not participate in any Yog practice.

Swami Ramdevji included the following Yog modules in daily Yog practise. 1, seven light exercises; 2, seven basic asana; 3, seven Pranayam; 4, yognidra and 5, meditation. Besides the session included mass prayers with devotional songs and health education. Different types of Pranayam and their scientific basis has been described in detail in the beginning of the book.

Analysis of Results Obtained

In case of healthy volunteers, personal measurement Anova was conducted repeatedly, which included factors in between one person (day -1 and day -8) and mutual factors in people (group -Yog and Control) was derived at using bonepherony adjustment on the basis of comparison of average total of day 1 and day 8 with day 1 in sequential manner.

Wilcockson paired signed ranks test: The percentage increase in finger plethysmogram

Amplitude and Insometric hand grip test was done followed by comparison of changes in blood level.

Metabolic Syndrome Group

Number 6 Cancelation Test

Separate combined tests were done in order to compare the values of day 1 and day 8 equal values with the help of symptom check list and tapping speed.

Results

For Healthy Volunteers

Autonomic and Respiratory Variables

Heart Rate: Repeated Anova measurements wherein non-significant difference was observed in factors between one person (day -1, day -8) and mutual factors in between people (group- Yog and control), (F=3.07, P>.05, Huynh-Feldt epsilon = 1.000), Group (F=.316, P>.05, Huynh-Feldt epsilon = 1.000) can be mutual in determinants and groups, (F=2.376, P>.05, Huynh-Feldt epsilon = 1.000).

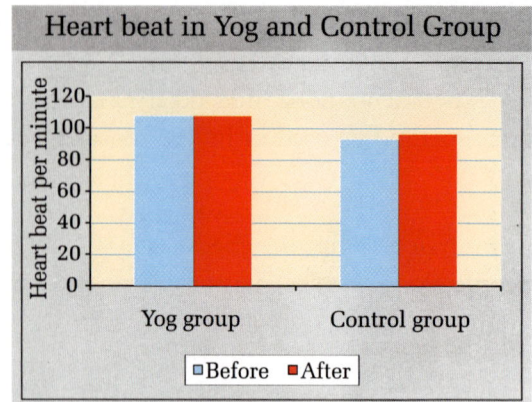

Heart beat in Yog and Control Group

Pairwise : Mutual comparison between day 8 and day 1 showed significant increase in heart rate after bonepherony adjustment (P<.05), whereas there was no difference in Yog group. (P<.05)

Galvanic Skin Resistance: Repititive Anova where significant difference was obtained in factors between one person (day -1, day -8) and mutual factor between people (Yog and control group) in determinants and groups (F=4.093, P<.05, Huynh-Feldt epsilon = 1.000). Similarly no significance difference was seen in mutual relation of determinants and groups (F=4.299, P<.05, Huynh-Feldt epsilon = 1.000) after using bonepherony adjustment (F=1.908, P>.05, Huynh-Feldt epsilon = 1.000) as per the total

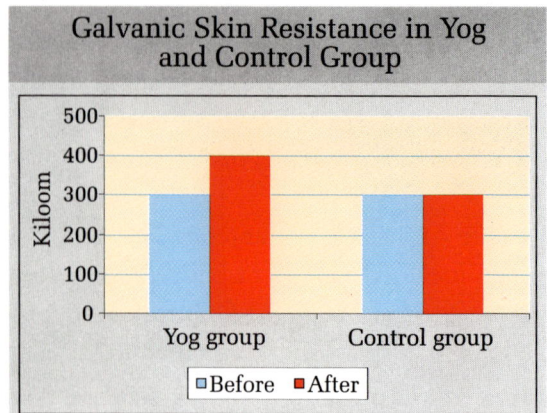

Galvanic Skin Resistance in Yog and Control Group

of Yog group, there was significant increase in galvanic skin resistance between values of day -8 and day-1 (P<.05) and there was no change in control group (P>.05).

Respiratory Rate: Repititive Anova wherein significant difference was obtained in factors between one person (day 1, days -8) and mutual factor between people (Yog and control group) (F=29.910, P<.001, Huynh-Feldt epsilon = 1.000), whereas there was no major difference between groups and (F=0.559, P>.05, Huynh-Feldt epsilon = 1.000) and similarly there was no significant difference between mutual relation of determinants and groups (F=0.424, P>.05, Huynh-Feldt epsilon = 1.000).

After bonepherony adjustment, as per the total of both groups, there was significant increase in respiratory rate between values of day -8 and day-1 (P<.001) and there was no change in control group (P<.001).

Finger Plethysmogram Amplitude: Comparison between values of day 8 and day 1 after insometric handgrip test showed significant increase in values of finger plethysmogram amplitude in both Yog (P<.01 Wilcockson paired signed ranks test) and control groups (P<.01 Wilcokson paired signed ranks test).

Blood Pressure

Systolic Blood Pressure: Repeated Anova measurements wherein significant mutual relation was noticed in between factors of one person (day -1, day -8) and mutual factors of people (Yog and control group) a significant mutual relation was noticed between determinants and groups (F=10.425, P<.01, Hugnh-Feldt epsilon =

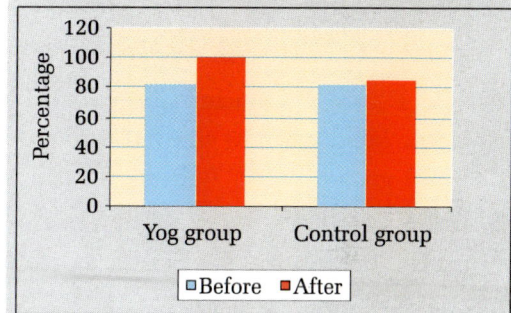

Respiratory Rate in Yog and Control Group

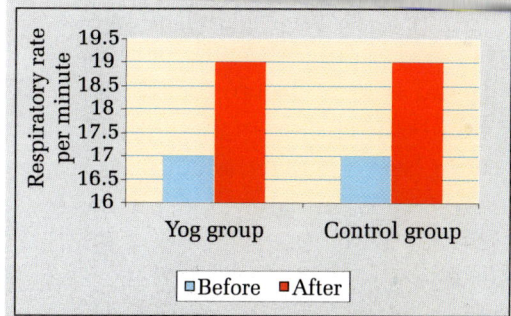

Change in Finger Plethysmogram Amplitude in both groups (per cent)

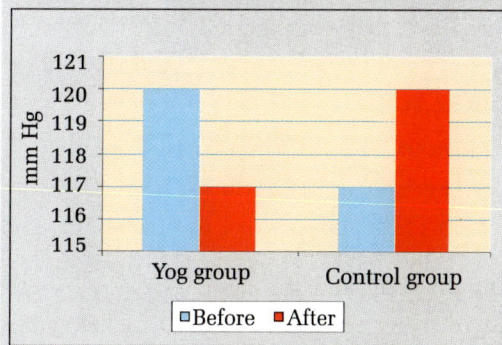

Systolic Pressure in both groups

1.000 and F=0.36 > P>.05, Huynh-Feldt epsilon = 1.000 respectively).

Comparison of mutual values of day 8 and day 1 after basic bonepherony adjustment showed significant drop in Yog group and increase in control group (P>.05).

Diastolic Blood Pressure: Repeated Anova measurements showed significant difference in factors between one person (day-8 and day-1) and mutual factors in between people (Yog and control group), (F=5.191, P<.05, Hugnh-Feldt epsilon = 1.000) and mutual relation between determinants and groups (F=12.66, P<.01, Hugnh-Feldt epsilon = 1.000, whereas there was no significant difference of groups (F=2.871, P<.05, Hugnh-Feldt epsilon = 1.000 respectively) comparison of total values of day-8 and day-

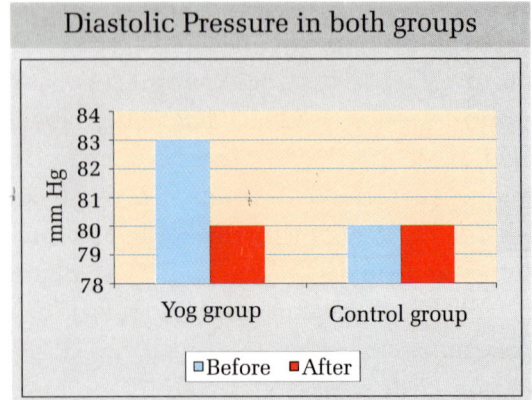

1 showed significant downfall in diastolic pressure after bonepherony adjustment (p<.001), whereas there was no difference of any kind in control group (p<.05).

Changes in Blood Pressure after Insometric Hand Grip Test

Systolic Blood Pressure: Comparison between the values of day-8 with day-1 after insometric hand grip test showed increase in percentage of total values of day 8 and day 1 in control group (p<.05 Wilcockson paired signed ranks test).

Diastolic Blood Pressure: Comparison between the values of day 8 with day 1 after insometric hand grip test did not show any difference in Yog and control group (p>.05 Wilcockson paired signed ranks test).

Motor Tasks

Motor Speed

Repetitive Anova obtained from tapping tasks on right circle where factors between one person (determinants day -1 and day -8) and mutual factors between one person (Yog and control group).

Insometric Hand Grip Test: Repetitive Anova measurements in right hand in which factors between one person (determinants day-1 and day-8) and mutual factors between one person (Yog and control group waiting list) showed significant difference between values, (F=7.285, P<.01, Huynlv-Feldt epsilon=1.000), whereas difference in mutual determinants and mutual relation of determinants and groups was not significant, (F=0.018, P<.05, Huynh-Feldt epsilon=1.000 and F=0.10>, P<.05, Huynh-Feldt epsilon=1.000 respectively).

There was a significant difference between the total values of day-8 and day-1 in tapping numbers after bonepherony adjustment in Yog group (P<.01) and there was no difference in control group (P>.05).

Comparison of total values of day-8 and day-1 and bonepherony adjustment there was no difference between hand grip strength in Yog and control groups.

Tapping Tasks on Left Circle: Repeated measurements in factors between one person (determinants day -1 and day -8) and mutual factors of people (Yog and control group) showed significant difference in mutual determinants (F=6.350, P<.05, Huynh-Feldt epsilon=1.000) mutual relation in determinants and groups (F=4.346, P<.05, Huynh-Feldt epsilon=1.000), whereas there was no significant change in between groups (F=0.071, P<.05, Huynh-Feldt epsilon=1.000).

Comparison of total values of day-8 and day-1 after bonepherony adjustment showed significant difference in tappings in Yog class (P<.01) and there was no difference in control group (P<.05).

Hand Grip Strength Test

Repetitive Anova measurements in right hand in factors between one person (determinants day-1 and day-8) and mutual factors between one person (Yog and control group waiting list) showed significant difference between values (F=7.285, P<.01, Huynh - Feldt epsilon = 1.000), difference in mutual determinants and mutual relation of determinants and groups was not significant (F=0.018, P>.05, Huynh - Feldt epsilon = 1.000 rFkk (F=0.107, P>.05, Huynh - Feldt epsilon = 1.000 respectively).

Comparison between values of day-8 and day-1 showed no significant difference in hand grip strength after bonepherony adjustment in Yog group and control group.

Hand Grip Strength Test : Repetitive Anova measurements in left hand in factors between one person (determinants day-1 and day-8) and mutual factors in one person (Yog and control group waiting list) showed significant difference between values (F=32.732, P<.001, Huynh-Feldt epsilon=1.000) and classes (F=4.645, P<.05, Huynh-Feldt epsilon=1.000), whereas mutual action was not significant in determinants and groups (F=.004, P<.05, Huynh-Feldt epsilon=1.000).

There was a significant increase in the total values of day-8 and day-1 in hand grip strength after bonepherony adjustment in Yog group, (P<.01 for comparison of both values) and there was increase in number of tappings of day-8 and day-1 after bonepherony adjustment in Yog group (P<.01) but there was no difference in control group (P<.05)

O' Connor Tweezer Dexterity: Repetitive Anova measurements in right hand in factors between one person (determinants day-1 and day-8) and mutual factors between one person (Yog and control group waiting list) showed significant difference between values (F=7.285, P<.01, Huynlv-Feldt epsilon=1.000), whereas there was no significant difference between determinants (F=7.862, P<.01, Huynh-Feldt epsilon=1.000) and groups (F=4.857, P<.05, Huynh-Feldt epsilon=1.000).

Comparison of total values of day-8 and day-1 after bonepherony adjustment showed significant difference in dexterity score in Yog and control group (P<.01 and P<.05 respectively).

Psychological Variables

Symptoms Check List

Repetitive Anova measurements in right hand in factors between one person (determinants day-1 and day-8) and mutual factors between one person (Yog and control group waiting list) showed significant difference between values (F=70.181, P<.001, Huynh-Feldt epsilon=1.000), whereas the mutual action was not significant between determinants and groups (F=.388, P<.05, Huynh-Feldt epsilon=1.000 and F=2.978, P<.05, Huynh-Feldt epsilon=1.000).

There was no significant difference between the total values of day-8 and day-1 in tapping numbers after bonepherony adjustment in Yog group and control group.

Six Letter Cancelation Test: Repetitive Anova measurements in left hand in factors between one person (determinants day-1 and day-8) and mutual factors between one person (Yog and control group waiting list) showed significant difference between values (F=.351, P<.05, Huynh-Feldt epsilon=1.000) difference in groups (F=2.241, P<.05, Huynh-Feldt epsilon=1.000) in the same way, whereas the mutual relation was not significant between determinants and groups (F=.988, P<.05, Huynh-Feldt epsilon=1.000).

Comparison of total values of day-8 and day-1 after bonepherony adjustment showed significant difference in dexterity score in Yog and control group (P>.05).

People with Metabolic Syndrome

Symptom Check List: There was significant decreases in net scores of day 8 and day 1 (P<.01 two tailed paired test).

Six Letter Cancelation Test: There was significant increase in net values compared between day-1 and day-8 (P<.01 two tailed paired test).

Motor speed

The tapping task on the right circle: There was significant increase in net values compared between day-1 and day-8 (P<.01 two tailed paired test).

The tapping task on the left circle: There was significant increase in net values compared between day-1 and day-8 (P<.01 two tailed paired test).

Description

The results have been presented in two main headings. They are : 1, for general healthy volunteers and 2, for those with metabolic syndrome (high level of BMI and cholesterol and obesity).

Volunteers with Normal Health: The participants were studied on the basis of three main factors. They are autonomic and respiratory variables, motor tasks and psychological factors.

Autonomic and Respiratory Variables: When recordings were taken on the basis of base-line it was found that there was significant increase in galvanic skin resistance in values at the beginning and end of Yog camp in Yog group but there was no change in control group. This was an indication of reduction in simulator of sweat glands. The description of this change is debatable. It is believed that sweat glands are helpful in natural galvanic skin processes as has been estimated according to the SRL recording. Human sweat glands are considered to be simulators of sympathetic cholinergic system. At the end of camp there was significant increase in heart rate in the control group, whereas there was no difference in Yog group. On the other hand the respiratory rate was even in both the groups (this shows that factor responsible for anxiety in body is not associated with practice of Yog). The systolic blood pressure had reduced drastically in Yog group. Average was 5.2 mmHg, whereas in control group the average increase in systolic blood pressure was 3.3 mmHg. The diastolic blood pressure reduced by an average 5.5 mmHg in Yog group. The changes in autonomic factors were done to put up with a challenge. Insometric handgrip strength that produces sympathetic rendition increased in both Yog and control group on the last day of the camp in finger plethysmogram amplitude. The results were higher in case of Yog group.

This shows that challenge leads to sympathetic activity in both groups. It is less on the last day compared to first day and proves that in both the groups the body is more efficient to face the challenge of insometric hand grip strength in the end.

Performance in motor tasks: Three motor tasks were performed, they were: 1, O' Conner hand dexterity test; 2, Handgrip strength test and 3, Tapping test.

There was considerable increase in hand dexterity in both groups on the last day compared to first day of the camp. Both the groups showed increase in scores. The values of second test done after the camp were less compared to values of the second test done before the camp; the difference between values of first and second tests were related to muscular weariness. This weariness was less after the camp compared to before camp. Similarly, practice improved hand dexterity and reduced the weariness of small muscles of hands.

Hand dexterity and speed tasks: Similarly the initial speed depends on the portion related to neck and spine. For example in case of a few American mammals (the superior quality of mammals include monkeys, human beings), the hand dexterity is considerably low. Dexterity and skill depend on the speed of movement of hands and shoulders, coordination of hands and reflexes of eyes and fingers. This study shows that Yog improves the O' Conner tweezer dexterity performance.

Peg board test used in speed tasks showed that excessive worry and weakness has an indirect relation with performance. Along with that lower efficiency of speed task tendency is co-related to mental worry. After six weeks of Yog practice there was considerable decrease in symptoms of worry in patients of depression. Hence the factor effective for reducing worry in present study can be responsible for improving the score in dexterity test.

In case of handgrip test, there was considerable improvement in grip of left hand after the Yog camp. Handgrip strength denotes the muscular strength and patience. Therefore, there was considerable improvement in both these factors after Yog. Not much change was observed in right hand which could be due to some fault in research planning. The fault was that all the blood samples of participants were collected from right hand; the handgrip strength test was completed before the Yog practice. Whereas the male educated adult volunteers showed improvement in hand grip strength, similarly those children who understand the importance of Pranayam in Yog also showed improvement. Patients of arthritis who participated in only one session a day also showed improvement. The improvement in hand grip strength was due to practice of Pranayam and reduction in oxygen requirement. The reason being that availability of energy and oxygenation of glucose affects the handgrip strength. But after practising other Yog increased the handgrip strength, along with determining factors and awareness.

The scores obtained from paper pencil task used for determining the hand dexterity (number/value) (round in left hand) showed increase only in Yog group. This test involves the coordination between hands-eyes and wrist-shoulder movement. The results show that Yog practice increases these qualities.

Psychological variables: This category includes two types of tests, a. Symptoms check list (SCL –90) and b. Six-letter cancellation test (SLCT)

a. SCL –90 one part of this list was selected on the basis of physical symptoms of mental disorders and those related to mental stress. In both the groups (Yog and control group) the scores of mental disorders and physical symptoms had decreased considerably.

b. No difference was found in SLCT score between Yog and control group at the end of Yog camp.

Metabolic syndrome: Three tests were done on people with metabolic syndrome, they are symptoms checklist, and six letter cancellation test and tapping speed task. There was significant down fall in SCL-90 symptoms score. Six-letter cancellation test was used because this task measures the concentration and scanning skills based on observation. Significant improvement was noticed in tapping speed and there was reduction in muscular weariness. This denotes greater effectiveness of Pranayam in comparison with medicines.

Effects of results and tests

1. Healthy volunteers showed lower level of anxiety after Yog practice in period of rest or when dealing with some problem. It shows that Yog module is helpful in reducing the stress in condition of mental worry measured against the base line.

2. Repeated improvement in speed tasks, fall in weariness, improved tolerance and handgrip strength. This shows that Yog practice can help in mitigating the effects of repeated use of hands and wrist.

3. The physical symptoms of mental disorders reduced in both Yog and control group of volunteers. This shows that this camp has been successful in reducing the feeling of stress due to surroundings, general atmosphere, food, session, routine etc.

Note: The above-mentioned effects were noted in the form of one part of test done on this voluntary group where participants of Yog and control group were divided. It was advised to use random sampling control test and repeat the results.

In people with metabolic syndrome

In case of people with Metabolic syndrome there was improvement in letter cancellation tasks, which proves that after Yog practice there is improvement in eye and hand coordination, visual scanning and in selected mental abilities. The tapping speed increased in case of repeated movements, which shows that weariness in hands, wrists and fingers got reduced.

The conclusion is that Pranayam is indisputably more effective and gives quick results when compared to other yogic processes and medicines.

Psychosomatic effects of Yog - A pioneering study based on large scale survey

Yog is an age-old tradition but its scientific aspect has almost become extinct. This was later followed by myths and illusions spread in the name of Yog or under the guise of Yog. Yog has a completely scientific basis but the modern civilization was hesitant to accept it even after seeing the results. The main objective of establishing Patanjali Yogpeeth was to eliminate the myths prevailing in the society against it. It was possible only when people were assured about its scientific basis. Patanjali Yogpith established Yog research and development department and began its work on a large scale. This department began documentation of Yog's psychological affects at a large scale and conducted a detailed study and analysis.

Methodology

For analysis and study of Yog's psychological affect around one lakh people were sent a questionnaire on random survey and were asked to provide information on the psychological affect of Yog. The participants of this survey were given a fully representative survey on the basis of age, sex, educational qualifications, occupation, income, residence etc. This was helpful in avoiding any type of doubts regarding the authenticity of affect of Yog. PatanjaliYogpeeth believes that this is the first survey of its kind conducted on not only Yog but also on any of the modern medical sciences. The task of analyzing the answers and reaching at conclusions was a cumbersome process. The participants have shown active involvement and the analysts and specialists of Patanjali Yogpeeth have strived hard in compiling the results.

Details of participants involved in the survey

Sample size

Around 84663* people from India and abroad participated in the survey .

Sex

Out of the total participants the ratio of male – female was 59.12 and 40.88 percent respectively. This ratio depicts the awareness and inclination towards Yog in females.

Age

This survey represents people of all age groups. It is also clear that highest number of participants were in the age group of 25-50 years, which is the most productive age. This shows that interest towards Yog is increasing among the youth.

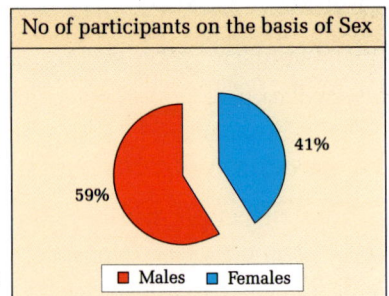

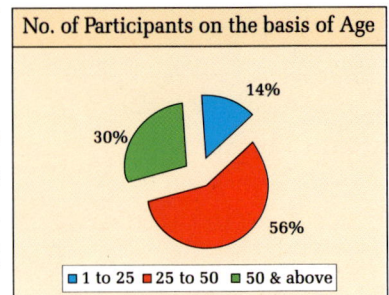

No of participants on the basis of Sex

41%

59%

■ Males ■ Females

No. of Participants on the basis of Age

14%

30%

56%

■ 1 to 25 ■ 25 to 50 ■ 50 & above

---

* We have compiled the feedback and reactions of more than one lakh people in this survey so far and it is an ongoing process. These conclusions have been derived on the basis of analysis of compilation and analysis of feedback of 84663 participants. These documents are kept at Research & Development department of Patanjali Yogpeeth.

Educational qualifications

The educational qualifications of the participant's makes it clears that all levels right from uneducated to highly qualified people have participated in the survey. It is to be noted that 85 percent of the participants are qualified up to 12th standard.

No of participants on the basis of Education

13.67% 14.44%
13.61% 29%

■ Illiterate ☐ 12th Std. ■ Graduate ■ PG ■ Ph.D

Occupation

A person's health is directly related to his income. People belonging to different occupations participated in it. As is clear from the list that on the basis of occupation, the highest number of participants (43 percent) were employed with the service sector. This group was more alert towards their well being and been proactive about it.

No of participants on the basis of Occupation

7%
23% 15%
3%
9%
43%

☐ Agriculture ■ Business ■ Labour ■ Service
■ Student ■ Unemployed

Residence

Around 65 percent of our population lives in villages. 42.19 percent of people who participated in this survey live in rural area and 57.18 percent live in urban areas. It appears that this survey is inclined towards urban areas but this aspect makes the survey even more effective. The reason is that cities are more prone to diseases and at the same time have better medical services. It is not that this survey is one sided, both the sides have been included in it. From the point of view of residence this survey is in the category of being a representative survey.

No of participants on the basis of Residence

43%
57%

■ Rural ■ Urban

Income level

The participants were divided into three categories on the basis of income – high, medium and low. This survey showed highest participation from middle class.

No of participants on the basis of Income

2%
45% 53%

■ High ■ Middle ■ Low

Awareness towards Yog

Television or electronic media has played an important role in Swami Ramdev's Yog revolution. It's interesting to note that same media which is blamed for cultural degradation and depreciation of moral values, extended the reach of Yog to large number of people.. Around 65.53 percent people watch television and gained awareness about Yog. Residential camps contributed by 8.33 percent and nonresidential

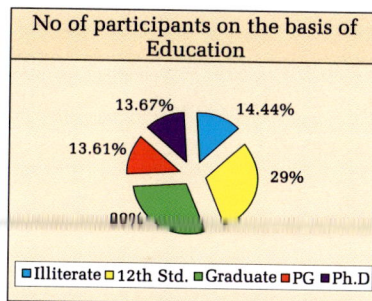

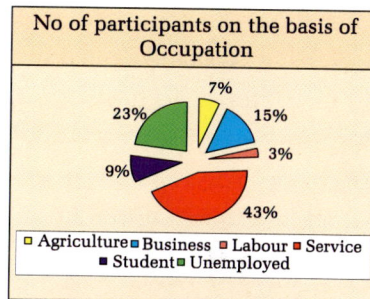

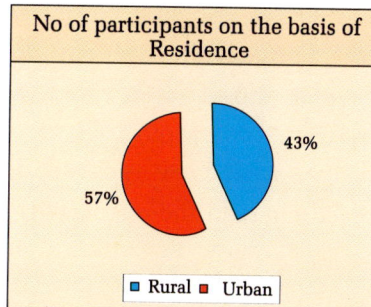

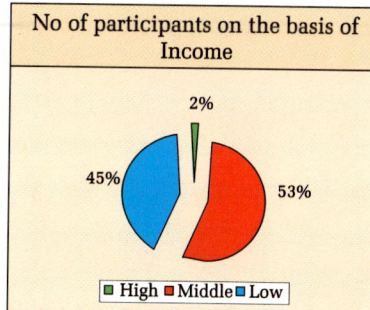

Yog camps contributed around 12.93 percent. Although Swami Ramdevji Maharaj spends most of his time in camps still it's television which has played a pivotal role is playing in extending the reach of Yog to every corner of the globe.

Regular practice of Yog

Out of the total participants 80.88 percent confirmed Yog practice. Rest 19.12 percent were not regular practitioners. This shows that people are assured of psychosomatic benefits of Yog and Pranayam and have adopted it as part of their lifestyle. Those who are unable to practice Yog despite being aware of its benefits, once they start practising Yog regularly then the world health scenario would be entirely different.

Time for practising Yog

The survey also showed that out of the total participants 76.18 percent practice Yog in the morning, 4.18 percent practice it in the evening and rest i.e., 19.64 percent in the morning and evening. As the morning time is ideal from the point of view of availability of oxygen. Therefore practising it in the morning is very beneficial.

Participant's states and countries

In this survey people from all the states were included so that the impact of Yog/Pranayam could be studied on the people living in places with varying climate, social and cultural scenario. The number of participants taking part in the survey from different states does not match with the population of that state. Leaving aside southern and eastern states, for other states the proportion of participants matched the to the population of the state. One unique feature of this survey was that the number may be less but participants from other countries like England, America, Thailand, Japan, Australia, Canada, Pakistan, Nepal, Bangladesh, Sri Lanka and UAE were also included. As a result this survey encompasses study of effects of Yog on people originating from much bigger spectrum of social, cultural and geographical backrgounds.

Benefits of Yog- Pranayam in different diseases

Obesity

Nowadays physical work has reduced to a great extent and eating habits are also poor. As

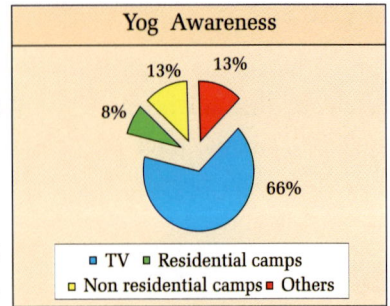

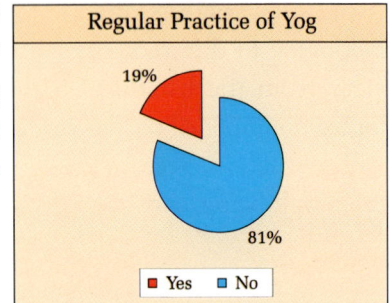

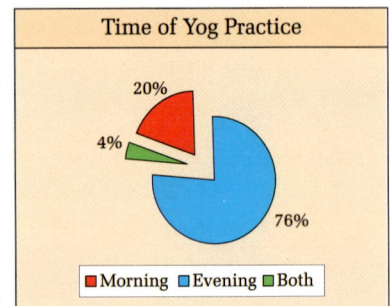

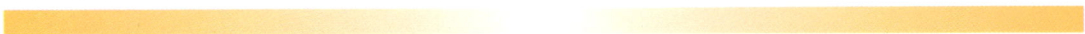

Yog Awareness

13% 13% 8% 66%

- TV - Residential camps
- Non residential camps - Others

Regular Practice of Yog

19% 81%

- Yes - No

Time of Yog Practice

20% 4% 76%

- Morning - Evening - Both

a result overweight problem is increasing. Yog is very effective for reducing weight. After this survey the conclusion was drawnYog is most effective for obesity in comaprison with its efficacy for all other diseases Out of the total participants included in the survey suffering from diseases, around 95.43 percent people got total or partial relief from obesity. The survey proved that 95.43 percent of participants definitely gained from Yog.

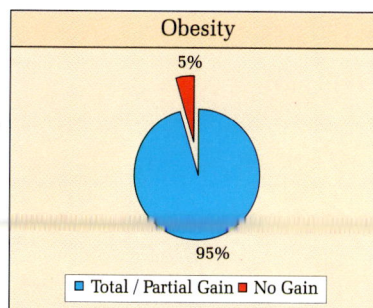

Obesity

5%

95%

◻ Total / Partial Gain ◼ No Gain

High blood pressure

Today a large section of the society is suffering from high blood pressure due to severe competition and hectic life schedule. Out of the total participants 18.46 percent were suffering from high blood pressure. 96.23 percent of participants confirmed positive effect of Yog and Pranayam in controlling blood pressure. Only 3.77 percent said that blood pressure increased after Yog practice. Positive effect of Yog and Pranayam on such a large number is miraculous. Yog is capable of curing blood pressure problem completely, there could be no better proof than above stated results of the survey.

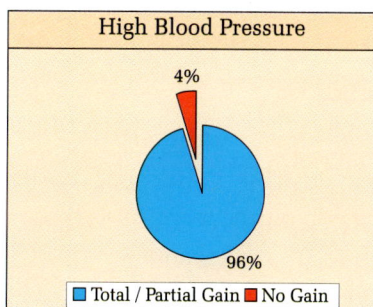

High Blood Pressure

4%

96%

◻ Total / Partial Gain ◼ No Gain

Arthritis

Irregular eating habits, lack of nutritious food and irregular life style leads to arthritis. 22.46 percent of the participants were suffering with this problem. 92.80 percent confirmed total or partial gain from Yog and Pranayam. Only 7.20 percent said that there has been no improvement even after practising Pranayam. This proves that Yog has played a major role in curing arthritis.

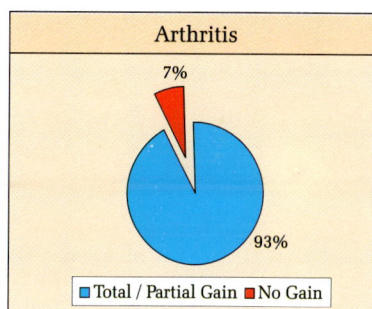

Arthritis

7%

93%

◻ Total / Partial Gain ◼ No Gain

Diabetes

Lack of physical exercise and eating high fat content food are some the reasons for diabetes. 28.42 percent of the total participants were suffering with this problem. 94.99 percent of participants confirmed partial or total benefit from Yog and Pranayam. Around 5.01 percent participants said that there has been no improvement even after practising Pranayam. We have personally experienced in thousands of cases that Pranayam has been able to control diabetes and

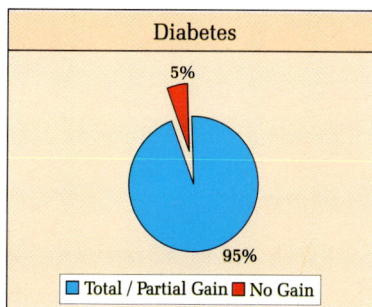

Diabetes

5%

95%

◻ Total / Partial Gain ◼ No Gain

its ill effects on body.

Heart disease

Stress, hectic schedule and cosmopolitan life style are increasing the number of heart patients. 13.48 percent of the participants were suffering with this problem. 94.36 percent of participants who gave their feedback said that Yog and Pranayam has given partial or total benefit. Around 5.64 percent said that their problem increased after practising Pranayam. Yog has played a major role in improving the health of heart patients.

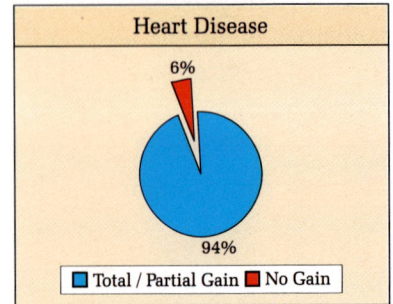

Heart Disease

6%

94%

☐ Total / Partial Gain ■ No Gain

Asthma

Pollution, unhealthy working conditions, lack of cleanliness results in asthma. 11.53 percent of the participants were suffering with this problem. 95.77 percent participants who gave their feedback said that Yog and Pranayam has given partial or total benefit. Around 4.33 percent said that problem has increased after practising Pranayam. According to a survey every fourth person in the world is suffering from some allergy

Asthma

4%

96%

☐ Total / Partial Gain ■ No Gain

(respiratory related disease) . Pranayam is a blessing for all of them. We can say that Pranayam can prove to be the final death blow to Asthama rather than death bringing an end to Asthma.

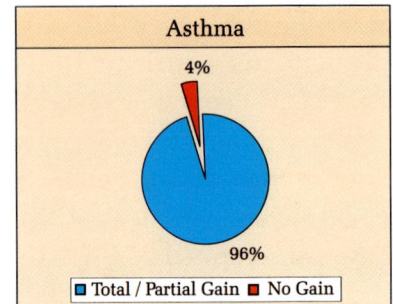

Kidney problem

Modern eating habits, pollution, and lack of cleanliness is increasing the number of patients with kideny problems. 18.45 percent of the participants were suffering with this problem. 93.67 percent participants who gave their feedback said that Yog and Pranayam has given partial or total benefit. Around 6.33 percent said that there has been no improvement even after practising Pranayam. Yog has played a major role in improving the health of the patients of kidney problems.

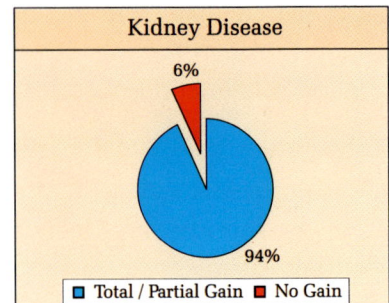

Kidney Disease

6%

94%

☐ Total / Partial Gain ■ No Gain

Spondylitis

Sitting in the same position for long hours, sedentary life style, lack of exercise is some of the problems that result in spondylitis. 15.48 percent of the participants were suffering with this problem. 94.91 percent of the participants who gave their feedback said that Pranayam has given partial or total benefit. Around 5.09 percent said that there has been no improvement even after practising Pranayam. This shows that Pranayam improves not only digestion and nervous related problems but also cures bone related diseases.

Skin diseases

Pollution, cosmetics, and lack of cleanliness result in skin diseases.13.25 percent of the participants were suffering with this problem. 91.71 percent of participants who gave their feedback said that Yog and Pranayam has given partial or total benefit. Around 8.29 percent said problem increased after practising Pranayam. This shows that Yog has played a major role in improving skin problems.

Liver and stomach diseases

Consumption of adulterated food, fast food culture, unhygienic life style results in liver and stomach related diseases. 30.80 percent of the participants were suffering with this problem. 93.67 percent of the participants who gave their feedback confirmed that Pranayam has given partial or total benefit. Around 6.33 percent said that problem increased even after practising Pranayam. Yog has played a major role in curing the liver and stomach

related diseases and people experience it immediately after beginning the practice.

Spondylitis

5%

95%

Total / Partial Gain ■ No Gain

Skin Disease

8%

92%

Total / Partial Gain ■ No Gain

Stomach Disease

6%

94%

Total / Partial Gain ■ No Gain

Change in mental condition with Yog and Pranayam

Yog and Pranayam are not merely physical exercises but they strongly influence our consciousness. They are effective in the treatment of those diseases which cannot be diagnosed or treated otherwise. Yog and Pranayam have a direct positive impact on our thinking. It has given a new life and energy to several people who had lost all hope and were highly disappointed and depressed. Yog and Pranayam has also led to lot of improvement in stress levels. The present life style and stress has adversely affected memory power of lot of people and they also got a chance to rejuvenate after coming into the shelter of Yog. During the survey the following results were seen on mental stress and thinking processes:

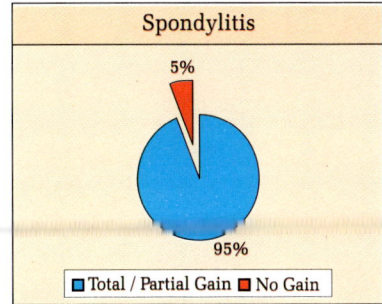

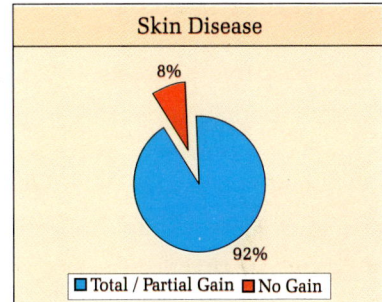

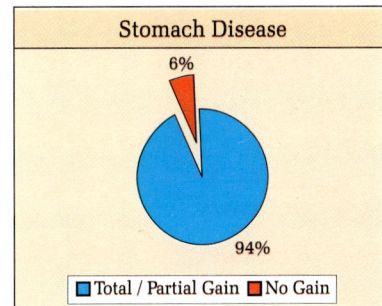

(a)   Mental stress

The results of the survey revealed that Yog and Pranayam reduced stress level in 48.07 percent people whereas 42.07 percent people did not have any affect on mental stress level with practice of Yog and Pranayam. 9.92 percent said that stress increased even after practising Yog and Pranayam. Yog and Pranayam have proved to be a blessing for the people suffering with mental stress even in the present modern world.

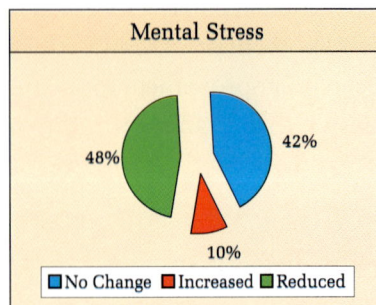

Mental Stress

48% · 42% · 10%

☐ No Change ☐ Increased ☐ Reduced

(b)   Positive attitude

When the person practices Yog and Pranayam he associates with the God present in his soul, and becomes successful in reaching his goals. As a result a totally frustrated person can lead a purposeful and enthusiastic life. The survey showed that practice of Yog and Pranayam has increased positive attitude in 61.77 percent people whereas 5.24 percent said the positive attitude reduced. 32.99 percent felt no impact. This survey shows that Yog and Pranayam increase positive thinking and our life becomes more objective and productive.

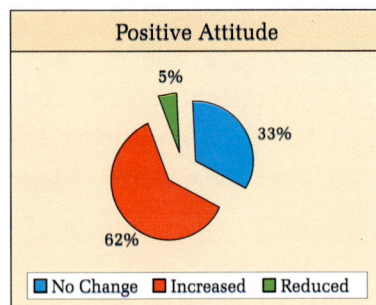

Positive Attitude

5% · 33% · 62%

☐ No Change ☐ Increased ☐ Reduced

(c)   Memory

Yog and Pranayam improve concentration power. As a result the memory power increases. Survey proves that memory power increased in 47.30 percent of the people and 48.73 percent felt no impact.

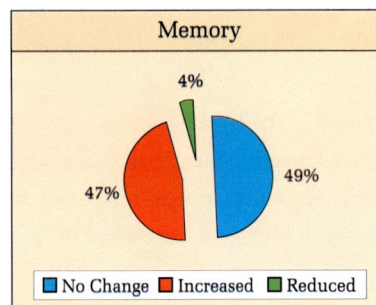

Memory

4% · 49% · 47%

☐ No Change ☐ Increased ☐ Reduced

Change in family life

Yog and Pranayam inspire us to see good qualities in every human being. It develops mutual love and affection in married life. Pranayam associates us with direct and indirect divine strengths and Gurus and makes us feel respectful towards them. As a result we develop reverence towards elders. Following are the changes seen in the lives of the participants.

Mutual Love

1% · 39% · 60%

☐ No Change ☐ Increased ☐ Reduced

(a)   Mutual love

59.54 percent of the participants agreed that Yog has

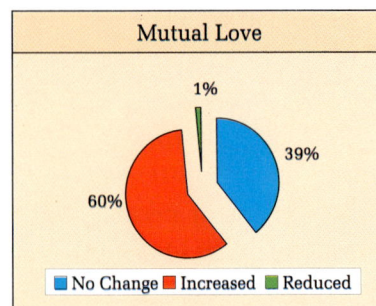

changed their family life and increased love in the family. 39.18 percent participants said that there has been no change in family life or mutual life. Whereas 1.28 percent said that mutual love reduced despite practising Yog and Pranayam.

(b) Happiness

Yog and Pranayam help us attain self-realization, it frees us from unknown fear and suffocation. It teaches us the art of living in the present. We feel happier and satisfied. 67.51 percent of the participants said that Yog and Pranayam increased the level of happiness, whereas 31.69 percent said that the level of happiness has not changed. Whereas 0.80 percent of the participants said that the level of happiness reduced in spite of practising Yog and Pranayam.

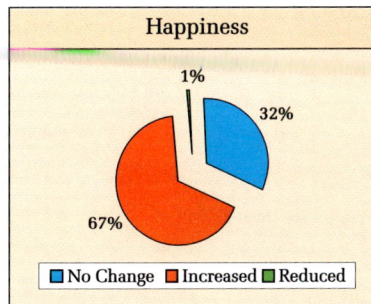

(c) Respect towards elders

61.98 percent of the participants agreed that Yog and Pranayam increased the level of respect towards elders. 37.98 percent said that there has been no change in this aspect. Only 0.74 percent said that the level of respect towards elders was reduced.

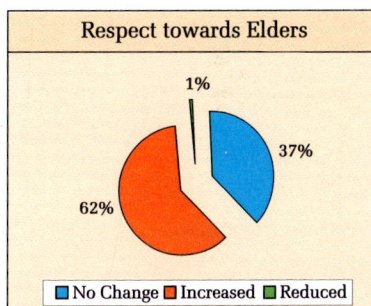

Change in social life

Yog and Pranayam make us sensitive towards social life and increase awareness. Regular practice helps us in fulfilling the social responsibilities to a great extent. Along with it we become sensitive towards the welfare of other living creatures. Following changes were seen in social inclinations in the survey:

(a) Interest in social work

The result showed that Yog increased the interest towards social work among 59.76 percent participants. 39.46 percent said that there was no improvement and a small percentage (0.78) percent said that the interest towards social work got reduced.

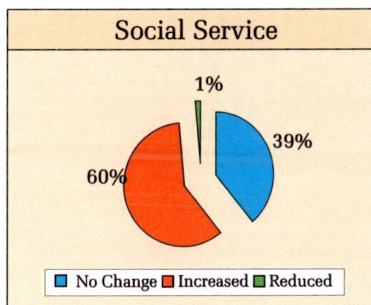

(b) Feeling of charity for poor and destitute

Practice of Yog increases feeling of doing charity for the poor and destitute. The survey showed that 66.29 percent

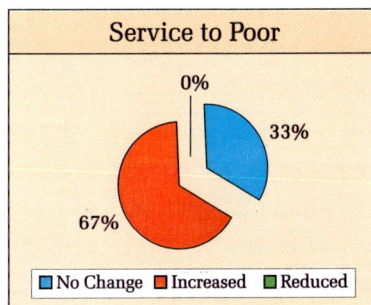

Happiness

1%
32%
67%

☐ No Change ☐ Increased ☐ Reduced

Respect towards Elders

1%
37%
62%

☐ No Change ☐ Increased ☐ Reduced

Social Service

1%
39%
60%

☐ No Change ☐ Increased ☐ Reduced

Service to Poor

0%
33%
67%

☐ No Change ☐ Increased ☐ Reduced

participants showed increase in the feeling of charity and public welfare. 33.30 percent showed no improvement in this area.

Changes in addictions and vices

Yog and Pranayam improve the good qualities within us. The eternal wisdom helps in quitting different kinds of addictions and vices. The survey analyzed the affect of Yog and Pranayam on different vices.

(a)   Vegetarian/Non-vegetarian

It is a scientific fact that human being's anatomy is suitable for vegetarian food. The person consumes non-vegetarian food for the sake of taste. Survey showed that 27.48 percent of the participants were non-vegetarians and out of them 72.60 percent quit non-vegetarian food. 15.65 percent could not quit non-vegetarian food even after practising Pranayam.

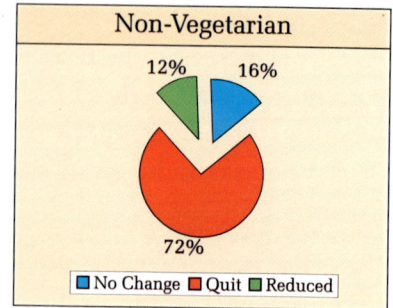

Non-Vegetarian
12%   16%
72%
No Change   Quit   Reduced

(b)   Alcohol

The survey showed miraculous results in people with alcohol addiction. It showed that 85.22 percent of people quit alcohol after practising Yog/Pranayam. Only 3.24 percent said that in spite of practising Pranayam they failed to quit this habit. Regular practice of Pranayam has changed the social, economic life of the people after they quit alcohol.

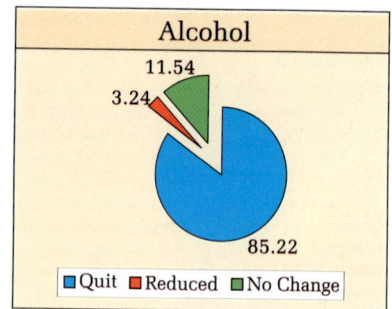

Alcohol
11.54
3.24
85.22
Quit   Reduced   No Change

(c)   Cold drinks

Now it has been scientifically proved that cold drinks are nothing but sweet poison. Even then attractive advertisements are luring millions and people are unable to quit it completely. Regular practice of Yog and Pranayam can be helpful in getting rid of the urge for cold drinks permanently. The conclusions drawn from the survey show that 63.23 percent of the participants were able to quit this habit after practising Yog and Pranayam and 30.15 percent people said that it reduced thier desire

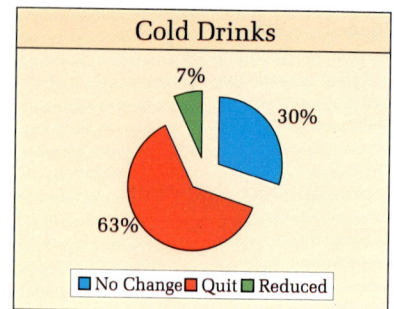

Cold Drinks
7%
30%
63%
No Change   Quit   Reduced

for cold drinks. Only 6.62 percent said that they could not leave the habit even after practising Yog and Pranayam.

(d)   Pizza / burger

The multinational companies are serving hot and spicy food with high fat content and making huge amounts of money. Pizza, burger are selling like hot cakes all over the world but it increases the risk of obesity, diabetes and even cancer. Those who quit this habit will definitely lead a long and healthy life. The conclusions derived from the survey show that 68.74 percent of participants practising Yog and Pranayam could quit this habit.24.60 percent reduced consumption of pizza/burger and only 6.66 percent people said that there was no impact even after practising Yog and Pranayam.

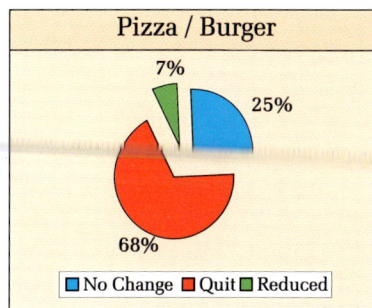

Pizza / Burger

7%

25%

68%

☐ No Change ☐ Quit ☐ Reduced

(e)   Multinational products

The multinational companies have spread their network all over the world. They are exploiting the poor countries ruthlessly. Sometimes the health parameters are also neglected. The survey clearly shows that after practising Yog, 67.84 percent people stopped purchasing MNC products and 21.17 percent people did not pay attention to this aspect. 10.99 percent said that there has been no impact. We can save our country's assets by quitting the use of MNCs products.

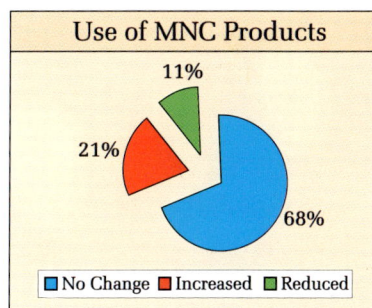

Use of MNC Products

11%

21%

68%

☐ No Change ☐ Increased ☐ Reduced

Role of Patanjali Yogpeeth in establishing Yog as science

Patanjali Yogpeeth was established to prove Yog scientifically. 83.16 percent participants said that the institute has played an excellent role in this direction. Whereas 11.41 percent said that the work done by Yogpeeth was very good. Only 2.56 percent said that the work of institution was satisfactory.

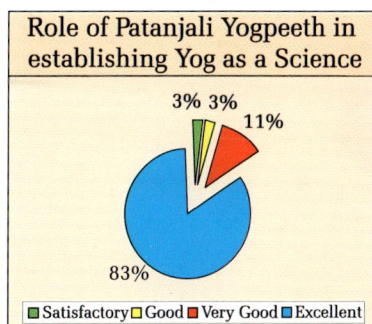

Role of Patanjali Yogpeeth in establishing Yog as a Science

3% 3%

11%

83%

☐ Satisfactory ☐ Good ☐ Very Good ☐ Excellent

Improving spirituality

Yog plays an important role in improving spirituality. It makes us capable of leaving the material comforts and lead a simple life. Our culture talks of attaining salvation with the medium of Yog. It teaches the importance of public welfare. The survey showed that 97.42 percent of the participants agreed that after practising Yog and Pranayam their spirituality level mproved. Only 2.58 percent said that negative thinking increased. This shows that Yog has played an important role in changing the attitude towards nation, culture and spirituality.

This large-scale survey has been remarkable with respect to its concept, method and representation. It has established the public opinion related to psychological impact of Yog on a scientific platform, which used to be questioned by the scientists. The specialty of this survey has been to analyze and compile the answers of all the participants with respect to the impact of Yog on physical body and our consciousness. The miraculous results of survey will establish Yog and Pranayam as a scientific knowledge and shall provide a new direction in the treatment of serious and incurable diseases. This is our hope and aspiration.

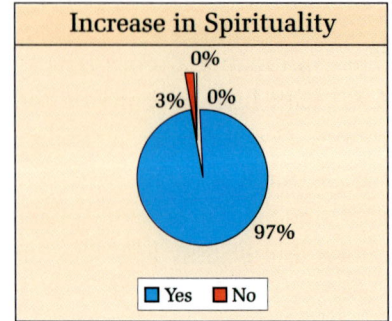

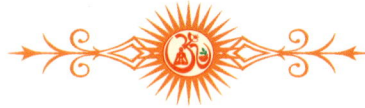

Chapter 7

APPALLING STATE OF HEALTH IN INDIA

India is a poor country from the angle of available economic resources. A number of people neither have sufficient economic resources nor are they physically and mentally healthy. There are many reasons behind this.

Around 26 per cent (1999-2000) of the population lives below the poverty line and this poverty line is determined on the availability of fixed calories per day. In rural areas, it is 2,400 calories and 2,100 calories in urban areas per day.

India has the highest number of poor people in the world. Around 40 per cent of world's poor people live here. India's population is 100 crore which is one-sixth of world's population. To maintain the health of such a huge population is not possible for any government or administration.

Increasing population is the major problem for India. In the last century worlds' population increased three times whereas India's population increased five times. About 50 per cent of world's population lives in cities, but only 30 - 35 per cent of India's population lives in cities. The health facilities are mainly available in urban areas; villages are still not having good medical facilities.

Health facilities are very important because India has the highest birth rate and hence the youth population is also high in our country.

Almost half of India's children have stunted physical and mental development due to malnutrition. Many are not able to work properly due to lack of nutritious food. The common health pattern of the people can be judged from the fact that around 37.4 per cent men and 39.4 per cent women are suffering from different kinds of deficiencies in rural areas. Every year around 24 lakh children below the age of five could be suffering from curable diseases due to the deficiency of resources.

Increasing life expectancy: increasing diseases

Life expectancy at birth has doubled during the past 50 years and this has increased the number of sick people in India unexpectedly. With the availability of better health facilities the life expectancy at birth has increased to 64.8 years. If the increasing population does not get proper health facilities, the productivity will reduce and the nation will become the place of diseased or land of sick people.

Population distribution according to age

Age	Population %
0-14	37.8
15-59	55.5
60 +	6.7

Present health scenario in India

It is interesting to note that with the increase in average life span in India the diseases are also increasing at a fast rate. It is shocking to note that life-style diseases are increasing which is natural. Besides contagious diseases and the diseases that can be cured with the help of technical development are still prevalent at large scale. As a result, the communicable and preventable diseases as well as noncommunicable and life-style related diseases are increasing in our country. The facts are very frightening. In India, the prevalence of both types of diseases is also high in comparison with developed countries and low and middle-income generating countries. According to WHO report of 1998, India is completely in the grip of such diseases (see table).

Treatment and its cost

The most shocking aspect of India's health scenario is that the patient has to spend around 80 per cent of the cost at the time of treatment itself. Only 20 per cent of the total expenditure is covered by the government or under insurance schemes. Expenditure incurred by the patients at the time of treatment is higher in Georgia (89.5 per cent) and Myanmar (82.6 per cent) compared to India. It is very difficult for the people of a poor country to spend huge amount on health.

Increasing diseases and expensive treatment

The medical expenses are also increasing at a very fast rate. As far as out patient care is concerned the cost has increased by 67.7 per cent in rural areas and 106.4 per cent in urban areas from 1986-87 to 1996-97. In the same period, the in-patient care expenses have increased to 436.3 per cent in rural areas and

Disease	Death (Percent)
1. Communicable, maternal, Prenatal and nutritional	**42.2**
Infectious and parasitic diseases	22.7
Respiratory infections	10.6
Maternal conditions	1.3
Prenatal conditions	6.6
Nutritional deficiencies	1.1
2. Non-communicable conditions	**47.9**
Malignant neoplasm	7.0
Other neoplasm	0.1
Diabetes mellitus	1.1
Neuropsychiatry disorders	0.0
Neuropsychiatry disorders	1.1
Sense organ disorders	0.0
Cardiovascular diseases	30.2
Respiratory diseases	3.0
Digestive diseases	2.6
Diseases of genitourinary system	1.1
Skin diseases	0.0
Musculoskeletal diseases	0.0
Congenital abnormalities	1.6
Oral diseases	0.0
3. Injuries	**9.9**
Unintentional	7.7
Intentional	2.1
Total	**100.0**

Source: World Health Organization 1998

320.1 per cent in urban areas.

There is a need to focus on this aspect that despite the increase in all types of diseases, the total government expenditure is higher than public expenditure on health. It is surprising that 80 per cent of the amount spent on various national health programmes is spent towards the salaries of the health workers engaged in these programmes.

Comparison of health expenses with other countries

The USA spends around 13 per cent of its Gross Domestic Product (GDP) on health services and in India it is only 5.6 per cent. Germany, England and USA spend 1.5, 76 and 196 times more on health services compared to India.

Availability of doctors in India - a comparison

India is lagging behind as far as availability of doctors per person is concerned. Germany has 350 doctors and 957 nurses per one lakh people. In America, it is 279 doctors and 972 nurses, while in India it is only 48 doctors and 45 nurses. The number of qualified doctors is very less in our country due to which around 10 lakh less or unqualified doctors are also working in our country. It is this group of doctors that provides preliminary consultation for almost 50–70 per cent of the health related matters.

Expenditure on health services by developed and other countries

Country	Amount of GDP spent (percent)	Amount of Government Expenditime (percent)
Bangladesh	3.8	7.1
Bhutan	4.4	9.2
China	5.3	11.1
Germany	10.6	17.3
India	4.9	5.3
Maldives	7.6	10.2
Nepal	5.4	9.0
Pakistan	4.1	4.0
UK	7.3	14.9
America	13.0	16.7

Availability of doctors and nurses per one lakh persons

Country	Doctors	Nurses
India	48	45
Germany	350	957
USA	279	972

Imbalance in medical facilities: rural areas neglected

A lot of imbalance is seen in the amount spent by the government on medical facilities. Around three-fourths of our population lives in rural areas but the amount spent by the government on medical facilities is only one-tenth of the total expenditure. This shows that people living in rural areas have to undergo a lot of difficulties with respect to medical facilities. In this context, Yog and Pranayam are the solution to cure their diseases.

Condition of various diseases in our country

The infant mortality rate in our country is 64 per 1,000. Death related to maternity is also very high. Around 570 per one-lakh (10,0000) women die due to pregnancy related problems. According to WHO out of 5 lakh, 29 thousand deaths take place during pregnancy all over the world, out of which 1, 36, 000 (25.7 per cent) take place in India, which is highest in the world. About 52 per cent Indian women are suffering from anaemia and 47 per cent children below the age of three are the victims of malnutrition. More than 20 lakh (over 2 million) malaria patients are seen every year. According to National AIDS Control Organization (NACO), 56 lakh people are suffering from AIDS, which is highest after South Africa. In 1995, three lakh people died due to AIDS. Even today many people die due to Diarrhoea. Around 30 lakh people die due to this problem all over the world and one-third of them die only in our country. Tuberculosis patients are also seen in large numbers and one-third of them are in India. According to an estimate, there are around 2.5 crore tuberculosis patients in our country and every year around 22 lakh new patients are added. Every year four-and-a-half lakh Indians die due to this curable disease. According to WHO, India will be the diabetes capital by 2025. In India, four per cent of rural population and 4–11.6 per cent of urban population is diabetic.

Availability of medicines

The poor health services available in the country can be known from the fact that there are only 48 doctors available per one lakh people. The World Bank report of 2006 titled 'Priorities in Health' shows that 65 per cent people do not have the facility for medicines. Only 60 per cent of the children below the age of 12 are being given vaccines. Such a large and poor population will have to adopt Yog for curing their diseases.

Diseases: The biggest reason for poverty in country

Several million people are under debt due to diseases. If one member of the family becomes the victim of some major illness then the whole family comes under debt and the loan keeps on rising because of high interest rate. The World Banks report of 2001 reveals startling facts:

- If an Indian gets admitted into hospital at least once then he has to spend around half of his annual income for hospital and medical bills.

- After getting admitted into the hospital around 40 per cent have to take loan for treatment or have to sell their property. Around 35 per cent of the patients that get admitted in the hospitals live below the poverty line.

Around 2.2 per cent of Indian population goes below the poverty line (BPL) every year due to expenditure (from their pocket) on medical facilities.

In a country where the average monthly income is Rs 1,000, diagnosis and treatment with allopathic system is impossible. The average annual income in 2000-01 was Rs10,306. The income in rural areas is very low and therefore the person is not able to cure even simple diseases like fever with the help of allopathic medicines. In Bihar, per person income is less than Rs 275 and treatment is very difficult for the common man.

The conclusion of this study is that the expenditure on treatment is the biggest reason for poverty in our country. The drug-manufacturing companies look at patients only as customers for the sake of their profit margins. In such a situation, the only silver lining in a dark cloud is Yog and Pranayam, which will not only cure diseases but also improve the general productivity of the person.

Main drawback in Western medical system

The main drawback of western medical system is that it generates other diseases in the process of curing one disease. The Western medical system is unable to cure the diseases and more suited to control the diseases. Besides, the medicine have many side effects and generate new diseases. On the whole, diseases are always a few steps ahead of new and better medicines developed to treat the same. The biggest evidence for failure of allopathic system of treatment is that after 1970 around 32 new infectious diseases came into existence.

Region-wise Sale of Medicines

World Audited Market	2003 Sales	% Global Sales
North America	229.5	49
European Union	115.4	25
Rest of Europe	14.3	3
Japan	52.4	11
Asia, Africa and Australia	37.3	8
Latin America	17.4	4
Total	**$ 466.3 bn**	**100**

Source: IMS World Review 2004

Medical research

The Western medical research is limited only to the developed nations. Out of 1,233 new medicines discovered between 1975 and 1999, only 13 are those that are useful in hot arid countries. Although the burden of diseases in middle and low-income countries is 92 per cent, whereas it is eight percent in high-income nations. Even then 95 per cent of amount spent on research is spent on diseases seen in developed nations and rest on low and middle-income nations. It is certain that the drug-manufacturing companies are concentrating on developed nations only for profits.

Expenses on new medicines

America spends around 250 million dollars (Rs1,125 crore) and 10 years to launch a new medicine in the market. Only 10 out of 10,000 new chemicals reach the pre-clinical stage.

Out of them, only five are found suitable for testing on humans and finally only one such chemical gets launched in the market in the form of medicine.

Production of medicines in India

In 2004-05, the Indian drug-manufacturing industry sold medicines worth four billion dollars (Rs 18,000 crore) in domestic market and exported three billion dollars (Rs 13,500 crore) worth of medicines. The total production was worth Rs 28,500 crore and in the same year it also imported medicines worth Rs 3,056 crore.

In 2005-06, the Indian drug-manufacturing industry sold medicines worth 4.5 billion dollars (Rs 20,250 crore) in domestic market and exported 3.8 billion dollars (Rs 17,100 crore) worth of medicines. The total production was worth Rs 37,350 crore and in the same year it also imported medicines worth Rs 3,500 crore.

This year medicines worth $602 billion have been sold all over the world, which is worth Rs 27,09,000 crore, which clearly indicates the spread of diseases. In northern America alone, $265.7 billion worth medicines were used which is equal to 47 per cent of world's share.

Study of cost involved in Treatment of various diseases with modern medicine

Yog can be helpful in saving a huge amount of money every year. Medicines worth crores of rupees are consumed in our country. India is a very lucrative market for medicines and all the

Sale of Allopathic Medicine in the World

Rank	Audited world therapy class	2003 Sales ($bn)
1.	Cholestrol and triglyceride reducers	26.1
2.	Anti-ulcerants	24.3
3.	Antidepressants	19.5
4.	Antirheumatic non-steroidals	12.4
5.	Atipsychotics	12.2
6.	Calcium antagonists, plain	10.8
7.	Erythropoietins, plain	10.8
8.	Anti-epileptics	9.4
9.	Oral antidiabetics	9.0
10.	Cephalosporins and combinations	8.3
	Total leading 10 ATCs at Level 3	**$142.8bn**

Source : IMS World Review, 2004

Sale of important medicine in 2003

Rank	Audited world product sales	2003 Sales ($bn)
1	Lipitor	10.3
2	Zocor	6.1
3	Zyprexa	4.8
4	Norvasc	4.5
5	Eprex/procrit	4.0
6	Ogastro/prevacid	4.0
7	Mexium	3.8
8	Plavix	3.7
9	Seretide/advair	3.7
10	Zoloft	3.4
	Total 10 leading products	**$48.3bn**

Source : IMS World Review 2004

Expected costs involved in the treatment of diabetic patients

Medicine	Rs 600 per month	Rs 7,200 per anum
Daily blood sugar test	Rs 600 pm	Rs 7,200 pa
Monthly tests	Rs 200 per visit	Rs 2,400 pa
Blood test	Rs 200 per test	Rs 2,400 pa
Glycocilated HB	Rs 300 (3 months)	Rs 1,200 pa
ECG	Rs 150 (3 months)	Rs 600 pa
Other tests	Rs 200 (6 months)	Rs 400 pa
Special tests	Rs 600 (3 months)	Rs 2,400 pa
3D echo and TMT		Rs 2,000 pa
Emergency admission and other serious problems		Rs 5,000 pa
	Total expenditure	**Rs 30,800 pa**

Expected cost of medicines given to insulin-dependent diabetic patients

Insulin	Rs 900 pm	Rs 10,800 pa
Blood sugar test	Rs 600 pm	Rs 7,200 pa
Monthly test	Rs 200 per visit	Rs 2,400 pa
Blood test	Rs 200 per test	Rs 2,400 pa
Glycocilated HB	Rs 300 (3 months)	Rs 1,200 pa
ECG	Rs 150 (3 months)	Rs 600 pa
Other tests	Rs 200 (6 months)	Rs 400 pa
Special tests	Rs 600 (3 months)	Rs 2,400 pa
2D echo and TMT		Rs 2,000 pa
Emergency admission and other serious problems		Rs 5,000 pa
	Total Expenditure	**Rs 34,400 pa**

Expected costs involved in the treatment of patients of bronchial asthma

Medicine	Rs 2500 pm	Rs 30,000 pa
Monthly tests	Rs 200 per visit	Rs 2,400 pa
Blood test	Rs 200 per test	Rs 2,400 pa
Special tests	Rs 800 per 3 months	Rs 3,200 pa
2D echo and TMT (Immunology / CT)		Rs 10,000 pa
Emergency admission and other serious problems		
	Total Expenditure	**Rs 48,000 pa**

Expected costs involved in the treatment of patients of high blood pressure

Medicine	Rs 1500 pm	Rs 18,000 pa
Monthly tests	Rs 200 per visit	Rs 2,400 pa
Blood test	Rs 300 per test	Rs 3,600 pa
ECG	Rs 150 (3 months)	Rs 1,800 pa
Other tests	Rs 200 (6 months)	Rs 2,400 pa
Special tests	Rs 1000 (every three months)	Rs 4,000 pa
2D echo and TMT		Rs 2,000 pa
Emergency admission and other serious problems		Rs 5,000 pa
	Total expenditure	**Rs 39,200 pa**

Expected costs involved in the treatment of patients of diabetes and high blood pressure

Medicines	Rs 1500 pm	Rs 18,000 pa
Daily sugar test	Rs 600 pm	Rs 7,200 pa
Monthly tests	Rs 200 per visit	Rs 2,400 pa
Blood test	Rs 300 per test	Rs 3,600 pa
Glycocilated HB	Rs 300 (3 months)	Rs 1,200 pa
ECG	Rs 150 (3 months)	Rs 600 pa
Other tests	Rs 200 (6 months)	Rs 400 pa
Special tests (lipid)	Rs 800 (3 months)	Rs 3,200 pa
2D echo and TMT		Rs 2,000 pa
Emergency admission and Other serious problems		Rs 10,000 pa
	Total Expenditure	**Rs. 48,600 pa**

Expected costs involved in the treatment of patients of coronary artery disease

Medicine	Rs 1,500 pm	Rs 18,000 pa
Monthly tests	Rs 200 per visit	Rs 2,400 pa
Blood test	Rs 300 per test	Rs 3,600 pa
ECG	Rs 150 pm	Rs 1,800 pa
Other tests	Rs 200 (6 months)	Rs 2,400 pa
Special tests	Rs 2,000 (every 3 months)	Rs 8,000 pa
2D echo and TMT		Rs 2,000 pa
Emergency admission other serious problems		Rs 10,000 pa
	Total expenditure	**Rs 48,200 pa**

Expected costs involved in the treatment of patients of arthritis

Medicine	Rs 3000 pm	Rs 36,000 pa
Monthly tests	Rs 200 per visit	Rs 2,400 pa
Blood test	Rs 300 per test	Rs 3,600 pa
Physiotherapy	Rs 2000 pm	Rs 24,000 pa
Rehabilitation	Rs 2000 pm	Rs 24,000 pa
Special tests (Immunological / CT)	Rs 5,000 (6 months)	Rs 10,000 pa
Surgery ((knee replacement)		Rs 2 lakh per surgery (approximately)
	Total expenditure	**Rs. 3,00,000 pa**

Expected costs involved in the treatment of patients of coronary artery disease and diabetes

Medicines	Rs 2000 pm	Rs 24000 pa
Daily sugar test	Rs 600 pm	Rs 7200 pa
Monthly tests	Rs 200 per visit	Rs 2400 pa
Blood test	Rs 300 per test	Rs 3600 pa
Glycocilated Hb	Rs 300 (3 months)	Rs 1200 pa
ECG	Rs 150 (3 months)	Rs 600 pa
Other tests	Rs 200 (6 months)	Rs 400 pa
Special tests	Rs 2000 (3 months)	Rs 8000 pa
2D echo and TMT		Rs 2000 pa
Emergency admission Due to some disease or complexity		Rs 10000 pa
	Total Expenditure	**Rs 59,400 pa**

multinational companies are trying to establish their business here. They are trying to increase the sales as much as possible and are ready to adopt both ethical and unethical methods to achieve their targets. They do not bother about the fact that the methods adopted for sale of medicines are ethical or not. If we conduct research on this point as to what is the percentage of useful drugs out of the medicines being sold in India, then on the basis of our experience it can be said that half of the medicines are prescribed unnecessarily and mainly to earn profits. And thus instead of benefiting, such unnecessary medication is adversely affecting the health of the masses. There is a need to focus on this point today in order to save the country and its people from serious side effects caused by these medicines. Besides side effects, crores of hard earned money is being wasted on medicines, which should have been actually used for the national development. The hard earned money of people is making the multinational companies richer instead of being used for developmental projects. The national wealth is improving the economy of foreign countries. Our objective is to change this trend. There is no point repeating that it is not possible to come out of the grip of MNCs. Everything can be changed, we need courage, willingness, honesty and sincere efforts. 'Nothing is impossible' all we need is dedicated efforts to achieve the goals. If we practise Yog regularly then there is no need to spend money on medicines. Yog is inexpensive and there is a need to understand the real situation and commit for the welfare of the mankind. The graphs given here show cost involved in treatment using modern medical systems which clearly speaks about the wastage of our national wealth while making the multinational companies richer by the day.

Our main objective of presenting these reports is to bring to light that the claims of available medical facilities and policies for bolstering public health is just an eye-wash. There is a need to analysse the merits of Swami Ramdevji Maharaj's Yog related research and make efforts to extend it to each and every individual of the country. This will give a new life to the poor who are unable to afford expensive medical treatment. We will be able to fulfil our dream of building a healthy, disease-free and prosperous India for everyone.

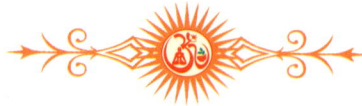

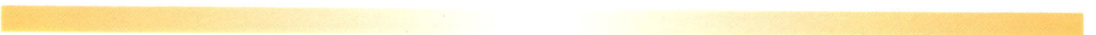

Chapter 8

FEEDBACK/TESTIMONIES OF PEOPLE WHO BENEFITED FROM YOG/PRANAYAM

In medical science two types of verifications are recognized, first is the controlled clinical trial and the second one is the factual documentation based on the medical experiments. In the fifth chapter of this book we have published the results of the controlled clinical trials. In this chapter, we have taken certain number of people as an example out of the millions of people who have benefited from Yog. Primarily, we have given complete factual evidence for those people whose ailments were considered incurable in the modern medical science.

It is an unprecedented research in the realm of health and its results shall certainly induce a sense of mystery and excitement and shall surprise the masses and the medical scientists across the world. Results of the medical tests done before and after the treatment of these sample patients demonstrate how it was possible to cure the diseases, which had been declared incurable by the modern medical science, with the combined force of Yog and Ayurved. Here we have refrained from using any superlatives nor we have talked about presence of any supernatural power and also we are not egoistic about what we do. Instead we have scientifically expressed the knowledge received from the saints and sages alongwith the scientific evidences. It is true that millions of people across the world have successfully cured themselves by practising Yog and Pranayam and have gained a new lease on life.

It was a tedious and complex task selecting people with incurable diseases out of the millions of people who have benefited from the practice of Yog; collecting their complete medical reports before and after the treatment; categorization of their diseases; and then verification of the proofs of the results obtained. All these reactions and acknowledgements on one hand highlight the truth behind the efforts of Swami Ramdevji and form a telling evidence of the usefulness and scientific veracity of Yog and Pranayam.

In conclusion we can say that our aim is very clear and that we have found a way to ensure that not even a single person shall die of illness or hunger in this world as we await Yog and Ayurved firmly established at the international platform. We are grateful to the people from whom we have received cooperation globally. But there is need of great amount of resources for the huge task of construction of Patanjali University, conducting clinical controlled trials and genetic research. In this work of world class standard of research and investigation, assistance of millions of people from around the world is expected. We again invite all those people who feel for the human race, who are willing to donate generously for the cause of protecting the lives of other people from deadly diseases and this holy job of making the world disease free. To make the world disease free we wish that the knowledge, which we possess, should reach each and every person and all of us be healthy and wealthy from body and soul.

CANCER

Blood Cancer (CML/AML etc.)

◆ I was suffering from fibrosancoma, I sought treatment from many doctors but I gained hardly any relief. On the contrary my problem aggravated. Then I started Yog and Pranayam exercises as told by Swamiji and now I am much better.

— **Ram Darshan Rai, Jhujjar, Patna**

◆ I was suffering from Non Hodkin's Limphoma from October 2004. I consulted many doctors but there was no relief. I am taking medicines from Divya Yog Mandir Trust and practising Pranayam regularly twice daily for one hour. Now I am totally healthy.

— **Chetram, Shimla, Himachal Pradesh**

◆ My daughter was diagnosed with having blood cancer two years ago. I have taken her to many big hospitals but got no relief. Her condition deteriorated. I came in contact with Swamiji and made my daughter to do regular Pranayam and gave her wheatgrass juice, Giloi juice and basil leaves. Slowly my daughter Hina's health started improving and her blood report is normal. Now she has completely recovered. I get regular check-ups done, doctors say she is completely alright. Swamiji mission of Yog and Pranayam is the ray of hope for incurable diseases.

— **Ghanshayam Jais for daughter Hina, Navi Sukurvari Mahal, Nagpur**

In this chapter, reactions of all the patients have been given who were suffering from incurable diseases. We specifically want to highlight this fact that we have tried our best to confirm the facts from the available sources and the reactions given by the patents. The reports of the patients from different laboratories are also being given here. They are not being published here in detail and also the phone numbers and addresses of the patients have been kept in safe custody of our research department. In order to safeguard privacy of the patients, we have not published their particulars. We also request other patients suffering from various chronic diseases, who have benefited by practising Yog and Pranayam, to send their reports and other complete details to us, so that they could be published in the second edition. This will help in encouraging millions suffering from similar diseases to get rid of the disease and shall help in developing their faith in Yog.

◆ I was suffering from blood cancer. My situation was very bad and all doctors lost hope on my ailment. Then I got myself treated from Patanjali Yogpeeth, Hardwar and since then I did Pranayam everyday. Now all my reports are normal and because of Swamiji's grace this miracle has happened. I devote my life to Swamiji.

— **Akshay Kumar, Volagiri, Orissa**

Before Treatment

After Treatment

The patient's PCR/AVL ratio before Yog practice was high, which became normal after Yog.

◆ After being unwell for almost two years, I got my blood test done which confirmed blood cancer. I consulted various senior doctors. The consultation and treatment did not help me much. Then I saw Swamijis programme on Aastha Channel and I started practising Pranayam. I also took medicines prescribed from the Ashram. Now, finally I am very healthy and all my blood reports are normal.

— **Pavan Kumar Jaiswal, Mohanpur, Godda, Jharkhand**

◆ I was diagnosed with cancer six months back and the blood test done on August 14, 2006 showed TLC at 259000, platelet count was 6,20,000 per microliter. I underwent chemotherapy and other treatments but there was no relief. My condition was worsening with each passing day and I felt that my death was certain. I visited Patanjali Yogpeeth and started practising Yog and Pranayam and also took Ayurvedic medicines. My health started improving with the practice of Pranayam and the TLC and platelet count were normal in medical tests done on December 15, 2006. Cancer was cured completely and Yog gave me a new life. I am thankful to Swamiji for giving me a new life.

— Madanpal Singh, Bahadarabad, Hardwar

Before Treatment   After Treatment

The blood test done before treatment showed WBC 2 lakh 59 thousand, platelets 6 lakh 20 thousand with enlarged spleen and liver. With regular practice of Pranayam and Ayurved treatment, WBC count came to seven thousand and platelets to 1 lakh 91 thousand. The spleen and liver regained their normal size.

Cancer of Urinary Bladder, Prostate etc.

◆ I was suffering from urinary problem since last one year. Medical tests showed cancer of prostrate gland. Doctors suggested immediate operation to be followed by hormone treatment. I was very worried and somebody told me about Pranayam. I started practising it regularly and took Ashram medicines. Now prostrate cancer is under control and I do not have any problem.

— **Hariram Garg, Faridkot, Punjab**

Before Treatment	After Treatment

The report before treatment showed cancer, whereas the present PSA report shows that cancer is under control.

◆ I was diagnosed with cancer of testicles in 2003. Doctors suggested operation. I came to know about Swami Ramdevji and I started practising Pranayam regularly and took Ashram's medicines. Now my condition has improved.

— **Mohd. Farudiq, Karaali, Meerut City, Meerut**

◆ I was diagnosed with cancer of urinary bladder in 2004, I took a lot of medicines but there was no relief. I started practising Yog and Pranayam as per Swami Ramdevji's advice and now all my reports are normal. I am practising Pranayam regularly and today I am totally healthy with the blessings of Swamiji and leading a normal life.

— **Manoj Kumar Singh, Nasik Road**

Before Treatment   After Treatment

The medical test done before treatment shows cancer in urinary bladder, which was normal after treatment.

◆ I was suffering from prostrate cancer and the weight of my prostate was 125.6 grams. Adenocarcinoma of prostate was found in my biopsy report. Since last three months I practised Pranayam in morning and evening for one hour each regularly and now I do not have prostate cancer. Now the weight of my prostate is 19 grams.

— **Chandramohan Rawat, Post Gugrali, Ashok Nagar (Madhya Pradesh)**

◆ I used to urinate with much difficulty. I got myself checked and was diagnosed with an enlarged prostate gland and PSA. Doctor suggested chemo-therapy. It was not possible to get a permanent cure with allopathy. I started doing Yog and Pranayam as told by Swamiji. Now I have completely recovered and my reports are normal.

— **Bajrang Lal Rathi, Ashok Vihar Phase-1, Delhi**

Cancer of Throat

◆ I was diagnosed with thyroid cancer three years back and came to know about Patanjali Yogpeeth from a close relative. I took treatment from Patanjali Yogpeeth, Hardwar and practised Pranayam as per Swamiji's guidance. Now thyroid gland is functioning normally and CT scan report was also normal. My condition has improved totally.

— **Pushpak Rani, PAC Road, Muradabad**

I was suffering from thyroid gland cancer. Chemotherapy was not beneficial and I was very worried. I am practising Swamiji's Pranayam since last one year after watching television programme. There has been a lot of improvement. Before practising Pranayam a lot of pus used to be formed in throat but now it has stopped. I am totally healthy and I have got second life with the blessings of Swamiji.

— **Santosh Kumar Soni, Boli Bagh Road, Reeva, Madhya Pradesh**

◆ I was having a tumour in throat for the last two years, which was detected as cancerous. I was operated one and half years ago at Kailash Hospital, Indore. Doctors suggested chemotherapy but I did not go for it. I visited Hardwar and the tumour was cured within three days with Ayurvedic medicine. This was a miracle and I started practising Pranayam after one month. I am not taking medicines since 8 - 10 months and Pranayam is giving me complete relief.

— **Kamla Soni, Bada Bazaar, Vidisha, Madhya Pradesh**

◆ I was suffering from cancer, because of it I was not able to speak properly and there were lumps in my tongue and cheeks. I was not able to move my right hand. I took many allopathic medicines and I was given chemo twice however it finaly did not work. My health detoriated. I lost my appetite and due to weekness I used to feel giddy. My haemoglobin level was also very low. I felt helpless, I used to pray for death. I started Yog and Pranayam for 3 months. I got unbelievable results and all my ailments got cured. I am doing Pranayam from last 8 months and I am not taking any kind of medicine.

— **Deepshikha, Kolkata**

Breast Cancer

I was suffering from breast cancer and was operated once. It recurred after three years. I started practising Pranayam since the last six months and there has been a lot of improvement. All my tests are normal and I have recovered completely.

— **Anjum Patel, UK**

◆ There was light and piercing pain with heaviness in my breast. While getting down from stairs or due to accidental pressure I used to get unbearable pain. I consulted various doctors and in the reports it was diagnosed as breast cancer. I am doing Pranayam from last one year and now I am absolutely healthy. I am able to have a normal daily routine comfortably. I do not have any pain or heaviness in my breast. I have been given new life all because of Swamiji.

— **Amitrani Banerjee, MB Road, Kolkata**

◆ I was suffering from hereditary cancer. My mother, sister and others have also died due to this dreadful disease. I was suffering from tumour in breast since last four years. I was very scared and had lost all hope. I consulted many specialists but they said it was incurable. I took chemotherapy a few times but it recurred. I took part in Yog camp of Swami Ramdevji and started practising Pranayam. I took wheat plant juice etc. and there was a lot of improvement in my condition. After a few months the tumour dissolved and now all the reports are normal. I am enjoying good health. There is no symptom of cancer after practising Pranayam. I have become an active member of Yog revolution. Swamiji's Pranayam has proven to be a blessing for everybody.

— **Shailaja Yadav, Mahendragarh, Haryana**

Intestinal Cancer

◆ I was diagnosed with cancer of large intestine and it spread into the liver. I took a lot of treatment but my condition did not improve and I was counting my days. For last one year, I started Yog and Pranayam as told by Swamiji. This has benefitted me a lot and my life is full of joy again.

— **Jetender Kumar Tewari, Hugali, Kolkata, West Bengal**

◆ I was suffering from intestine cancer, I got myself treated from various doctors however I did not get any benefit. It seemed that my life had come to an end. I started Yog and Pranayam as told by Swamiji. Now I am absolutely healthy because of Pranayam.

— **Shivrav Madhavrav Patil, Guru Nanak Colony, Etanagar, Latur**

◆ I was diagnosed with intestinal cancer which started spreading. I got operated followed by chemotherapy and radiotherapy. In my second operation, about 1.5 feet part of intestine was removed. I am doing Pranayam regularly since February 2005. I tested negative for cancer in August 2005. For last 8-10 months, I am not taking any medicine and I am totally healthy.

— Smt. Nirmala Srimali, Khargon, MP

◆ I was suffering from intestine cancer and after operation tumours developed in liver. Treatment was not beneficial and cancer started spreading in whole body. I lost all hope and then I went to Divya Yog Mandir and took medicines. I am practising Pranayam regularly and now I am healthy. I am also going for regular medical check up and all the pathological reports are normal. I am grateful to Swamiji.

— **Natkishore Mishra, Sundargarh (Orissa)**

Before Treatment	After Treatment

Cancer detected in CT Scan before treatment and it was normal after treatment.

Uterine and Ovarian Cancer

◆ I was detected with uterus cancer three years ago. I took a lot of medicines but there was no improvement. Finally I started practising Pranayam regularly and positive results started showing. I have underwent all types of cancer tests and consulted doctors. Now the reports are normal and I am enjoying good health.

— Jessy Roy, Jhambad Estate, Chetnanagar, Aurangabad

Before Treatment　　　　　　　　　　　　After Treatment

Before practice of Pranayam patient's CA 125 was 159,
which became normal after Pranayam.

◆ I was suffering from uterine cancer. Allopathic treatment scared me and I took refuge in Yog and Pranayam. For last one year I am practising Pranayam earnestly and now I am totally cured of disease. I believe, Swamiji is here to shower us all with the blessing of the Almighty.

◆ I was suffering from high BP and I had cancer in uterus. After I consulted doctors at AIIMS, I was told to get Chemotherapy done. I have deep faith in Swamiji and Pranayam, because of this faith even while taking chemotherapy I did Pranayam and took medicines prescribed by Ashram. It is all due to Pranayam, side effects of chemotherapy got reduced and I have less pain. My CA 125 level reduced to 2.79 in April 2007 as compared to 1062.8 in July 2006. Now I am absolutely healthy due to Pranayam, I have completely recovered and got a new life.

— **Sheela Upadhyay , Sarita Vihar, New Delhi**

Before Treatment   After Treatment

The test report before treatment showed CA 125 level as 1062.8 and later after Pranayam exercises it was found CA 125 level 2.79.

Brain Cancer

◆ I was suffering from brain tumour from the past four years. I went into coma after taking chemotherapy. Doctors told me that my chances of survival are very slim. I took two months' medicine dose from Patanjali Yogpeeth. I came out of coma after several months. After coming out of coma, now I am regularly practising Pranayam. I have recovered completely and I am leading a normal life. Swamiji has blessed me with second life.

— **P.K.Pathak, Village - Pousar, Yamunanagar**

◆ I was detected with cancer of Pituitary gland two years ago. The doctors at SGPGI, Lucknow, said it was incurable and refused treatment. I went to other hospitals but did not get suitable answer. One of my friends told me about Swami Ramdevji's Ashram. I took medicines and started practising Pranayam regularly and tumour got cured within six months. Now I am totally healthy and CT Scan report is normal.

— **Ms Priyanka, Kanpur (UP)**

Before Treatment	After Treatment

The tumour size in Pituitary gland as per CT Scan report was 15.4 * 20.1*20 in supra sellar region and 15.2-11.2 in left parasellar region before the treatment. The CT Scan report was normal after the treatment.

Lung Cancer

◆ I was diagnosed with lung cancer. I consulted many hospitals and was advised by many people that it was pointless. Also I thought it would be impossible for me to go for such expensive treatment. Just because of this reason I was not able to get my treatment done. Then after I took medicines prescribed by Swamiji's Ashram and I also started doing Pranayam, which helped me to cure my ailment. After 10 months now there is no cancer in my lungs. I am absolutely healthy.

— **Shivnandan Vadkaghar, Hazari Bagh, Jharkhand**

◆ I was detected with lung cancer two years ago. I was told that it was incurable and I felt that I was nearing death. Finally I started practising Pranayam and took Ashram medicines regularly, which gave considerable relief. Now I am totally healthy and all pathological reports are normal. I am going to Tata Memorial hospital for regular check ups and the condition is normal. I am grateful to Swami Ramdevji.

— **Subhash Garg, Delhi**

Before Treatment	After Treatment

The FNAC test done before treatment confirmed cancer, whereas CT Scan report was normal after treatment.

Gall Bladder Cancer

◆ I was diagnosed cancer of gall bladder and my condition had deteriorated. The cancer had spread in large area. I was operated and then given chemotherapy. But there was no improvement. Then I took medicines from Patanjali Yogpeeth and started practising Pranayam. Gall bladder and liver cancer was cured. I got a new life with the blessings of Swami Ramdevji.

— Mohd. Shafagat Ali, Old City, Itawa, UP

◆ I offen used to get light pain in upper part of the stomach. It started worrying me and I consulted doctors. Ultrasound showed tissue growth in gall bladder. Another ultrasound done after a few days showed further growth.Doctors at PGI, Lucknow, found that this tissue was growing by 1 mm by a day. I lost all faith in doctors and started doing Pranayam and started using medicines prescribed by the Ashram. Gradully my health and my thinking took a positive turn. The tissue growth in my gall bladder started getting reduced. Now I feel totally recovered. No hope was left for me in allopathy, Yog and Pranayam proved to be miraculous for me. My whole family is filled with gratitude towards Yog and Swamiji.

— P. K. Choubey, Aishbagh, Lucknow

Other Cancer

◆ I was troubled with cancer. I feel totally defeated in body and soul. I discovered a ray of hope in Pranayam and now after practising it, I am totally recovered.

— Rajender Kapoor, Noida (UP)

◆ I was suffering from cancer from a very long time. I saw Swami Ramdevji's prograame on Aastha Channel and started practising Pranayam and also took medicines as prescribed by the Ashram. Now I am completely free from this terrible disease and I have stopped taking any medicine.

— Ranjan Roy, Seenimuri Houston, Texas

◆ I have appendix cancer. I got myself tested in 2004. I used to have pain in the stomach and used to vomit. Despite getting allopathic treatment, my health did not improve. I started doing Pranayam and started consuming wheatgrass juce, neem and Basil leaves. I got myself checked again in October 2006 and I have recovered completely. Now I am completely healthy.

— Mahesh Sharma, Gonjarhahr Rd. Bikaner, Rajasthan

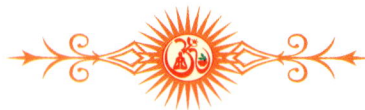

HIV Positive

◆ I had become very weak five years back and my weight reduced to 40 kilos. Blood tests revealed HIV positive. I consulted many doctors but there was no relief. I took Ayurvedic medicines from Patanjali Yogpeeth and practised Pranayam. There has been a lot of improvement in my condition.

— **Prashant Kumar, Gujarat**

Before Treatment	After Treatment

DEPARTMENT OF MICROBIOLOGY
NATIONAL HIV/AIDS REFERENCE CENTRE
A.I.I.M.S , NEW DELHI

LAB REF. NO. : 111975   SOURCE : MOPD   CR NO.: 26600

NAME   : PRASHANT KUMAR   AGE :29   SEX (M/F) : M

RISK GROUP   : NOT KNOWN

TREATMENT :   NIL

TEST PERFORMED:-

CD 4 COUNT   25   CD 4 %   0.84
(cells/ul)

CD 8 COUNT   2570   CD 8 %   86.73
(cells/ul)

CD4/CD8   :   0.01

WBC (m/mm3)   LYMPH %

COMMENTS

(DR. MADHU VAJPAYEE, MD)
ASSOCIATE PROFESSOR
INCHARGE, IMMUNOLOGY DIVISION
DEPTT. OF MICROBIOLOGY
AIIMS, NEW DELHI-110029

E: 18/08/2005

DEPARTMENT OF MICROBIOLOGY
IMMUNOLOGY LAB
A.I.I.M.S, NEW DELHI

Dated:- 15.05.2006

LAB REF. NO. : 231   SOURCE: ART-288   CR NO. 26600/04

NAME   PRASHANT KUMAR   AGE 29 M

TREATMENT : YES

TEST PERFORMED

ABSOLUTE COUNTS: CELLS/ ul.

CD 4 COUNT   338

CD 8 COUNT   1755

TOTAL CD 3 AVERAGE   2424

presently on leave

(DR. MADHU VAJPAYEE, MD)
ASSOCIATE PROFESSOR
INCHARGE, IMMUNOLOGY DIVISION
DEPT. OF MICROBIOLOGY
AIIMS, NEW DELHI- 110029

The patient's absolute CD count was 4 and weight was 40 kilos before Pranayam. After Pranayam the count was 338 and weight increased to 63 kilos.

◆ I was HIV positive for the last three to four years. I took lot of medicines but there was no relief. I did not get any kind of assurance from doctors instead I became more afraid. I used Ayurvedic medicines and practised Pranayam, there is a lot of improvement in my condition and I feel much better. I am positive that HIV positive will become negative one day.

— **Kaushalya Devi, Dehra Dun**

◆ I was very weak since the past two to three years. I used to have mild fever, headache and weakness. The blood tests showed HIV +. I was depressed, treatment was not beneficial and I thought my life was coming to an end. Then I practised Swamiji's Pranayam and Ayurved and there has been a lot of improvement in my condition. Now I am leading a stress–free life and this is all because of blessings of Swamiji. I have discontinued allopathic treatment.

— **Surjeet Singh, Amritsar, Punjab**

Before Treatment   **After Treatment**

The absolute CD count was 74 before Pranayam and it was 132 after Pranayam.
There is a lot of improvement in this patient's condition.

◆ I was diagnosed HIV positive four to five years back. I consulted various allopathic doctors but there was no relief. I was very disappointed and wanted to commit suicide. Then I took treatment from Swamiji. Regular practice of Yog, Pranayam and use of Ayurvedic medicines has improved my condition. Now I feel very healthy.

— **Krishnabhai Patel, Kutch, Gujarat**

◆ I was very weak since three years and had mild fever. Blood tests revealed that I was HIV positive. I took a lot of medicines but there was no relief. Then I took Ashram medicines and practised Pranayam regularly. My condition is improving gradually.

— **Kantaben, Gujarat**

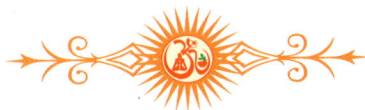

Before Treatment — After Treatment

The absolute CD4 count was 173 before practice of Pranayam. After Pranayam it increased to 513 improving overall health of this patient.

HEART DISEASES

Coronary Artery Disease, Angina Pain, Myocardial Infarction, Rheumatoid Heart Disease

◆ I was suffering from breathlessness since 2003. I had heart disease and could not sleep for several nights. I could not even turn on my side. I had tumours on hands, legs, and spinal cord. I was very furstrated and was tired of consulting doctors and taking allopathic medicines. My health has improved since the day I started practising Pranayam. Pranayam has become the basis of my life. I thank God and Swamiji for everything.

— Tara Babbar, Kankarkheda, Meerut (UP)

Before Treatment

After Treatment

The blood test before treatment showed cholesterol -242, triglycerides - 925, HDL cholesterol - 39. Regular practice of Yog and Pranayam for one year showed cholesterol -189, triglycerides - 161, HDL cholesterol - 47.

◆ I suffered from heart disease and chest pain in December 2001 and doctors suggested TMT and angiography. The tests revealed blockage in arteries. The RCA and LCA had 100 and 80 percent blockage respectively. Doctors advised immediate operation and it was to be done after 20 days. I deposited some amount but I started practising Pranayam and Yog as per Swamiji's guidance. I took gourd juice and went to Allahabad on scheduled date for operation. The angiography showed that arteries had opened completely. This was nothing less than a miracle. Angioplasty was avoided and now I am practising Yog and Pranayam regularly.

— **Ramesh Kumar Sharma, Neemuch Cantt. M.P.**

Before Treatment	After Treatment

The RCA was 100 percent before Pranayam which opened after treatment.

◆ I was suffering from hereditary problem of CAD. I am having hemiplegia and Veins aphasia in my right hand since one-and-a-half years. I am feeling much better with the practice of Pranayam and Ayurvedic medicines. My weight had reduced from 122 to 89 kilos. There is 95 percent improvement in Hemiplegia and in my voice. I have regained health with the blessings of Swamiji.

— **Kaviraj Panjwani, Vijaynagar, Bhavnagar, Gujarat**

◆ I got first attack on May 8, 2003 and angioplasty was done in July 2003. I am having 80 percent blockage since two years. I started practising Pranayam and taking Ayurvedic medicines. The blockage has opened completely and there is a lot of improvement in the heart condition. Revered Swamiji is like a God for me. Now I am absolutely fine and I am teaching Pranayam to others.

— **Balkrishna Shamrao Goswami, Pune**

◆ I was very disappointed due to Rheumatic heart disease and could not walk even two steps. After various medical tests doctors told that heart valves were damaged and the heart had become very weak. The doctors told that valve replacement was the only option left out but it was not possible due to weak heart. Swamiji's Pranayam has brought a new ray of hope in my life. I started practising Yog and Pranayam and took Ashram medicines. Regular practice of Pranayam for one year and Ayurvedic medicines have cured my heart disease.

— Sudesh Rao, Temple Lane, Gurgoan (Haryana)

Color Doppler Eco-cardiography test done before treatment showed left ventricular ejection fraction at 53 percent, whereas after one year of Pranayam the second test showed it at 74 per cent. Besides there was positive improvement in other parameters as well.

◆ I suffered heart attack in May 2005. My weight was 116 kilos at that time and EF was 20-25 percent. I started using Ayurvedic medicines and practice of Pranayam in August 2005. My condition started improving and weight reduced to 90 kilos. The EF was 46 percent and blockage had opened. I got a new life with the blessing of Swamiji.

— Vinod Choube, Chandannagar, Hugli, W B

◆ I suffered from heart attack in 2002 and the medical tests showed arterial blockage. I was also having high blood pressure and high cholesterol level. Modern medication did not prove to be beneficial. Then I practised Yog and Pranayam and took Arjun quath and other medicines from Ashram. Yog and Pranayam improved my hearing power, and I could enjoy sound sleep. Eyesight also improved and weight reduced by five kilos. Now I am totally healthy and I am able to do my work normally. Swamiji has blessed me with new life.

— **Virendra Kumar Kulshreshtha, Udhamsingh Sanai, Siliguri, W B**

Before Treatment   After Treatment

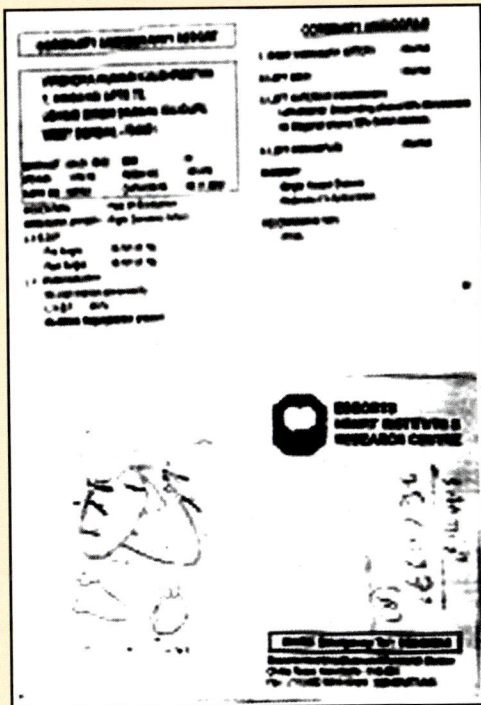

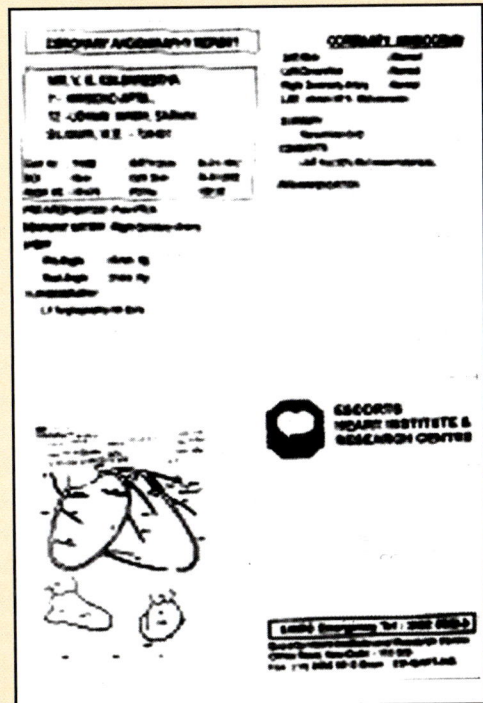

The coronary angiography report before treatment showed left anterior descending with 90 percent mid stenosis. Whereas after practice of Pranayam it reduced to 30 percent. Besides there was significant improvement in left ventricle irregularity.

◆ I suffered the first heart attack in December and had severe chest pain and palpitation. I have been practising Pranayam regularly and taking Ayurvedic medicines. I am feeling healthy and active. I am was unable to walk before but now I can walk easily. Revered Swamiji has filled a new ray of hope in my life.

— **Balveer Singh, Ambala, Haryana**

I was suffering from Rheumatic Heart Disease and urinary diseases. I consulted many doctors and took medicines but there was no relief. Doctors told me that medication would be necessary for life long. I am practising Pranayam from last four years, and now I am not taking any medicines. I am relieved of both the problems and it has been possible only with Pranayam.

— **Indra Rani, Dharmashala, HP**

◆ I had angina pain in May 2004 and TMT was positive and everybody advised me for angioplasty. I was all alone and internal bleeding had shocked me. I shouted for help and managed to get medical attention otherwise I would not been alive today. On May 17, while returning home I watched your programme on Astha channel and started practising Pranayam regularly. I had become anaemic due to excessive bleeding and had become weak. I was also a chronic patient of constipation, migraine and acidity. There was ringing in my ears, my all problems have relieved with Yog practice. Pranayam has indeed given me a new life.

— **Dr. B.R. Baru, Udaipur, Rajasthan**

◆ I was suffering from heart blockage since January 2004, I used to have severe pain in hands and could not walk. Dr Sanjeev Sachdeva of Yamunanagar referred me to AIIMS, New Delhi, for operation. My fasting blood sugar level was 360 and doctors gave me medicines to control sugar level. In the meantime I started practising Yog and Pranayam as taught to me at Divya Yog Mandir Trust. The sugar level came down after 27 days and I felt like being 25 years old at the age of 40. Now I can run 10 kilometres and I do not take any medicines as well. I am practising Pranayam regularly and have been relieved of all the diseases.

— **Suresh Kumar Malik, Old Hamida, Yamunanagar, Haryana**

I developed high blood pressure in 2004. Angiography showed 100 and 95 percent blockage in both arteries. I started practising Pranayam with the inspiration of Swamiji and have been doing it for the last one-and-a-half years. Now heart blockage has opened and I have stopped taking medicines completely. I feel much better.

— **Vilas Shankarrao, Yavatmal, MS**

◆ I got heart attack in June 2004, Angiography showed 70–90 percent blockage. I was advised bypass surgery but I was also a diabetic. I started practising Kapalbhati and Anulom-vilom Pranayam along with Yog asana. The sugar level became normal and weight has decreased by around 10 kilos. TMT was done again on February 4, 2005 and after the reports doctors said that operation was not required.

— **Pradip Kumar Harsola (Jain) Piplani, Bhopal (MP)**

I suffered heart attack in December 2003 and was admitted into Norvik Hospital in Kathmandu. I was unconscious for five days and Dr Bharat Rawat of Escorts Hospital in New Delhi checked me. After investigation he informed my relatives and family members that the chance of my survival was just nine percent. At that time Norvick and AIIMS doctors along with doctors at Spandan Heart Institute, Nagpur, suggested a bypass surgery. Dr Bharat Ravat and K.K. Talwar, Cardiologist, AIIMS had written in the prescription that the mitral valves were not functioning and advised replacement. On the advice of a saintly person I refused operation and started practising Yog. Four years have passed and I am hale and hearty. Not only that, new black hair is growing on my head, a new glow can be seen on face and body. I have also gone for tracking in mountains twice. The same doctors at Norvick hospital are saying that it is a miracle and have totally dismissed the effect of Yog, Pranayam, Asana and meditation on my body as just a miracle. They also say that your example cannot be given to other patients because it is a rare incident.

— **Ramashish, Sitamarhi, Bihar**

Before Treatment   After Treatment

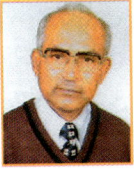

◆ I was suffering from arterial blockage and heart disease since three years and suffered two attacks on account of that. My LVEF had dropped to 28 percent and I could not walk two steps even. I took Ayurvedic medicines from Ashram and started practising Pranayam. LVEF became 36 percent and I am feeling better. Now I do not have any problem while walking or doing my work.

— **Omprakash Arya, Adarshnagar, Bokaro, Jharkhand**

◆ Angiography was done in January 2002 and 80 percent blockage was detected. Angioplasty was done according to the advice of doctors. They suggested by pass surgery but I was not ready. I started practising Pranayam as per Swamiji's advice and also used some home remedies along with Ayurvedic medicines. There was a lot of improvement in health. Stress Thelium test done in January 2003 showed normal heart condition. This has happened because of Swamiji's blessings.

— **Santosh Prakash Johari, Rangpur, Road No.3**

◆ I am suffering from Asthma Bronchitis from the last 13 years and Inferior Myocardial Ischemia was detected in February 2004. I am practising all the seven types of Pranayam since September 20, 2004 and have gained a lot of improvement. The medical test done on October 13, 2004 showed that the disease was cured. It is your blessing that today I am able to walk and do my work.

— **Major M.L.Sharma (Retd), Adarshnagar, Gurudaspur**

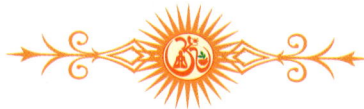

Hepatitis B, Hepatitis C, Liver Cirrhosis

Hepatitis B

◆ I was suffering from liver problem from the last two years and was detected with Hepatitis B. I took Ashram medicines and practised Pranayam regularly. Blood tests done after four months showed negative reports and now I am totally healthy.

— R.G.Verma, Jawalapur, Hardwar

Before Treatment	After Treatment

The patient had Hepatitis B positive before Pranayam and treatment, which became negative after treatment and Pranayam.

◆ Hepatitis B was detected in 2005 and there was no hope despite taking a lot of treatment. Doctors said that Hepatitis B cannot be cured and then I came to know about Swamiji and Ashram medicines. I visited Patanjali Yogpeeth and started treatment. Regular practice of Pranayam and medicines cured the disease. I was once again a healthy person.

— Akhilesh Kumar Dube, Kunji, Ramnagargarh, Dhanbad, Jharkhand

Before Treatment   After Treatment

Hepaptitis B was positive before Pranayam and treatment, which became negative along with liver function test after treatment and Pranayam.

◆ I used to fall sick frequently due to jaundice. Tests revealed Hepatitis B. I was very upset and somebody told me about Swamiji's Yog and Pranayam. I thought it is better to practise, I got some benefit and took Ashram medicines. I practised Pranayam and next reports showed negative results. I am indebted to Swamiji for life.

— S. S. Soni, Ambala City, Haryana

◆ I was suffering from Hepatitis B, doctors told me that it is an incurable disease. I faced a lot of physical weakness and I was also mentally disturbed. No one was able to help me. I was very depressed in my life. I was frustrated taking pills again and again. Then I took treatment from Patanjali Yogpeeth and started practising Yog and Pranayam. With Pranayam and medicines my Hepatitis B is negative now. With the grace of Swamiji I have got a new life.

— **Kailash Kumar Mishra, Mubarakpur Road, Delhi**

Before Treatment   After Treatment

When the patient was examined before treatment his test reports indicated symptoms of Hepatitis B but post-test reports indicated negative Hepatitis B.

Hepatitis C

◆ I was diagnosed Hepatitis C Genotype -1 an year ago. Then I suffered from liver cirrhosis. My weight reduced suddenly and doctors said it was incurable. I was very disappointed and I came to know about Patanjali Yogpeeth. I visited the place and took Ayurvedic medicines, which cured Hepatitis and now it is negative. I am totally healthy.

— **Narendra Kumar Yadav, Maternagunj, Haryana**

Before Treatment   After Treatment

The patient had Hepatitis C positive and liver cirrhosis before Pranayam and treatment. After Pranayam and treatment it became negative and there has been significant change in cirrhosis of liver.

◆ I was suffering from Hepatitis C, because of this my health was deteriorating down day by day. I lost my appetite and after taking food I was not able to digest it properly. I was very depressed in my life and doctors told me that it is an incurable disease. I was frustrated taking pills again and again. Then I took treatment from Patanjali Yogpeeth and started practising Yog and Pranayam. With Pranayam and medicines I regained my appetite and there was a remarkable improvement in my health. With continuous practice of Pranayam and medicines now my Hepatitis C is negative. I found a ray of hope in my life.

— **Vinay Kumar, Kamla Nehru Nagar, Ghaziabad**

Before Treatment	After Treatment

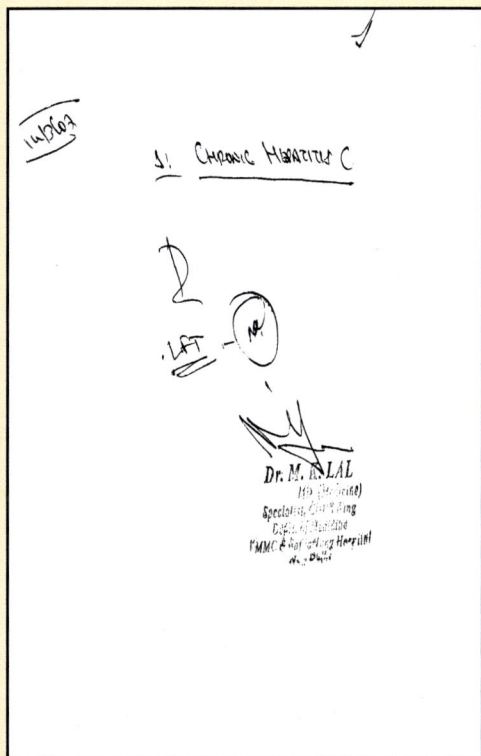

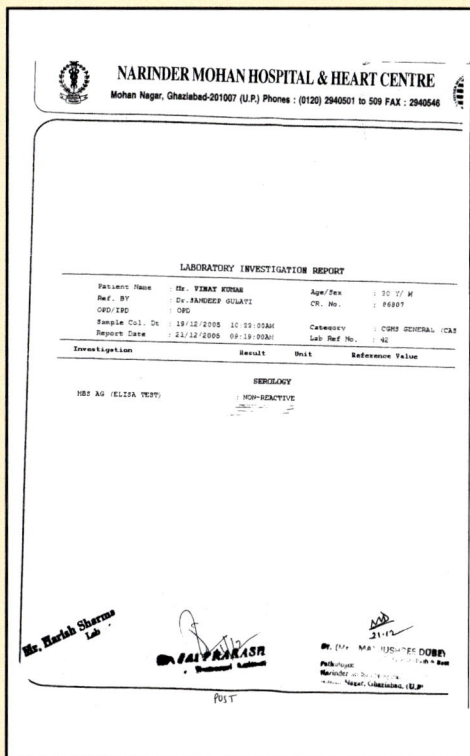

The patient's test reports reflected Hepatitis C before medication but after doing Yog and Pranayam they found it had become Hepatitis C negative.

Liver Cirrhosis

◆ I was suffering from liver cirrhosis and my condition was worsening day by day. Jaundice had reached maximum level and I had swelling on hands, legs, stomach, along with weakness, and dark skin. I had boils on my face, eczema. I used to get sudden shivering with fever, stiffness in body, pain in neck and back side of head. Pain and other symptoms had given rise to a lot of mental tension. I first took some traditional medicines and then went for good allopathic treatment. Regular blood tests were done under the supervision of senior hepatologist, expensive medicines were taken but I had to be admitted in hospital and finally in November 2004 I went to pre-coma condition and I was totally disappointed.

I took Bhui Amalaki quath and practised Anulom-vilom, Kapalbhati, Udgeet and other Pranayam in morning and evening after seeing Swamiji's programme. There was gradual improvement. Doctors said that liver was damaged up to 60-65 percent and transplant was the only solution. It involved several lakh rupees and complete recovery was not guaranted there was no guarantee for recoupment. On the other hand regular practice of Pranayam strengthened my liver and there was a sort of regeneration. The blood tests done in March 2005 gave miraculous results. Now the condition has improved without operation.

— **Vivek Kumar Mishra, Bhayendar (W), Mumbai**

◆ I was detected cirrhosis of liver and diabetes. Well-known doctors gave up. I visited Patanjali Yogpeeth and took Ayurvedic medicines after consultation. Now I am totally healthy and taking some Ayurvedic medicines. I am also practising Pranayam regularly.

— **Premprakash Bhatia, Lajpat Nagar, Kanpur**

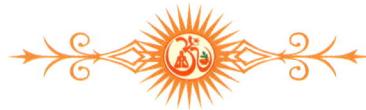

Jaundice

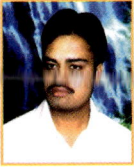

I was suffering from jaundice since last one year. Renowned doctors treated me but there was no relief. I was on death bed. The serum bilirubin in blood was 43.67. Doctors said it was incurable and I lost all hope. I consulted Acharya Balkrishna Ji and started practising Pranayam. I was also taking Ayurvedic medicines and slowly I started recouping. The serum blirubin started reducing and I got a second life with the blessings of Acharya Ji.

— **Ashish Kumar, Bahadarbad, Hardwar**

Before Treatment	After Treatment

The total bilirubin, direct bilirubin, and indirect bilirubin were 43.67, 25.30 and 18.37 respectively before treatment and Pranayam. After three months of practice and Ayurvedic treatment the levels dropped to 2.02, 0.7 and 1.32 respectively.

Cholelithiasis

Cholelithiasis

◆ I got stone in my gall blader since last 7-8 months, doctors told me to get operated. I took medicines prescribed by Swamiji and also started practising Pranayam. After 2-3 months when I got my ultrasound done the reports were completely normal. After knowing that I do not have any stone in my gall bladder, I felt extremely happy.

— **Mayanarayan, Vikasnagar, Lucknow**

Before Treatment   After Treatment

At pre-Pranayam stage the patient's ultrasound reports verified presence of gall stones but post-Pranayam reports were quite normal.

◆ I was very disturbed because of stone in my gall bladder, for this I got my ultrasound done which indicated that the stone size was about 14.7 mm. I started practising Pranayam as told by Swami Ramdevji and after some time in sonography reports showed that the size got reduced to 11.2 mm and 0.9 cm. In this way the size of my stone, in my gall bladder got reduced.

— **Uttam Kumar Shah, Pratapnagar, Agartala, Tripura**

◆ I was suffering from obesity and later it was found that I had stone in my kidney. After this I also got stone in my gall bladder. I saw Swami Ramdevji's programme on Aastha Channel and I started practising Pranayam. Now I am doing Pranayam for the last six months. I have also reduced fat from my body and the stone in my kidney is also cured. The size of stone in my gall bladder has been reduced from 1.23 to 0.4 cm.

— **Mousuni Das, Dharalsavar PO Agartala , Tripura**

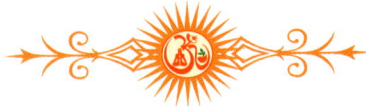

Gynaeological Disorders

Uterine Fibroid and Ovarian Cyst

◆ I had ovarian cyst and doctors suggested operation. I refused and at the same time I came to know about Swamiji's Yog and Pranayam. I also started practising Pranayam and took Ashram medicines. The tumour was cured completely and now I am totally healthy.

— Sumitra Kumari, Chakradharpur, Sinhbhoom, Jharkhand

Before Treatment   After Treatment

The size of ovarian cyst was 5cm X 4cm before Pranayam. After Pranayam and Ayurvedic treatment reports came out normal.

◆ For last many years I was suffering from uterine fibroid, paralysis and lumps in muscles. I practised Pranayam and Yog as told by Swamiji and now I am absolutely healthy.

— Medha Alkari, 3 Cross Road, Mumbai

◆ Ovarian cyst was detected and doctors advised operation. I refused for the operation and at the same time somebody told me about Swami Ramdev Baba's Yog and Pranayam. I also practised Pranayam and took Ashram medicines and cyst got cured. Now I am enjoying good health.

— Priyanka Priyashri, Bhoorkunda, Hazaribagh, Jharkhand

Before Treatment   After Treatment

The patient had poly cystic ovaries before Pranayam and treatment. The ultrasonography report was normal after the treatment and Pranayam.

◆ I had uterine fibroid in my womb, I used to face acute pain and menstruation was also too high. I was not getting results from any medical treatment. Doctors recommended me to remove my womb because of which I had terrible depression. Then I started doing Pranayam as guided by Swamiji and the disease of my womb got cured. My depression and unhappiness was also over. I also had skin diseases and I got relief from it as well. I am living very happy life by the grace of Swamiji.

— Shrimati Maya, Rohini, Delhi

◆ I was suffering from several problems. I used to experience pain in my uterus and ultrasound reports showed swelling in uterus and fibroid growth. Doctors advised operation and said that uterus has to be removed. But I had lot of faith in Swami Ramdevji and started practising Yog and Pranayam. I also took Ashram medicines and the latest medical tests showed normal condition of uterus and there was no tumour or pain. Yog and Pranayam proved to be beneficial.

— **Shankuntala, Hamirpur, U.P.**

Before Treatment　　　　　After Treatment

Ultrasound reports before treatment and Pranayam showed fibroids in uterus and cystitis which were cured after practice of Pranayam.

◆ I was suffering from joint pain and lumps in my womb. Doctors adviced me to undergo surgery but I was very scared of getting operated. I started consuming medicines prescribed by the Ashram and also started practising Pranayam; now after 10 months I am absolutely healthy and I am not even taking any medicines.

— **Priyanka Vashist, Pawan Puri, Bikaner**

◆ I had ovarian cyst and uterine fibroid. Gynecologist adviced me to get operated and suggested to remove my utreus. I saw Aastha Channel and started practising Pranayam as told by Swamiji. After 4 months my ultrastonography report is absolutely normal. Before doing Pranayam my weight was 38 kg and now it is 45.5 kg. Now I am absolutely healthy.

— **Beena Pani, Debta, Nadia, West Bengal**

The patient was having uterine fibroid before doing Pranayam and now it is completely cured.

◆ I was suffering from uterine fibroid and migraine since long time because of that I used to get headache and ache in stomach. I was depressed in life. I was advised to get operated. I am doing Pranayam as told by Swamiji from last 4 years and now I am feeling absolutely healthy. Before I used to take pain killers and now I do not need them. My uterine fibroid is completely cured.

— **Durga Mishra, Vinayak Nagar, Mary Kalvi, Chandarpur**

◆ Since last one year I had uterine fibroid because of this I suffered a lot. Doctors advised to get operated and to remove the womb. One day I saw Swamijis programme on Aastha Channel since then I started doing Pranayam regularly. After doing Pranayam the fibroid in my womb is cured. The ultrasound reports are also normal.

— Renu Haldar, Hughli, West Bengal

Before Treatment   After Treatment

The patient was having Fibroid stone in womb before doing Pranayam and later after doing Pranayam the ultrasound report is normal.

◆ I was suffering from uterine fibroid since long time, I was taking allopathic medicines and doctors were advising me to get operated. One day I saw Swamiji's programme on Aastha Channel and started practising Pranayam, after doing Pranayam for about 8-10 months I am absolutely healthy. Swamiji has saved me from surgery.

— Mithilesh Bhardwaj, Air Force Station, Barakachpora, Kolkata

Since last one year I had pain in my left side of the stomach, my monthly cycles were also irregular. Doctors told me after check up that I have cyst in my left ovary for which I will have to get operated. I started practising Pranayam as told by Swamiji, now I am doing Pranayam since last 6 months. I got my ultrasound done after 3 months of Pranayam practice and I found that there was no cyst. I am absolutely healthy now. Swamiji has saved me from surgery. I am very grateful to him.

— **Aarti Sahu, Koyal Nagar, Raurkela**

Before Treatment	After Treatment

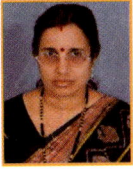

The patient was having cyst in womb before doing Pranayam and later after doing Pranayam the ultrasound report is normal.

◆ I was suffering from tumor from a very long time, doctors told me to get operated but I started practising Pranayam instead of getting operated. After doing Pranayam for 5-6 months I got myself checked, my tumor had disappeared. I was extremely happy. Swamiji has saved me from surgery.

— **Sudha Tiwari, Azad Nagar, Jabalpur**

◆ I was suffering from stone in uterus because of which I was not able to stand for a long time and my menstruation cycles were also irregular. When I consulted few doctors they advised me to remove my womb. Then I started practising Pranayam after seeing Swamiji on Aastha Channel, now I am practising Pranayam from last 3 years. After doing Pranayam my stone in uterus is cured and my menstruation cycles are regular. My ultrasound report is also normal.

— Krishni Singh, Korba, Chattisgarh

The patient was having Fibroid in womb before doing Pranayam and later after doing Pranayam the ultrasound report is normal.

◆ I had stone in my womb since last 3 years, there was a lot of trouble due to excess bleeding during my menstruation cycles. Doctors advised to remove uterus. Then I started practising Pranayam as guided by Swami Ramdevji. After regular practice of Pranayam my Fibroid (tumor) in womb is completely cured. Now I am absolutely healthy.

— Poonam Aggarwal, JC Mallike Road, Hira Pur, Dhanbad

◆ Since last 2-3 years I used to have excess bleeding during my menstruation cycle. Doctors advised to remove uterus. I got scared as I already had three operations done before. I kept consuming allopathic medicines. After 4-5 months when there was no relief; my lady doctor suggested me to go to Swami Ramdevji. On February 2006 I took treatment from Ashram and started doing Pranayam regularly, 1-2 months later I started getting relief and I got very confident that I can get cured without operation. When I got myself checked in July 2006 then I actually found that there was no tumor in my uterus. I am really obliged to Swami Ramdevji that he helped me to get cured without operation in very short time.

— **Saroj Gupta, Janak Puri, Delhi**

Before Treatment   **After Treatment**

The patient was having Multiple Fibroid in womb before doing Pranayam and later after doing Pranayam the ultrasound report is normal.

Infertility and Fallopian Tube Blockage

◆ Since last many years my menstruation cycle used to occur after 4–5 months and there was no ovulation of egg in my ovaries. After getting a lot of treatment I was not getting any benefit from anywhere. Then I started practising Pranayam as guided by Swami Ramdevji. After regular practice of Pranayam my menstruation cycle got regular. Then I got ovulation study done and I found that there was timely ovulation in my ovaries. I am very obliged to Swamiji.

— **Soniya, Salapar, Himachal Pradesh**

Before Treatment   After Treatment

The patient had problems of ovulation in ovary before doing Pranayam and later after doing Pranayam the ovulation is normal.

◆ I got married 8 years back but we do not have any child till now. I got myself treated from several places however I got no positive relief from anywhere. When I came to know about Swamiji and his Ashram then after consulting we started taking medicines. Along with medicines we also started doing Pranayam. After regular practice of 3 months Pranayam and medicines I came to know that I am pregnant. I will always be grateful to Swamiji.

— **Neena, Panki, Kanpur**

Before Treatment

After Treatment

The patient was having non secretory endometrium with acute endometritis. Doctors told that she will never be able to get pregnant but after tests the patient found positive in pregnancy tests.

◆ My fallopian tubes were blocked and there was no relief even after allopathic treatment. I consulted many doctors but in vain. Regular practice of Pranayam and Ashram medicines opened fallopian tubes and other health problems were cured automatically.

— Pooja Goswami, Kanpur, UP

Before Treatment	After Treatment

The above pathological report shows clearly that both the fallopian tubes were blocked, which opened after treatment.

◆ I am a Political Science Professor, for better health I used to do Yog before. I got married in the year 2000 and even after 4–5 years of marriage we faced problems having a child. We did whatever possibly we could but there was no positive result. Since May 2006 we started consuming medicines from Divya Yog Mandir Trust, Hardwar and we also started practising Pranayam and Yog. In June 2006, my wife got pregnant. In 2007, we were blessed by a child. You are a hope for childless couples like us whom you have blessed with Pranayam, Yog and Ayurvedic medicines.

— Dr Surendra Meena, Durgapura, Nagad, Madhya Pradesh

◆ I was married 13 years back but we were not blessed with children. After three years of marriage life I was detected tumour in ovary and doctors suggested me to adopt a child. They did not advice operation with a saying that tumour would not affect getting pregnant. In the meantime I underwent laproscopy four times and the body had become weak. I was also suffering from other ailments like severe stomachache, choked throat, and doctors were suggesting operation for these problems. All I could think about was having a child and everything alse reemed minor. I was very upset and managed to keep a smile on my face. I used to do Yog from childhood but started doing Pranayam after watching Swamiji's programme. I did not realize when I conceived. and according to doctors everything is normal. My ankle and throat problems have also been cured.

— **Archana Mishra, Armament Section, 32 Wing Air Force, C/o 56 APO**

◆ For the past so many years my menstruation cycle used to occur once in 4-5 months and there was no egg formation in the ovaries. Even after taking a lot of treatment my condition did not improve. Then I started practising Pranayam and Yog taught by Swamiji. After a few months my menstrueal cycle regularized and I got ovulation study done and I found that eggs are being formed regularly in the ovaries. Swamiji, I am grateful to you.

— **Sonia, Salapar, Mandi (Himachal Pradesh)**

◆ I used to feel low due to childlessness. After visiting Swamiji's camp I started practising regular Pranayam, due to which I conceived. I am very happy with this miracle of Pranayam. Now my home will also be filled with the pleasing voice of a child. By the miracle of Pranayam taught by Swamiji and the Ayurvedic treatment from the Ashram I am lucky enough to become a mother.

— **Indu Yadav, Birdopur, Varanasi**

Irregular Menstrual Cycle

◆ About two and a half years ago, excessive menstruation discharge started. When the blood discharge did not stop with the help of medicines then I under went TCRE (in which uterus endometrium's small pieces are taken out of the body, because of which the bleeding stopped). But I felt irritated and tired all the time. After practising Pranayam for two years my menstruation cycle began again and now I do not feel irritated or tired. Endometrium has again developed and at the age of 47 years now my menstruation cycle has again started.

— **Smt. Gyanprakash, Jagritivihar, Meerut**

◆ I faced the problem of Irregular menstruation cycle since a long time. My harmones were imbalanced. I used to take harmones supplements for that. After practising Pranayam for 6 months every thing is alright and now I am absolutely healthy. It is all because of your blessings and you have lit the lamp of Yog in the world.

— **Sameeta R. Aneek, Vidyanagar, Chandrapur**

Breast Tumor

◆ I had tumor in my breast. I started practising Yog and Pranayam taught by Swamiji. After practising Pranayam the tumor of breast is fully cured. Swamiji, you are spreading the light of Yog and Pranayam in the world and by which people like us are getting rid of their diseases.

— **Anjana Das, Rajarahat Chekpur, Kolkata, West Bengal**

◆ I had breast tumor. I consulted many doctors but got no relief. I contacted Divya Yog Mandir Trust and was advised to do Pranayam and take Ayurvedic medicine. I started doing regular Pranayam and using Ashram's medicines. Now I have fully recovered. Swamiji, you are like God for me.

— **Hema Kutega, Kolkata, West Bengal**

◆ I had tumor in both breasts. I got one tumor removed by operation in Mumbai. Doctors suggested me to get second tumor to be removed as well. Now after doing regular Pranayam, my second tumor has disappeared.

— **Sheela Rai, Baxer, Bihar**

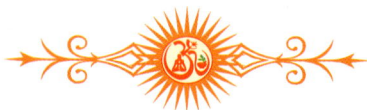

Renal Calculi / Renal Failure

Renal Calculi

◆ I used to have slight stomach ache and medical tests revealed that I had fatty liver and stones in kidney. I was very upset and I practised Pranayam and took Patharchatta medicine as per your advice. After two months of Pranayam practice, test report showed normal liver.

— Sandeep Bansal, Nazarbagh, Lucknow UP

The ultrasound test done before treatment showed 4 mm kidney stone and fatty liver, which was normal after Yog - Pranayam practice.

◆ There was a 8 mm stone in my kidney. Allopathic medicines were not beneficial and pain used to recur. I took Ayurvedic medicines from Patanjali Yogpeeth, which cured kidney problem and now I am not taking any type of medicine. I am completely healthy.

— Gopal Prajapati, Apna Nagar, Gandhidham

◆ I had a stone and infection in my kidney. Due to acidity, I had lost my apetite. I got allopathic treatment including injections it helped me for a while but problem recurred. Then I started doing Yog and Pranayam as told by Swamiji. I am doing Pranayam for last two years. Now I have good digestion and my blood pressure has become normal. Size of stone has also reduced. Now I am totally off the allopathic medicines.

— **Jagdish Chandra Sharma, Indra Puri, New Delhi**

I had stone problem since birth and was operated twice but there was on relief. I could not go for operation due to economic constraints and I have been practising Pranayam since last two years. The stone problem has been cured and now I am totally healthy.

— **Sarvottam Chintamanrao Godse, Latur, Maharashtra**

◆ I had kidney stone and some tests were done when the problem recurred. The reports showed that kidney stones had formed. Doctors suggested immediate operation. I was very upset and started practising Yog and Pranayam regularly. Tests were done again after two months and there was no sign of stones. Doctors were also surprised to see the results. I am deeply inclined towards Yog.

— **Kamla Sharma, Nishatgunj, Lucknow (UP)**

Renal Failure

◆ I was suffering from kidney problem, My serum creatinine was 7.2, serum protein was 6, SGPT was 63 adn SGOT was 84. Allopathic medicines cured fever but burning sensation in urine continued. I took Ayurvedic medicines from Divya Yog Mandir Trust and got a lot of improvement. I started practising Pranayam and now I feel much better. The reports are also normal.

— **Dharamveer, Guhana, Sonipat**

◆ I was admitted into hospital due to accumulation of water in stomach. Excess medication had increased urea and creatinine level. Then I took Ayurvedic medicines and practised Pranayam as per Swamiji's guidance. Now I am totally healthy. The creatinine, urea and potassium level is also normal.

— **Amit Giri, Daltongunj, Jharkhand**

◆ I was suffering from urinary infection. Passing urine was painful and it passed at a slow pace. Due to accumulation of urine in the urinary bladder, it caused acute pain in abdominal region. Investigation revealed that I had an enlarged prostrate gland. Allopathic medicines did not help much and then I started taking medicine from the Ashram and also started practising Pranayam. I am cured of all my problems. Ultrasound report showed considerable improvement. Along with there has been an improvement in my behaviour and my attitude is positive. After practising Pranayam I have stopped taking all the allopathic medicines.

— **Chandreshwari Bhagat, New Ashok Nagar, Delhi**

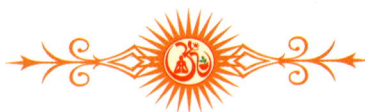

A positive difference can be seen in the patient's ultrasound test before and after the treatment.

Obesity and its Complications

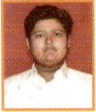

I was obese and used to feel embarrassed in attending social functions and gatherings. I have been practising Pranayam for the last three months and my weight has reduced by 20 kilos. I feel much better and I would like to thank Swamiji a million times.

— **Akhilesh Kumar Gautam, Ghaziabad**

◆ I was suffering from insomnia due to obesity and lacked efficiency at work place. I started practising Pranayam from January 2007 and my weight reduced by several kilos. I feel active and healthy and I am able to sleep properly.

— **Lisa Amure, Glasgow, Scotland, UK**

◆ I used to be stressed due to obesity. I started practising Yog and happiness had come back into my life. Sleeplessness, obesity, stress started reducing and my breathing improved. Pranayam indeed is the new mantra of my life.

— **Louise Kelly Glasgow, Scotland, UK**

◆ I was suffering from arthritis, obesity and blood pressure for the last 15 years. I consulted many doctors but did not get any relief. I was extremely disappointed. One day my daughter saw your programme on Astha Channel and inspired me to do Yog. After a few days of practice I noticed considerable change in my life. My weight reduced from 83 to 61 kilos and waist size reduced by eight inches. I was very short tempered before but now I am very calm. My wife is also obese and after practising Yog her weight reduced from 109 to 83 kilos. My daughter also lost 22 kilos weight. Besides my daughter also had thick tumours in body, which are gradually reducing.

Before Treatment   After Treatment

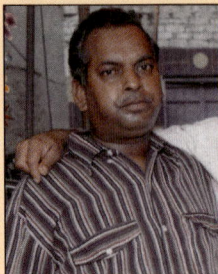

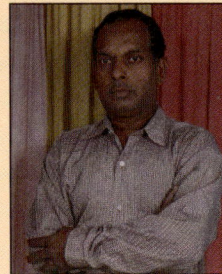

— **Om Prakash Sharma, Badla Chowk, Jalandhar, Punjab**

◆ Obesity was a major problem for me and I used to feel tired and I had lost interest in doing any work. I took part in Yog and Pranayam classes conducted by Sunita Poddar. My weight reduced by seven lbs within one month. This was indeed a great experience.

— Josephine MacGregor, Glasgow Scotland, UK

◆ My work was very tiring and it caused a lot of stress. I became obese and suffered from sleeplessness, backache, sciatica, joint pain and cancer. I was stress free within two weeks of Yog practice and I was able to enjoy sound sleep. My body has become active and Yog has shown miraculous results.

— Mourine Atkil, Glasgow, Scotland, U.K

◆ I saw your programme in the last week of March on Doordarshan and started practising all types of Pranayam like Bhastrika, Kapalbhati, Anulom-vilom, Bahya, Ujjayi etc. My weight was 105 kilo and now it has reduced to 71 kilo. I am enclosing both the photographs. I was also a patient of high blood pressure and joint pain, which is under control with regular practice of Pranayam. Now I am healthy and active.

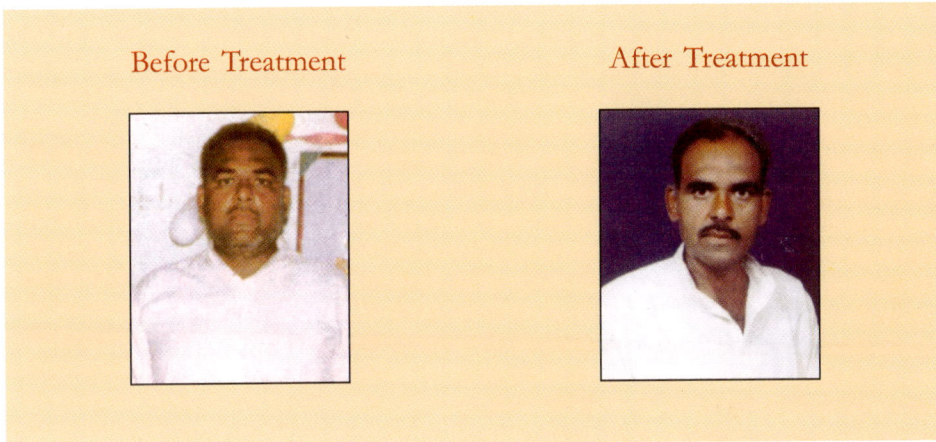

Before Treatment   After Treatment

—Rajdev Dhiman, Roorkee, Hardwar

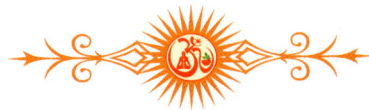

Diabetes

Genetic Diabetes

I was suffering from diabetes for last four years and my blood pressure was at 150/100. I took allopathic medicines, diabetes and blood pressure became normal for a few days but it started increasing after a few months. I am practising Pranayam regularly and now my blood sugar and blood pressure is normal. I am not taking medicines presently.

— **Tapasi Pohar, Narottam Park, Kolkata**

I was a diabetic and my fasting sugar level was 162 and PP was 395. I used to take 27 units of insulin in the morning and 18 in the evening. I used to feel weary and tired but after practising Pranayam there is no need to take insulin and my body has become active. I feel much better and energetic.

— **Dipankar Das, Hugli, West Bengal**

I was a diabetic patient and before practising Yog I used to take 35 and 22 units of insulin in the morning and evening respectively. I have been practising Pranayam for the last two years and have stopped taking insulin. I just take one tablet, I am very happy and do not have any kind of problem.

— **Santosh, Khanpur, New Delhi**

Diabetes and acidity are both hereditary in my family. Medicines were unable to control my sugar level. I am practising Pranayam regularly from April 4, 2004 and now PP sugar level is 96, fasting is 114 and acidity has been cured completely. All the problems have been relieved with the blessings of Swamiji.

— **Fakirchand, Nabha, Dist - Patiala**

◆ I was a patient of diabetes and blood pressure. The blood sugar was between 250-300 and blood pressure also used to be high. After practising Pranayam and using Ayurvedic medicines blood sugar and blood pressure are normal. Regular practice of Pranayam for last 40 days has been helpful in controlling my health problems.

— **B.S. Kuber, Mahalakshmipuram, Bangaluru, Karnataka**

◆ I was suffering from diabetes for the past several years and my sugar level had reached 660 on May 25. I was taking allopathic medicines. I started practising Pranayam for last one month and there has been tremendous improvement. Sugar level is 150 and I am taking just five units of insulin. I am confident that there will be no need to take insulin soon. Swami Ramdev is like a God for me.

— **Makar Singh, Umarpura, Gurdaspur, Punjab**

◆ I was suffering from diabetes for last so many years. My blood sugar used to remain above 300. I did not benefit by taking any medicine. Only the quantity of the medicines started to increase. In the investigation, the amount of C-Peptide used to be very high. Then I started practising Pranayam as taught by Swamiji. After practising Pranayam for a few months when I got my blood sugar examined, I was surprised to see that factors came out as normal including the level of C-Peptide. Now I am not taking any kind of medicine and I no longer have a sugar problem.

— **Anup Chakravarti, Village Rahra, 24 Pargana, Kolkota**

◆ I am suffering from diabetes for last six years and allopathic medicine have not given any relief. Diabetes is in my family and both my father and grandfather are diabetic. After practising Yog and Pranayam and taking ayruvedic medicines my sugar level has become normal. I am not taking any other medicine at present.

— **Gulab Bhai, GIDC, Bhuj, Gujarat**

◆ I was suffering from diabetes and because of this my weight had also increased and my eyesight had gone weak. From the time I have started practising Pranayam as taught by Swamiji, I have been benefited in all the diseases. Now diabetes is also cured and the weight has reduced. The eyesight is also improving.

— **Vinay Kumar Sharma, Muzafarnagar**

◆ I was suffering from diabetes, obesity and respiratory disorder and I had gained a lot of weight. I was very disturbed due to this. Now for the past three years I am practising Pranayam. Due to this my diabetes and respiratory disease is completely cured and my weight has also reduced by 38 kg, and my mind has become so peaceful and stable that I have given up non-vegetarian food.

— **Abdul Ali, Alidabad, Andhra Pradesh**

◆ I was suffering from diabetes. Earlier sugar level used to be 470 and my knee joints became useless. I kept on taking painkillers and a number of allopathic medicines. But neither the sugar could get under control nor I could get rid of pain. Now after practising Pranayam, I have benefitted a lot and I take much less of allophathic medicines.

— **Vijay Baburao Chandavaar, City Post Officer, Chandrapur, Maharashtra**

◆ Since a long time I was suffering from hereditary diabetes, high BP and obesity. I was frustrated of consuming allopathic medicines. Now I have started practising Pranayam by attending Swamiji's camps since last four months. Now my sugar and high BP is normal and my weight has also reduced. I feel absolutely alright and I am also not taking any medicine.

— **Arjun, Hanumantrao, South Sadar Bazar, Solapur**

◆ For the past so many years I was suffering from High BP and diabetes. My parents also suffered from this disease. I was taking allopathic medicine for this. But I was not getting any relief so I started practising Pranayam and Asans. Now I am relieved of the problem of diabetes and high BP. I do not need to take any medicine. I am getting regular check-ups and my reports are always normal.

— **Rajeshwari Chakravarti, HRBR Layout, Bangalore**

◆ I suffered from sugar and high BP for the past 15 years. One day I watched Swamiji's programme on Astha Channel and after that I started practising Pranayam on regular basis and since the time I have started practising Pranayam my sugar and high BP are under control. I am not taking any kind of medicine and I am absolutely healthy.

— **Vinay Kumar Singhal, Kachha Katra, Shahajanpur**

◆ I was suffering from diabetes and my sugar level was between 300 and 400. I used to take 30 units of insulin each in the morning and evening. I have been practising Pranayam for the last two years and now my sugar level is around 150. I do not take insulin. I am trying to cure the diseases of people by organizing Yog classes with the inspiration of Swami Ramdevji. My weight was 150 kilos, which has reduced to 93 kilos.

— **Bharat Singh, Patel Nagar, Patna**

◆ My blood sugar was always on the higher side, and when checked after meals it used to be very high. I am practising Pranayam taught by Swamiji for the last 6 months in morning with empty stomach. Now my blood sugar is normal and after meals it is 135. I have also reduced my weight by three kg and I have stopped taking allopathic medicines. My parents too suffered from sugar problem..

— **Mahesh Malviya, Kakasan Complex Phase-2, Koijia, Bhopal**

◆ I was suffering from IDDM. For which I had to take insulin. I was very much disturbed by this. Then I started practising Pranayam and Asan as taught by swamiji and also started taking medicines from the Ashram. With the regular practice of Pranayam the insulin intake has slowly come to an end and now the blood sugar report is also normal.

— **Trilochan Sahu, Kamakhya Nagar, Dekhanal (Orissa)**

◆ I was suffering from diabetes. For which I had to take insulin. I started practising Pranayam after watching Swamiji's programme on Astha Channel and after the practice of Pranayam I have stopped taking insulin. Now I do not take any other medicine also. I only practise Pranayam. I am healthy. When tested, my report shows normal sugar levels.

— **Meera Nayyar, Green Avenue, Amritsar, Punjab**

Diabetic Retinopathy

I was suffering from urinary problem and used to wake up several times in the night due to this problem. I saw Swamiji's programme on television and have been practising Pranayam for the last two years. I had lost vision in one eye after operation. Pranayam has reduced diabetes to a great extent and I have reduced the medicine intake as well.

— Savita Rani Gandhi, Kalkaji, New Delhi

I became diabetic eight years ago and developed eyesight problem. I took a lot of medicines but there was no relief. I felt compeltely helpless. I have been practising Pranayam for the last one-and-a-half years. Now I can see clearly and feel very healthy and active.

— Sunanda, Naka Madar, Ajmer (Rajasthan)

I was a diabetic and had very weak eyesight. I felt I was going to become blind and consulted doctors. They diagnosed the problem as Diabetic Ratinopathy and said it was incurable. I came to know about Swamiji and I have been practising Pranayam for the last two years. Pranayam has reduced diabetes to a great extent and my eyesight has also improved. I have discontinued medicines and I am practising Pranayam regularly. I have got a new life with the blessings of Swamiji.

— Rajesh Shrivastava, Mukherjee Nagar, Vidisha, MP

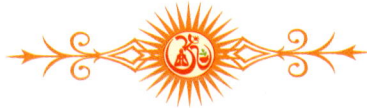

High Blood Pressure

Chronic Hypertension

My blood pressure was 180 /60 and I used to suffer from headache and excessive prespiration. I saw Swamiji's programme on television and have been practising Pranayam for last two years. Now the blood pressure is 110/70 and headaches are gone. I am very happy.

— **Lakshman Rao, BHU, Varanasi**

I was having high blood pressure from the past 30 years and used to take medicines everyday. The blood pressure used to increase when I did not take a tablet. I am practsing Pranayam from the past three years by watching television. Pranayam has improved eyesight and blood pressure is normal. I do not take any kind of medicine and feel better.

— **Shankuntala Goyal, Adarsh Colony, Jabalpur**

My blood pressure was 170/110 before practising Yog, I took lot of medicines but there was no relief. I am practising Pranayam since last two years and now blood pressure is 110/80 and I do not require any medicines..

— **Madan Kumar, Madhubani, Bihar**

◆ I was suffering from hereditary problem of blood pressure. Doctors said that this would be a life-long problem. I lost all hope and thought that I would have to live with this problem. I started practising Pranayam for last two years and this hereditary problem has been cured completely. I do not take any medicine any more, Pranayam alone was sufficient. This is like a miracle for me.

— **Poonam Bhatnagar, South Malaka, Allahabad**

◆ My blood pressure was 250 / 120 before practising Pranayam which was very high and I used to have severe palpitation and used to feel restless. I saw Swamiji's programme on television and started practising Pranayam. Now my blood pressure has reduced to 150/ 100 and I have lost weight as well. I feel better.

— **Harkeval Singh, District Patiala, Punjab**

◆ I was a patient of high blood pressure, which was a hereditary problem. Medicines were unable to control it. I started practising Pranayam and now my blood pressure is 150 /90. My weight has also reduced from 85 to 74 kilos. I am feeling much better.

— **Mahesh Chandra Agrawal, Vivekanand Nagar, Ghaziabad**

I was having high blood pressure for the last three years. The blood pressure used to be 210/120 and I suffered a paralytic attack as well. I am practising Pranayam since three months and now the blood pressure is normal. I am working for 12 hours in the office and feel healthy.

Mahendra Dutt Sharma, ILL Colony, Bhopal

◆ My immune system had become very weak. I started practising Pranayam from January 14, 2007 along with Yog and Asana. My blood pressure became normal within three weeks and backache also decreased. My immunity has improved and now I feel healthy and discuss the benefits of Yog with others.

— George Gray, Glasgow, Scotland, UK

I used to suffer from high blood pressure and this was hereditary. I had to take medicine everyday. I started practising Pranayam from September 22, 2006 and now my blood pressure is normal at 120 /80. I am cured of this hereditary problem.

— Rajvinder Singh, Fatehgarh Sahin, Punjab

◆ I was suffering from hereditary blood pressure. I was inspired by Swamiji's discourses and started prasticing Pranayam for the past four years. Now my blood pressure is normal and I am not taking any medicine as well.

— Ashok Kumar Pal, PO Nabo, Paragana

Genetic Hypertension

◆ I was suffering from diabetes, cholesterol, high BP and other diseases. All of my diseases were genetic. For which I had to take many medicines which gave only temporary relief. I was very upset for not able to get a permanent cure. I started practising Pranayam by attending Swamiji's camps and within three weeks of practising Pranayam I started to benefit. Now my high BP, cholesterol level has become normal. I do not take any kind of medicine any more. I have also stopped using inhaler and now I feel much better.

— Dr Meera Parikh, Boletone BLI 5 DB, UK

◆ I was suffering from hereditary hypertension for the last 15 years. My father and grandfather had also suffered from this disease. Their high BP was not getting controlled with allopathic medicines. Then I started doing Pranayam and thereafter my BP was fully under control. I have completely stopped taking medicines. Pranayam has given me all-round relief - physically, mentally and spiritually.

— Dr P. L. Kaul, SK Nagar, GAU, Gujarat

◆ I had been suffering from CAD (Coronary Artery Problem) and high BP These diseases were hereditary. My father also suffered from it. For this, I had been taking allopathic medicines. I started doing Yog and Pranayam from October 2006 which gave me great relief. Now I have stopped taking any medicine. After doing Pranayam I have been keeping very well.

— Ratan Kumar Pandey, Ramakrishan Palli, Malda (West Bengal)

◆ I had been suffering from pain in joints, skin disease, and high BP for last many years. I was not getting cured even after prolonged treatment. I started doing Pranayam regularly as advised by Swamiji. Now I am feeling healthy and I am free from medicines. With Pranayam, I have again started enjoying life.

— Shri Ram Singh Rathi, Distt. Hamirpur

◆ I had been suffering from high BP and Asthma for last 9 years. Due to this I had difficulty in walking and speaking. My weight got reduced to 57 kg but my stomach hung out Now after following Swamiji's advise I am doing Yog and Pranayam and I am cured of my health problems. I have stopped taking any medicines. With your kindness, my life has changed for better.

— Gulab Domaji, Near Jai Mahal, Bajrang Nagar, Nagpur

◆ My parents and my elder brother died because of high BP It was a hereditary disease. With regular practice of Pranayam and with the blessings of Swamiji, I am now alright. Now my BP is normal and I donot take any medicines. I get my BP checked regularly. If I had known about Pranayam taught by Swamiji earlier, my other family members would not have died of this hereditary disease.

— Kanta Sharma, New Colony, Hoshiarpur

◆ I was very disturbed and very upset due to hypertension and severe knee pain for last many years. I got many side effects from the regular use of allopathic medicines. Then I started doing Pranayam as shown by Swamiji on Astha Channel and started taking medicines from their Ashram. Now I am fully relieved of hypertension and knee pain and I am not taking any medicines now. I feel quite healthy at present.

— Madhu Sharma, Hira Mandi, Ferozepur

◆ I had been suffering from hereditary high BP and acidity for the last six years. I had seen Swamiji on Astha channel since then I have been regularly practising Yog and Pranayam. Now my BP and acidity problem has been cured completely. I have stopped taking any medicines. Now, I feel rejuvenated and I have started thinking positively.

— Seema R. Radhakrishnan, Vanvari, Pune

◆ I had been suffering from high BP and psoriasis for last 15 years. I took treatment from various places but all was in vain. I was depressed. Encouraged by Swami Ramdevjii, I was determined to heal myself. Now with the help of Pranayam and Ayurved I have been living a healthy life for last 3 years. I advise others also to practise Yog.

Jagdish Bhai Patel, Vidya Nagar Road, Anand

◆ I had been suffering from high BP, Sciatica and Skin disease and also Migraine for the last 24 years. I got treatment from various physicians from various places but could not get cured. Then with full determination I started doing Pranayam. After 8-10 months of doing it I am fully cured and I got rid of the medicines.

— Jai Prakash Mani Tiwari, Priya Nagar, Jharsugarh

◆ I was suffering from hypertension and heart problems. After taking prolonged treatment I didn't not get cured. For the last 3 years I am doing Yog and Pranayam regularly. As a result, my hypertension is 100% cured. I feel a lot of improvement in my heart problems. My eyesight has also improved. I have stopped taking medicines.

— Pritam Singh Saini, Vill. Sarora, Akalpur, Jammu

◆ I was suffering from high BP, heart problem and diabetes. I was facing lot of difficulties. I benefited a lot with regular practice of Yog and Pranayam. My BP and heart problems are over now. I have stopped taking BP and cardiac medicines. Now I do only Yog and Pranayam.

— Vishwanath Malhotra, Amritsar

◆ I had been suffering from hereditary hypertension. In my family, my mother and other family members also suffered from hypertension. I have been doing Pranayam for the last two years as instructed by Swamiji. I am absolutely healthy now. I am not taking any allopathic medicine for hypertension.

— Pushpa Hastir, Noida

◆ I was suffering from hereditary hypertension. I had been regularly taking allopathic medicines. Since I started doing Pranayam as guided by Swamiji, my hypertension is under control. Now I am not taking any allopathic medicine.

— Brij Kishore Naina, Angeergodis, Balasore, Orissa

◆ I suffered from genetic high BP for last few years because of which I was worried. Now, I have been practising Pranayam for the last one-and-a-half year. I am not taking any medicines any more. With the grace of Swamiji my chronic high BP is now in control

— Keshav Shalik Sheikh

◆ I had been suffering from hypertension for last many years. I used to feel heaviness in the eyes, physical weakness and used to have severe headache. Since, I started doing Pranayam as guided by Swamiji, I have stopped taking all allopathic medicines. Now I am healthy. All my family members have benefited by doing Pranayam.

— **Manvari Singh, P.O. Chandra, Bullandshahar**

◆ I was suffering from hypertension, due to which I used to get headaches, sleeplessness, dizziness and irritation. On being adviced by a friend I started doing Pranayam. Earlier I was not able to practise it regularly. Slowly and gradually I started feeling its benefits and I became confident about its usefulness. Now I do not have complaint of hypertension. I feel energetic and healthy.

— **Virender Singh Thakur, Taima, Chiradwara**

◆ For last many years I had high BP problem. My mother also had this disease and she died because of it. Initially I was able to control it with allopathic medicines. For last 8-10 months I am doing regular practice of Pranayam and I no longer need to take any medicines.. I am now relieved of this terrible problem.

— **Santosh Payal, Delhi**

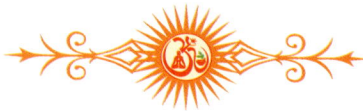

DISORDERS OF NERVOUS SYSTEM

Multiple Sclerosis

◆ I was diagnosed with Multiple Sclerosis ailment in December 2004. After this I got treatment from the best of the best medical centers of the country but it did not help. Slowly I started losing my eyesight and I was not able to walk. I got depressed and thought of committing suicide. Doctors prescribed medicines and thought that their duty was done. I was not satisfied with all this. As a last resort, I came to Swamiji with full faith in him. I started doing Pranayam. I started feeling a wonderful improvement in all my ailments. Multiple sclerosis, which the doctors found incurable, got completely cured with Yog. I regained my eyesight. Once again I felt rejuvenated. With the blessings of Swamiji once again I started to live life.

— **Kavita Gupta, Sarita Vihar, New Delhi**

◆ I was suffering from Multiple Sclerosis since 1991. Medical treatment has not given desired results. The neurologists declared it as incurable. I saw Swamiji's programme on Astha Channel and started practising Pranayam since April 2004. I also took wheatgrass juice, Giloy and there has been significant improvement in my problem. Now I am a totally healthy person and do all the household work myself. I am teaching Yog and Pranayam to others so that I can become a source of inspiration for them. Multiple Sclerosis Society of Pune has honoured me for this initiative. Swamiji's Pranayam is blessing for any patient.

— **Pratibha Amarje, Abhinav Apartment, Pune**

Parkinson's Disease and Cerebral Atrophy

◆ I was suffering from Parkinson's disease. I had cramps, my teeth bled and my whole body used to tremble. I had to take many medicines however I was not getting any benefit from them. I started Yog and Pranayam for last 5 months and took medicines from the Ashram. Now I feel a lot of relief and I hope that I shall be fully cured with Yog and Pranayam.

— **Lata Devi, Salapad Colony, Salapad Sunder Nagar, Mandi**

◆ I was suffering from Parkinson's disease. My hands, feet and head used to tremble. I was not able to do any kind of work, there was no improvement from any treatment. Then I started doing Yog and Pranayam as guided by Swamiji. I have been regularly doing it since last year. There has been noticeable improvement. I do not take medicines now and I am feeling better these days.

— **Promila, P.O. Khagariya**

◆ I was suffering from Cerebral Atrophy. As shown on TV, I started doing Yog and Pranayam for about two months. Gradually I have started feeling a lot of improvement. Doctors have stopped all medicines. Now I do only Yog and Pranayam.

— **Ajay Kumar Jain, Mahatma Gandhi Marg, Maheshwar**

◆ I was suffering from Parkinson's disease. My jaws were very weak. I was getting treatment from AIIMS, New Delhi. There was not much improvement. Doctors said it is an incurable disease and medicines can only give some relief. I was depressed. I followed Swamiji's Yog and Pranayam exercises as shown on Aastha Channel and I feel better now. I had been taking medicines since last two years and now from the last two months I have not taken any medicine.

— **Bhagwati Hans, Rishi Nagar, Faridabad**

◆ I was unable to speak and walk and doctors had diagnosed it as Cerebral Atrophy. I started doing Pranayam from September 2004. After doing Pranayam for about a year now, I do not need any of those allopathic medicines that I was using. Earlier when I was in your camp I could walk with support, now I can walk without any support. There is an improvement in my speech as well.

— **Suraj Shukla, Varasivni, Balaghaar (MP)**

Epilepsy

◆ I have been suffering from Epilepsy for the last 5-6 years. I used to have attacks after intervals of 3–4 months. I was fed up with allopathic medicine Epton. The disease was not getting cured. I have been doing Pranayam for the last one year now. With Pranayam, my disease is getting cured. I am now not taking any medicines. With the blessings of Swamiji I am now all right. May God bless you and take you to the pinnacle of glory!

— **Sanjiv Sharma, Mahavir Road, Bir Ganj, Nepal**

◆ I was suffering from Degenerative Cysticercosis. As a result of it I used to have attacks. I got all sorts of treatment done but it resulted in vain. I regularly started doing Yog and Pranayam after I saw Ramdevji on TV in year 2005. Now I feel very healthy and also had no attacks. I have stopped taking all allopathic medicines. I do only Yog and Pranayam.

— **Reema Kaushal/Chaman Lal Kaushal, IPL Township, Virbhadra**

◆ I used to get Epilepsy attacks from the age of 7. I got all types of treatment done but I got no relief from anywhere. Three months ago, I saw Swamiji's programme on Astha Channel and I started doing Pranayam. In just three months I got a lot of relief and I do not need to take much of medicines.

— **Nitin Kumar Jain, Mungana, Tehsil Dhariabad, Udaipur**

◆ I used to get trembling, cramps and stiffness in the left portion of my body. After 10-12 attacks in a day I used to feel lifeless. I felt like committing suicide sometimes. Doctor gave some medicines, after using these medicines I used to feel better for some time however the attacks continued to recur. I had side effects like physical weakness, insomnia, listlessness, sleeplessness etc. I got very frustrated in life. After seeing Swamiji on TV, I started doing Pranayam. I started feeling better physically, mentaly and spiritually. I have stopped taking any medicines. There are hardly any attacks. Now I am quite healthy and happy.

— **Harish Chander Pandey, Mayur Vihar Phase-I, Delhi**

◆ I had been suffering from Epilepsy attacks since the age of eight. My hands and feet twitched, mouth foamed, and I had irregular urine discharge. I consulted many small and famous doctors, all claimed to cure my ailment however no one was able to cure it. After seeing Swamiji on TV, I started doing Pranayam and used medhavati from the Ashram pharmacy, I got cured in just 2 weeks. I feel fully rejuvenated and happy now. I have also stopped taking allopathic medicine. With the blessings of Swamiji I am now relieved of the life of hell which I was living earlier. I offer my heartiest greetings to Swamiji.

— **Vaishali K. Makwana, Broadwell, Komal Milton, Kitni M.K.B.8**

◆ I had been suffering from Epilepsy since 1981, because of it I had to face a lot of difficulties. The attacks were very frequent because of which my life became miserable. Encouraged by Swami Ramdevji, I started doing Pranayam with full determination. I consulted the physicians at the Ashram and started taking Ayurvedic medicines from there. I am doing Pranayam from the last three years and since then I did not get any seizure.

— **Baldev Dhingra, East Bonair Road, Nawada**

◆ I was very upset because of Epilepsy and because of this disease I used to become unconscious anytime, foam oozed out of the mouth, my hands and feet twitched. Whenever I had to go out I had to take somebody with me out of fear because of seizures. I have been doing Pranayam from the last one-and-a-half year and now I feel fully cured with the Ayurvedic medicines which I got from the Ashram. Every member of my family has full faith in Pranayam.

— **Samir Saxena, Rispana Pul,Cement Road, Dehra Dun**

I was a chronic patient of Epilepsy since childhood, my father was also a patient of the same disease. I am practising Pranayam for the past four years and my 30 year old problem has been cured along with asthma, cervical spondylitis. Swamiji has blessed me with a new life.

— **Shweta Arpita, Anand Vihar, Andheri, Mumbai**

I was suffering from Epilepsy for the past 10 years. Initially I used to get the attacks every alternate day or once in two days and I used to be unconscious for a long time. I have started practising Pranayam and now I am totally free from this problem.

— **Satnam Singh, Radhu Palace, New Delhi**

Paralysis

◆ I had Facial Paralysis, saliva used to come out of my mouth and I could not even laugh properly. I was very much worried about my ailment. I was not getting any relief because of its chronic nature. After seeing Swamiji's programme on Astha Channel I felt encouraged and confident, I started doing Pranayam with full determination. Today I feel that 90% of my disease is cured. Now I do not have any difficulty. With your blessings Swamiji I did Pranayam and I am very healthy now.

— **Pushp Lata Narayan Rao Godge, Nandeh**

◆ Swamiji, I could not hear well, walk or speak before. I attended the Yog camp at Gurgaon. Thereafter, I did Pranayam regularly. I got fully cured after a few days. I did not take any kind of medicine. I can now run like any other normal person. I express my gratitude to you for giving me a new life.

— **Jagdish Yadav Vill/Mohalla Heda, Gurgaon (Haryana)**

I was suffering from high blood pressure for the last several years and one day I went into coma due to this problem. The condition continued for eight days and I suffered paralysis attack. I lost all hope and was under stress. I started practising Pranayam as a last resort. Now my blood pressure is under control and I feel healthy. Paralysis has also been cured and there is no need for any medication.

— **Devendra Jagannath, Satara, Maharashtra**

I suffered from paralysis attack on December 25, 2005 and the right side was completely paralysed. I was feeling helpless and disappointed. I saw Swamiji's programme on television and started practising regularly. I recouped health and also stopped taking medicines.

— **Rampravesh Sharma, Allahabad**

◆ I had an attack of facial paralysis at the age of 14 as a result of which my eye and mouth became uneven. I got only 50% relief from the treatment done. I have been doing Yog and Pranayam from last 2 years, as a result of it the unevenness of my eye and mouth is corrected. During this period I have not taken any medicine. I am fully cured with Yog and Pranayam only.

— **Prasant Kumar Upadhaya, Sonar Para, Raigarh**

◆ During the last 1-2 years, due to numbness in my feet I had paralysis type disease. I got no cure even after consulting the well-known doctors available. Tired of all treatments, I started doing Pranayam in Swamiji's Ashram. I have been doing Pranayam from the last 5 months. I am highly benefited and now I can run freely. I have stopped taking all allopathic and Ayurvedic medicines. With the blessings of Swamiji my foot is all right now. I will remain grateful to you, Swamiji.

— **D.K. Singh, P.O. Mahanwa, Champaran, Bihar**

Polio

◆ I had polio since my childhood, because of which my feet were very weak. In the beginning the doctors said that it was a case of a major operation and success of this operation was also not guaranteed. Therefore operation was not possible. Due to weakness in my feet I could not park my two-wheeler at the stand. I started doing Pranayam as guided by Swamiji. I have been doing it from the last 8 months. Now I can park my scooter easily at the stand. My feet has regained the lost energy. Now I am healthy to a great extent. I am very grateful to you.

— **Amarjit Singh Rathi, Mohadipur, Gorakhpur (UP)**

◆ I was suffering from polio, gastric, depression, overweight, etc. I took many allopathic medicines but there was no sign of improvement. Later on after seeing Swami Ramdevji's programme on Astha Channel I started doing Pranayam. My feet gained new strength, depression got over. Gastric problem reduced to a large extent. Doctors stopped all my medicines. Now I am very healthy.

— **Surender Narayan Pandey, Gorakhpur (UP)**

Lumber, Cervical Spondylitis and Slip Disc

◆ I suffered from Spondylitis for a long time. Allopathic medicine gave some relief but only for a short while. I saw Swamiji's prorgamme on TV and started practising Yog and Pranayam has given me a new life and I am totally cured. I have stopped taking allophatic medicines.

— **Saurabh Das, Sidpur, Kolkota**

◆ I had a lot of problem in walking due to pain caused by slip disc and for last 5 years I have been suffering epilepsy seizures. I saw Swamiji's programme on TV. I have been doing Pranayam for the last two years now. I do not have any pain from slip disc and epilepsy attacks are also over with Pranayam. I am not taking any medicine. I am perfectly healthy now.

— **Krishan Chand Uppal, P.O. Noorpor, Kangra (Himachal Pradesh)**

◆ I suffered back ache and was almost bed ridden for last nine months. I consulted many doctors but it was not of much use. I felt totally dejected. I started doing Yog and Pranayam which gave me a new hope and now I am completely healthy and I do all my tasks myself.

— **Pushpa Kumari, Basikya Street, Sawakarpet**

◆ I suffered from lack of saliva in my mouth. I was unable to eat and my tongue used to get caught between my teeth causing bleeding in the mouth.After a while, I developed problem of gout, spondylitis and cataract. I took allopathic treatment for some time but it did not help much. One of my friends told me about Pranayam and I started practising it and I started feeling better. My faith in Pranayam grew and I started practising Pranayam twice a day. Now I have fully recovered and no longer take any allophatic medicines.

— **Vranti Sharma, PWD Hamirpur, Himachal Pradesh**

◆ I used to have a lot of pain in my back. I was not able to do any work, bend or lift heavy weight. I was not able to do any work independently. I was left dependent on others. From MRI and CT Scan I came to know that there is some problem in my back bone. Doctors said it could not be cured completely, only medicines could be prescribed to reduce the pain. Allopathic medicines caused a number of side effects. I lost my appetite. There was a burning sensation in my stomach and throat. I preferred death. After losing all hope I adopted Pranayam. I used to sit before TV and do Yog and Pranayam as guided by Swamiji. Gradually, my pain subsided and I stopped taking medicines and with time I got rid of the side effects of allopathic medicines. Now I enjoy a healthy life.

— **Sunita Pandey, Greater NOIDA (UP)**

Depression and Migraine

Two years ago I was under great strain, I was not able to sleep properly. Because of depression I could not breathe properly and due to bodyache I was not able to walk properly. I was also given electric shocks in a Delhi hospital. I have been doing Pranayam from last two years. Now I feel a lot of relief. In a way I got a new life.

— **Upma Trehan, Paschim Vihar, New Delhi**

◆ I was suffering from migraine for last 10 years. My headache was so severe that I could not tolerate it. I could not get relief even from pain killer injections. I had started gaining weight to 90 kg. I have been doing Pranayam for last one year. During last six months I had no pain and my weight has also reduced. With the grace of Swamiji happiness has come back to my life once again.

— **Smt. Mahadevi, Beejapur, Karnataka**

◆ I was suffering from depression from last five years. I was not able to sleep properly and I was not able to take interest in any work. I consulted many doctors, who prescribed allopathic medicines which made me more frustrated. One day I saw Swamiji's programme on Astha Channel and I started doing Pranayam. Now, I have been doing Pranayam since last six months. With Pranayam I have got a lot of relief from depression, I get sound sleep now and I am able to enjoy working again.

— **Ramesh Chand, Bank Colony Road, Madoli Extn, Delhi**

◆ Right from my childhood I was suffering from migraine. I used to get headache and vomit. I also suffered from constipation and acidity. I gained good weight. I saw Swamiji's programme on TV since then, I have been doing Pranayam. I do not have migraine now and my weight has reduced. At present, I do not have any constipation or acidity.

— **Nirmal Rana, Thana Ganj, Rampur**

I suffered from depression, hypertension and also from hereditary headache. I used to have severe headache. I have been doing Pranayam for last one year and half. Now my BP is 130/80. My intake of medicine is reduced considerably. Now I am perfectly all right and my life is filled with joy again.

— **Sudesh Kamboj, Model Town, Karnal**

◆ I had migraine for last 25 years, High BP and eye problem. I was not getting any relief from allopathic medicines. After seeing Swamiji's programme on Astha Channel in 2005, I started doing Yog and Pranayam. Regular practice of Yog and Pranayam cured my migraine, helped me to get rid of my spectacles. I do not take medicines now. I do only Yog and Pranayam.

— **Gurbuksh Kaur, Stat Fort Road Hall Green**

◆ I suffered from migraine and eczema. I tried to get the best treatment but it did not help much. Then I started practising Yog and Pranayam. I have been regularly doing Yog and Pranayam since last eight months. As a result, my migraine and eczema problems are almost over. Doctors have stopped my allopathic medicines.

— **Krishna James, A.N.E. Canton Haro Medix**

◆ I had been suffering from migraine for last many years. I used to have such a severe headache that even the pain killers were of no use. I have been doing Pranayam for last 12-14 months. Now I am perfectly all right and I do not get migraine seizures. For helping me to get relief from this painful disease, I will always remain grateful to Swamiji.

— **Savitri, Adarsh Colony, Chirava, Jhunjhunu**

POLYMYOSITIS

◆ I had problem of polymyositis. Due to which I used to feel weakness in my upper and lower limbs. I also felt pain in my muscles; besides it I also had other problems as weakness, tension, and sleeplessness. I took long treatment to get relief from all these diseases but I got no benefit. Then I started practising Yog and Pranayam regularly as guided by Swamiji. I am absolutely healthy now.

— Direndra Behra, Sasi Niwas, Post Tulsipur, Katak (Orissa)

Before Treatment   After Treatment

Before Treatment	After Treatment
CURE WELL LABORATORY Dr. (Mrs.) Basanti Mishra, MD. (Path & Micro) Regd. No. 17/1998 (Under Clinical Establishment Act) Mangalabag,Kathagola Road, Cuttack - 753 001, ☎ : (0671) 2306114, 2306344 E-mail : cure_well @yahoo.com	**CURE WELL LABORATORY** Dr. (Mrs.) Basanti Mishra, MD. (Path & Micro) Regd. No. 17/1998 (Under Clinical Establishment Act) Mangalabag,Kathagola Road, Cuttack - 753 001, ☎ : (0671) 2306114, 2306344 E-mail : cure_well @yahoo.com

Before Treatment:

NAME : DHIRENDRA BEHERA   SL. NO. : 20C22
AGE : 41   DATE :- 20-Oct-2005

TEST PARTICULARS	RESULT	UNIT	REFERENCE RANGE
S G O T (AST)	51	u/l	(5 - 40) u/l
Serum LDH	701	u/L	(225 - 450) u/L at 37 d.c
Serum Creatine Kinase	417	u/L	(15 - 190) u/L at 37 d.c

After Treatment:

NAME : DHIRENDRA BEHERA   SL. NO. : 06B13
AGE : 41   DATE :- 06-Feb-2006

TEST PARTICULARS	RESULT	UNIT	REFERENCE RANGE
Fasting Plasma Glucose	77	mg/dl	(65-110) mg/dl
Post Prandial Plasma Glucose	110	mg/dl	(75 - 140) mg/dl
S G O T (AST)	23	u/l	(5 - 40) u/l
Serum LDH	435	u/L	(225 - 450) u/L at 37 d.c
Serum Creatine Kinase	56	u/L	(15 - 190) u/L at 37 d.c

Before treatment Serum Creatine Kinase of the patient was 417 while it was 56 after Yog practice which is normal level.

◆ I had severe problem of Ankylosing Spondylitis for the last seven years. I was unable to walk properly. I had to take steroid injections every month that gave me little relief for some time and then again later I had to face the same problem. I am practising Yog and Pranayam from last two years. From the last fourth months I increased the time period for exercise and I feel tremendous improvement in my ailment. I have not used any steroid injection for last four months. I can easily walk now. My blood circulation has also improved.

— Nirmit Goel, Roma Road, Aadarsh Nagar, Delhi

LUNG DISEASE

Genetic Asthma

◆ I was a patient of asthma (hereditary). I was very weak and was frequently given oxygen and medicines but asthma attack was common with change in the season. I started practising Pranayam and took some medicines from Divya Yog Ashram. Now I am healthy and I have stopped taking medicines. My weight has increased from 40 to 45 kg. I am practising Pranayam regularly for the past one-and-a-half years.

— **Smt Kamlesh Jain, Gurgoan**

I was suffering from hereditary problem of asthma. Injections were necessary every three to four days but relief was temporary. I started practising Pranayam for last four months, now I do not require injections. I have become active and enthusiastic.

— **Mahendra Singh Dahiya, Sonipat, Haryana**

I was suffering from palpitation from the last three years, which used to increase on climbing stairs or exposure to dust etc. The problem got cured with three months of Pranayam practice. I have discontinued medicines and developed positive attitude.

— **Rajshri Vashisht, Shiv Vihar, Saharanpur**

I was overweight and had cough problem. I attended Yog camp for one month in June and got good results. Cough has been cured and my weight has also reduced with regular practice of Pranayam.

— **Sargam Bhangu, Ludhiana (Punjab)**

◆ I was a chronic patient of asthma. Allopathic medicines were not useful. I started practising Pranayam and now I am completely healthy. I am practising Pranayam regularly and would like to state that Swamiji is working on a global mission.

— **Nand Gopal Dikshit, Sundargarh, Orissa**

◆ I was suffering from asthma, joint pain and liver related diseases. I had difficulty in breathing, pain in hands and feet and digestion problem. Due to all these diseases I was not able to do my daily home work properly. Now I have been doing regular practise of Pranayam from last six months. Day by day I am getting relief from all my diseases. Now every one in my family practises Pranayam regularly.

— **Manbhavati, Bhatnagar Colony, Jind**

◆ I am suffering from hereditary asthma for the last 30 years. I have not suffered an attack for the last two years with regular practice of Pranayam. The whole world is reaping the benefits of Pranayam through Baba Ramdevji. We cannot repay his debts at any cost.

— **Amarjeet Tandon, Tilaknagar**

◆ I was suffering from asthma and heart disease. I was not able to breathe easily. During the night, especially in winters, sometimes it seemed as if my breath had stopped. Then Pranayam gave me new hope and I am able to give my comments here. I am proud to say that Pranayam has helped millions of Indians to get relief from this incurable disease and made them mentally fit. I am free from all diseases because of Pranayam and I am leading a healthy life.

— **R.B. Verma, Sarghana Road, Kankerkhera, Meerut**

◆ I had been suffering from respiratory problem for last 15 years. Due to this it was very difficult for me to do any work. It was not possible to walk. Now I have been doing Pranayam for the last two years. After doing Pranayam, I have got complete relief from breathing trouble. Now I have no problem in taking breath. Now I do all my work myself.

— **Anindita Kumari, South Ramnagar, Agartala**

◆ I had been suffering from genetic asthma since last 15 years. I consulted many specialist doctors but I could not get any relief. I had to go on steroids and used inhailer everyday. I have been using medicines given by the Ashram and doing regular practice of Pranayam from last two years now. I feel absolutely healthy. I have stopped taking allopathic medicines now.

— **Raman Bala Puri, Nehru Colony, Meerapur, Allahabad**

◆ I was suffering from genetic asthma and I have been doing Pranayam since last two years. After doing Yog I have benefited beyond expectations. My genetic disease asthma and ovarian cyst is now absolutely under control. My digestion has improved. I do not have any physical problems any more. Now I am totally fine from last two years. I am not taking any allopathic medicine. I have developed deep faith in God, Yog and Pranayam.

— **Devleena Vasu, Serebarahan Palli, Post Jhaka, Kolkata**

◆ Since childhood I have been suffering from breathing trouble, especially when the weather changes. My voice used to get heavy and for this I had to take inhaler. I had to face asthma fits about 10 times in a year. Then I started practising Yog and Pranayam as guided by Swamiji. After doing Pranayam I do not have breathing problems any more. I am feeling quite well now.

— **Vipin Bihari Ram, Nawabgarh, Dhanbad**

◆ I suffered from asthma when I was only 15 years old. For this I had to take inhaler regularly but since the time when I had started doing Pranayam as guided by Swamiji and medicines given by Ashram I feel much better. Now I do not use inhaler.

— **Prathibha Jain, Charajat, Priyadanshi, Katak (Orissa)**

◆ Asthma is a genetic disease in my family, due to asthma I was very much troubled to breathe. I did not get any relief despite taking so many medicines. I feel unexpected benefit since I started Pranayam. After doing Pranayam regularly for the last six months, my asthma is completely cured. Now I am leading a healthy life without using any allopathic medicines.

— **Saroj Tyagi, Housing Board Colony, District Ferozpu**

◆ I had been suffering form asthma and heart disease since last 15 years. In 2005, I faced PTC (stent) operation of heart, due to this my two veins were blocked and due to asthma I could not even walk properly. I was not able to breathe freely. My mother who has died now, she also suffered from asthma. I am working in Neurosurgery Operation Theatre of AIIMS as a Technical Assistant. I am doing Yog and Pranayam from about half hour to an hour regularly since September 2005. After doing Pranayam I have relieved my problems to about 80 percent. I am very active now. I was also suffering from pyorrhea. My gums used to bleed but now I am totally free from this disease.

— **Ved Prakash, Panchal Vihar, Karaval Nagar Delhi**

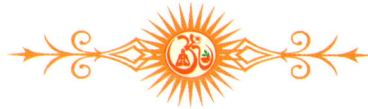

EYE, EAR AND THROAT DISEASES

Myopia, Metropia, Retina Disease and Cataract

◆ My retina was damaged and I was also suffering from migraine and joint pain. I have been doing Yog and Pranayam from last one year. I have benefited a lot after practising Yog and Pranayam regularly. My eyesight has also improved. I do not have migraine problem any more. My joint pain has also reduced. I am taking medicine in less quantity now. My retina has also improved now.

— Devika Makwana, 30 The Seding Bolton, UK

◆ I was facing eye disorder. My eyesight was too weak that I could not see anything properly. I watched Swamiji's programme on TV and then I started practising Yog and Pranayam everyday. After practising it regularly my eyesight is improving day by day. Now my eyesight has improved.

— Harish Jawaharmani, Nawahar Road, Mumbai

◆ I had allergy since my childhood. It did not get better even after a prolonged treatment. I have heard about Pranayam but there was no one to guide me on how to do Pranayam. One day I watched Swamiji's programme on Aastha Channel and then I decided firmly to practise Pranayam regularly. I have been doing Pranayam for last two years. I am completely fit now.

— Mukesh Kumar, Gandhi Nagar

◆ I was suffering from photophobia disease from several years. I took homeopathic cure. Allopathic physicians said photophobia being a genetic disease was incurable and they refused to cure it. I felt hopeless, worried and depressed and filled with inferiority complex. One day I watched Swamiji's camp programme on Astha Channel. After watching and hearing about Yog and Pranayam, I was filled with confidence and hope. I started doing Pranayam regularly and my disease was cured to a great extent. When I went to the eye specialist for check up, he was also surprised to see so much improvement. Now I practise Pranayam regularly. I have deep faith in God and I have a relaxed mind now.

— Aaditya Budhdev, Raipur, Chattishgarh

◆ I have been facing eye disorders from many years. My eyesight was very weak. Sometimes my eyes used to become dry. After doing Pranayam from last one year, I feel some improvement in my eyesight. Now tears have started forming again in my eyes. Eyesight has also improved.

— Dashrath Vishvakarma, Post Sidholi, Verdhman (West Bengal)

◆ I was facing several problems as there was a hole in my retina, irregular menstrual cycle and thyroid related problems. My weight was also increasing. There was no relief despite taking a lot of allopathic medicine. I have been doing Pranayam from last two years now. My weight has reduced at present. There is no complaint of thyroid now and the important thing is that my retina is quite well now.

— **Savita Agarwal, Dunlop Road, Durga Ghat Bandar Ghat Deenajpur**

◆ I was facing eyes disorder since my childhood. I could not see distant things clearly. My eyes used to get watery and red. I have benefited a great deal by doing Pranayam as guided by Swamiji and after taking medicine given by the Ashram. Now my eyes are quite well.

— **Shaliendra Kumar, Dhanbad**

◆ I lost eyesight of my left eye from 1 February 2007. There was severe pain in my head but after doing the Pranayam as guided by Swamiji my eyesight has improved a lot. For this I took no medicine.

— **Neeta Pandey, Ibrahim Gali, Bhopal**

I was unable to work without using glasses and used to suffer from headache. My eyesight was deteriorating day by day and specs were inevitable. I am practising Pranayam for the last two years and now I do not need specs. I do not have any problem in reading or writing.

— **Pushpa Arora, Udhamsingh Nagar, Khatima**

I was suffering from cataract problem since 2002. Doctors suggested operation as I had lost vision completely. I started practising Pranayam, my eyesight has improved with the blessings of Swamiji. Now I do not have any vision problem.

— **Smt. Tapeshwari, Shahpura, Bhopal**

◆ I am practising Pranayam for three months and my 40-year-old problem has been cured. My ear drum has started functioning normally and diabetes is also under control. The body has become disease-free. I have overcome my restlessness. Now I have a comfortable life. I practise Pranayam regularly.

— **Naresh Mishra, Jhansi Road, Bhind, Maharashtra**

I was suffering from problem in both eyes. I consulted reputed doctors in Delhi and Bihar but did not get any relief. I am practising Pranayam for the last three months and have been free of attacks since then. Now I am totally healthy and I have stopped taking medicines as well.

— **Gita Bhushan, Mujaffarpur, Bihar**

◆ Besides Asthma I was also suffering from Intra-ocular pressure. Due to this I was very much tensed. I went several places for treatment but I could not get any relief. One day, I saw Swamiji's programme on Aastha Channel after watching the programme, I started doing Yog and Pranayam. I did practice Yog and Pranayam for six months, and the result is that my intra-ocular pressure is normal while asthma is completely cured.

— **Dr Jyoti Yanket Rao, Sai Kirpa Niwas, Pushpa Nagar, Nanded**

◆ I am 65 years old. I am using glasses since 1965. Since then my spectacle lens numbers has increased many times. After some time, I was not able to read any book. One of my friends adviced me to practise Yog and Pranayam as guided by Swamiji. Then I started to attend the Yog camp for practising Pranayam. It has been four months since I am doing Pranayam. There is improvement in my eyesight. Now I am telling everyone about the benefits of the Pranayam.

— **Ramkhilan Tiwari, Phoolwari, Bilaspur**

◆ I have been suffering from several diseases for a very long time. My ear had disorders, so I had have a surgical operation for it but all was in vain. My eyes were weak and also I had complaint of piles and obesity. For all these diseases I was taking allopathic medicines. But all these medicines were not very effective and then I attended Yog camp run by Swamiji. I have been doing Pranayam since December 2006, after doing Pranayam I have got much relief in my all diseases to a great extent. Now I am not taking any kind of medicine.

— **Asharam Chaudhary, Tehsil Behrod, Alwar (Rajasthan)**

I was suffering from cataract and knee pain along with pain while walking. There was no relief even after retina operation. I saw Swamiji's programme on Astha Channel and started practising Pranayam. All my problems have been cured within 10 months. Pranayam has proved to be nectar for me as I had lost hope of improving eyesight. It makes me feel young and active.

— **Mohan Das Tilwani, Ajmer, Rajasthan**

I was very upset due to poor eyesight, allergy and baldness. I have been practising Pranayam for the last two-and-a-half years. My hairs have grown again and I can read and write without specs. I have stopped taking medicines and I feel several years younger. This is indeed miracle of Pranayam.

— **Prayag Mahato, Patna, Bihar**

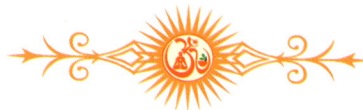

INCURABLE SKIN DISEASES

Psoriasis, Eczema etc.

I was suffering from serious skin ailment below the knees in both legs for the last 20 years. I used to experience severe itching and bleeding. My skin had become white, I consulted various doctors and took a lot of medicines but in vain. I lacked proper sleep but Pranayam has cured my problem up to 90 percent and I have discontinued medicines.

— **Virendra Singh Yadav, Mahendragarh, Haryana**

I had small boils on my whole body. Allopathic medicines did not prove beneficial. I stopped taking medicines and started practising Pranayam. Now the problem has been cured completely. Revered Swamiji is giving a new life to people like me.

— **Balveer Verma, Karnal, Haryana**

◆ Four years ago my skin began to break at various places. When I consulted a doctor, he told me that I was suffering from psoriasis and it was incurable and to keep it under control regular intake of medicine was required. I was worried. I was taking allopathic medicines for the past 3 years without getting any benefit from it. But a year ago I started practising Pranayam taught by Swamiji and stopped taking medicines. With Pranayam practice, I could see surprising results. Today I am alright and I do not take any medicine. I am grateful to Swamiji, because of him I could get rid of this incurable disease.

— **Amita Sehrawat, Gurgaon, Haryana**

I am suffering from Superative Hyudronitis for the past 10 years. Due to this large sized nodes have formed all over my body and there was always pain in my body and I underwent surgery many times. Then after watching Astha Channel I started practising Yog and Pranayam. The nodes that had formed after practice of Pranayam automatically dissolved. Now, new nodes are not forming and I am absolutely fine.

— **Shwati Kelwar, Bilaspur, Chattisgarh**

I was suffering from skin ailment since 1987. The disease had spread all over the body except face. I consulted a number of doctors and took a lot of medicines but there was no relief. I am practising Pranayam for the last one year. I have recovered up to 99 percent with the blessings of Swamiji and I have stopped taking medicines.

— **Pushkal Verma, Reeva, MP**

◆ I was suffering from skin disease and high BP. I consulted many doctors but could not get rid of the disease. Then I started practising Yog and Pranayam taught by Swamiji and took medicine from Patanjali Yogpeeth. Now I am alright and I am out of the clutches of the allopathic medicines.

— **V.K. Sinha, Rohtas, Sasaram**

I was suffering from psoriasis and had eruptions at different places on the body. I used to experience severe itching and faced difficulty in passing stools. It used to bleed, but there is no problem from the day I started practising Pranayam. Piles have been cured along with constipation and gastric trouble. I have discontinued medicines as well.

— **Jyoti Navhal, Mandsoar, MP**

◆ I was suffering from psoriasis. Even after taking a lot of treatment it was of no use. Then I took refuge in Swamji's Yog and Pranayam. Now with regular practice of Yog and Pranayam my psoriasis problem is completely cured. I have stopped taking all allopathic medicines. I only practice Yog and Pranayam.

— **Vijay Kumar Das, Taalchar Teerma, Orissa**

◆ I was suffering from numbness in my hand for a long time for which I took treatment for a very long period, but it was of no use. Later on I came to know that it was leprosy. I took medicine from Swamiji's hospital and regularly practised Pranayam, and with the blessings of Swamiji I have got a second chance to live. Earlier people used to avoid me and looked at me with hatred. Now I am alright. I bow my head before Swamiji.

— **Abhimanyu Behra, Rupakhand Bayabana Bhola Saur, Orissa**

◆ I was suffering from psoriasis , for which I took a lot of treatment but it was useless. I listened to Yog and Pranayam programme of Swamiji on TV on Astha Channel and started watching the programme and then after that I started practising regularly Yog and Pranayam. Now after 2 months of continuous practice of Yog and Pranayam, problem of psoriasis is cured to much extent. Earlier I was taking allopathic medicines. Now I have stopped taking them. Now I am only practising Yog and Pranayam.

— **Riti Bhattacharya, Lake Side, Kolkata**

◆ I was suffering from psoriasis for the last 15 years. It had spread all over the body. I was very much disturbed because of this. I took treatment from many renowned doctors but it was useless. After watching Swamiji's programme on Astha Channel I started practising Pranayam regularly. After the practice of Pranayam the liver functioning also improved and my psoriasis is cured.

— **Shiresh V. Reddy, Anand Nagar, Karnataka**

◆ I had eruptions all over the body along with itching. I took a lot of medicines but there was no relief. I consulted a lot of doctors but could not get permanent cure for this problem. I started practising Pranayam and now I have gained very much relief. My complexion has improved and I have stopped taking medicines completely.

— **Ajit Singh, Rohtak, Haryana**

I was suffering from hereditary eczema since childhood. I used ointments to and control it but in vain. I saw Swamiji's programme on television and started practising Anulom-vilom and Kapalbhati Pranayam. Eczema has been cured completely and now I am enjoying total health.

— **Ashish Kumar Sinha, Kankar Bagh, Patna, Bihar**

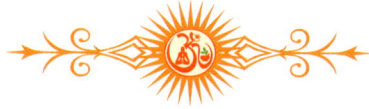

LEUCODERMA

◆ My whole body was covered with white patches. I used to feel ashamed because of this. I used to hesitate in going out and also avoided changing my clothes in front of other people. Now I am practising Yog and Pranayam since one-and-a-half years. With the practice of Pranayam the number of white patches on my body have reduced. Now I am much better than before.

— Shumbhangshu Dey, Kumar Ghat, North Agartala

◆ I was suffering from white patches for past many years. I took lot of treatment. Then after watching Swamiji's programme on Astha Channel I started practising Pranayam. Slowly I began to benefit from it and then encouraged by the result, I increased practice of Pranayam. Now I am alright. I pray that the work Swamiji is doing for the welfare of others, may god bring him all the success.

— Sitaram, Nangloi, Delhi

◆ Since 1998 I had the problem of white patches on my body and there used to be patches all over the feet, the back, and the face. I consulted many renowned doctors of Kolkota, but it was useless. Also because of using steroids as prescribed, I had developed diabetes and other digestive disorders. I became hopeless. Then I came in contact with the revered Swami Ramdevji Maharaj and adopted Pranayam in my life-style. With regular practice of Pranayam the white patches started to cure slowly. Now all the white patches have been cured. Now I am alright. Leucoderma being an incurable disesase got cured by miracle of Pranayam. I shall be grateful to Swamiji for the rest of my life.

— Shashidhar Chowdhary, Pulia, West Bengal

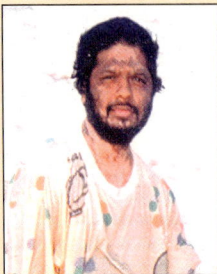

Spread of white
patches before Pranayam

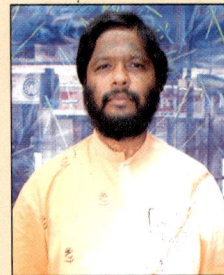

Spread of white patches after
the practice of Pranayam

◆ I was suffering from the problem of white patches since many years. I took a lot of treatment but it could not be cured. I am regularly practising Pranayam, the white patches have been cured and my weight is also under control. I was also suffering from diabetes and this has improved too. Pranayam is meant for incurable diseases. I bow my head to Swamiji.

— **Bimla Joshi, Hanumangarh, Rajasthan**

◆ I had problem of white patches for many years. I took lot of treatment but it did not help much. I am doing regular practice of Yog and Pranayam as told by Swamiji for a while and it has helped me a lot. I have lost weight. I also suffered from diabetes and I am feeling much better now. I send a million salutations to Swamiji.

— **Sagar Chandrashekharvad, Sagar Madhya Pradesh**

◆ I had the problem of white patches for a long time. I took a lot of treatment for this but it was of no use. Then I started practising regularly Yog and Pranayam as taught by Swamiji and also took medicines from the Ashram. Now I am alright.

— **Rajkumar Srivastav, C.P. Colony, Gwalior (MP)**

◆ I was suffering from the problem of white patches for about four years. My body had turned white all over. I used to feel shy while going out in society. I took treatment from the renowned doctors but my disease kept on spreading. Then after watching Pranayam on Astha Channel, I started practising Pranayam regularly. Slowly white patches began to cure. Now all the white patches have disappeared from body and it has become normal as before. Only a few patches can be seen on the body. Pranayam proved miraculous for me. I bow my head to Swamiji.

— **Smt. Heena S. Mehta, Nagtaalwadi, Distt-Navsaari, Gujarat**

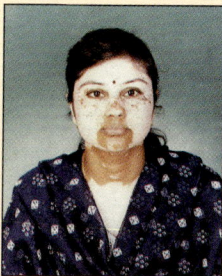

The condition of white patches before Pranayam

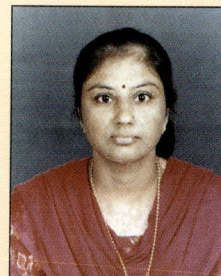

The condition of white patches after the practice of Pranayam

GIT DISORDERS

Colitis & Ulcerative Colitis

◆ I am a patient of Ulcerative colitis since 1984, which was diagnosed at AIIMS, New Delhi. I was prescribed medicines. Excessive bleeding used to occur in every attack and I was literally on my death bed. I got transferred to Jagdishpur unit. I consulted doctors at SGPGI, Lucknow, and was treated for a long time. The body became immune to medicines and the dose had to be increased. I was forced to take steroids (Predenisolone). The attacks became frequent and steroids were necessary to control the problem. This resulted in serious side effects and I had almost died. I used to be admitted to the hospital for long periods of time. Now the doctors at SGPGI are thinking of operating my large intestine. I was worried and I used to become depressed during this long period of 20 years. There is a probability of Chronic Ulcerative Colitis converting into cancer. I am working as a technician in the pathology department. In such a situation Swami Ramdevji has descended on this earth in the form of God himself. His Yog and Pranayam have made me physically and mentally healthy. I have not taken steroids since August 2004 till date. I practise Pranayam regularly.

— **Jaiprakash Singh, BHEL Hospital, Jagdishpur, Sultanpur, UP**

◆ I was facing problem of piles from long times. My weight was increasing. I am also a diabetic. My blood sugar level never used to reduce even after taking a lot of medicines. To get relief from piles and bhagandar, doctor advised me for operation. Seeing Swamiji's programme on TV, I started practising Pranayam and found that my blood sugar got under control within one month. My weight also reduced. I am cured of piles and bhagandar. Now I am quite healthy. Swamiji has changed my life. I practise Pranayam regularly now. I hope to have Swamiji's blessing always.

— **Manoj Jain, Bomikhal, Bhubneshwar**

◆ I was suffering from fistula in the anus for the past three years and have been operated thrice. But there was no relief and problem persisted. I was very depressed and after practising Pranayam I have become-disease free and have no problem whatsoever.

— **Govardhan Chabbalval, Shiv Colony, Jaipur**

◆ I was a patient of Ulcerative colitis from five years. I took lot of allopathic medicines but there was no improvement. Regular practice of Pranayam and Ayurvedic medicines have been beneficial. Now I am totally healthy and do not take any medicines.

— **Jagdish Patel, Ambika Nagar, Chandigarh**

◆ I had stomach disorder for several years. I was much disturbed because of gas and indigestion. I was feeling weak day by day. My appetite was also decreasing regularly. After doing Pranayam for the last three months I am feeling much improvement in my health. All diseases related to stomach are now over. My weight has also increased and the appetite is also good.

— **Patel Jagdish Chandan, Ambika Nagar, Highway, Gandhi Nagar**

◆ One day I felt a lot of pain in my stomach and I started vomiting blood. I went to a Kanpur Hospital for treatment. After the check up they found ulcer. The doctors advised me to undergo an operation for the same. I took treatment for a month however there was no improvement in my health. I was also facing joint pain. I was not able to walk properly at that time as my left hip was replaced. I had problem of Ankylosing spondylitis. Then I came to Swamiji's Ashram, at Hardwar for cure. There I practised Yog and Pranayam from the very first day. I was given some Ayurvedic medicines from the Ashram. Today after three month long treatment my wounds are healed. Now I do not have any problem of spondylitis. I am completely healthy now. Swamiji's cure system through Yog and Pranayam is very beneficial. This system is much cheaper than allopathic cure system.

— **Ashwani Sood, HBTI West Campus Colony, Kanpur**

I was suffering from bleeding piles from 1986. I used to experience severe burning sensation and pain in rectum along with giddiness. I took lot of medicines but there was no relief. I started practising Pranayam for the last three years and there has been lot of improvement. Now I am totally healthy and medication is not required.

— **Anand Kumar Pandey, Sant Kabir Nagar**

◆ I was facing problems of piles and prostate from a very long time. I faced much difficulty during defecation. I had to sit for long time in the toilet. Then I started practising Pranayam seeing Swamiji's programme on Ashta Channel. After two years of regular practice of Pranayam, I have recovered completely. I am quite well now. I do not have any disease now.

— **Mohit Ghosh, Agartala, Tripura**

◆ I was suffering from fistula from a long time. My clothes were spoiled by puss, blood and water. After operation there was no positive relief. Then I started doing Pranayam as guided by Swamiji for four years and then I felt that my fistula has dried mysteriously. The doctor to whom I went for operation was also surprised to see me healthy. Now I am not taking any medicine. I practise Pranayam only and want to be always fit.

— **Damodar Khadka, Keloli, Sudoor Pachim Nepal**

◆ I was suffering from fistula since a long time. I got it operated upon many times but it was not cured. Even after getting operated upon, fistula used to recur. One day I saw Swamiji's Yog and Pranayam programme on Astha Channel and started practising Pranayam. Because of practice of Pranayam the wounds of fistula started to heal. Now fistula is completely cured. Pranayam is a boon for incurable diseases.

— **Vishnu Sombhavse, Vaibhav Nagar, Latur**

◆ I was suffering from anal fissure for the last 22 years and I had low blood pressure. It used to bleed heavily and I used to bear a severe pain. Even after taking treatment from various places I could not get any relief. By practising Pranayam for just two months I got 100% relief and my BP also remains normal now. Revered Swamiji has saved my life from severe problems, therefore I shall remain grateful to him for my life.

— **Dr Jaishree Dwivedi, Gyanpur (Varanasi)**

I was suffering from piles and fistula for the last 15 years. On the advise of the doctors I got it operated upon but it was useless. Then after watching Swamij's TV programme, I started practising Pranayam. After practising Pranayam for two years now I am completely healthy and along with the piles, fistula has also been cured without any surgery.

— **Shashi Kushwaha, Allapur, Allahabad (UP)**

◆ I was suffering from bleeding piles. While passing stool my rectum used to come out and my blood pressure used to be 210/130. By practising Pranayam taught by Swamiji for one year, now the problem of piles is completely cured and my blood pressure remains 130/90 and I do not take any medicine.

— **K. P. Sharma, Ten Astha Sevohi (MP)**

◆ I was suffering from Ulcerative colitis since 1993 and consulted the doctors at AIIMS, New Delhi. I used to get frequent urge for bowel movement and sometimes used to experience pain and heaviness in stomach. Now I am practising Pranayam and I feel active and energetic. I am totally healthy and I have stopped taking medicines.

— **Shivcharan Rawat, Faridabad**

◆ I had been suffering with hyper acidity, body pain and obesity for several years. I had to take medicines to get relief from acidity. I started to practise Pranayam for last six months. My weight reduced by 9 Kg and there is no pain in the body now. Now I do not take medicine for acidity. I am absolutely healthy now.

— **Saleem Jiwani, Adilabad, AP**

◆ I am a patient of Ulcerative colitis since 1984, I took a lot of medicines but there has been no improvement. I started practising Pranayam regularly and small health problems like headache, pain etc. have been cured since last four months. Now I am totally healthy.

— **K. Gangadhar, Vencation Colony**

◆ I had acute piles and always suffered constipation. I took prolonged treatment but I could not get any relief. Now I practise Yog and Pranayam guided by Swamiji regularly. As a result my pile problem is over.

— **Amitabh Mishra, Bhanipada, Mayapuri, Orrisa**

◆ I was suffering from ulcerative colitis from the past 10 years. Doctors prescribed some allopathic medicines but there was no relief. I visited Ayurvedic hospital at Patanjali Yogpeeth and started practising Pranayam. Ayurvedic treatment and Pranayam have cured my problem completely and there is no need for any medicines.

— **Rajrani, Sonipat, Haryana**

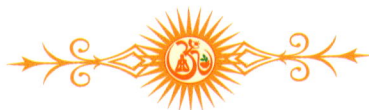

PANCREATITIS

◆ I kept on consuming alcohol continuously for 18 months due to which I started vomiting, I started to suffer from loose motion and acidity. On getting examined by a doctor, I was told that I was suffering from chronic panecreatitis. The proper cure for which is not available at present. After knowing this I was upset. Then I watched Swamiji's programme on Ashtha Channel and I continuously started practising Pranayam and I also started taking Ayurvedic medicine from the Ashram. Now I am absolutely healthy and the ultrasound report of my ailment is completely normal.

— Vijay Kumar Garg, Sirsa (Haryana)

Before Treatment	After Treatment

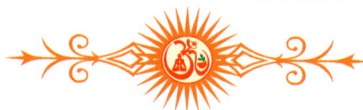

The serum amylase of the patient before the practice of Pranayam was 272.00. After the beginning of practice of Pranayam serum amylase report was 74.00, which is at normal level.

ARTHRITIS AND RHEUMATOID ARTHRITIS

Arthritis, Rheumatoid Arthritis and Spondylitis

◆ I was suffering from arthritis, slip disc, thyroid and other diseases, I took treatment from various doctors and took a number of allopathic medicines but it was of no help. Then I went to Divya Yog Mandir Trust, here I took some Ayurvedic medicines and started practising Pranayam. I felt much better by practising Yog and Pranayam, my arthritis has improved a lot. There used to be acute pain and swelling in my knees and it was difficult to walk. Now all these problems are cured and I have stopped taking allopathic medicines.

— **Mahua Shah, Nabhanagar, West Bengal**

◆ I was suffering from pain in the knees for the last 3-4 years. For this I used to take allopathic medicines but it was of no use. From 4 March, 2007 I started practising Pranayam and other vital exercises for one-and-a-half hours daily and now I am completely healthy and I am not taking any medicine.

— **Syeed Shaukat Ali, Ballarpur**

◆ I was suffering from arthritis and heart disease since many years. My life was disturbed due to joint pain and heart disease. Treatment from elsewhere only gave me a temporary relief. Now I am absolutely fine after practising Pranayam taught by Swamiji and also with the help of Ayurvedic medicines. Now even at the age of 73 years I am able to accomplish all my daily tasks without anybody's help.

— **Swaraj Sharma, West Patel Nagar, New Delhi**

◆ I was suffering from arthritis and spondylitis since a long time. None of the treatment was spared. I had lost hope and due to arthritis there used to be a lot pain in my hands. Because of spondylitis my hands used to get numb. Pranayam brought a ray of hope in my life. I am practising Pranayam for the past 18 months. Even after spending thousands of rupees on allopathic medicines I have not benefited. But now without spending a penny and just practising Pranayam I am absolutely healthy.

— **Nirmit Goya, Adarsh Nagar, Delhi**

◆ I was suffering from joint pain for the past ten years. Doctors advised knee replacement as I could not sit properly. I am prasticing Pranayam for the past two years and there has been a lot of improvement within three to four months of practice. Now I am totally healthy and do not have any problem in sitting or doing my work. I have stopped taking medicines.

— **Smt. Poonam Singh, Ravatpur, Kanpur**

◆ I was always unhappy due to arthritis. Despite taking treatment from various places my disease was aggravating. As advised by one of my friends I started practising Pranayam. Slowly I realized that my disease was being cured. Earlier my hands used to develop cramps and unbearable pain which gradually eased off. Now after practising Pranayam for a year and taking Ayurvedic treatment from the Ashram, I have recovered completely.

— **Meena Ben, C.P. College Complex, Anand**

◆ I was disturbed due to joint pain for past few years. I was tired of visiting doctors and taking allopathic medicines. It was of no use. All the doctors declared my illness as incurable and just prescribed pain killers. At last I was advised to take treatment from Patanjali Yogpeeth. I consulted Vaidji at the Ashram and he gave me some medicines. I took medicines for 4-5 months continuously and practised Pranayam for one-and-a-half hours to two hours daily. My RA factor had turned negative. Now I am feeling absolutely healthy.

— **Sangeeta, Kinaur, Himachal Pradesh**

The RA factor of the patient which had increased to 35, reduced to 17 which is normal due to practice of Yog and Pranayam.

◆ I was suffering from Rheumatoid arthritis and weakness for the last few years. Despite taking a number of allopathic medicines the intensity of the diseases was not decreasing, instead the body was becoming weak day by day. I am practising Pranayam for the last two-and-a-half years. Now I am feeling alright. I have stopped taking medicines also. By grace of God I got a new life.

— **Manju Shrivastav, Nazari, Rohtas**

◆ I was suffering from arthritis for the past five years but medicines were not giving desired results. I was not able to walk properly, then I started practising Yog and Pranayam as told by Swamiji. I also took Ayurvedic medicines from Patanjali Yogpeeth which gave me immediate results. I am practising Pranayam regularly and it has given me miraculous results.

— **Jyoti Kumar Mishra, Ara, Bihar**

◆ I suffered from severe pain in hand in May 2002 and doctors treated me for muscular pain for one year. But different tests for ESR, TLC, DLC, RA factor were done in June 2003 when there was no improvement in the condition. Arthritis specialist at Jaipur diagnosed rheumatoid arthritis, which is incurable. My fingers had bent and I became helpless like a paralysed patient. I could not walk or move my fingers or even hold a spoon with my hand. I was facing the worst condition of rheumatoid arthritis that cannot be expressed in words. I started taking Ayurved, homeopathy, natural therapy and the medical reports in January 2004 showed that ESR had increased to 70 to 72 Eq. I saw your television programme in February 2005 and started practising Bhastrika and Anulom-vilom Pranayam on the bed. I used to practice it at the night whenever I woke up due to disturbed sleep. After a few days I was able to sit on my own. Ayurvedic doctor told that this improvement is the result of Pranayam. From that day onwards my husband and I have thrown out all the medicines and just practising Pranayam. I used to take six types of quath and 15 doses of medicines daily. I started practising Kapalbhati Pranayam for 15-20 minutes since July 2004. Besides this the ankle and neck bone had enlarged and doctors suggested operation. But I did not realize when I had overcome this problem. I regained my health and started walking. My blood pressure used to be very low and I was wearing spectacles for eyesight (-2 power). These problems were cured within one month of Pranayam practice.

— **Sangita Devendra Saxena, Vigyan Nagar, Kota, Rajasthan**

◆ I was suffering from arthritis and spondylitis. These diseases filled my life with difficulties. Due to unbearable pain in my feet and whole body, me and my family had to bear a lot of hardships. Ayurvedic treatment from the Ashram and Pranayam has helped me recover completely. Now I am absolutely alright and I practise Pranayam daily.

— **Sandhya Dev, Bidhan Niwas, Kolkota**

◆ I was suffering from arthritis since one year. My fingers got deformed. Due to pain in the knees I could not walk. I was very much disturbed. Then I started practising Pranayam taught by Swamiji on regular basis because of which my fingers also got straightened up. I do not have pain in the knees anymore. Now I am walking without any difficulty.

— **Kaushalendra N. Singh, Usbridge UB 8 BIY**

◆ I was suffering from nodes in my body for the last 7 years. On examination it was found that the bones in my body had enlarged. It was difficult for me to perform routine tasks and to be able to walk. The hands and feet became numb. The Pranayam taught by Swamiji and also the Ayurvedic medicines from the Ashram cured my disease completely. Pranayam has brought a new energy into my life. Now I can perform my daily chores easily.

— **Sulochan Chauhan, Shivalik Nagar, BHEL, Hardwar**

◆ Regular practice of Yog and Pranayam has cured my five year old arthritis problem. Prior to that I had taken all kinds of medicines and consulted allopathic doctors but I was told that the problem was incurable. I am practising Pranayam and feel that Swamiji is the God of this age.

— **Sukomal Shah**

◆ I was suffering from Rheumatoid arthritis for last 8-10 years. I took treatment from a number of doctors but it was of no use. Now I am practising Pranayam for last one year regularly and I am healthy. I am also not taking any kind of medicine.

— **Tapeswari Devi, Akash Ganga, Sahapur, Bhopal (MP)**

◆ I was suffering from arthritis for so many years. I found it difficult to climb stairs and also had difficulty in getting up after squatting. I am practising Pranayam taught by Swamiji for the past one year. I am also not taking any medicine. I still do not have any problem now.

— **Veena Gautam, Pitampura, Delhi**

◆ I was a patient of arthritis for the past several years and I was unable to walk or do routine work. Pranayam has given me a lot of benefit and I am practising it regularly. Now I able to do my routine work without any difficulty, I thank Swamiji a million time.

— **Neeru Garg, Garg Sales Corporation, Sangrur**

◆ I was having acute pain in the knees. I consulted a number of doctors and took a variety of medicines, but it was of no use. Now I am practising Pranayam as told by Swamiji on regular basis. I am cured off the disease completely.

— **Mahendra M. Parmar, Selai Road Silvassa**

HYPER AND HYPOTHYROIDISM

◆ I was suffering from thyroid problem for the past several years along with restlessness, discomfort all the time. Allopathic medicines were not beneficial and doctors asked me to take medicines for life long. I started practising Swamiji's Pranayam and took Ashram medicines. Now thyroid level is normal.

— **Dashrath Pal, Vanila, Fatehpur**

Before Treatment	After Treatment

Before Treatment

पतञ्जलि योगपीठ, हरिद्वार
PATANJALI YOGPEETH, HARIDWAR
[दिव्य योग मन्दिर ट्रस्ट का बहुआयामी सेवा प्रकल्प]
(MULTIDIMENSIONAL SERVICE UNIT OF DIVYA YOG MANDIR TRUST)
रोग परीक्षण एवं अनुसन्धान विभाग
Diagnostics & Research Department

Reg. No. __7336__   Date: ....
Name of Patient: Mr./Mrs./Ms. __DASHRATH__   Age/Sex: __10/12/06__ __43yrs/M__
Address ....
Refferd by: ....

TEST	VALUE	NORMAL RANGE
T3	0.7ng/ml	(0.8-1.9 ng/ml)
T4	144.0ng/ml	(50-130 ng/ml)
TSH	21.3µIU/mL	(0.4 – 8.9µIU/mL)

REPORT IS NOT FOR MEDICO LEGAL USE

Pathologist

दिल्ली-हरिद्वार राष्ट्रीय राजमार्ग, निकट बहादराबाद, हरिद्वार Delhi-Haridwar National Highway, Near Bahadarabad, Haridwar (U.A.)
Phone: 01334-244107, 240008, 248755 Fax: 01334-244805 email: divyayoga@rediffmail.com website: www.divyayoga.com
Note: Not for Medico Legal Purpose

After Treatment

पतञ्जलि योगपीठ, हरिद्वार
PATANJALI YOGPEETH, HARIDWAR
[दिव्य योग मन्दिर ट्रस्ट का बहुआयामी सेवा प्रकल्प]
(MULTIDIMENSIONAL SERVICE UNIT OF DIVYA YOG MANDIR TRUST)
रोग परीक्षण एवं अनुसन्धान विभाग
Diagnostics & Research Department

Reg. No. __8220__   Date: ....
Name of Patient: Mr./Mrs./Ms. __DASHRATH__   Age/Sex: __09/01/07__ __43 yrs/M__
Address ....
Refferd by: ....

TEST	VALUE	NORMAL RANGE
T3	1.76ng/ml	(0.8-1.9 ng/ml)
T4	25.5 ng/ml	(50-130 ng/ml)
TSH	0.44 µIU/mL	(0.4 – 8.9µIU/mL)

REPORT IS NOT FOR MEDICO LEGAL USE

Pathologist

दिल्ली-हरिद्वार राष्ट्रीय राजमार्ग, निकट बहादराबाद, हरिद्वार Delhi-Haridwar National Highway, Near Bahadarabad, Haridwar (U.A.)
Phone: 01334-244107, 240008, 248755 Fax: 01334-244805 email: divyayoga@rediffmail.com website: www.divyayoga.com
Note: Not for Medico Legal Purpose

Before practice of Pranayam and treatment TSH was 21.3, it became normal after practice.

I was obese and had thyroid problem. I took lot of medicines and consulted SGPGI doctors at Lucknow but there was no relief. I am practising Pranayam for the past two years. Now TSH is normal and my weight has also reduced. Thyroid level is becoming normal and now I do not have any problem.

— **Amita Gupta, Shyamnagar, Kanpur**

◆ I am a patient of thyroid since 1990 and my TSH level continued to increase. I took treatment at renowned hospitals like PGI but there was no improvement. The relief was temporary and thyroid used to be normal when I took medicines, but no therapy could cure my problem permanently. Finally I started practising Pranayam and Asana from last six months after watching Swamiji's programme on Astha Channel. I am also following home remedies, which has shown significant improvement. Besides, I was also suffering from ear secretion, which has also been cured and blood pressure is also normal. I reduced five kilo weight after practising Pranayam.

— **Shanti Gupta Snehanagar, Lucknow, UP**

Before Treatment   After Treatment

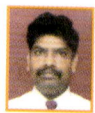

The TSH level was 22.61 before the treatment whereas after six months of Pranayam practice the second test showed TSH level at 0.08, which is normal.

My weight was increasing due to thyroid problem and appetite had increased. Weight reduced to 52 kg after practice of Pranayam and appetite is also normal. Now I feel much better and I have discontinued all medicines.

— **Vijay K. Sonkuser, Nagpur**

◆ I was suffering from thyroid due to which my body had become heavy and there was swelling all over the body. I could not even climb up the stairs. Due to this I was under depression. I started practising Pranayam as taught by Swamiji. Slowly I started to recover. Today I am absolutely healthy and I am also not taking any medicine. This miracle has taken place because of Yog only

— **Kuldeep Singh, Nanglul, Delhi**

Before Treatment	After Treatment

The thyroid profile of the patient was on the higher side before the treatment. There has been a considerable change in it by the practice of Yog and Pranayam.

◆ I was suffering from thyroid due to which my body had become heavy and there was swelling all over my body. I could not even climb up the stairs. Also menstruation discharge was sometimes low or it never used to occur. By practice of Pranayam I have started to benefit. Today I am absolutely healthy and I am not taking any medicine. It has been possible only due to the miracle of Yog.

— **Bipasha Pal, Muhuni, Agartala, Post Tripura**

◆ I was disturbed by a number of diseases like thyroid, tumor in uterus, joint pain etc. for many years. All the doctors used to prescribe me medicine for thyroid and told me to reduce my weight. I was tired of taking allopathic medicines. I was going under depression. Then I consulted the Vaidji at Divya Yog Mandir Trust, and took medicines for 4-5 months regularly and practised Pranayam daily and also practicised a few aasans. I also strictly followed the dietary instructions given to me by the Vaidji. I was surprised to see that after all this when I under went the tests for ultrasonography and thyroid profile, all the reports were normal. Hence I started to see a ray of hope for a healthy and disease-free life. Now my life is filled with joy.

— **Rita Singh, Badar Ghat, Agartala**

Before the treatment the thyroid profile of the patient was on higher side. There has been a considerable change in it by the practice of Yog and Pranayam.

◆ I had thyroid problem for last 11 years. Neither allopathic nor homeopathic treatment was of much help. I used to feel giddy, suffer headache, insomnia, overweight, irregular menstruation and other problems. I started doing Pranayam from January 2005 after watching Swamiji's prorgamme on TV. My problems slowly started getting reduced. I stopped taking thyroid medicine for 15 days and when tested my report was normal. Later as advised by the doctor, I stopped taking medicine and I am cured of thyroid problem. I also got cured of giddiness, insomnia, and irregular periods. I lost weight from 78 to 69 kg. Now I am living a completely healthy life.

— **Mahadevi I. Pujari, Shakti Nagar, Raichur, Karnataka**

Before Treatment	After Treatment

Before Pranayam, this patient's T3, T4, TSH level was abnormal and in the test done after practice of Pranayam the results showed T3 1.21, t4 105, TSH 2.55 which is normal.

◆ Since a long time I was a patient of Hypothyroid. For this I had to take allopathic medicines, but it was of no use. I started practising Yog and Pranayam taught by Swamiji and now I do not take any medicines. I have been greatly benefited. My thyroid profile has also become normal.

— **Rashmi Sudhir Dalal, Madhav Nagar, Akola**

I have been a patient of thyroid for the past 20 years and have been taking medicines since then. My palpitation used to be high and medicines were not giving any permanent relief. I started practising Pranayam and now the problem has been cured up to 90 percent. I am on the verge of discontinuing all the medicines.

— **Jyoti N. Singh, Dhandeli, Kakhar, Karnataka**

◆ I saw your programme on television and I am practising Pranayam regularly since May 7, 2004. This has given surprising results and reports are being enclosed for your perusal. The first thyroid test was done on March 9, 2004 at Metropolis Health Service (India) Pvt Ltd, Borivili (W), Mumbai and the TSH level was CLIA 91.75 UIU / ml and after three months the medical test done at Hindustan Health Point, 2406, Garia Main Road, Kolkata it had dropped to 0.35 UIU / ml. The doctors had initially asked me to take medicines for rest of my life. Doctors were surprised to see my first report. This miracle has happened only because of your blessings. My whole family practices Yog and I am teaching my neighbours also.

— **Dipti Rai, Garia, Kolkata**

◆ I was suffering from Hypthyroidism. On 1 November, 2003 it was confirmed that I was suffering from Hodgkins Lymphoma, for which various tests were done. The doctors advised chemotherapy. After chemotherapy I had many other problems. The colour of my skin began to change and the cancer had spread to whole of my skin. Even after taking treatment I had not recovered completely so I had started practising Yog-Pranayam as taught by Swamiji. After which the improvement began to take place slowly. The problem of thyroid is completely cured. In the case of cancer also I have benefited a lot. Now I have stopped taking all the allopathic medicines. I was a non-vegetarian and after practising Yog I have absolutely given up consumption of non-vegetarian food. Patanjali Yogpeeth is a heaven on earth, it is a centre of spiritual and medicinal healing, everybody should take advantage from it. If there are four Dhams (pilgrimage) then Patanjali Yogpeeth is the Fifth Dham. Yog has come out of the caves and has spread to each and every home, it is a great achievement in itself.

— **Sheela Shah, Noida (UP)**

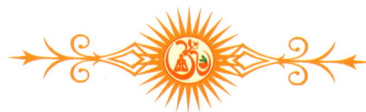

OTHER INCURABLE DISEASES

Alopecia

I was suffering from lack of hair and hair loss. I became bald and my hair turned gray. I am practising Pranayam regularly from June 2002, the hair growth has started, and it is turning black again.

— **Dinesh Kisanrao, Yavatmal, MS**

Varicose Veins

I was suffering from varicose veins for the past several years. I took many medicines but there was no improvement. I felt that I would never be able to recover from this problem. I saw Swamiji's programme on television and I am practising Pranayam for the past three-and-a-half months. There is a lot of improvement and now I have stopped taking medicines.

— **Ravindra Kaliravana, Bhiwani, Haryana**

◆ I suffered from high blood pressure, deep vein thrombosis, backache, arthritis and hypothyroid. I got to know that Pranayam can cure all the diseases. I saw Swamiji's prorgamme on TV and started doing regular pratice of Pranayam. Now I have fully recovered and motivate others also to do Pranayam.

— **Santosh Kumari Gupta, Vikas Marg, Delhi**

Aplastic Anaemia

◆ I was a patient of Aplastic anaemia and diabetes due to which haemoglobin had dropped to 4 and platelets count had reduced to 12 thousand. Regular practice of Pranayam and Yog increased haemoglobin to 8.5 and platelets count increased to 54 thousand. The sugar level is also normal.

— **Dr G.P. Agarwal, Kanpur Road, Lucknow (UP)**

◆ I was suffering from aplastic anaemia and haemoglobin used to be 3.4 normally. Platelet count had reduced to 32 thousand. Regular practice of Yog and Pranayam increased haemoglobin to 13.4 and platelet count to 94 thousand.

— **Savitri Devi, Saharanpur (UP)**

Before Treatment   After Treatment

The patient's haemoglobin used to be between three and four due to aplastic anaemia. The haemoglobin increased to 13.4 after the treatment.

Sickle Cell Anaemia

◆ I am a patient of sickle cell anaemia. I had lot of problems and often had lack of blood and once my haemoglobin was 9. Since then I have started doing Pranayam, my condition has improved a great deal. Now my haemoglobin is 15. I have recovered completely from Pranayam and Ayurved.

— **Ananta Kumar Patra, Balepal, Balasor**

◆ I was suffering from anaemia for the last five years and the haemoglobin level used be low. This resulted in weakness and I used to be hospitalized frequently due to blood loss. The sickle cells were more than 50 per cent. I consulted several doctors but there was no relief. Then I started practising Pranayam and Yog and took Ayurvedic medicines. Regular practice and medication proved to be beneficial. The haemoglobin increased to 10 and now I am completely healthy.

— **Krishna Sahu, Darbhanga (Bihar)**

Before Treatment	After Treatment

Sickling test was positive (70 per cent) before practice of Yog and Pranayam, which became negative after treatment.

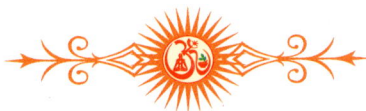

BONE TB

◆ I was a patient of bone TB and the spinal cord had bent due to this problem. I was unable to walk and used to suffer from severe pain. I consulted doctors, they operated and placed rods, but there was no relief. The I visited Swamiji's Ashram and took some Ayurvedic medicines and started practising Pranayam. There has been miraculous improvement and now I am totally healthy. I can walk freely without any problem.

— Aruna Raghuvanshi, Maharana Pratap Enclave, Delhi

Before Treatment   After Treatment

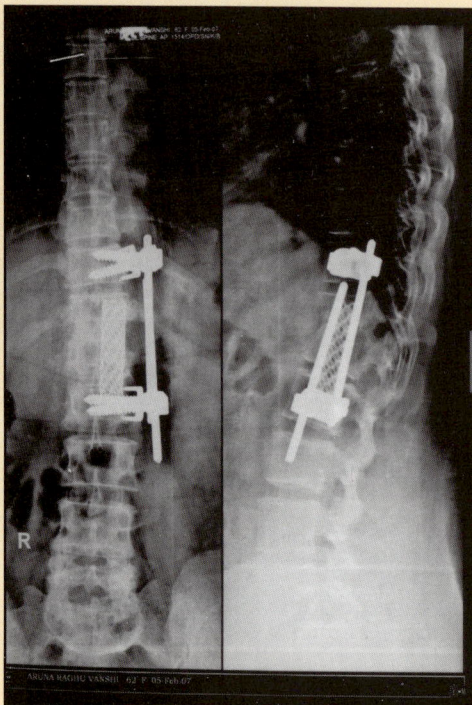

The spine bone D12-L1 had disorder before treatment but the X-ray taken after practice of Pranayam and treatment shows normal bone.

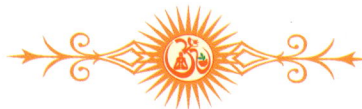

PITIUTARY MICROADENOMA AND OTHER DISEASES

◆ I have a 15-year-old son. Because of malfunctioning of pitiutary gland the level of the harmone and the male harmone testosterone were found to be negligible in the test. My son started behaving like girls and his body was not growing. I took medicinal and Pranayam consultation by going to Patanjali Yogpeeth. After 6 months of treatment the growth harmone testosterone starting increasing. Before the treatment GH 0.1 and testosterone was 20. After the treatment GH became 0.48 7, testosterone became 541.5. I had consulted renowned doctors in famous hospitals for treatment of my son. But I felt totally hopeless. By blessings of the Swamiji my son has become absolutely normal. This is no less than a miracle.

— **Shekhar Tyagi, Muradabad (UP)**

Before Treatment — After Treatment

The level of growth harmone of the patient before the treatment was 0.1 and testosterone was less than 20. After the Pranayam and treatment the growth harmone has become 0.45 and testosterone has become 541.50.

◆ In the year 1995, Pitiutary Microadenoma was detected. The level of prolactin was high in my blood. I used to have headache and I used to feel giddy. Sometimes I used to get fits. I took treatment from various specialist doctors but it was of no use. It was of help only till the time I took medicine. Then I started feeling that I may never get cured. Then I started practising Yog and Pranayam taught by Swami Ramdevji. It is the result of Pranayam only that in the last 9 months the Prolactin level has come down to normal. Now in the CT Scan test the condition of Pitiutary gland comes across as normal. By the blessings of Swamiji the disease Pitiutary Microadenoma is fully cured. Today I am absolutely fine.

— **Sangeeta, Central Road, New Delhi**

The higher level of prolactin can be clearly seen in blood test and also Pitiutary Microadenoma can be seen in the CT Scan before the treatment. Whereas CT scan test taken after practising Yog-Pranayam the level of Prolactin and also the condition of Pitiutary gland be seen as normal.

◆ I was suffering from migraine, Sinositis, Dysmenorrhoea, Harmone imbalance and other similar diseases. After consulting the doctors it was found that IgE level had increased to great extent. Allopathic treatment could not provide any benefit. My menstruation cycle used to be very painful. There used to be excessive bleeding. Later by practising Yog and Pranayam as told by Swamiji I got cured of my diseases slowly and steadily. Before the treatment my IgE level was 426, and Haemoglobin was 10.4, in just 5 months of practice of Yog IgE level was 181 and Haemoglobin became 12.5. Now I am completely healthy. All the troubles relating to my menstrual cycle are cured.

— **Sharmila Dutta, Mayur Vihar Phase 2, Delhi**

IgE level of the patient before the treatment was 426 and Haemoglobin was 10.4, after just 5 months of practice of Yog IgE level became 181 and Haemoglobin level became 12.5.

CHRONIC FEVER

◆ In 2007, I suffered from malaria, which could not be diagnosed by the doctors and they considered it to be typhoid and gave me treatment for typhoid. Even after giving me antibiotic continuously for one month my fever never came down. After that I have to be admitted to hospital. After coming back from there the body temperature remained at100 degree. After this my health started deteriorating. Suddenly one day I had severe pain in my chest, then the doctor advised me to go for ECG. ECG report was normal, thereafter I got test done for HB which was 5.6, after that for investigation purpose all the other tests were done, but nothing could be diagnosed. Slowly my digestive system got disturbed. I lost appetite, and the food consumed could not be digested. I could not sleep for weeks, the body had high temperature, when I lied down it was difficult to breathe. I am a lecturer of

Before Treatment	After Treatment

The HB level of the patient was 5.6 Gms. before the treatment whereas after the treatment his HB level was found to be 6 Gms.

Economics in Swami Vivekanand Saraswati Vidya Mandir. It was difficult to teach the students. I used to forget the figures while teaching. I found life difficult to manage. At that time my son was 6 years old. I was always worried about him. I was going into depression and kept thinking that I might be having liver cancer. I thought so because my mother had liver cancer, due to which she had died while I was a kid. My father was a heart patient and he also died at an early age, at that time I was just 12 years old. By just taking one allopathic pill my stomach used to get upset and because of this I took homoeopathic and Ayurvedic medicines, but it was of no use. By going on special diet for one month the HB level went up to 8 and it came down to 5.6 in just one week. On the advise of the doctor I got bone marrow test done, but nothing could be found so another test was advised which I did not get it done. On his advise I did Pranayam and got examined by the Vaidyaji at the Ashram. The first miracle happened after consuming Giloy juice for one month when my fever normalized and after that by practising Pranayam HB level started rising. Today HB is 11.6. I have taught Yog and Pranayam to 1,300 students regularly. Today what I am, I am because of your blessings only.

— Kavita Rastogi, Sahibabad

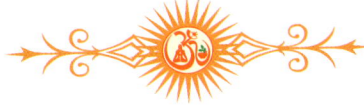

FILARIA

◆ I was suffering from Filaria for a long time. I had taken treatment from a number of doctors, it initially used to be helpful, but later on the problem aggravated. The doctors declared it as incurable disease. But by the blessings of Swamiji the above disease was cured in just 3 months due to practice of Yog and Pranayam. Now my self-confidence has increased and I practise Pranayam regularly. By the blessings of Swamiji my life is full of joy. May you be praised all over the universe and the science of Yog may be admired all over the universe.

— **Deendayal Radheyshyam Agarwal, Chanakyapuri, Vadodra**

SCOLISIS AND AVASCULAR NEOROSIS

◆ In 2002 I suffered from Avascular Neorosis. Even after a lot of treatment it was not cured. At last I took treatment from Swami Ramdevji's hospital and started practising Pranayam in morning and evening. Now I am alright. I send million salutations to Swamiji.

— **Meena Chauhan, FPUI, Gurgoan**

◆ My daughter Arti Chopra's spine had a deformity (scolisis). We immediately consulted Dr Ram Bahadur at Chandigarh he advised immediate operation. We were nervous and in August 2006 we consulted Acharaya Balkrishnaji at Divya Yog Mandir Trust, Hardwar. He gave us a few medicines from his Ashram and advised to practise Pranayam. By regular practice of Yog and Pranayam, Arti's spinal deformity was cured to a great extent. Earlier right shoulder's bone was quite raised but due to regular practice of Pranayam her condition has improved quite a lot. We are grateful to Acharya ji.

— **Pradeep Rai Chopra, Chandigarh (Punjab)**

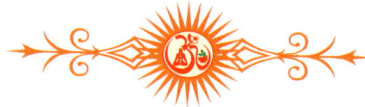

LOW BP AND UNDER WEIGHT

◆ I always used to have low BP. Due to which I always felt giddy and sometimes I fainted also. But with regular practice of Pranayam taught by Swamiji my BP is 120/80 and weakness is also cured. Now I am alright.

— Asha Sharma, Trilang, Bhopal

◆ By your blessing I have achieved a new life, my life is filled with enthusiasm when my weight increased, which otherwise never increased from 53 kg despite my best efforts. It has increased to 63 kg. and my intestine is powerful enough to digest the food and also new teeth developed for chewing the food. It was astonishing, we had heard of increase and decrease of weight but development of teeth for the third time is a miracle. It has been possible with the blessings of Swamiji, Yog and Pranayam. I am highly obliged.

— Yog practioner, Bharwar, Allahabad

◆ I was suffering from hernia and low BP for the last 5 years. When I consulted doctors they advised me operation. I did not want to get the operation done. At that time I started practising Pranayam as taught by Swami Ramdevji and also took Ayurvedic medicines from his Ashram. Very soon hernia and low BP and other ailments of my stomach were cured absolutely. Now I regularly practise Pranayam.

— Mahesh Modi, Mathura Chowk, Kathmandu

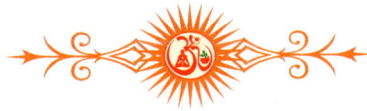

With the help of Pranayam a tooth stuck in the throat came out

◆ I was using artificial teeth. Once while I was eating, these teeth got stuck in my throat. Despite all the efforts they could not be taken out of the throat and due to this a number of problems started to rise. In those days I started practising Pranayam taught by Swamiji on TV. With the practice of Pranayam the stuck teeth started coming out of the throat. It was surprising for me. It has all been possible because of Kapalbhati. I have sent my teeth to be kept in a museum.

— **Samir Kumar, Jharkhand**

The glass pieces which got embedded into my head during an accident came out without an operation with the help of Pranayam

◆ I met with an accident on 12 December 1996. During the accident I was unconscious for one-and-a-half hour. On the right side of my face there was acute pain. On 19 December 1996, a CT scan of my head was done. In the CT scan, on the frontal side of my face Haemorrhagic Lesion could be seen, in addition to this some bone enlargement could also be seen. I was very upset because of this. One of my friends advised me to watch Swami Ramdevji's programme on Astha Channel. After watching the programme I started practising Pranayam. Now it has been two years since I started practising Yog and Pranayam. I have benefitted quite a lot from the regular practice of Yog and Pranayam. The embedded pieces of glass in my head have come out without any surgery. Earlier I could not walk and was bed ridden, now I can walk. Pranayam has filled new energy in my life. Now I practice Yog and Pranayam regularly.

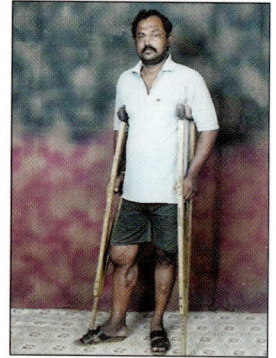

— **Pushparaj, Bhilai**

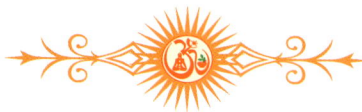

Chapter 9

REDISCOVERING YOG, RISING PUBLIC AWARENESS AND ROLE OF MEDIA

Swami Ramdev Ji's indepth study and research on Yog, Pranayam, Ayurved, and other ancient health-building systems has made everybody take notice. Some call it a miracle, some take it as divine power and some consider it an heavenly act. Swamiji is a great soul and his Yog revolution has proved to be a Sanjivani or life-saving device for the sick and suffering people. His divine foresight presents the body as a temple and has filled new energy and spirit in the people.

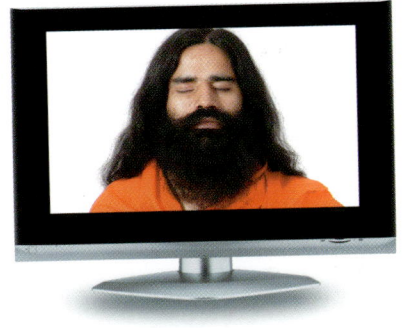

It will not be an exaggeration to say that media and public communication have played a major role in establishing Yog culture among the masses.

Media has changed its outlook, recognized the utility of Yog, played a responsible role and became a major source of communication for the great mission propounded by Swamiji in the public interest. If we analyze the facts mentioned below then we can understand the depth and scope of this mission which is re-establishing the culture of Yog and bio-agriculture.

Role of Electronic Media in Yog Revolution

Electronic media has played a major role in extending the reach of Yog to each and every household. Today, people are able to see and experience the benefits of Yog in the privacy of their homes through this medium. The number of people reaping its benefits by watching the programmes and learning is many a times higher than those who attend the camps. The most important contribution of electronic media is that the Yog revolution is spreading very fast in the foreign countries also. Astha and other channels are telecasting the programmes abroad. Now, Yog is beyond the geographical boundaries and we are assured that the whole world will be disease-free and inclined to lead a spiritual life very soon. This mega success would not have been possible without the positive role of media. The media is contributing continuously. The second aspect of its advantage is that people are learning Yog and following the path of righteousness. A nation's progress is dependent on the ideals of its citizens. It is a matter of pride that 100 crore population who have embraced

Yog have brought in new optimism in their lives.

Here we would like to highlight Pakistan as an example of role played by electronic media. The Yog awareness among the Pakistanis has been possible only because of this media.

The Financial World conducted a survey in five major cities of Pakistan. According to the survey results, Swami Ramdevji left behind the megastar of the century, Amitabh Bacchan and topped the popularity rank. Forty-two percent of the Pakistani people in the age group of 45 - 60 years believed that Swami Ramdev was the most popular personality of India. Yog awareness in an Islamic country is possible only with the help of electronic media. Print media has played a major role in propagating Yog, but faster and broader reach of electronic media is appreciable and desirable. Role of media in propagating Yog is a big service to the society, nation and the world.

Swamiji's Yog Revolution - a Message of leading a positive life through TV Channels

India is a good example of fast rate of globalization taking place all over the world. In the past one decade India's interest in developing technical facilities in different areas became stronger and it continued to make all possible efforts to achieve its goals. People's life-style changed either voluntarily or involuntarily. Nothing remained unchanged either at home or office. The pace of progress in the past 10 years has increased and it cannot be denied. But the negative impact was that the people were losing their mental peace. The question was raised that this progress might move Indians away from their culture, deep faith towards religion and spiritualism. The desire to find a solution to such problems of modern life, attain mental peace and lead a stress-free life inspired people to get on the path of Yog and Pranayam. People felt the need to establish a synergy between progress and mental peace. The most important point is that good health was extremely necessary. People felt confused. Strong need was felt to go back to our old traditions and that together with modern technology it will enable us to have deep devotion towards God, spiritualism and still be part of the world progress. How could the person manage everything so that he would not lag behind in worldly matters and also attain mental peace? In the midst of this confusion and dilemma Swami Ramdev Ji Maharaj came up with Patanjali Yog Science as an answer to the complex problems cited above. His path showed the correct way to the people and they were successful in making progress, attaining mental peace and also leading a disease-free life. People started developing faith in him and the number of people participating in his camps kept on increasing and so did Swamiji's popularity.

Electronic media played a major role and this needs to be mentioned especially. Swamiji could reach to the masses and express his views only with the help of this media. He opened the gateway to good health through this media. It also needs to be mentioned that on whichever channel Swamiji's Yog programmes was telecast it gained popularity. Whether it is Astha, NDTV, Sahara One or Sahara Samay, the Yog program's telecast on these channels increased the viewership of these channels.

The biggest advantage of telecasting Yog programmes on electronic media is that the places where the camps are not being organized or the print media is not able to contribute in a big way, there also people are able to learn Yog through this media. It is not easy to reach each and every place through camps. India is a huge country and it is possible to reach every corner of the country with the help of electronic media only. Swami Ramdev informs people about Yog on these channels and people gain insight into ancient knowledge. It is well-known that in the race of modernization the western countries are much ahead of us but the people of those countries also seek mental peace, stress and disease-free life through Patanjali Yog.

People experience a divine feeling when Swamiji says boldly that we will fulfill the dream of healthy world through Yog. Today, people are spending their hard earned money on medicines which they can save by practising Yog. They will also be free from corruption, crime and other negative tendencies. A person who adopts Yog in life becomes stress-free, gains mental peace, becomes tolerant, and adopts ethical behaviour. As the number of ethical minded people increases, corruption and injustice will reduce automatically. Swamiji's Yog revolution is a beautiful blessing for the entire humankind. It has been successful in drawing the attention of the people in a very short time due to television channels. Channels broadcasting Swamiji's programmes are much ahead of other channels in their TRP rates. Their business and popularity are increasing. Hence it can be said that Swamiji's programmes are a blessing even for the television channels.

Role of Television

♦ Today, national and international channels are telecasting seven-and-a-half hours of Yog science programmes of Swamiji regularly. Astha channels telecasts Swamiji's programmes from 5.30 to 8 AM and again from 8 to 9 PM. India TV telecasts half-an-hour programme from 6.30 to 7 AM and again from 5.00 to 5.30 PM. Sahara Samay telecasts his programme from 6.30 to 7 AM, while Sahara One from 6.30 to 7.00 PM. Besides Yog programme on Astha International channel is telecast from 5 to 7.30 AM and 8 to 9 PM. Star News telecasts Swamiji's Yog programme from 6.30 to 7 AM (IST).

♦ Since the beginning of television in India no individual has been telecast at this large scale other than Swamiji. Till now Swami Ramdev's total recording has exceeded 5,000 hours (including Yog camps) in 3-4 years, something of rare occurrence in world broadcasting.

♦ India Today published a survey report on 21 August, 2006. According to that report an

Indian watches television programmes for two hours a day on an average. The Yog programme of Swamiji is telecast for four times a day. This is the reason that every individual belonging to every sector is able to associate himself or herself with Yog programmes. The Yog revolution has reached even the interior villages of the country.

* Out of the total channels shown in India, around 51 have a keen eye on Swamiji's Yog related programmes. The related news is telecast from time to time.

* Almost all the channels telecast special programmes on Swamiji.

* After year 2000, the number of news channels has increased from 13 to 51, while the number of Yog channels from two to 11. There has been 168 percent increase in the number of total channels but Yog channels increased 11 times within a period of six years. *India Today* magazine published a report recently. According to it in 2000, there were only 112 channels, which have now increased to 300.

* About 51 percent of 108 million Indian population watch television currently. Swamiji's programme gets telecast on such a wide spread system, reaching 65 crore people that clearly shows that today Yog, family values and culture is being nurtured in minds of the Indian people. They are becoming aware of the feeling of national pride, self-respect, disease-free life and humanity.

* The channels based on Yog, health and spiritualism have increased manifold and clearly indicate increasing interest of people towards Swamiji's Yog revolution. His Yog programmes on Astha channel are on top in viewership ratings. Swamiji's programmes are viewed by more than 20 crore people in India and the latest survey says that only 2.3 crore people only watch movies on television everyday. This means the number of people watching Swamiji's Yog programmes is 8.7 times higher compared to those who watch films.

* Swamiji's programme tops the list of programmes which is watched for the longest duration. Analysis shows that it has created a world record.

Role of Print Media

Print media has also given a lot of coverage to Yog programmes, which was never done before. Previously print media used to publish Yog related news without much importance but we can see a clear change in this attitude. When efforts were made to extend the reach of Yog to the last person and that too with a different approach then this was a matter of curiosity for everybody. Print media is not an exception. It felt the necessity to not only know about such successful issue but also give it prominent position in the newspapers.

This paradigm shift in print media is due to the positive role of Swami Ramdev with his Yog revolution, who taught people the yogic life-style, who were otherwise resistant. Print

media began to give good coverage and importance to Yog related news. It has also tried to keep away from the popular notion of people who used to consider Yog to be some kind of communal subject. Nowadays we find news related to Yog in prominent position in any newspaper, magazine etc. Many newspapers have started a special Yog column. This change was not seen till Yog was not proved scientifically. This is the reason that Swamiji has begun a mission to put up with the challenge of science. Today people will accept a thing only when it has been proved and tested scientifically as per modern standards.

As the popularity of Yog grew, print media started giving more and more coverage to Yog related news. Swamiji has tried to present Yog in such a manner that anybody can adopt it without difficulty. This is the reason that those who showed resistance before are not embracing Yog with all seriousness. The real Yog revolution has begun five to six years back and now it has taken the form of global Yog revolution. This proves that in today's age of commercialization, Indian print media is giving importance to social issues instead of only commercial issues. Before Independence Indian freedom fighters had projected their thoughts with the help of newspapers, it gave a momentum to Indian freedom struggle and became the major weapon for Independence. Swami Ramdev Yog revolution has also begun with the same momentum. Print media has completely changed the old ideologies prevailing with respect to Yog.

It is not possible to describe other advantages of print media in propagating Yog revolution, but the advantages derived by Yog revolution need to be mentioned. Previously Yog and other such issues were opposed by secularists but Yog revolution has changed the scenario. Truth cannot be masked with secularism or any other ideology. Truth cannot be concealed either. It cannot be destroyed. This is hard fact and so is the truth of Yog. It cannot be denied. Print media has not changed its thinking overnight. It was hesitant in the beginning but its curiosity increased with increasing popularity of Yog. Print media which soon changed into faith, efforts and healthy cooperation. It also played a major role in extending the reach of Yog in interiors of the country.

Majority of the people begin their day with newspaper. Magazines are also popular as they not only give information but also change the life-style and have a deep impact. Newspapers cover the Yog camps organized in various cities and inform people. People come in large numbers to attend the camps after reading the news items. People living in cities get tired of leading a mechanical, boring, monotonous, stressful life and search mental peace through Yog. Print media has changed reading habits of rural people by informing them about Yog and its advantages. People are accepting Yog and following the right path. People have become more aware of healthy eating habits and its effect on body. They are also developing positive thinking.

Present scenario of Print Media in Yog Revolution

♦ Around 60,413 registered newspapers and magazines with a circulation of 156,719,209 have prominently carried articles and news related to Swami Ramdevji.

♦ Newspapers and magazines are being published in 22 regional languages other than English and have a readership of 67 crore. The news published in these regional newspapers has aroused the feeling of patriotism, ideal life-style, humanity and importance of leading a disease-free life.

♦ Swamiji's Yog revolution is getting mass publicity through the word of mouth from educated readers to other citizens of the nation.

♦ Previously crime and negative news used to get prominence in print media but now positive news related to Swamiji, his thoughts and guidance are published prominently. Local, regional and national newspapers and magazines carry special pullouts on Swamiji's Yog camps. Till now more than 100 seven-day Yog camps have been organized under the guidance of Swamiji from Kashmir to Kanyakumari and Kutch to northeast. Each camp had a participation of more than 60,000 people and one crore people have directly learnt the mantra to lead a disease-free life.

♦ Besides, around 17 residential camps, two hormone test camps and two other medical test camps have also been organized, which included a lot of documentation and important research work to prove Yog on a scientific platform. Print media has published the results prominently and presented the significance of Yog in our day-to-day life. It also presented a topic of discussion for the learned and ordinary people.

♦ Apart from this Yog, Pranayam, Ayurved and Indian values were established with a mission of making the world disease-free, which crossed the national boundaries and reached UK. Four Yog camps were organized on the request of Indian origin UK residents. Around 50,000 people took part in this camp and got direct benefit. This was astonishing for the whole Western world. The most interesting fact is that out of the total number of participants, 14 percent were Britishers and had never participated in a large social activity like this ever before. The media of that country gave prominence to Yog revolution. Besides the participants, 23,000 people were addressed by Swamiji about Yog.

♦ During the seven-day Yog camp, it was seen for the first time that journalists not only took part in the camp with their families but also used to be present at the venue in the wee hours for press coverage. Swamiji's speech was also covered in detail despite the fact that journalists tend to avoid early morning assignments.

♦ The main topics covered were Swamiji's speech, number of participants, arrangements at the venue, participants' reactions, method of Pranayam, home remedies, curing incurable diseases, message given for arousing national feeling, and social issues that were discussed in the camps.

◆ Today slogans given by Swamiji like 'Cold drink means toilet cleaner', 'Burger is destroyer' etc. are popular among children.

◆ Almost all the leading newspapers, magazines and publications have included cover story on Swamiji. It shows that Yog is today the most favourite, interesting, useful, informative and widely read topic among the people. This has given rise to a sort of competition among various publications to publish work of Swamiji.

◆ During last six years, newspapers and magazines publishing articles on Yog, duty, Ayurved, family values and spiritualism has increased to a considerable impact. The figures obtained from Registrar of Newspapers of India reveal that out of 209 magazines published on Yog and related topics, 111 are registered in the name of Indian residents and 28 in the name of foreign nationals.

◆ Today the number of related magazines and newspapers circulation has touched the magical figure of 20 million, which is 12.76 percent of total circulation of print media.

◆ Swamiji has attained celebrity status but he still meets the press with modesty, simplicity and in a casual and informal manner. In the past three years, Swamiji has spent around 3,94,200 minutes for media at the rate of six hours per day on an average. This has helped in bringing people closer to revered Swamiji's transparent life.

Role of Radio

Radio has the maximum reach in India with more than 18.57 crore listeners. A common man listens around 90 minute of radio programmes everyday. Swamiji's Yog revolution and related news is the topic of discussion and other programmes broadcast by radio. The cities, which happen to be buzzing with popular Bollywood songs on FM channel, inform the listeners about Swamiji's Yog camp from time to time. They also inform about the diversions in routes at the time when Yog camps are organized in that particular city, what are the modes available to reach the venue, how many people are participating, what are the reactions of participants etc. Besides, Swamiji's message is also broadcast under 'Thought for the day'.

Role of other Mass Communication Media

◆ Audio cassettes on Yog, health and spiritualism are becoming an important source of infromation. There has been a tremendous growth in the sale of audio cassettes released by the Yogpeeth in the past three years. Divya Sadhna, Publication Department of Divya Yog Mandir Trust, Hardwar, has released around 16 cassettes containing Swamiji's discourses and devotional songs.

- According to an estimate the market of CDs / DVDs on Yog, spiritualism and heath has increased 33 times within six years. The audio-visual production department of Divya Yog Mandir Trust has released around 64 cassettes on Swamiji's Yog, Pranayam and Ayurved, which talk about cure and remedies for different diseases.

- There has been an unexpected increase in the number of websites launched on Yog, health and spiritualism. A study conducted by a non-governmental organization (NGO) has revealed that awareness about Yog and its benefits has increased in the world. There are around seven lakh pages available on net that give complete information on Yog.

- Around 50,000 teachers have been trained with an objective of fulfilling the dream of 'Healthy India Healthy World' under Swamiji. These teachers have taken the message of Yog throughout India & abroad.

- Various books and literature published by Divya Prakashan like Yog Sadhana Evam Yog Chikitsa Rahasya, Aushadh Darshan, Vedic Nityakarma Vidhi, Ayurvedic Jadi - Booti Rahasya etc. have registered fantastic sales. These publications have played an important role in popularising Yog.

- The monthly magazine 'Yog Sandesh' published in 11 different languages by Divya Yog Mandir Trust has a total readership of 31,50,000 persons. This has proved to be an effective medium of communication. It contains a lot of information regarding Swamiji's messages, research results, Ayurvedic and yogic applications and readers wait eagerly to read it. This magazine also informs people about Swamiji's Yog revolution.

- More than 2,000 - 3,000 patients visit the OPD of Patanjali Yogpeeth located in Bahadarabad, Hardwar where they are given free consultation. Besides, 150 service centres are operating in different parts of the country and centrally managed by Patanjali Yogpeeth give free consultation and treatment to around 20,000 patients. This huge system is proving to be a tree of plenty for the sick and suffering people.

- Divya Yog Mandir Trust receives more than 1,300 letters everyday, which means around 4,75,000 letters in a year. A special cell has been created, which takes care of giving answers for the readers' questions and letters. The information centre located at Hardwar answers around 1,175 calls everyday on an average, which guides more than 5,00,000 people every year.

In conclusion, one can say that average Indian and people of the whole world now have greater degree of awareness about Yog and its benefits. This is mainly because media globally has taken a positive, balanced approach towards Yog and related issues.

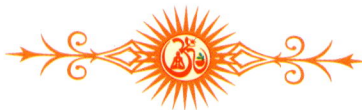

Chapter 10

PATANJALI YOGPEETH

Concept

Divya Yog Mandir Trust and Patanjali Yogpeeth are the institutions working for the world health through scientific basis of Yog and Ayurved. Swami Ramdev Ji Maharaj had conceptualized this mission along with Acharya Balkrishna, Swami Muktanand and other friends in his small office but it is a mega success today. Swamiji had a dream to establish Vedic knowledge of Yog and Ayurved with scientific approach and provide health and prosperity to the mankind which has now been given a new direction with large-scale research conducted on these health-building systems.

Today, the concept of healthy world is serving the mankind in different ways through different services. The Out Patient Department (OPD) of Patanjali Yogpeeth has given a momentum to this mission. This department is equipped with latest modern techniques and testing facilities suitable for research and health. The world class facilities available include Ayurved Medical and Research Department, Yog Training and Research Department, Clinical Test and Research Department, Panchkarma and Shatkarma Medical and Research Department, world's premier latest Ayurved and Surgery and Research Department, Medical and Research Department for Eyes, Pharmacy and Research Department, world class Ayurved Dental Clinic and Research Department through Yog and Ayurved, Vedic Yagyashala, Annapurna (kitchen and dining hall), excellent accommodation facilities need special mention. Our other services include state-of-the-art facilities and international standard techniques and laboratories (GLP), India's first Ayurvedic Pharmacy – Divya Pharmacy, Herbal Research Department, Patanjali Nursery, Cow Shed and Panchgavya Research Department having ISO 9001, ISO-1400 and ISO – 18001 certification are functioning at various premises of the institute situated at Hardwar. Sadhna Ashram situated at Gangotri and Gurukul running at Ghaseda village in Revadi district of Haryana are other major institutions of Divya Yog Mandir. Patanjali Yogpeeth carries on various other programmes in public interest. This includes scholarship plans for children of volunteers and staff, taking care of marriage expenses of poor girls, free medical facilities for poor, rehabilitation schemes in case of natural disasters, providing basic amenities for the needy, co-operative plans for lepers, destitute and orphan children, encouraging blood donation camps, providing health facilities in interior areas are included.

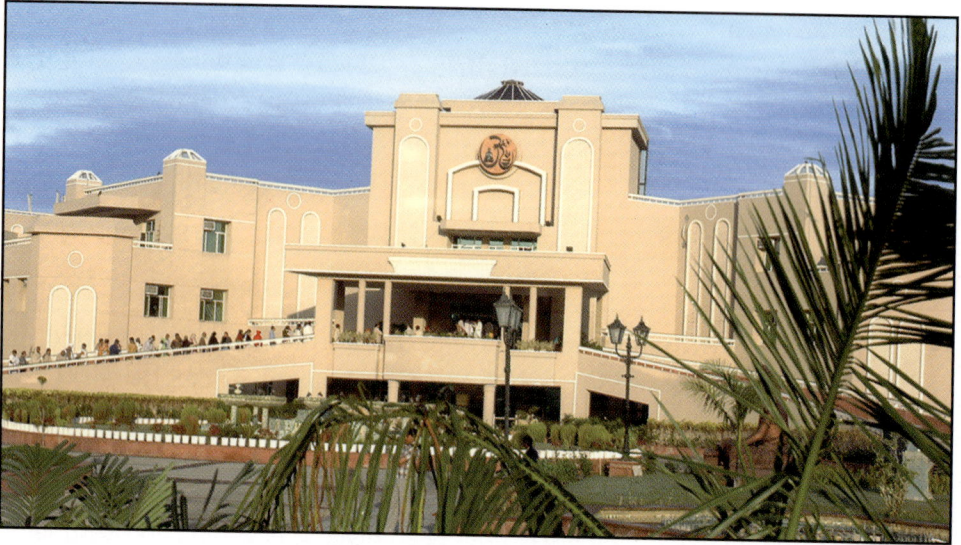

Patanjali Yogpeeth, Hardwar

Future plans

Establishing Patanjali University

The concept of building Patanjali University with the inspiration of Swami Ramdevji in now is in full swing. The Uttarakhand government has passed the legislation in this regard. Following plans are associated with the establishment of university:

♦ To begin a PhD, Post-Graduate, Graduate degree and diploma courses in Yog for 5,000 students of the world in Atharvaveda, Charak, Sushrut, and other traditional systems. To begin PhD, MD, MS, BAMS and other degree courses in Ayurved on the lines of modern medical science and also start hostel facilities for students.

♦ To begin BSc, MSc, BCom, MCom, MA, BA, D-pharm, B-pharm, Yogic Physiotherapy, Acupressure and other vocational and job–oriented courses along with Yog and Ayurved, Vedic and spiritual values in curriculum. This aims to become an ideal institute in the field of academics.

♦ To provide world–class medical and research facilities to all students along with education.

♦ Clinical control and research on genetic (hereditary) diseases, cancer, heart disease, asthma, diabetes, arthritis and other incurable diseases and establish Prana or vital life energy as evidence based medicine internationally, thereby accomplishing the mission of sages to make the people of world disease–free.

- Continuous research and development on herbs and medicinal plants and encourage the herbal based agriculture in order to eradicate poverty and build a healthy and prosperous nation.

- Scientific research on Agnihotra (sacrificial fire), cow urine and nature therapy, Vedic system of stages of life, Vedic ceremonies, and all traditional cultural knowledge to bring to light scienfic aspects of Vedic culture and achievements.

- Research on celibacy, household, living in forest and ascetic stages of life under Vedic system and show the path of health to the world.

- About 25,000 Yog teachers are visiting each and every village and city in all countries propagating Yog education. We propose to have one lakh Yog teachers by the end of 2007 and 10 lakh by the end of 2008, accomplishing the mission of 'Healthy India Healthy World.'

- Construct a huge indoor stadium for Yog training, which can accommodate 5,000–10,000 people.

- Begin Yog education in schools, hospitals, police, administration, defense, industry and commercial institutes, and build a healthy, prosperous, spiritual, sensitive and responsible nation.

To Set up a world class research institute

Patanjali Yogpeeth and Divya Pharmacy has independently set up a huge pathology laboratory, a Botany, Chemistry and Microbiology Laboratory which is carrying on different types of research and also associating with various institutes and universities to take forward the research work.

Study on Ayurved, Yog, medicinal herbs and plants along with large-scale research on Prana or vital life energy as medicine, to prove the scientific basis of Pran as medicine for the treatment of both curable and incurable diseases. Deep and in-depth study of the constitution of physical body, etheric body, astral body, mental body, and causal body and curing genetic diseases through Yog, Ayurved and especially Pranayam. This will be helpful in curing hereditary diseases and in preventing serious diseases without Ayurvedic medicines and fulfill the dream of creating a disease–free, healthy and prosperous society.

Establishment of modern genetic laboratory

A state-of-the-art genetic laboratory will be established in Patanjali Yogpeeth in order to provide momentum to genetic research. It is clear that hereditary, infectious diseases have been increasing along with the progress of science. Even today science is ineffective in the treatment of hereditary and genetic diseases. Yog and Pranayam are highly effective in these cases, and Swamiji has proved it through various experiments and tests. Today, there is a need to prove this fact as per modern scientific standards, so that our ancient scientific health building system gets scientific recognition. Large-scale genetic and clinical research will be conducted in order to establish new milestones in the treatment of cancer, thalassemia, multiple sclerosis, cerivelar Ectesia and other serious conditions.

Research on Scientific background of Vedic Traditions

Vedic traditions like conservation of different breeds of cows, looking into the medicinal importance of Panchgavya (cow, urine, cow dung, milk, curd and clarified butter), construcion of huge cow shed, development and research plan, to get the yield of cow milk, clarified butter, urine and other products.

Besides, there is a provision for performing sacrificial fire for overcoming anguishes and purification of environment and to attain physical happiness along with spiritual progress. To present the scientfic importance of sacrifical fire (yagya) and construct a huge yagyashala and research centre for the purpose.

Promote Herbal based agriculture and encourage Ayurved

Medicinal plant nursery, exhibition and research

The future institution will shine with spiritual beauty on one side and the external view will be beautified with different varieties of herbs, medicinal plants, flowers, creepers, beautiful trees and gardens. People will be mesmerized with the natural beauty surrounding the institution and would like to get lost in the enchanting beauty. Both rare and common herbs of India and the Himalayan region will be grown on a large-scale. This will help in the conservation of herbs, which are on the verge of extinction. The plants conserved in this manner, the flowers, leaves, skin, roots etc. can be used for the purpose of research and treatment. The mild fragrant breeze flowing from the herbal garden will relieve the pain of the diseased. The fresh herbal juice available from the garden will be given to the patients depending on the physical condition. The rare herbs and medicinal plants will be grown and analyzed for their germplasma conservation. There will be a provision for research and study on the main factors and qualities of herbs and medicinal plants. The research will be advantageous for the farmers engaged in herbal farming. This will also improve the financial condition and also encourage herbal farming. The economically weak farmers will become self-reliant and nation will become prosperous, and we could probably eradicate poverty and reduce unemployment.

Several millions have been encouraged to grow herbal plants in flower pots, which include Harad, Baheda, Myrobalan, Neem, Parijat, Arjuna etc. People are being encouraged to grow these plants on streets, schools, gardens and other common places. Besides, people are being inspired to grow Basil, Giloy, wheat, Ashvagandha, Mahua, Ghritakumari and evergreen plants in pots and plans for setting up herbal gardens in villages is also a proposal under consideration. A project will be made for encouraging herbal gardens at national and regional levels after discussions with administration and government. Besides, farmers will be motivated to begin herbal farming through cooperative institutions and organize programmes and seminars for providing required information. Plan is being made to purchase herbs at reasonable prices.

Plan to purchase herbs and manufacture pure medicine and supply at nominal prices

We have to increase prosperity of the country and raise 33 percent of the population above poverty line. We have to provide employment to all and for this we need to develop cultivation of herbs as the 'the medicine for the nation' with this aim in view, we have established an Ayurvedic pharmacy in Hardwar.

Other plans of the institute

- Form a large group of volunteers and set up a permanent relief fund for rehabilitation work during natural calamities.
- Plan to provide scholarships to poor and deprived students.
- The institution is now registered in UK and many projects are underway to build a healthy, happy and disease-free world.

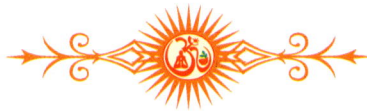